MENTAL ILLNESS AND SOCIAL POLICY

The American Experience

MENTAL ILLNESS AND SOCIAL POLICY

THE AMERICAN EXPERIENCE

THE INSTITUTIONAL CARE OF THE INSANE IN THE UNITED STATES AND CANADA

EDITED BY

HENRY M. HURD

VOLUME II

ILLUSTRATED

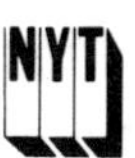

ARNO PRESS
A NEW YORK TIMES COMPANY
New York • 1973

Reprint Edition 1973 by Arno Press Inc.

Reprinted from a copy in
The University of Illinois Library

MENTAL ILLNESS AND SOCIAL POLICY:
The American Experience
ISBN for complete set: 0-405-05190-5
See last pages of this volume for titles.

Manufactured in the United States of America

Library of Congress Cataloging in Publication Data

Hurd, Henry Mills, 1843-1927, ed.
The institutional care of the insane in the United States and Canada.

(Mental illness and social policy: the American experience)
Reprint of the 1916-17 ed. published by Johns Hopkins Press, Baltimore.
1. Psychiatric hospitals--United States.
2. Psychiatric hospitals--Canada. I. Title.
II. Series. [DNLM: WM27 DC2 H9 1917F]
RC443.H852 362.2'1'097 73-2404
ISBN 0-405-05210-3

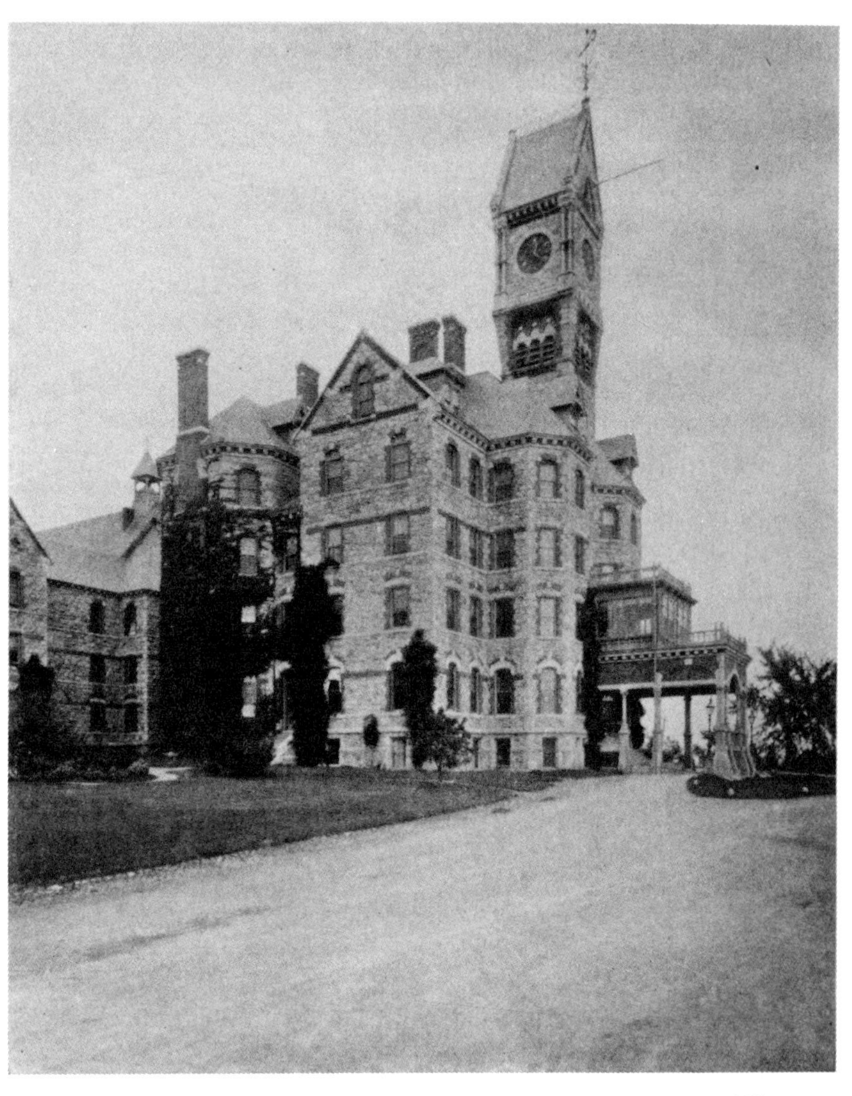

ADMINISTRATION BUILDING, WORCESTER STATE HOSPITAL, MASS.

THE INSTITUTIONAL CARE OF THE INSANE

IN THE

UNITED STATES AND CANADA

BY

HENRY M. HURD, WILLIAM F. DREWRY, RICHARD DEWEY,
CHARLES W. PILGRIM, G. ALDER BLUMER
AND T. J. W. BURGESS

EDITED BY

HENRY M. HURD, M.D., LL.D.

Emeritus Professor of Psychiatry, The Johns Hopkins University; formerly Medical Superintendent of the Pontiac State Hospital; Secretary, The Johns Hopkins Hospital

VOLUME II

ILLUSTRATED

THE JOHNS HOPKINS PRESS
BALTIMORE, MD.
1916

The Lord Baltimore Press
BALTIMORE, MD., U. S. A.

CONTENTS.

ALABAMA.

ARIZONA.

ARKANSAS.

CALIFORNIA.

COLORADO.

CONNECTICUT.

DELAWARE.

DISTRICT OF COLUMBIA.

FLORIDA.

GEORGIA.

IDAHO.

ILLINOIS.

INDIANA.

IOWA.

KANSAS.

KENTUCKY.

LOUISIANA.

MAINE.

MARYLAND.

MASSACHUSETTS.

MICHIGAN.

MINNESOTA.

MISSISSIPPI.

MISSOURI.

ILLUSTRATIONS.

PART III

STATE, CORPORATE AND PRIVATE INSTITUTIONS IN THE UNITED STATES

THE CARE OF THE INSANE IN ALABAMA.

There are two institutions for the state care of the insane in Alabama, under the corporate name of "The Alabama Insane Hospitals"; one is located at Tuscaloosa, and is known as "The Bryce Hospital"; the other is located at Mt. Vernon, and is known as "The Mt. Vernon Hospital." The Bryce Hospital is devoted to the care of the white insane, with a few negroes; The Mt. Vernon Hospital is devoted exclusively to the care of negroes.

An exceptional feature with the Alabama hospitals is that they are under the same management. They have the same board of seven trustees; three from the neighborhood of The Bryce Hospital; two from the neighborhood of The Mt. Vernon Hospital and two from the state at large. This Board of Trustees was originally appointed by the Legislature in 1901, and is a self-perpetuating body, filling its own vacancies. The term of one trustee expires every year. Their elections are subject to the approval of the Senate. There is also the same superintendent for both institutions, with an assistant superintendent at each hospital. The finances and general business are conducted from one office by the steward and treasurer at Tuscaloosa, with an assistant steward at Mt. Vernon.

State care for the insane dates back in Alabama to the year 1852. A wave of reform in favor of state care as opposed to other kinds had extended over the country and reached Alabama in turn. State care would most probably have been initiated in 1849—there being indications in the state and in the Legislature to that effect—had not the capitol building at Montgomery burned, which delayed matters until 1852. The subject had been agitated by the medical profession, and Miss Dix had addressed an eloquent and effectual appeal to the Legislature in the session of 1849. In the session of 1851-2 a memorial from the State Medical Association, of which Dr. A. G. Mabry was president, which had been adopted by the Association in 1847, and again in 1851, was presented to the Senate by Senator Gunn and urged by a special committee of the Medical

Association, of which Dr. A. Lopez was chairman. A favorable report followed and a bill "To Establish a Hospital for Insane Persons in Alabama" passed the Legislature and was approved by the Governor, February 9, 1852.

The establishment of The Mt. Vernon Hospital was provided for in the legislative session of 1900-01.

The admissions into the insane hospitals in Alabama, as in all the states, have steadily increased from year to year, at a more and more rapid rate. In the ten years prior to 1912 the state's population increased about 16 per cent; in the same period the admissions into the insane hospitals increased about 45 per cent. The whites have increased 30 per cent and the negroes 60 per cent.

The maintenance of the Alabama insane hospitals rests upon a continuous appropriation by the state—an amount not to exceed $3.50 per capita per week, payable quarterly. At present (1912) the rate is fixed by the trustees at $3.25 per capita a week. For a number of years there has been no appropriation otherwise for improvements or additions; all of these have been made out of the regular fund.

Physicians are frequently exchanged from one hospital to the other, as well as employees and patients. The superintendent spends about one-fourth of his time at Mt. Vernon. Most of the employees at Mt. Vernon are white.

The Resident Committee of Trustees, three at Tuscaloosa and two at Mt. Vernon, have frequent supervision of the hospitals and the full board holds annual meetings at both hospitals, besides called meetings.

In Alabama all classes of patients are admitted to the state hospitals except simple, harmless, incurable dements, dotards or idiots.

Private Patients.—No provision by statute exists for the admission of private or pay patients.

Legal Procedure.—An application for admission to the judge of probate of the county of residence, who in turn is directed to make application to the superintendent of the hospital to ascertain if the patient can be admitted. If he can be admitted the judge of probate calls witnesses, at least one of whom must be a physician, and investigates the facts of the case, either with or without a jury and with or without the presence in court of the person in question.

If the judge or jury believe the patient to be sufficiently defective in mind to be sent to the hospital, the judge must make two copies of the certificates of the fact, one to be filed in his office and the other to be sent to the hospital.

Appeal from commitment may be taken by the patient or his next friend within 10 days after the order is made. The probate court summons a jury and after trial may revoke the order or dismiss the case.

Cost of commitment is borne by the county of residence in case of an indigent person.

THE BRYCE HOSPITAL.

TUSCALOOSA, ALA.

Under the provisions of the act of February 9, 1852, "To Establish a Hospital for Insane Persons in Alabama," a joint committee from the Senate and House, consisting of one member from each judicial circuit, with Governor Collier as chairman, selected the County of Tuscaloosa in which to locate the hospital. Five commissioners, appointed by this joint committee, selected the site two miles east of Tuscaloosa, and adopted the "Kirkbride plan," recommended by the Association of Superintendents of Hospitals for the Insane.

The name adopted by the Legislature was "The Alabama Insane Hospital." Dr. A. Lopez, of Mobile, had previously been appointed by the Governor to visit other hospitals and report to the committee with plans.

The committee of three trustees, after some changes, finally composed of James H. Dearing, A. C. Gooch and A. S. Nicholson, all residing in Tuscaloosa, was appointed by the Governor to take charge of the erection of the buildings. Five per cent of the state's income was appropriated for the work. Three hundred and twenty acres of land were at that time purchased, and the erection of the main building was begun in 1852.

Owing to some opposition and difficulty in obtaining material, the erection of the main edifice, a four-story center building, with three-story wings, in three sections of three wards each, was continued through eight years. In the fall of 1860 parts of the hospital were sufficiently complete to receive patients.

In 1857 the Governor nominated to the Senate the following seven gentlemen, whose names were confirmed, as trustees to control the hospital: Dr. Reuben Searcy, president; Dr. James Guild, Dr. A. G. Mabry, R. T. Nott, J. C. Spencer, Porter King, and Rev. B. Manly.

The trustees held their first meeting in Tuscaloosa in July, 1858. They reviewed their duties and determined on a general plan of work. In 1860, upon the recommendation of Miss Dorothea L. Dix, they elected Dr. Peter Bryce, superintendent. He was a native of South Carolina and was assistant physician in the hospital at Columbia, S. C. He was 26 years of age.

Dr. Bryce was elected for a term of eight years from October 1, 1860. At the time of his death, in August, 1892, he had been elected to four terms of office, and a few weeks lacking had been continuously superintendent for 32 years.

Dr. Bryce began his duties in troublesome times. The Civil War was just beginning and during the long four years of its history and the period of reconstruction that followed he was greatly embarrassed. With a depleted state treasury, it required great tact and administrative ability to care for and support his hospital during that time. During the 32 years of his administration he lived to see the institution grow in the confidence and esteem of the state. He died in 1892 noted, honored and respected in his own state and over the whole country. The Legislature to his honor incorporated his name into that of the hospital.

Dr. J. T. Searcy in October, 1892, was elected to succeed Dr. Bryce and still holds the position. In the 51 years of state care of the insane in Alabama there have been but two superintendents. The "political victors" in changes of state administrations have not counted the control of the insane among their "spoils."

The Tuscaloosa Hospital has connected with it about 1500 acres of land, lying in an irregular shape some three miles along the south bank of the Warrior River. The colony, to accommodate 75 white men, is about two miles from the main building. These patients do the farm work and are most satisfied, seldom wishing to return to the main hospital.

The buildings at The Bryce Hospital, with two or three exceptions, are of brick or cement. With the labor of a few hired carpenters and workmen and the help of patients, buildings of cement are being successfully built. A cement building for 250 women, the materials of which, except iron and glass, were prepared on the premises, has been recently erected. The saw and planing mill of the hospital furnished the lumber and woodwork—sash, doors, flooring and all.

The original building has a center building four stories high and wings of three stories, extending on each side to a total length of about 1100 feet. This building accommodates about two-thirds of the patients. There are to-day, April, 1912, 1441 patients, 1377 whites and 64 negroes, in this hospital. There are a few more women than men. There have been, to this time, 13,066 patients treated in The Bryce Hospital.

This hospital has separate psychopathic wards for new patients, and separate wards and buildings for the violent, the demented, the tubercular and the pellagrin patients.

Cases of pellagra come in increasing numbers, and constitute a most serious problem. Pellagra generally prevails in summer months and gets well or better during the winter. The psychic and the skin symptoms show themselves generally following two or three seasons of salivation, anorexia and diarrhœa. Patients exhibiting the psychopathic results of the disease are coming into the hospital generally from over the state. The back-country furnishes the greater number, few coming from towns and cities.

The days of reconstruction rendered necessary the employment of patients in many ways. Since then out-of-door employment is found to be far the most efficient remedy. Men and women patients are employed in one way and another in as large proportions as practicable. Work upon the farm and gardens takes the larger portion of the men. Most of the women do needle and laundry work. An out-of-door life is encouraged for as many as possible, which, in this climate, can be enjoyed most of the year.

Out of 1500 acres of land, about 400 are cultivated in field crops and about 100 in gardens.

SUPERINTENDENTS.

Dr. Peter Bryce	1860-1892
Dr. J. T. Searcy	1892-in office

ASSISTANT SUPERINTENDENTS.

Dr. E. D. Bondurant	1892-1896
Dr. W. D. Partlow, Bryce Hospital	1908-
Dr. E. L. McCafferty, Mt. Vernon Hospital	1908-

ASSISTANT PHYSICIANS.

Dr. J. H. Murfee	1867-1869	Dr. G. C. Boudousque	1898-1900
Dr. John Little	1869-1875	Dr. George R. Reau	1899-1901
Dr. R. P. Huger	1872-1886	Dr. W. S. Sowell	1899-1900
Dr. H. P. Cochrane	1875-1881	Dr. M. L. Winn	1899-1899
Dr. B. L. Wyman	1881-1884	Dr. M. L. Molloy	1900-1900
Dr. F. H. Sims	1882-1889	Dr. C. M. Rudolph	1900-1908
Dr. E. D. Bondurant	1885-1892	Dr. T. F. Huey	1901-1901
Dr. W. G. Somerville	1889-1891	Dr. W. D. Partlow	1901-1908
Dr. R. A. Wright	1890-1896	Dr. George H. Searcy	1901-1905
Dr. W. B. Hall	1891-1893	Dr. R. D. Spratt	1901-1902
Dr. P. T. Vaughan	1892-1895	Dr. E. L. McCafferty	1902-1908
Dr. H. B. Wilkinson	1893-1897	Dr. Joseph Leland	1902-
Dr. J. S. Musiat	1893-1896	Dr. W. M. Dupree	1903-1904
Dr. Burgett Woodcock	1894-1896	Dr. T. F. Taylor	1904-1907
Dr. C. W. Hilliard	1895-1895	Dr. J. A. Lanford	1905-
Dr. S. J. Purifoy	1895-1895	Dr. J. H. Somerville	1906-1908
Dr. W. M. Faulk	1896-1902	Dr. M. L. Tisdale	1907-
Dr. Sydney Leach	1896-1898	Dr. R. R. Ivey	1909-
Dr. Hardee Johnson	1896-1896	Dr. N. T. Davie	1909-
Dr. J. B. Killebrew	1896-1898	Dr. T. S. McDiarmid	1909-1910
Dr. J. E. Wiley	1897-1898	Dr. B. A. Burks	1910-

TRUSTEES.

Dr. Reuben Searcy	1857-1887	Dr. B. H. Moren	1865-1873
Dr. James Guild	1857-1873	Judge Wm. Miller	1870-1875
Dr. A. G. Mabry	1857-1874	E. F. Jennings	1870-1874
Capt. R. T. Nott	1857-1867	J. DeF. Richards	1870-1872
J. C. Spencer	1857-1859	E. F. Bouchell	1870-1871
Porter King	1857-1878	A. F. Given	1872-1875
Rev. B. Manly	1857-1868	O. Berry	1873-1875
M. L. Stansel	1861-1863	N. H. Browne	1876-1890
Judge A. B. Clitheral	1861-1863	W. S. Mudd	1876-1877
J. W. Payne	1863-1867	H. M. Somerville	1876-1893

Dr. J. J. Dement........	1876-1891	B. Friedman............	1894-1896
Dr. J. C. Hamilton......	1876-1887	J. Manly Foster........	1896-1907
J. W. Inzer.............	1878-1900	Dr. J. L. Williamson....	1896-
Dr. George D. Norris...	1878-1890	Samuel Will John.......	1899-
Dr. J. T. Searcy........	1887-1892	E. M. Robinson.........	1900-1908
Dr. J. B. Gaston........	1887-1908	Dr. E. D. Bondurant....	1902-
Dr. Elisha Young.......	1890-1898	C. B. Verner............	1907-
A. C. Hargrove.........	1890-1896	Dr. W. M. Wilkinson...	1908-
R. T. Simpson..........	1892-1905	J. C. Rich..............	1909-
Dr. Wm. G. Somerville..	1893-	Dr. W. M. Falk.........	1912-
Prof. Alonza Hill.......	1893-1894	Dr. F. A. Webb.........	1912-

OFFICERS OF BOTH HOSPITALS (1910).

Dr. J. T. Searcy..............................Superintendent
Dr. John Little..............................Treasurer
W. C. Harris..............................Steward

THE MT. VERNON HOSPITAL.

(For Negroes)

Mt. Vernon, Ala.

In the session of 1900-01, the Legislature set apart for the use of the insane the old military reservation at Mt. Vernon, Ala., which a few years before had been ceded to the state by the United States Government to be held for public purposes. The trustees devoted it to the care of the colored insane. The same act of the Legislature incorporated the two institutions, The Bryce Hospital at Tuscaloosa, and The Mt. Vernon Hospital, at Mt. Vernon, with the name, the Alabama Insane Hospital, under the control of the same board of trustees, having one superintendent and one treasurer. The single management of both hospitals simplifies and unifies the control of the two institutions. There is no rivalry between them for appropriations and they reciprocate with each other in many particulars.

The Mt. Vernon Hospital is about 30 miles north of Mobile on the Mobile River, and on the Birmingham and Mobile branch of the Southern Railway system.

Most of the buildings have been built by the hospital employees and are one-story cottages; no one of them holds more than 150 patients. A large acreage of the best Southern pine on the place furnished from the hospital saw-mill and shops the material for building at a very low cost.

In May, 1901, after remodeling the old building and the erection of a number of others, the place was made habitable for patients. Three hundred and twenty negro patients were moved from Tuscaloosa to Mt. Vernon in one train in one day, without accident. There were, in 1912, about 700 patients at Mt. Vernon, and about 1500 at Tuscaloosa.

Separate buildings for all classes of patients are provided here. The pellagrins and the tubercular are separated from the others.

The negro insane are increasing at a more rapid rate than the whites. Lineal deterioration of general health is the first predisposing cause for it.

THE CARE OF THE INSANE IN ARIZONA.

The Arizona State Hospital for the Insane, located at Phoenix, is the only state institution for the care of the insane in Arizona.

It was opened for the admission of patients on January 10, 1887, prior to which time the insane were cared for in a private asylum at Stockton, Cal.

The institution is under the direction of the Board of Control, which is composed of the Governor, State Auditor, and a citizen member.

All persons are entitled to admission to the State Hospital. Pay patients may be received under rates established by the Board of Control.

Legal Procedure.—A sworn application to the judge of probate because the person is dangerous to be at large.

The insane person is brought before the judge of probate for examination and two or more witnesses who are acquainted with the patient are examined. Two reputable physicians must examine him and make written statements under oath as to his mental condition, as to his safety to be at large and prospect of recovery. If the judge of probate is satisfied the patient is insane he directs his confinement in the hospital until restored to reason.

Appeal from Commitment.—Every patient may procure a writ of *habeas corpus* by a petition signed by himself or friend.

Cost of commitment must be borne by the patient if he has sufficient estate; if indigent, by the county.

ARIZONA STATE HOSPITAL FOR THE INSANE.[1]

PHOENIX, ARIZ.

The State Hospital for the Insane is situated about three miles east of the City of Phoenix, and consists of 160 acres of land, together with administration building, hospital, cottages and other buildings necessary for the needs of such an institution.

It was established in 1886, at an original cost of $100,000, and had, at that time, a capacity of 200 patients. Since that date more

[1] By Thos. E. Farish, Arizona Historian.

than double the original cost of the institution has been expended in the erection of new buildings, etc.

Prior to the establishment of this institution, insane patients of the Territory of Arizona were taken to Stockton, Cal., where they were cared for in a private institution. In 1887, when the hospital was ready for the admission of patients, there were brought back from California and placed in the institution 61 patients, 49 males and 12 females.

The first government of the hospital under territorial rule consisted of a Board of Directors composed of three members, and the construction of the first buildings was, unfortunately, attended with some scandal.

The first superintendent of the institution was Dr. O. L. Mahoney, who was followed in 1888 by Dr. I. S. Titus.

In 1896 Dr. H. A. Hughes was superintendent and resident physician of the institution.

In 1898 Dr. J. Miller was superintendent, and the number of inmates was: male, 119; female, 48; total, 167.

During the 18 months next preceding June 30, 1900, extensive repairs were made to the buildings then existing, and new buildings were erected, all at a cost of $14,000. The number of inmates at that time was: males, 135; females, 40; total, 175.

At this time the government of the institution was vested in the Board of Control of the Territory of Arizona, consisting of the Governor, the Auditor, and a citizen member, the latter being the secretary of the board.

In 1902 Dr. H. H. Ward became superintendent, and on June 30 the number of inmates was: males, 173, females, 33. The number of inmates on June 30, 1914, was: males, 211; females, 43.

In 1906 Dr. Ray Ferguson became superintendent. There were 266 patients in the institution—215 males and 51 females. At this time the institution consisted of one main building, with six wards and two detached cottages, with the necessary outbuildings, etc.

In 1907 the institution was crowded beyond its capacity, there being 289 patients—231 males and 58 females.

In 1908 Dr. Ray Ferguson was succeeded by Dr. J. A. Ketcherside. During the year a new hospital building was constructed, and two cottages were also built. The total number of patients was 309.

In 1910 a new hospital building was completed, furnished and occupied. The number of inmates on June 30 was 367—290 males and 77 females.

On June 30, 1911, the number of inmates was 370, and the superintendent was Dr. H. K. Beauchamp.

On June 30, 1912, the number of inmates was 375, and the superintendent was Dr. A. C. Kingsley.

On June 30, 1913, the number of inmates was 409, and on June 30, 1914, the number had increased to 442.

The institution was originally a territorial institution, and was, as above stated, established and organized in 1886. When Arizona was admitted into the Union as a state, the institution became the property of the state, and much has been done since that time for the benefit of the patients. New buildings have been added and appropriations have been made for more. Appropriations have also been made for other improvements, such as musical instruments, a moving picture machine, etc., for the amusement and recreation of the patients. Agriculture is carried on to quite a large extent, those of the patients whose condition permits being engaged in working the farm. The climate of Arizona being such that outdoor work and exercise are practicable nearly every day in the year, opportunity is found for the patients to be in the open much of the time, which contributes largely to the general health and often-times to the ultimate cure of the patients.

The comparatively large number of inmates of the institution may be ascribed to the fact that the State of Arizona has no institutions for the care of the epileptic, the feeble-minded and the alcoholic and drug habitue, and in consequence these classes are taken into this institution.

BOARD OF CONTROL, 1914.

George W. P. Hunt............................Governor.
James J. Callahan............................Auditor.
Charles R. Osburn............................Secretary.

RESIDENT OFFICERS, 1914.

Alfred C. Kingsley, M. D................Superintendent.
Harlan P. Mills, M. D...................Pathologist.
Francis F. Malone, M. D.................Assistant physician.

THE CARE OF THE INSANE IN ARKANSAS.

Up to 1883 the insane of Arkansas were confined in so-called poorhouses and jails. In that year the Arkansas State Hospital for Nervous Diseases was established at Little Rock, largely through the influence of Dr. P. O. Hooper, subsequently its superintendent. The Arkansas State Lunatic Asylum, as it was first called, was opened for the reception of patients on March 1, 1883, and remains to-day (1915) the only state institution for the care of the insane in Arkansas.

The institution is under the control of a Board of Trustees, consisting of six members, appointed by the Governor for a term of two years, one from each Congressional district; the Treasurer of the state is ex-officio president of the board. This board has charge of the state charitable institutions, as well as the insane hospital.

All indigent patients are maintained at the State Hospital at the expense of the state.

The Legislature of 1913 passed an act which provides that the superintendent, in his discretion, may parole patients for a period of six months, and upon application extend the parole for an additional period of six months, at which time the patient must be discharged.

Any insane citizen or resident of the state may be admitted to the State Hospital for Nervous Diseases as a patient upon proper proof and proceedings according to law.

Legal Procedure.—A written statement is made and filed by any reputable citizen with the county and probate judge alleging that the person should be admitted to the state hospital for the insane. The judge appoints a time to hear the testimony of witnesses and must cause the insane person to be examined separately by two reputable and disinterested physicians, who must present a sworn statement of the result of their examination. If the judge of probate finds the person insane he transmits his decision in writing with copies of the original statements and the results of the examination of the physicians to the superintendent of the State Hospital. The superintendent notifies the judge of probate of his willingness to admit the patient if there is room. If there is no room he must notify the judge and return him the documents in the case and must record at the Hospital the name and county of the insane person, who then becomes entitled to precedence in admission over all who apply later.

An insane person wandering at large must be arrested by any peace officer and taken before a magistrate, who may keep him in restraint until he can be sent to the hospital. If he has no friends the magistrate may order that he be confined in the county or city jail and must give immediate notice to the county judge or city attorney, whose duty it is to take the proper proceedings to have him sent to the Hospital.

Expense of Commitment.—Each county in the state is responsible for all expenses of committing and removing to the State Hospital insane persons resident in the county.

STATE HOSPITAL FOR NERVOUS DISEASES.[1]

LITTLE ROCK, ARK.

According to the laws of Arkansas, approved February 20, 1838, each family was liable for the maintenance of its poor and impotent members and for the confinement of its insane. This responsibility extended to the third and fourth generations. The law further stated: "If there be no person having charge of a person of unsound mind, any judge of a court of record, or any two justices of the peace of the county, may cause such insane person to be apprehended, and may employ any person to confine him in some suitable place. The "suitable places" for the dangerous insane were the county jails, where many unfortunates spent their lives. The harmless frequently wandered off into the woods, and lived as wild people. This was the condition of affairs before the State Hospital for Nervous Diseases, or Arkansas State Lunatic Asylum, as it was first called, was opened March 1, 1883.

On the 11th of January, 1873, a bill appropriating $50,000, to be used in purchasing grounds and erecting buildings for an insane asylum, was introduced in the Arkansas Legislature by H. M. McVeigh, of Mississippi County, and D. P. Baldwin, of Hot Springs. Because of the wild extravagance of that period, public finances were in a terrible condition and the treasury was bankrupt. As a result, the asylum bill was reported back from the Committee on Ways and Means of the House with the recommendation that it do not pass. But it was too popular a measure to fail. All classes of people had commended it, and the bill was passed by an overwhelming majority, and approved by the Governor April 19, 1873.

This bill owed its existence largely to Dr. P. O. Hooper, for many years the leading physician of Arkansas, and later the superintendent of the asylum. He appreciated the great need for such an institution and worked hard for it. During the session of the Legislature he devoted much of his time to lobbying for the bill. H. M. McVeigh, George Thronburg and James Rutherford

[1] By Mrs. Adolphine Fletcher Terry, daughter of John G. Fletcher, a member of the Board of Trustees at the time the Institution was opened.

were members of the General Assembly who contributed to its final successful passage. The bill provided that the Governor should nominate, and with the consent of the Senate appoint five persons to be trustees of the lunatic asylum, to manage and direct the affairs of the institution, hold and purchase property and erect buildings. At this time, owing to the exigencies of reconstruction, Arkansas had two Governors, Brooks and Baxter, and was practically in a state of civil war. Baxter was finally declared Governor, but was too much occupied with militant matters to do anything more than approve the bill for the asylum, and it was left to his successor, Governor Garland, to appoint the first Board of Trustees. His appointments were entirely non-partisan. Dr. Hooper was the chairman and directing spirit; among others Dudley E. Jones, H. C. Caldwell, later United States Circuit Judge, and Gordon Peay, of Little Rock. Dr. Hooper and Judge Caldwell took up the matter of a site for the institution, and finally selected 80 acres of land on an elevation west of Little Rock. The chief problem to be solved was that of an adequate water supply, but the board was assured by engineers that the springs in this particular land would be sufficient. The tract was bought from Judge G. C. Watkins, who was so interested in public improvements that he sold the land to the board at a low price.

Dr. Hooper personally inspected all the large institutions for the insane in the United States, and under his direction plans were made for a building by Joseph Willis of Memphis, Tenn.

The work so far had been done quietly, as the board was anxious to have the institution located near Little Rock. But during the administration of Governor Miller a bill was introduced and passed by the Legislature appropriating money to buy Snow Springs, a dilapidated summer resort, composed of a number of ramshackle frame houses, about four miles from Hot Springs. The Legislature evidently thought that the place could be used just as it was. Governor Miller vetoed the bill, and was publicly burned in effigy in Hot Springs.

Nothing else was accomplished until 1881, when a board was appointed by Governor Churchill, composed of Dr. P. O. Hooper, G. R. Welch, John G. Fletcher, J. M. Hudson and J. W. Stayton. The Legislature of that year appropriated $150,000 for an asylum building. The board met, elected Dr. Hooper president, and let the contract to Thalman & Clask for an institution to be erected according to plans and specifications furnished the previous trustees.

The board wrote in advance to the sheriffs in the various counties asking for the number of insane known to them. The estimated number was 366, more than enough to fill the original building, which was designed for 250 inmates. Within half a year after the opening of the building the wards were filled beyond their original capacity. Three hundred and five were admitted during the first eight months, and it was evident that a new building was necessary. The board recommended a house for negroes, as there was trouble on this score.

The institution was opened March 1, 1883. The central part of the building was 62 feet in front by 104 feet deep, four stories high, surmounted by a tower. From this wings extended north and south 40 feet wide and 120 feet long, three stories high. At the end of each of these wings was a transverse wing 36 feet front by 66 feet deep, projecting 10 feet in front of the others. It contained 212 rooms. In addition a rear building was built, containing the kitchen, laundry, store room, bake room, ovens, steam engine, boilers, engineer's waste room and sleeping rooms for employees. The entire cost was $149,750.37.

Dr. C. C. Forbes, who had made an excellent reputation in connection with the treatment of the insane in Louisville, Ky., was elected to the position of superintendent. He accepted the appointment and entered upon his duties December, 1882, continuing in office until May, 1885, when he resigned because of failing health. During his administration the grounds were enclosed, apple and peach orchards planted and new grounds opened for gardening. Much grading and road building was done and a barn, smoke house, coal house, shed, carpenter shop, tool and pump house erected, in the main without the employment of a laboring force. The patients were all employed as far as their well-being would permit—the men out of doors, the women in the sewing room, laundry and kitchen. As little restraint as possible was used. In a report on this subject Dr. Forbes said: "There is not what is known as a lodge or strong room in the building. There is not a crib bed here. On the other hand, there are lockless doors. The camisole, wristlets, mittens and anklets are the restraints sometimes resorted to; but only with the violently maniacal or the violently destructive of clothing." He also reported that games and music were furnished the patients for pastime, that occasional dances were given, and once a month religious exercises were held in the chapel, with 60 per cent of the patients in attendance.

When Dr. Forbes resigned the Board of Trustees prevailed on Dr. Hooper to become superintendent. He held office until 1893, John G. Fletcher succeeding him as president of the board. These were years of constant growth. In 1885 over $77,000 were expended on a building which accommodated 200, and increasing the capacity of the institution to 450. In 1891 an appropriation of $85,000 was made to erect three new buildings, a chapel, located west of the main building, a female annex, north, and a male annex, south of the main building. The female annex was built two stories in height, in the shape of a letter L, each arm being 185 feet by 37 feet, containing four wards and two dining rooms. The male annex measured 158 feet by 87 feet, three stories high, and contained three wards and one dining room. The contract was given to James R. Miller, of Little Rock. During the period of construction there was no money in the treasury to meet the expenses incurred. Nevertheless, Mr. Miller continued the work, taking the warrants of the board and holding them until they could be paid.

The water supply proved from the first to be insufficient. Originally it came from wells and cisterns on the grounds. Later six lots one and three-quarter miles from the asylum, containing valuable springs, were purchased, and the water conducted through iron pipes to cisterns near the buildings. A residence was built contiguous to the pump house for the engineer who had charge of the machinery for pumping the water. Eighty additional acres west of the asylum were purchased during this period and a storehouse was built. The weekly per capita cost of maintenance of the patients, including the salary of officers, was $3.

Many difficulties were experienced by the management. According to law, each county was permitted to send a certain quota of patients, based on the population of the county. But the law also provided that "no person shall be refused admission, as long as there is unoccupied room for patients in the asylum." Some of the counties, not sending their full number, others speedily overran theirs. As there was never sufficient room for those seeking admittance, it frequently happened that patients, unimproved, had to be returned home to make room for those from other sections of the state. Many persons regarded the institution as a place of punishment for those sent to it and a degradation to their families. So families often kept their insane members at home until all chances of effecting a cure had passed. Two-thirds of all the patients had been insane over two years at the time of their admittance. Others regarded the institution as a mammoth poorhouse. Idiotic and epileptic children were constantly sent by county judges who expected in this way to get rid of them. Old, harmless, incurable people, who should have been cared for at home, were constantly being admitted on the sworn statement of relatives that they were violently insane and dangerous to the community.

In the spring of 1893 the method of appointing the Board of Trustees was changed by an act of the Legislature. The Treasurer of the state became the ex-officio president of the board and six members were to be appointed by the Governor, one from each Congressional district. This board has charge of the three state charitable institutions: the insane asylum, blind and deaf mute schools. In September of that year Dr. Hooper resigned and Dr. J. J. Robertson, of Malvern, Ark., was elected to fill the unexpired term—until November 1, 1894, when he was re-elected for four years. The appointment was a political one, and his administration was not a success. In 1896 he resigned.

The year 1894 was a particularly disastrous year. During the summer the institution suffered from serious epidemics of erysipelas and dysentery. There were 132 deaths. Few patients or attendants escaped the latter illness. For a part of the time there were not enough well persons to wait on the sick. On the night of October 2, 1894, a cyclone destroyed six wards of the south wing of the main building. The center building was entirely unroofed, the tower thrown down, stables, servants' houses, furnace buildings and fences all ruined.[1] Two years later the laundry, valued at $2000, was burned, there being no insurance. The springs which had supplied the institution gave out early in 1894 and the question of water supply became a serious one. The board then contracted

[1] Dr. J. F. Ingate, assistant physician, was killed during this cyclone.

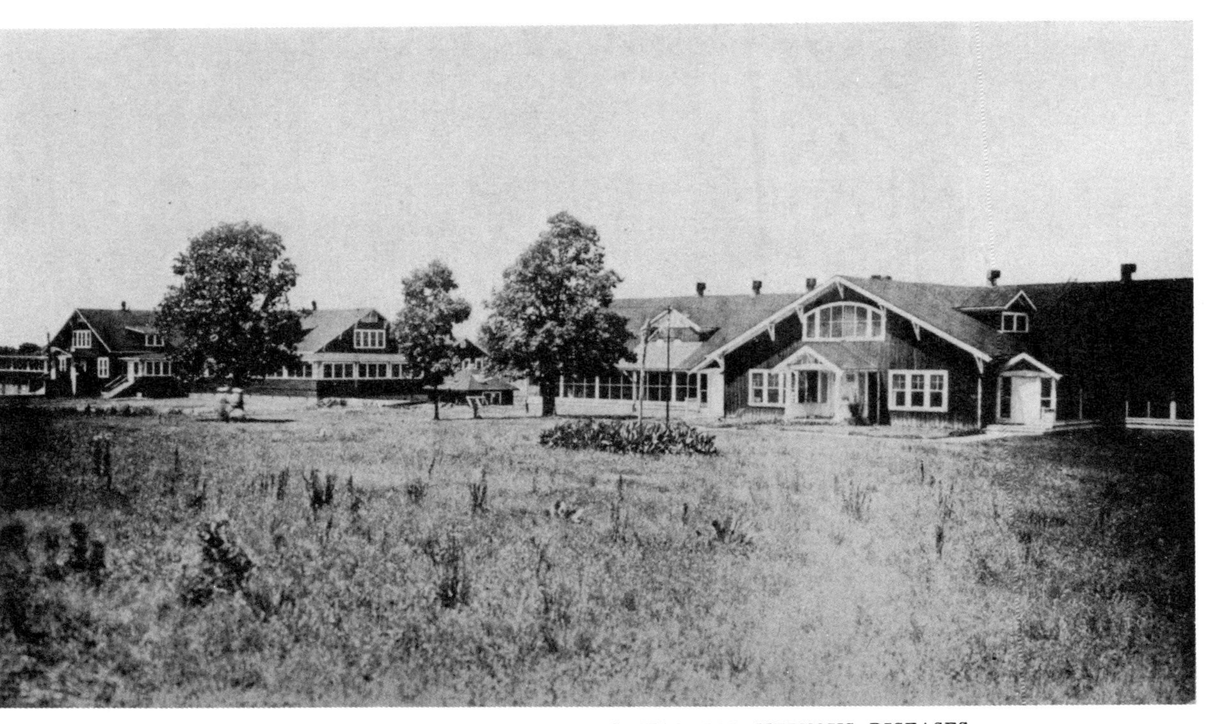

INFIRMARY, ARKANSAS STATE HOSPITAL FOR NERVOUS DISEASES.

with the Home Water Company to supply 45,000 gallons a day from the Arkansas River, at a monthly cost of $195.

The question of the disposal of sewage also gave much trouble.

During the first year of Dr. Robertson's administration the average cost per capita was $117.93. In 1895 the Legislature, in a sudden fit of economy, stipulated that the amount expended should not exceed $100 per patient per annum. Dr. Robinson reported that this had been insufficient, and the patients had been denied many luxuries and even necessities.

Following Dr. Robertson's resignation, Dr. Hooper was re-elected, serving through 1900. During this time a new cold storage plant, an additional dining room, kitchen and an infirmary were built. The infirmary cost $22,000 and accommodated 40 patients—20 males and 20 females. The average number of patients was 613; the average cost of each patient per annum $97.88.

Dr. Hooper's death occurred suddenly July 29, 1902, while aboard a train on his way to California in search of health.

Dr. H. C. Stinson, an Arkansas physician, succeeded Dr. Hooper. Upon his retirement he was put in charge of the Confederate Home, which had been placed under the control of the Board of State Charitable Institutions. At the session of the Legislature in 1909 an appropriation of $200,000 was made for the erection of a second hospital for nervous diseases (the name of the institution having been changed). This appropriation was not available, however, because of a lack of money in the treasury. It was thought that some city in Arkansas, in order to secure the institution, would offer to the state an amount in lands and available money equal to the appropriation made by the Legislature. No offers worthy of consideration were made and the plan was abandoned.

When Dr. James L. Greene, the present superintendent, took charge, September 1, 1911, he undertook the thorough reorganization of the institution. Earlier in the year the Legislature had appropriated $100,000 for annexes, in the hope that this amount would provide sufficient room for those then being denied admission. The appropriation was vetoed by the Governor. Dr. Greene, through rearranging the wards and reconstructing an unused building, not only made room for all the insane in the state, but provided for future growth, at a cost of only $47,364. It was found that the property was in a very bad state of repair, and the buildings were taken in hand in a systematic way, overhauled and put in order. All insane persons are now received without delay; for the year ending August, 1912, 619 were admitted. Although the institution was provided with an infirmary, it had not been used for that purpose. The patients who became physically ill were allowed to remain in whatever room they occupied before the advent of the illness. There was also a very large number of cases of tuberculosis, with no effort toward isolation in practice. Arrangements were made at once by Dr. Greene to care properly for the sick and to isolate those suffering from and suspected of tuberculosis. Investigation showed that records of patients had not been kept at all in many cases, or, if kept, were entirely inadequate. In some cases even the commitment papers had been lost. A card index system was inaugurated and one ward set apart in each wing of the main building as a receiving ward, where patients should be received, examined and registered. Dr. Greene also determined to have all the patients examined and classified. The work was begun January 1, 1912, with 1124 patients in the institution and completed by September 1. Surgical equipment of the best variety has been purchased; a laboratory and a department for the use of hydrotherapy established.

The hospital grounds contain 160 acres. The tract was purchased for $16,000 and is now estimated to be worth $176,000. There are 11 buildings on the ground, all built in a substantial way. These buildings now have 1718 beds for the accommodation of patients, and funds are available for additions to the infirmary that would increase the capacity of that building to an extent that will bring the total capacity of the institution to 1788 patients. On May 19, 1914, there were in the institution 1584 patients.

Dr. J. L. Greene resigned as superintendent in November, 1914; he was succeeded by Dr. F. B. Young, who assumed office on December 1, 1914.

ASSISTANT PHYSICIANS.

Dr. J. M. Buchanan.
Dr. H. B. Williams.
Dr. D. C. Carroll.
Dr. J. C. Crenshaw.
Dr. W. L. Worcester.
Dr. J. L. Blakemore.
Dr. J. F. Baum.
Dr. H. Wells.
Dr. J. F. Ingate.[1]
Dr. W. B. Barner.
Dr. J. C. Crenshaw.
Dr. R. L. White.
Dr. C. Arkebauer.[2]
Dr. W. F. Saner.
Dr. D. W. Roberts.[2]
Dr. W. S. Woolford.
Dr. G. B. Fletcher.
Dr. C. R. Doyne.[2]
Dr. J. C. Davis.[2]
Dr. W. P. Moore.[2]
Dr. W. C. Dunaway.

CLINICAL DIRECTORS.

Dr. G. W. Dishong.
Dr. R. F. Darnall.[2]

PATHOLOGIST.

Dr. L. O. Thompson.
Dr. D. C. Lee.[2]

DENTIST.

Dr. J. T. Starnes.

[1] Was killed during the cyclone mentioned in the body of the history.
[2] Now in the service of the institution (1914).

THE CARE OF THE INSANE IN CALIFORNIA.[1]

The first asylum for the insane to be established in California was that at Stockton, which was opened in 1853. In 1875 the Napa State Hospital was opened at Napa. In 1888 the Agnew State Hospital, located at Agnew, near San Jose, was opened as a chronic asylum. In 1893 the Mendocino State Hospital, located near Ukiah, Mendocino County, and the Southern California State Hospital, located in San Bernardino County, were opened for the reception of patients. In 1889 the Agnew Asylum was changed from an asylum for the chronic insane to one for the reception of all classes. In 1903 the Folsom State Hospital for the care of the criminal and convict insane was established on the grounds of the Folsom State Prison; this hospital is as yet unfinished, owing to lack of available funds. Contracts are about to be let (1915) for the construction of a new hospital (Norwalk) in Los Angeles County. In addition to the above mentioned hospitals, the Legislature of 1885 established at Eldridge the Sonoma State Home "for the care and treatment of feeble-minded children."

From the beginning California had made the care of the insane a state proposition. There is no county care, as such, with the one exception of Los Angeles County, which has made provision for a few insane on its poor farm. There are no city hospitals for the insane.

For many years after the organization of the state hospitals they were each conducted by a separate Board of Directors, or Managers, who were responsible for the conduct of the institution, for the purchase of supplies, and the general running of each institution.

In 1897 a State Commission in Lunacy was created, consisting of the Governor, the Secretary of State, the Attorney-General,

[1] The material for this chapter, together with the histories of the individual institutions, with the exception of Mendocino, was furnished by F. W. Hatch, M. D., general superintendent California State Commission in Lunacy.

the secretary of the State Board of Health and an appointed officer for General Superintendent of State Hospitals. The Board of Managers' actions and estimates for expenses were subject to review by this commission, who had also supervisory charge of the hospitals and their conduct. In 1911 a State Board of Control, governing the state institutions, was created, whose functions mainly were the final supervision of contracts and expenditures, the auditing of institutional accounts, and the creation of a system of accounting for each state institution. The local boards are still in existence, but in the case of the hospitals they are subject to the State Commission in Lunacy and the Board of Control, the latter exercising mainly a business function.

The main buildings of the hospitals were erected from 20 to 50 years ago and generally followed the plan of a central or administration building, with three-story ward buildings on each side. About 1900 the state began to make enlargements along the cottage system, which plan is being continued. Agnew, which was originally built on the lineal plan, was, after its destruction by the earthquake in 1906, rebuilt as an entire cottage system, no cottage exceeding two stories in height. All the state hospitals, with one exception, have fully equipped receiving buildings. They are fitted up with complete operating rooms and an up-to-date hydrotherapy installation, the latter being in constant use, with trained operators in attendance. Much work has been done in the hospital system in the sterilization of proper cases of chronic insanity. The plan pursued is first to get the consent of near relatives where it is possible to do so, then the history of the case is referred to a commission consisting of the secretary of the State Board of Health, the General Superintendent of State Hospitals and the local hospital superintendent, for consent or refusal. Since the commencement of the work operations have been done in something like 400 cases.

The medical staffs are at present appointed after civil service examinations. There are at present two special medical officers working along pathological and bacteriological lines, and one specially employed physician is doing Wassermann work for the hospitals that are not supplied with workers in that line.

There is a state dentist who covers four of the hospitals, and a regularly appointed dentist in each of the two largest hospitals.

In 1914 there was established an after-care physician, located in San Francisco, whose work is meeting with much success.

An eugenics field worker from Cold Spring Harbor, L. I., is now (1915) making a survey of the state under the general direction of the State Commission in Lunacy.

It has been found very difficult to establish satisfactory training schools in the California hospitals, owing to the long hours necessarily enforced upon attendants.

The first general law in California regarding the insane was enacted about May 17, 1853. It provided that the county judge of any county in the state should, upon the application of any person under oath, setting forth that any person by reason of insanity was unsafe to be at large, or was suffering from mental derangement, forthwith cause the said person to be brought before him and cause to appear two reputable physicians, to examine the alleged insane person, and if they found such person to be insane, to certify under oath that the charge of insanity was correct, and if the judge was thereupon satisfied that the insane person was unsafe to be at large, he should order him placed in an insane asylum of California.

Another section of the law provided that the state should in all cases be chargeable with the expense incurred by the conveyance of the indigent insane to and from the asylum and for their maintenance during their residence in said asylum.

Another section provided that paying patients should pay according to the terms directed by the trustees of the asylum, but that the insane poor should in all respects receive the same medical care, treatment and good and wholesome diet from the institution.

According to section 18 of the law then passed two-fifths of all monies received in computation of bonds, in accordance with an act concerning passengers arriving in the ports of California, approved May 3, 1852, was set apart as a fund for the insane asylums of California.

In 1854 the law regarding commitments was slightly modified in the respect that it required the county judge to make inquiry into the ability or inability of the insane person to bear the charge or expense for the time he might remain in the asylum. Another modification reads as follows: "The county sending the insane person to an asylum shall, in all cases where the person be indigent, pay the expense of such conveyance and, in the event of the death of such person, be chargeable with the funeral expenses."

The laws under which commitments are made remained practically unchanged until 1897, at which time the present lunacy law became a law. The purpose of the present lunacy law was based upon the proposition that the hospitals were intended to care for the poor and indigent, and that the state should appropriate sufficient money to maintain them. It recognized that there was a class, additional to the poor and indigent, who would become inmates of a hospital and it provided that this class should be made to pay for their support as stated in section 6, part 3, of the lunacy law.

In section 6 the State Commission in Lunacy is charged with the collection of the costs and charges of the commitment and transportation of insane persons to a state hospital and it may bring action to recover such charges.

The law of 1897 provided that counties should establish quarters for the alleged insane outside of a jail proper, and that examiners in lunacy should be appointed by the superior judge after filing their appointments with the Commission in Lunacy. It also tried to make the committal proceedings more of a medical than a legal proceeding. It was carried on successfully for a time, but certain provisions of the law were attacked on *habeas corpus* proceedings and were declared unconstitutional.

Under the laws it is the duty of the hospitals, and in case of their failure, the commission, to collect from father, mother, husband, wife or children, or the estate, or the individuals, if they have sufficient means, a certain monthly sum for their maintenance in the hospital. This is closely followed. The collections made under this method are placed in what is known as the "contingent fund," deposited with the State Treasurer monthly and placed to the credit of the hospitals, where it may be used for permanent improvements—buildings, lands and other improvements as are required for the best interests of the hospital and for such supplies and expenses as may be necessary. The "contingent fund" collected in 1911 for all the hospitals amounted to $168,372.35.

The commission, on the application of the superintendent of the hospital, may remit or reduce the amount demanded of the relatives of a patient in order that no hardship may be inflicted upon such relatives or on the individual.

The state hospitals are supported by appropriations made every two years by the Legislature. The appropriations are of two general characters, one covering strictly maintenance or support, the other salaries and wages. Under the general appropriation law the amounts are appropriated for two years and not more than one twenty-fourth can be drawn out in any one month, excepting where a surplus has been created, when it can be drawn upon. Contracts are let yearly for the staple supplies of the hospital. Monthly estimates are required of the Board of Managers of each hospital for both contract and non-contract supplies and for salaries and wages. On approval by the commission and the Board of Control, they can proceed to expend.

All insane persons are entitled to admission to the state hospitals except cases of idiocy, imbecility, epilepsy, chronic mental unsoundness, feeble-mindedness or *mania a potu.*

Voluntary patients may be admitted to any hospital except the Folsom State Hospital by an application to the medical superintendent for admission. Such patient may not be detained more than seven days after he has given notice in writing of his desire to leave.

Pay patients may be received under special agreement with relatives, guardians or friends.

Medical examiners, not less than two of whom must be in each county, receive certificates from the superior judge of each county, or city and county, that they are reputable physicians, graduates of incorporated medical colleges and in actual practice for five years.

Legal Procedure.—Whenever an affidavit is filed with a magistrate that a person is so disordered in mind as to endanger health and personal property the magistrate must order him taken before a judge of the superior court of the county.

A copy of the affidavit and warrant of arrest must be previously delivered to the alleged insane person and the judge must inform him that he is charged with insanity and has the right to make a defense. The judge must also state the time and place of hearing, which must be in open court.

The judge may also order a notice of the arrest to be served upon relatives residing in the county.

At the hearing two medical examiners must be present to listen to the testimony and to make a personal examination of the insane person and testify before the judge. The judge must examine any other proper witnesses who have knowledge of the mental and financial condition of the person. The alleged insane person must be present at the hearing and if he has no attorney the judge may appoint one.

If the medical examiners believe him to be dangerously insane they must make out a certificate to that effect, whereupon the judge must declare him insane and issue an order for confinement in the hospital. The certificate of examination accompanying the statement must be filed with the county clerk. If the judge refuses to grant an order any one aggrieved may demand a jury trial of the question.

The Commission in Lunacy is empowered to inquire into the reason why an insane person is not confined in a hospital and may apply to the judge of the superior court for his commitment.

An indigent insane person without residence in the state for at least one year may be returned to the county or state to which he belongs. Each hospital superintendent must, within three days, thoroughly examine the patient's physical and mental condition, and thereafter periodically, and note the condition upon blanks.

Appeal from Commitment.—If a person ordered to be committed is dissatisfied with the order he may, within five days, demand that the question be tried in the superior court of the county before a jury. The cause against the alleged insane person must be represented by the district attorney, and unless three-fourths of the jury render a verdict that he is insane, the alleged insane person must be discharged. Any one in custody is entitled to a writ of *habeas corpus.*

Costs of commitment are paid by the county or city and county in the case of an indigent person; if not indigent by his estate. If the patient is adjudged not to be insane the judge may charge the cost of the proceedings to the person making the application. Husband, wife, father and mother or children of the insane person and the guardian of his estate are liable for the charges for commitment and transportation to the hospital for the insane.

STOCKTON STATE HOSPITAL.

STOCKTON, CAL.

The Legislature in 1853, realizing the necessity for the proper care of persons so unfortunate as to become mentally unbalanced, established the "Insane Asylum of California," to be located in or near the City of Stockton. Through the generosity of Chas. M. Weber the site for this institution was deeded to David S. Terry, Isaac S. Freeborne, B. F. Lee, Samuel Purdy, H. A. Crabb and Nelson Taylor, trustees of the Stockton State Hospital. The Stockton State Hospital is located in what is now the residence district of the City of Stockton; it comprises 9 or 10 city blocks and has become very valuable. In recent years the hospital has acquired by purchase 220 acres of rich farm land about two miles from the city, on which has been erected buildings for the convalescent insane, the object being to afford employment for this class of patients. The buildings erected consist of the original structure made of brick, which still stands and is in use; the male department of similar construction, which contains the administration office, and the female department, located about one-third mile to the north of the male department.

In addition to the above is the receiving building, constructed of reinforced concrete, one story in height. Here all patients are first entered and given the hydrotherapy treatment, the equipment for same having been installed in the last few years. These buildings are surrounded by lawns and gardens, which afford pleasant recreation for convalescent patients. The medical superintendent and assistant physicians are comfortably housed in dwellings situated on the main avenue.

The disposal of sewage is cared for by the City of Stockton at a monthly rate of $65.

The water supply for domestic purposes is obtained from artesian wells. For irrigation at the farm, water is purchased from private parties.

Electricity is generally used for lighting purposes, being purchased on contract. Until recently natural gas, produced by wells belonging to the hospital, has been used for illuminating purposes. The supply of natural gas has been diminished for some time, and about two years ago electricity was installed.

The institution is governed by a Board of Managers consisting of five members, appointed by the Governor. The Board of Managers appoint the medical superintendent, and the medical superintendent appoints the subordinate officers and employees.

The medical staff consists of the medical superintendent, four assistant physicians, one of whom is a woman, and a resident dentist.

Numerous industrial pursuits are maintained, chief of which is the shoe shop; here are manufactured all shoes and slippers for the inmates. The main industries are mattress-making, broom-making, tin shop and general repairs.

The farm of 654 acres is now being productively maintained, the principal crops being potatoes and beans, all of which are consumed by the inmates and employees. Considerable alfalfa hay is raised and some wheat. Eggs in sufficient quantity to give the inmates a liberal supply come from the poultry yard. The dairy herd consists of 118 head of Holsteins, producing on the average 7500 gallons of milk per month.

In the fall and winter months dances are given weekly, accompanied by moving pictures.

On January 1, 1915, the population of the hospital consisted of 1356 males and 799 females, making a total of 2155. To administer to and care for these patients require 262 officers and employees.

Since the organization of the institution $1,231,065 has been appropriated for buildings and improvements, together with $345,-924.58 from special funds raised by direct tax. In addition to the above $413,330 has been expended from the contingent fund for improvements and repairs. The sources of revenue are as follows: Appropriations by the Legislature for improvements, maintenance and salaries, and the contingent fund. The latter is derived principally from paying patients and averages, for the past four years, about $30,000. The present yearly appropriation for maintenance is $203,310 and for salaries $162,530.

BOARD OF MANAGERS.

Name	Term
Nelson Taylor	1853-1854
P. E. Jordan	1853-1854
Andrew Lester	1853-1854 1857-1858
J. K. Shafer	1853-1854
Enoch Gore	1853-1854
S. A. Hooker	1855-1855
P. E. Connor	1855-1855 1857-1858
Dr. Grattan	1855-1855
Judge Barnes	1855-1855
J. W. O'Neal	1856-1856 1859-1860
J. W. Buffington	1856-1856
Dr. G. A. Shurtleff	1856-1856 1861-1863
R. Fowler, Jr.	1856-1856
J. R. Hobbs	1856-1856
J. T. Huggins	1857-1858
W. H. Lyons	1857-1858
Thomas Marshall	1857-1858
B. W. Bours	1859-1861
L. R. Bradley	1859-1862
A. C. Bradford	1859-1859
W. M. Lannis	1859-1860
Lewis Dent	1860-1861
Rev. John A. Anderson	1861-1861
T. R. Anthony	1862-1865
Austin Sperry	1862-1865
H. B. Underhill	1862-1863
E. S. Holden	1863-1869
Rev. J. G. Gasman	1863-1865
R. B. Parker	1865-1869
Wm. A. Baggs	1865-1869
A. J. Spencer	1867-1869
Newton Booth	1867-1869
N. D. Popert	1867-1869
Timothy Paige	1867-1869
Edward Moore	1871-1874
John B. Hewson	1871-1872
Edward Twitchell	1871-1872
E. E. Thrift	1871-1874
Henry S. Austin	1871-1874
Donald McLennon	1873-1878 1880-1885
Obed Harvey, M. D.	1873-1878 1880-1885 1888-1893
L. M. Cutting	1875-1876 1882-1885
W. R. Cluness, M. D.	1875-1876
J. K. Doak	1875-1876 1880-1889
Frank T. Baldwin	1877-1879
Calet Dorsey	1877-1879
Robert Watt	1877-1891
S. A. Holmes	1879-1879
Frank Stewart	1879-1881
J. D. McDougald	1886-1889 1894-1897
O. H. Randall	1886-1889
Dr. H. N. Rucker	1886-1887
H. T. Dorrance	1890-1893
R. S. Johnson	1890-1893
Arthur Thornton	1892-1897
A. McDonald	1892-1901
H. O. Southworth	1894-1897
Joseph Steffens	1894-1901
John N. Woods	1898-1901
John T. Doyle	1898-1901
John C. Thompson	1898-1901 1910-1911
Frank E. Lane	1902-1907
George W. Langridge	1902-1905
J. W. Thompson	1902-1909
L. E. Doan	1902-1903
C. D. Fontana	1902-1913
C. M. Keniston	1904-1909
N. F. Peikle	1906-1913
J. F. Dietrich	1908-1909
F. D. Dietrich	1910-1911
J. H. McLeod	1910-1914
W. B. Nutter	1912-1914
F. J. Dietrich	1912-1914
E. Harbert	1914-1914
B. F. Pache	1914-1914

MEDICAL VISITORS.

J. P. Whitney, M. D.	1865-1871	John F. Morse, M. D. ...	1865-1871
Lorenzo Hubbard, M. D..	1865-1871		

RESIDENT PHYSICIANS.

Robt. K. Reid, M. D.	1853-1855	W. D. Aylett, M. D. (Supt.)	1857-1860
Samuel Langdon, M. D. (Supt.)	1856-1856	W. P. Tilden, M. D.	1860-1863
		G. A. Shurtleff, M. D. ...	1863-1884

MEDICAL SUPERINTENDENTS.

W. T. Brown, M. D.	1884-1885	Asa Clark, M. D.	1894-1907
W. H. Mays, M. D.	1884-1885	Fred. P. Clark, M. D. ...	1908-
Hiram N. Rucker, M. D..	1888-1893		

NAPA STATE HOSPITAL.

NAPA, CAL.

Owing to the rapid increase in population, due to the discovery of gold and the opening up of a new country, the Asylum at Stockton became so crowded as to attract the attention of the Legislature. By an act approved March 27, 1872, a new institution for the care and treatment of the insane was created, to be located as follows: "Confined to the central and western portion of the state, embracing the central coast counties and the counties bordering on or near the Bays of San Francisco, San Pablo and Suisun, and lying west of the Valley of the Sacramento and San Joaquin rivers."

The commission appointed by the Governor selected a site comprising 208 acres situated one and a half miles southeast of Napa. Additional land has been purchased from time to time until 1899 acres now comprise the holding of this institution.

The principal water supply is Lake Marie, a reservoir constructed in the foot hills to the rear of the hospital, supplemented by smaller reservoirs lower down, and wells.

Electricity supplied by the Bay Counties Power Company is now used for lighting and power. Gas is manufactured and is used for cooking, in a small way, on the wards.

Sewage disposal is by gravity system, emptying into the Napa River, which is affected by the tides.

The building scheme comprises the following: A center building contains the offices; extending north and south are the wings for male and female patients. Here is found the cottage system, begun many years ago, and recently enlarged by new groups, all of brick construction. Located on the main drive near the entrance to the grounds the receiving building is found. As in the case of Stockton, the appliances for hydrotherapy treatment are installed in this building. The dwellings of the medical staff are also located on the main drive and are of very substantial brick construction. The landscape is improved with flower gardens and lawns, affording desirable recreation for certain classes of patients. A recreation hall has just been completed and supplies a long felt want. It is large and roomy and will enable a great number of patients to enjoy the dances and moving pictures.

A Board of Managers of five members appointed by the Governor makes monthly visits to the hospital. The chief medical and executive officer is the medical superintendent appointed by the managers. The medical staff consists of the medical superintendent and five assistant physicians, one of the assistants being a woman and one a bacteriologist.

The tailor shop and sewing room, in which is made all the clothing for the inmates, constitute the principal industrial enterprise. The carpenter shop and mill, tin shop and others, while of lesser importance, turn out large quantities of work necessary to the proper upkeep of the hospital.

While this institution possesses about 1900 acres, a large portion of it is not suitable for farming purposes, only 300 acres being available for farm use. Fresh fruit in liberal quantities and varieties is raised, which affords a desirable change in diet for the patient population. Several hundred tons of grain hay are produced yearly, the larger portion of which is sold and alfalfa hay purchased for the dairy. The dairy consists of 160 cows, producing about 10,000 gallons of milk monthly. The poultry ranch produces eggs in sufficient quantity to provide a liberal diet for the patients. Several years ago the state purchased a tract of 375 acres lying along the Napa River. This land had been subject to overflow at high water and only a small portion of it was cultivated. The soil is very rich and has never been tilled. The Legislature was induced to see the practicability of appropriating money for the reclamation of this land and the project has been completed. The land is now being worked and in the course of two years will produce more than sufficient alfalfa hay to supply the needs of the institution. Garden truck will also constitute a part of the crop of this land and its purchase will prove very valuable.

Cool weather prevailing, weekly entertainments are given, at which dancing is permitted patients. These affairs are usually accompanied by moving pictures. Band concerts and baseball constitute the outdoor amusements.

Beginning the year 1915 the population at this institution was 2136—1221 males and 915 females. Engaged in the care and treatment of these unfortunates were 259 officers and employees.

The Legislature has been extremely liberal in providing for this institution, having appropriated $1,651,505 and authorized by special tax the sum of $241,047.70. In addition, $270,644 has been expended from the contingent fund. Practically all of this money has gone into buildings and improvements. The income of the institution, other than appropriations made by the legislature, is derived from pay patients, amounting in the average for the last four years to $45,000.

BOARD OF MANAGERS.

John F. Morse	1873-1873	H. H. Harris	1896-1899
J. H. Jewett	1873-1876	E. E. Washburn	1896-1901
James H. Goodman	1873-1876	Raleigh Barcar	1896-1901
Chancellor Hartson	1873-1876	Robt. P. Lamdin	1896-1901
R. H. Sterling	1873-1876	E. Z. Hennessey	1900-1909
Abner Doble	1874-1876	J. L. Martin	1900-1901
F. E. Johnston	1877-1881	R. M. Swain	1902-1907
A. G. Boggs	1877-1881	F. W. Bush	1902-1907
George C. Perkins	1877-1881	W. V. Stafford	1902-1905
John Boggs	1877-1881	Max Boldberg	1902-1907
P. Van Bever	1877-1881	J. H. Steves	1906-1911
Benj. Shurtleff, M. D.	1880-1895	Richard Belcher	1908-1911
J. C. Martin	1880-1895	H. M. Meacham	1908-1911
N. D. Rideout	1880-1883	Emmett Phillips	1908-1914
J. F. Lamdin..1882-1885;	1888-1895	Thomas S. Dozier	1910-1911
D. L. Haas	1882-1885	John S. Chambers	1912-1913
John Q. Brown	1884-1895	David Rutherford	1912-1914
G. N. Cornwell	1886-1889	J. N. Clark	1912-1913
W. F. Henning	1886-1887	C. J. Corcoran	1912-1914
G. M. Francis	1890-1895	H. J. Widerman	1914-1914

MEDICAL SUPERINTENDENTS.

Edwin Bentley, M. D.	1874-1876	Elmer E. Stone, M. D.	1904-1912
E. T. Wilkins, M. D.	1876-1892	A. E. Osborne, M. D.	1912-1914
A. M. Gardner, M. D.	1892-1902	A. W. Hoisholt, M. D.	1914-
L. F. Dozier, M. D.	1902-1904		

AGNEW STATE HOSPITAL.

Agnew, Cal.

In the decade following the establishment of the Napa State Hospital the population of California had increased by 304,000, thereby creating the need of more accommodations for the insane. By act of the Legislature approved March 9, 1885, this need was provided for by the establishment of an asylum for the chronic insane.

The Santa Clara Valley was selected as the site for the location of this institution and, at a cost of $55,000, 276 acres of land were purchased at Agnew, a small town on the Southern Pacific Railroad, six miles northwest of San Jose. In 1896, at a cost of $8500, 57 acres were purchased from the contingent fund.

An artesian belt extending through the portion of the Santa Clara Valley in which the institution is located gives an abundance of water. These subterranean streams have been tapped by wells, the water is pumped into large tanks and distributed by gravity to the several buildings and departments. At first electricity generated at the hospital plant was used for illuminating purposes. At present the supply is obtained by purchase. The sewage is disposed of by a gravity system to tide water.

Under appointment by the Governor five members constitute the Board of Managers. The medical superintendent, appointed by the managers, is the chief medical and executive officer. The medical staff is composed of the superintendent and two assistants. No special industry is maintained. The general repair and upkeep of the hospital is taken care of by competent mechanics.

Owing to the limited acreage owned by this institution no large crops are produced. Truck gardening produces sufficient fresh vegetables to supply the inmates and employees. The hospital is fortunate in having a well-established poultry yard, which produced during the fiscal year ending June 30, 1911, 15,314 dozen eggs. Swine are also raised and supply the hospital with sufficient pork, thus avoiding the necessity of purchasing this article of food.

Band concerts and theatrical entertainments and dances afford indoor amusements, while baseball and other sports provide recreation in the open air.

On January 1, 1915, the roster showed 1425 patients enrolled—801 males and 624 females. To look after the needs and welfare of this village there are 179 officers and employees. Prior to the disastrous earthquake of April 18, 1906, the population was 1108. Of this number 101 lost their lives in the destruction of the buildings and 99 were transferred to Stockton. By reason of death and discharge and that no new cases were admitted the population was reduced to 758 on June 30, 1909. Within the last year (1914) the completion of the new buildings has enabled the authorities to receive patients and from now on the roster will show a gradual increase.

The original plan of construction was similar to the asylums previously erected, viz.: administration building, with wings for ward purposes. In 1897 it became manifestly necessary to provide further accommodation, notwithstanding the fact that two new asylums were in course of construction, one in the south in San Bernardino County, and the other in the north in Mendocino County. No appropriation for this purpose being available, the contingent fund was utilized and the cottage system was inaugurated. Subsequently more cottages were added and the contingent fund had built and furnished four commodious structures when the disaster of 1906 leveled all, destroying in a minute what hard work and conscientious endeavor had taken years to create. After providing temporary quarters for the patients who had survived, the management began to plan an institution inferior to none and up to date in every respect. At present the institution consists of the modern cottage system, so-called, with separate buildings allowing for proper classification and treatment. The buildings are of reinforced concrete, one and two stories in height, scientifically ventilated, plumbing modern and sanitary, and architecturally simple but pleasing to the eye. The landscape, owing to the reconstruction work, became practically obliterated. Now, however, the grounds are being improved under the plan and direction of experts and in a few years will be more beautiful than ever.

The Legislature by special appropriation has provided $2,378,449 for buildings and improvements. This is a large sum, but it should be borne in mind that $1,322,375 of this amount was appropriated to rehabilitate the institution. Up to the time of the earthquake the contingent fund was in a flourishing condition and even now is in fairly good condition, notwithstanding the unusual expenditures incident thereto and the loss of pay patients.

The general scheme of the new hospital is as follows:

1. A central receiving or acute group; this is called the hospital group and consists of a central treatment building, which contains offices for the assistant physicians, laboratories, hydrotherapy, dispensary, operating, dental, eye, ear and throat, X-ray, photograph and electrical rooms; and other equipment. 2. On either side of this building are the receiving wards, connected to it by an arcade. There are three receiving wards for each sex, each ward accommodating 25 patients; also a hospital ward for each sex for the acute sick, cases under operation, and cases requiring very special nursing. This group, of course, is a great workshop of the physicians. 3. Outlying on either side of this group for either sex is an infirmary for the old, paralytics, etc., a convalescent home and various cottages, each arranged for a special class. 4. More to the rear are cottages for demented and the chronic-disturbed patients, so that this class can be quite segregated from the more acute and better class. 5. The administration or office building is to the front, where it can be visited for business purposes without entering the hospital proper. To the front also is a building utilized as a social center for both patients and employees and as an assembly hall, etc. 6. In the immediate rear of the hospital group is a dining building for officers and employees, and immediately to the rear of this is a domestic group consisting of kitchen, flanked on either side by bakery and commissary, and still to the rear the power-house, laundry and shops.

The buildings are entirely without window guards and windows can be freely opened, with the exception of two buildings on either side. During the day the doors are also open. The institution is practically an open one, which at first was feared to be unwise for acute cases, but which experience has proved to be very satisfactory with a minimum of elopements.

The following changes have been wrought at Agnew: Twenty years ago all windows were barred, all doors locked; only heavy tables and benches were permitted in the wards; no pictures or flowers, no shades or curtains; restraint of all kinds freely used, including staples in floors to which patients were strapped; dining tables supplied only with tin cups, plates and spoons; nothing done in the way of investigation and little in the way of treatment. Now there are few screens on the windows, open doors; well-furnished wards everywhere, attractive and homelike; restraint practically abolished with active hydrotherapeutic and other treatment substituted; Agnew is now an advanced and modern mental hospital, with an efficient medical staff, which is endeavoring to keep abreast of the times as regards the care and treatment of the insane.

BOARD OF MANAGERS.

E. F. Delger............ 1888-1889
J. W. Gally, M.D....... 1888-1889
C. H. Maddox.......... 1888-1889
A. McDonald........... 1888-1891
W. D. Tisdale.......... 1888-1891
B. D. Murphy.......... 1890-1893
O. A. Hale............. 1890-1907
V. Koch................ 1890-1891
W. W. Montague....... 1892-1895
H. V. Morehouse....... 1892-1895
Isaac Upham........... 1894-1907
J. T. Porter............ 1894-1895
J. R. Curnow........... 1896-1901
F. H. Gould............ 1896-1899
Edward White.......... 1896-1914
A. Greeninger........... 1900-1907
Jas. K. Wilson......... 1902-1909
F. H. Bangs, M.D...... 1908-1914
T. S. Montgomery...... 1908-1914
David Rutherford....... 1908-1911
Horace Wilson......... 1910-1914
Duncan McPherson..... 1912-1914

MEDICAL SUPERINTENDENT.

W. W. Macfarland, M.D.......... 1888-1889

MEDICAL DIRECTOR.

F. W. Hatch, M. D................ 1890-1897

MEDICAL SUPERINTENDENTS.

F. M. Sponogle, M.D... 1898-1899
J. A. Crane, M.D....... 1900-1903
Leonard Stocking, M.D... 1904-

4

MENDOCINO STATE HOSPITAL.[1]

TALMAGE, CAL.

In the year 1889 the Legislature of the State of California passed "An Act Entitled an Act to Establish a Branch Insane Asylum for the Insane at Ukiah, to be known as the Mendocino State Insane Asylum, and Appropriating Money Therefor." This act was approved by Governor Waterman on February 20, 1889, and he soon after appointed a Board of Directors, whose duty it was under the act, to select a site, to erect buildings and to furnish and prepare them for the reception of patients. This Board of Directors was composed of the following gentlemen: Archibald Yell, T. L. Carothers and Dr. E. W. King, of Ukiah, as local members, and J. B. Wright, of Sacramento, and Cornelius O'Connor, of San Francisco, members from the state at large. Messrs. Wright and O'Connor were appointed for four years and Messrs. Yell, Carothers and King for two years. This board organized by electing Archibald Yell as chairman, and J. H. Seawell as secretary and treasurer of the board. On September 7, 1889, the Board of Directors accepted the offer of a tract of land, consisting of 139.08 acres, about three miles east of Ukiah, as a site for the asylum, together with the unobstructed flow of the waters of South Mill Creek, which furnished an ample and abundant supply of pure fresh water for all purposes of the asylum.

In June, 1890, plans and specifications for the asylum buildings were presented by Messrs. Copeland & Pierce, of San Francisco, and accepted by the Board of Directors. On October, 1890, contracts were let for the construction of a male ward building, connecting corridor, kitchen building, laundry and bakery building and a boiler and engine house; the total contract for the erection and completion of the above buildings was $182,520. On the 26th of January, 1891, the Board of Directors let contracts for the erection of a female ward building for the sum of $89,025. On the 2d of April, 1891, the board accepted a contract for furnishing

[1] By Robert Lewis Richards, M. D., medical superintendent.

iron pipe and laying same for water supply for the sum of $3865, and subsequently allowed for extra material and work $294.60, making a total of $4159.60. On the 21st of April, 1891, the board elected R. M. Garratt superintendent of construction, at a salary of $8 per day until the further order of the board.

The work of construction proceeded steadily from this time and on September 14, 1892, the secretary of the board reported "that the contracts heretofore let will complete the male ward building, the connecting corridor, the kitchen building, the laundry and bakery building and the boiler and engine house. That the contract for the female ward building will enclose and roof said building, but that there are not sufficient funds to complete same. All the buildings under construction, except the female ward building, will be completed by January 1, 1893, and the contracts let on the female ward building will be completed on that date. The contract already let will exhaust the appropriation for the construction of the asylum, namely, $350,000. To this sum must be added $790.38, indebtedness incurred by permission of the State Board of Examiners to construct a retaining wall for the front of the building."

The total cost of construction, including water supply, etc., and purchase of site, September 14, 1892, was $350,790.38, and by an act approved March 3, 1893, there was appropriated the sum of $100,000 for the completion of the female ward building, for furnishing the several buildings, to construct a dam for a water supply, and for other purposes necessary to prepare the asylum for the reception of patients. The sum was expended under the direction of the Board of Directors.

From the foregoing statement it will be seen that the entire cost of the site and water supply, the erection of the buildings, lighting plant, construction of dam and laying pipe for water supply, heating and plumbing, and for everything necessary for the reception of patients on December 12, 1893, amounted to $450,790.38, to which must be added $60,000 for the administration building, just completed, making a gross amount under appropriation of $510,790.38.

On December 12, 1893, patients were received, to the number of 60, by transfer from the Napa Asylum; on December 14, 1893, 60 from Stockton Asylum, and on March 25, 1894, 30 from Agnew Asylum.

The Legislature of 1897 made an appropriation of $60,000 for the erection of an administration building. Plans and specifications for this building were drawn by Cunningham Bros., of San Francisco, and contracts for the construction of the building were let by the Board of Directors. This building was practically completed on June 30, 1900.

During the previous three years the Board of Directors had constructed, by means of the contingent fund, a stable, which cost $4500, and had built a new dam, which made a reservoir containing about 5,000,000 gallons of water, and laid a new pipe line of 12, 13 and 14-inch steel pipe, at a cost of about $12,000 for both dam and pipe line.

The Legislature of the year 1901 appropriated a sufficient amount of money to purchase 270 acres of land to be added to the hospital tract. A large portion of this land was first class river bottom; well adapted to raise grain and all kinds of garden vegetables; also the small and large fruits; in fact, almost everything necessary in the line of fruits and vegetables for the hospital. The purchase of this land also enabled the hospital to procure a dairy herd of 30 cows, which furnished milk at a minimum cost.

This Legislature also appropriated the sum of $2500 for sewer pipe. This pipe was used for conducting the sewage from the hospital to land recently purchased, where it was used for irrigation and fertilization after passing through septic tanks.

About the 1st of March, 1902, a contract was let to Charles F. Sloane & Co., of San Francisco, to put in an electric plant and wire the hospital buildings for same. This plant was of a capacity of 450 lights. The motive power was water and steam, the water power generated by a Pelton wheel of 45 horse-power, and the steam power by an engine of the same capacity. The water to run the Pelton wheel was taken from the supply pipe which furnished the hospital. This pipe was 12 inches inside diameter at the hospital, and increased in size from 12 inches to 13, then 14 and finally near the dam to 24 inches. The water in the reservoir at the head of the pipe line was about 300 feet above the hospital buildings, giving a pressure on the wheel of 135 to 140 pounds to the square inch. On June 30, 1902, the hospital was lighted with electricity generated by water power, with a large amount of water flowing over the dam. The expense of running the plant by water was practically nothing. The cost of wiring the buildings and putting in the lighting plant was $6050, paid from the contingent fund. A brick building 24 by 50 feet was built by the patients and employees to house the plant, at a cost of about $900, also paid out of the contingent fund.

In the fall of 1904, by advice and consent of the State Commission in Lunacy, there was constructed a small plant for the outdoor treatment of the tubercular cases. This consisted of seven tents as follows: three small dormitories capable of holding five beds each, a sitting room, a dining room and pantry, a tent for attendants, and one for a lavatory and bath room. On November 11, 1904, 15 tubercular cases were taken from the wards to the tents and put in charge of two attendants and a night watch. All of these cases were suffering from some form of insanity, except one, which was a case of drug (morphine) habit as well as tuberculosis. January 1, 1905, the number of cases was increased to 37. Of these 37 cases treated in the tents, 19 were tuberculous and suffering from various forms of insanity. Most of them were in the second and third stages of tuberculosis and considered hopeless cases, yet most of them were benefited by the open-air treatment. Five died from phthisis, two from dementia paralytica and two from heart disease; a total of 9. Notwithstanding a heavy rainfall during the winter most of the patients soon showed a marked improvement in appetite and many increased in weight, and quite a number of patients, who had been bedridden for months, improved so as to be up during the day and sit under the trees. There were no cases of grip and no cases of severe colds among the patients in the tents, while there were many cases on the wards in the main building.

On June 30, 1906, this tent plant, which consisted originally of seven tents, was enlarged by the addition of five wooden structures, built of 2 x 3 surfaced studding, covered with double surfaced rustic, so as to be painted on both sides. These wooden structures were nine feet high on the sides, the roof being shingled. They were built with ventilators of sufficient capacity so that when open the air of the room would be pure and fresh. One of these buildings was used for a sitting room, one for a dining room, one for a dormitory, one for a hospital and one for the attendants.

The wooden buildings were somewhat more costly, averaging $60 per bed, but they would last much longer than the canvas ones, and were better adapted to the class of patients (chronic insane) which was under treatment there. Around the whole there was a six-foot smooth woven wire fence, inclosing about 2 1-2 acres of ground. This camp was conveniently located near the hospital and was connected with water, electric light, steam and the sewer system. Food was furnished from the main kitchen. Within the inclosure were plenty of shade trees, sunlight and pure fresh air.

There are in this camp at present (1914) 102 patients, which is more than it was designed to hold. But the results have shown that outdoor life is better not only for the tubercular patients, but also for those who are mentally unsound, and the chronic insane have been given the advantage of this method of treatment, while the tubercular insane have been maintained in a more restricted and separate area.

The Mendocino State Hospital was without an assembly hall until the year 1903, when the Legislature made an appropriation of $30,000 to build and furnish an assembly hall, but the money was not made available until July, 1904. Plans and specifications were procured and adopted and this building was completed in July, 1905.

The Legislature at the same time appropriated $7500 to purchase land on each side of Mill Creek in order to preserve and protect the water supply of the hospital. The purchase of this land became a necessity, as the cutting of the timber along the banks of the creek would have very materially affected the amount of water, which in dry seasons was only sufficient for the present hospital use.

During the year 1905-1906 a roomy hothouse for the propagation of plants was built by the patients and employees at a cost of $846.13.

In July, 1905, it was deemed advisable to increase the capacity of the reservoir by an addition of six feet to the height of the dam. This work was commenced at once and was completed before the fall rains at a cost of $1,075.42. This addition nearly doubled the capacity of the reservoir, enabling the impoundment of from 10,000,000 to 11,000,000 gallons of water.

During this year there was also a notable increase in the products of the farm and garden and there was an abundant supply of vegetables of all kinds. The dairy furnished an abundance of fresh milk and the chicken yards eggs and chickens for the table.

As a result of the earthquake which visited the west coast of California in 1906 the buildings were damaged, but no person was seriously injured. The administration building was badly damaged and it became necessary to remove the patients from a ward in this building. The Legislature at its special session appropriated $30,000 for repairs and for a water tower, it having been found necessary to remove all tanks from the buildings, as their great weight in the towers was a constant menace. The towers at the north and south ends of the ward buildings were also taken down one story, all of the heavy stone ornamentations dispensed with and the water tanks removed. The tower in the administration building was taken down to the roof line.

In the year 1907 the Legislature appropriated the sum of $30,000 for the purpose of building a cottage to accommodate about 91 female patients and this cottage was completed during 1908. There was also appropriated the sum of $42,500 for the purpose of erecting a cottage for male patients. Both of these measures were necessary to provide for the increase of patients.

The hospital was constructed, as far as the ward building, kitchen and laundry were concerned, and made ready for occupancy by patients in 1893. The bill which passed the Legislature establishing this hospital called for a building that would accommodate not to exceed 500 patients. On June 30, 1908, there were in the hospital 846 patients, and at this rate of increase in three more years the number would reach 1000 patients. As the kitchen and dining rooms as originally built were found to be entirely inadequate for their needs the Legislature authorized the expenditure of $10,000 for the purpose of enlarging the kitchen and dining room.

The sum of $2500 was also appropriated for the purpose of purchasing laundry machinery, and the sum of $5000 for the purpose of erecting and constructing a dairy barn and this work was completed during the years of 1909 and 1910. A strictly modern, sanitary, reinforced concrete dairy barn and milk room was erected.

It was also found advisable that the first and second assistant physicians have a residence outside of the hospital, but on the hospital grounds, and for this purpose there was taken from the contingent fund the sum of $4270, the cost of the residence of the first assistant physician, and $3500, the cost of a residence for the second assistant physician. The residence of the first assistant physician was completed in 1909 and that for the second assistant physician in 1912.

A male cottage which will accommodate 91 patients was completed during the year 1910.

The water supply proved inadequate, owing to the large increase in population, and an additional appropriation of $25,000 was granted by the Legislature for the purpose of constructing a storage dam and reservoir estimated to hold 30,000,000 gallons of water in addition to which wells were sunk on the hospital grounds, the water from which is used for the purpose of irrigating the vegetable gardens.

The cold storage plant was also thoroughly overhauled and enlarged. Milk and butter rooms have been constructed where these arcticles can be kept free from contamination.

The ranch land of 300 acres has proven very profitable and the yearly gross income is $30,000. The introduction in this section of irrigation from wells was due to this hospital and the large returns are largely due to irrigation. During the year there are five cuttings of alfalfa and an average of 10 tons per acre is secured.

The usual carpenter, mattress, painting, plumbing, laundry, bakery and shoe repairing departments are maintained, as well as an unusual amount of construction work with patients' labor. Indeed, an unusually skilled steward and the careful use of a great deal of patients' labor accounts for the remarkably low cost of construction work at this hospital for the past 10 years.

Occupational work in addition has been established in the past two years without cost to the state, since the sale of articles made, which was divided into three parts—one-third for the patient, one-third for the cost of material and one-third for the amusement fund—provided enough for the maintenance of the work and purchase of a piano, etc. The hospital has had the usual success with patients' individual work in this connection.

Weekly moving picture and musical entertainments, weekly Protestant and Catholic religious services and occasional dances for attendants have given a home atmosphere for patients and employees. The patients respond to such influences and show appreciation by better care of clothing and furniture, and thus help to establish improved conditions of living.

The original design of the hospital was that especially adapted to chronic insane and the wards were large, accommodating 70 to 100 patients. Subsequently the male and female cottages were built with small wards and single rooms, permitting segregation of quiet and convalescent patients. More than 30 per cent of the women have in the past two years been placed on free parole, and the female cottage is an open ward. There has been no serious abuse of this privilege.

A farm or ranch cottage, costing $14,000 for the building and equipment, with a capacity for 52 male patients, has been completed this year (1914) and is also an open free parole ward for men. There remains the especial necessity for an acute receiving building, where the new cases may be more satisfactorily studied and treated and where the acute excitements may be provided for. There is every reason to expect that plans for a two-story building with four wards of 25 beds, hydrotherapeutic department (at present the male and female hydrotherapeutic equipments are in the male and female cottages), operating room, etc., will be included in the state budget and an appropriation by the Legislature made effective.

The single and sound-proof rooms and the continuous bath on each ward will make possible the care of acute mental conditions, which is now defective because of the large wards which cannot be subdivided. The prospect is that the hospital will be increased from the present population of 1072 to the state standard of 2000 patients and in the construction of the required additional buildings the feature of segregation of patients can be given the emphasis required by the present methods of treatment of the insane.

There is now a complete record of ward history, correspondence, etc., of each patient, with card index of cases. Each patient is received by a doctor, is bathed, fed and put to bed. Preliminary history and a study of the case is presented within two weeks and tentative diagnosis made. The medical conference considers also subsequent developments in the case, changes of status, deaths, etc. Besides a complete study of the case and valuable scientific records, this has led to earlier discharge and consequently less net increase in the hospital population.

The system of accounting now in use means that all transactions pass over the medical superintendent's desk; purchases are made on competitive bidding; the storeroom is charged with everything entering the hospital and credited only by issues on properly signed requisitions; besides hospital approval, all transactions are audited and approved by the local Board of Managers, State Commission in Lunacy and the State Board of Control.

Civil service governs all employees except the medical superintendent and the pay-roll must be approved by the Civil Service Commission before it reaches the State Controller.

After-care is provided for by correspondence from the hospital and by an after-care physician in San Francisco Bay section, from which is received more than half the patients.

The central kitchen and ward dining rooms are working very satisfactorily. The rear parole ground walls have recently been transformed by building a mission cloister, 12 feet wide, with cement pillars and arches and red tile roof.

A new gas plant at a cost of a little more than $10,000 provides an ample supply of gas for reserve lighting, power, heating purposes, ward diet, kitchen, etc.

A new female tubercular cottage, costing $3500, with a capacity of 30 beds, is nearing completion.

One other need will be requested of the Legislature at its next session, *i. e.*, nurses' and night attendants' homes. At present all attendants sleep on the wards and this is manifestly undesirable.

Dr. E. W. King, who was appointed medical superintendent on July 1, 1893, served in that capacity continuously until May 1, 1912, on which date, owing to ill health, he resigned. Dr. G. D. Marvin, at that time first assistant physician, became acting medical superintendent, and acted until October 1, 1912, at which time Dr. Robert Lewis Richards, the present medical superintendent, was appointed.

STATEMENT GIVING AS NEARLY AS POSSIBLE VALUE OF EACH BUILDING AND STRUCTURE WITH EQUIPMENT NOW ON THE STATE PROPERTY AT THE MENDOCINO STATE HOSPITAL AND THE YEAR OF ITS CONSTRUCTION.

Building and Structure.	Year Constructed.	Cost.
Main building Laundry and bakery Engine room Morgue	1890-91-92-93	$413,224.18
Dam No. 1	1892	4,500.00
Dam No. 2	1898	9,500.00
Barn	1898	5,000.00
Water supply, main pipe line	1898	5,500.00
Administration building	1900	60,000.00
Sewer	1902	2,500.00
Poultry yards and houses	1903-1913	1,500.00
Assembly building	1904	30,000.00
Hot house and conservatory	1905	856.13
Outdoor tubercular colony	1906-07-08-09	6,000.00
Isolation building	1906	333.77
N. & S. brick walls for male and female yards	1906-08	1,291.41
Fencing and improving front grounds	1906-07	4,500.00
Repairing buildings after earthquake	1907	8,265.54
Female cottage	1907-08	35,391.82
Furnishing female cottage	1908	5,000.00
Water tower and tank	1908	7,691.21
Building for ranch hands, mechanics, etc	1908	4,615.70
Oil tanks and pumps at unloading station, Ukiah	1908	3,283.30
Hay sheds at the ranch	1908-09	1,364.35
Residence first assistant physician	1909	4,270.43
Electric light plant and line	1909	3,257.69
New laundry machinery	1909	2,500.00
Remodeling kitchen and dining room	1910	12,024.94
Barn, dairy, concrete		6,474.65
Male cottage	1910	46,236.09
Furnishing male cottage	1910	2,500.00
Wagon sheds	1911	800.00
Pumping plants	1911-12-13-14	7,500.00
Stand at baseball grounds	1911	250.00
Apple and vegetable house	1911	180.00
Dam No. 3	1912-13-14	25,000.00
Residence second assistant physician	1912	3,500.00
Repairs to plumbing	1912	3,000.00
Farm cottage for male patients	1913-14	14,500.00
Furnishing and equipping same	1914	4,000.00
Mattress shop	1913	679.55
Shelter corridors in male yard	1914	2,250.00
Total		$749,212.76

January 1, 1915, there were in residence, 762 males and 323 females, a total of 1085; officers and employees 132; total population 1217.

BOARD OF MANAGERS.

Name	Years	Name	Years
Archibald Yell	1889-1891	A. H. Foster	1898-1899
T. L. Carothers	1889-1895	B. Fehnemann	1900-1903
E. W. King, M. D.	1889-1892	T. A. Templeton	1900-1901; 1904-1905
J. B. Wright	1889-1892	E. B. Martinelli	1900-1909
Cornelius O'Connor	1889-1897	A. Hockheimer	1900-1905; 1910-1914
J. H. Seawell	1891-1899	A. B. Truman	1902-1907
W. D. White	1893-1895	G. D. Clark	1906-1914
M. Gardner, M. D.	1893-1903	J. L. McNab	1906-1914
Charles Cunningham	1895-1895	W. A. S. Foster	1906-1914
J. C. Ruddock	1896-1899	A. J. Fairbanks	1908-1914
J. Q. White	1896-1899		

MEDICAL SUPERINTENDENTS.

Name	Years	Name	Years
E. W. King, M. D.	1893-1913	Robt. Lewis Richards, M. D.	1914-

SECRETARY AND TREASURER.

Name	Years	Name	Years
J. M. Manion	1891-1895	W. W. Cunningham	1895-

SOUTHERN CALIFORNIA STATE HOSPITAL.

PATTON, CAL.

In 1890 the population of the territory comprising the counties of Los Angeles, Orange, Riverside, San Bernardino, San Diego, San Luis Obispo, Santa Barbara and Ventura was 217,424 and in 1910, a lapse of two decades, there were 757,102, or about one-third the population of the State of California.

In 1889 the Legislature, by act approved March 11, recognized the necessity for an institution for the insane in Southern California, and the rapid increase in population has more than justified the establishment of the same. In providing for the location of the institution the selection of the site was confined to the following counties: Los Angeles, San Bernardino, Ventura, Santa Barbara and San Diego. San Bernardino drew the prize and a tract of land lying along the foot hills in the shadow of the Arrowhead, about six miles northeast of the City of San Bernardino, was purchased. The Santa Fé Railroad runs through the property within a quarter of a mile of the main building, affording ample transportation facilities.

Water for domestic purposes is obtained from springs in the mountains adjacent to the hospital. This supply was developed by running a tunnel about 100 feet. For irrigation water is obtained from the Bear Valley Water Company. This supply is guaranteed by reason of original and preferred rights purchased by the state and has proved a valuable investment. In 1901 twenty acres adjoining the state property, on which a good well has been developed, were purchased and a pumping plant installed. This plant is purely of an emergency character, to supply water in dry seasons and for fire protection.

Electricity for light and power is purchased at a monthly expenditure of $400. Gas for cooking is purchased at a cost of $240 per month.

A farm is utilized for sewage disposal. Septic tanks are provided, the liquid matter being used for irrigation and the solid matter for fertilizer. The system has recently been overhauled and improved and is giving satisfaction.

A board of five members constitutes the governing body. The chief executive and medical officer is the medical superintendent, who is appointed by this board; all other appointments are made by the medical superintendent, subject to confirmation by the Board of Managers. The medical staff is composed of the superintendent and four assistant physicians, one of whom is a woman.

Shops are maintained to care for the general repairs, no particular line being specialized. Particular attention is given to the manufacture of shoes in a shop equipped with modern machinery and the product turned out cannot be excelled for the purposes intended.

The hospital is located in what is known as the "Highlands Citrus Belt." The soil is of a sandy character, but with proper fertilizers and irrigation can be and is made very productive. Citrus fruits of all kinds are successfully produced in the locality, especially the orange. Thirty-two acres are devoted to this crop, producing a yearly income of about $6000. Deciduous fruits of all kinds are cultivated, which supply the inmates with a very desirable article of diet. A truck garden produces a liberal supply of fresh vegetables throughout the year. Hogs are successfully raised, thus avoiding the purchase of staple articles. The dairy herd numbers 84 head, giving a monthly supply of 5500 gallons of milk.

Moving pictures, band concerts and dancing constitute the principal amusements for patients. The hospital has collected quite a library of fiction, history and periodicals for the use of inmates who are able to and care for reading. Outdoor recreation in the form of walks, hay rides and use of the lawns and gardens is extended to trusted patients. The circus, which visits the state annually, is enjoyed by fifty or more of the better class of patients at the expense of the state.

On January 1, 1915, the inmate population was composed of 1369 males and 811 females, making a total of 2180. The corps of officers and employees numbered 239, with 9 others as members of the families of the officers, making in all a village of 2428 inhabitants.

The original plan adopted was accomplished by the completion in 1908 of the central ward building, the first floor of which was arranged for the executive officers. To provide for future enlargement, the cottage system was adopted and numerous buildings, some of brick and others of concrete, have been added from time to time. The group includes receiving buildings equipped with the latest appliances for the hydrotherapy treatment. Here we find separate quarters for the female help which are greatly appreciated by those whose employment keeps them in close association with the inmates from 12 to 18 hours of the day. The grounds are improved with lawns, flower gardens and evergreen shrubbery, the latter affording grateful shade from the fierce rays of the sun during the summer. From a scenic point of view a better site could not have been chosen. The buildings stand on rising ground facing the Valley of San Bernardino, with a commanding view of Redlands, Highlands and the numerous small hamlets in the vicinity. Snow-capped mountains in winter add their grandeur to the view.

The State of California has been extremely generous to this institution, having provided for buildings and improvements the sum of $1,248,081.41. Further sums have been expended from the contingent fund which is given in detail in the table, given as an appendix.

The climate is strictly Southern Californian. It is safe to say that but two seasons prevail during the year, summer and winter, with the former predominating. As a rule the winters are very mild, with hardly sufficient rain in the lowlands to insure early crops. Artificial irrigation is absolutely necessary and by long experience has been brought to a high plane of efficiency. The summer season is long and dry, with hot weather prevailing, but when one becomes acclimated and adjusts his mode of living to conform therewith, the San Bernardino Valley is a health resort, as is evidenced by the rapid increase in population.

BOARD OF MANAGERS.

H. L. Drew............. 1892-1899
John Anderson.......... 1892-1893
M. A. Murphy.......... 1892-1893
H. A. Palmer........... 1892-1893
James A. Gibson........ 1894-1899
I. K. Fisher............. 1894-1895
George Cooley.......... 1894-1895
Frank A. Miller........ 1894-1895
T. B. Van Alstyne...... 1896-1897
John McGonigle........ 1896-1907
H. W. Patton........... 1896-1899
James C. Kays.......... 1898-1903
E. P. Clarke............ 1900-1913
D. R. Seeley............ 1900-1903
T. A. Lewis............. 1900-1903
J. W. A. Off............ 1904-1907
H. B. Wilson........... 1904-1911
H. T. Hays............. 1904-1905
G. P. Adams............ 1906-1907
Geo. L. Hasson.......... 1908-1911
H. McPhee............. 1908-1914
Francis M. Parker...... 1908-1911
E. W. Burke............ 1912-1914
Austin T. Park.......... 1912-1914
A. B. Paddock.......... 1912-1913
W. A. Avery............ 1914-1914
E. C. Merryfield......... 1914-1914

MEDICAL DIRECTOR.

M. B. Campbell, M. D......................... 1894-1905

MEDICAL SUPERINTENDENTS.

A. P. Williamson, M. D... 1906-1909
E. Scott Blair, M. D..... 1910-1911
John A. Reily, M. D..... 1912-

FOLSOM STATE HOSPITAL.

Represa, Cal.

For many years the medical authorities of the several hospitals for the insane have called attention to the vicious system in vogue in California of permitting the association of criminal and convict insane with those of a milder type. Both the criminal and convict insane are refractory and, while mentally unbalanced, do not seem to lose their vicious cunning. They are a disturbing element among the other patients and are continually scheming to obtain their liberty. For these reasons it was deemed proper that a separate institution should be provided. In order to provide this necessity at the smallest expense to the state it was decided to locate the hospital on the grounds of the Folsom State Prison. By this procedure purchase of land was avoided and access had to cheap building material and labor. The prison operates a large granite quarry which gives employment to many of its inmates. In 1903 the sum of $25,000 was appropriated for the purpose above outlined, but owing to defects in the act no progress was made. The Legislature of 1905 passed a more comprehensive act and added $15,000 to the former sum, making $40,000 available. In January, 1906, the construction work was begun and has progressed slowly. In 1909 $39,000 was provided and it was estimated this amount would complete the building. The sum proved insufficient and at present the work is at a standstill owing to lack of available funds. As the building stands all the rock work is completed and is covered with a temporary roof. The building stands on a high bluff overlooking the American River and it is hoped the next Legislature will provide the necessary funds to provide for its completion and occupancy.

SONOMA STATE HOME.

ELDRIDGE, CAL.

The Legislature, at its session of 1885, at the urgent request of a group of citizens who had, by their personal donations, been supporting a private benevolent society in Alameda County, known as the "Home for the Care and Treatment of Feeble-Minded Children," provided the means for the establishment of a state institution for the care, treatment and education of feeble-minded and idiotic children. In conformity with the provisions of this act, at a cost of $14,000, 50 acres of land with a building thereon, located at Santa Clara, were purchased. Additions and improvements were made to properly care for the inmates. By reason of the crowded condition of the Home and insistent demand of those unable to gain admission, the Legislature of 1889, by act approved March 6, authorized the purchase of a permanent site to "consist of not less than 300 acres at a cost not to exceed $51,000. A commission, appointed for the purpose, selected the Wm. McPherson Hill rancho, comprising some 1670 acres, situated about one-half mile from the Town of Glen Ellen, in Sonoma County, paying therefor $50,000. After careful research as to proper method of construction, plans and specifications were prepared and building was begun during the summer of 1890. November 24, 1891, marks an epoch in the history of this institution, for this was moving day. It is easy to imagine the surprise and delight of the children on the arrival at their new home. Here they found themselves in the country, surrounded by hill and dale, well timbered and watered by nature. The home is favored by good transportation, the Southern Pacific and California North Western Railroad passing within one-quarter of a mile.

Numerous springs, having their origin in the range of foothills just back of the institution, supply water for domestic and irrigation purposes. Concrete tanks, with a reservoir to store the overflow, constitute the system of conservation. With normal rainfall the system will provide sufficient supply.

With crude oil as fuel the Home maintains its own light plant, generating electricity to light the buildings and grounds.

Septic tanks solve the problem of sewage disposal. The effluent is used for irrigating a small patch of alfalfa in the immediate vicinity of the tanks.

A Board of Managers of five members constitutes the governing body. The medical superintendent, appointed by the managers, is the chief medical and executive officer. The medical superintendent appoints all other officers and employees, his medical staff being two assistant physicians, one a woman.

Under the direction of the shoemaker a number of the male inmates are employed in making shoes and slippers for the institution. The boys are employed throughout the various mechanical departments and on the farm. The girls devote their time to the sewing room, where various articles of clothing are made and kept in repair.

While the home possesses a large acreage, the larger portion of it is fit only for dairy and pasturage. However, fresh fruits in abundance are produced and large quantities are dried and preserved for use the year round. Vegetables of all kinds are cultivated, supplying the inmates in generous quantity. The poultry yards give a plentiful supply of fresh eggs. The home is fortunate in possessing a modern dairy. It has been unfortunate with its herd, having to combat tuberculosis. This has been eradicated, a new herd is being acquired and in a short time milk in plenty will again be supplied.

Much thought and time is given by the management to amusements. Various games, both indoor and outdoor, are indulged in. The institution has a band, which is very creditable, giving concerts at frequent intervals. Books and magazines are supplied and are well patronized and enjoyed.

All inmates are compelled to devote some part of each day to school. The Slyod system is utilized and a corps of five teachers employed during nine months of the year to instruct the children.

On January 1, 1915, the population consisted of 558 males and 478 females, 174 officers and employees, and 14 others, the latter being members of the families of the officers, making a total of 1224. During the 29 years this institution has been open to the public the inmate population has increased from 20 to 1036. Many more would now be on its roster if the proper accommodations were available, as the Home has had for a long time a large waiting list.

The original building plan adopted for the Home was similar to that of institutions of like character prevailing at that period, namely, large dormitory buildings with central building for officers, etc. The management, however, was quick to perceive the evils of this mode of habitation, especially for the class of unfortunates under their charge, and soon began the construction of smaller buildings, where proper classification could be had. The " cottage system " has since been followed and numerous buildings of plain but commodious design now dot the landscape. A modern hospital with up-to-date equipment has recently been provided and fills a long felt want. Within the last few years a gymnasium has been erected. The home is situated in one of the small vales of the Sonoma Valley, surrounded by foothills fairly well timbered. The view is inspiring and in the spring presents a charming picture. The landscape around and about the buildings is improved with lawns, flowers, orchards and vineyards.

Situated within 20 miles of San Pablo Bay, at an elevation of 278 feet, climatic conditions are similar to the counties surrounding San Francisco Bay, excepting a little higher temperature during mid-day in summer.

As one of the pioneer states in the erection and maintenance of institutions of this character the state has been very liberal, having provided by appropriation the sum of $895,410.66 for purchase of land and erection of buildings and improvements thereon. The contingent fund has been called upon from time to time to provide improvements of a more or less permanent nature.

BOARD OF MANAGERS.

Name	Years	Name	Years
Kate B. Lathrop	1885-1892	W. S. Wood	1893-1894
Lucy E. Higgins	1885-1886	W. T. Eldridge	1893-1894
Caroline F. Bigelow	1885-1886	R. A. Poppe	1893-1894 1900-1901 1904-1914
E. B. Hartson	1885-1886		
William Harney	1885-1891		
Julia M. Judah	1887-1891	John T. Harrington	1895-1901
Abram Block	1887-1888	R. R. Reibonstine	1895-1898
John Widney	1887-1888	T. P. Woodward	1895-1901
Charles A. Murdock	1889-1889	J. J. O'Brien	1895-1898
J. W. Findley	1889-1889	A. B. Ware	1895-1896 1900-1901
A. P. Overton	1890-1894		
George W. Gibbs	1890-1894	H. F. B. Mobist	1897-1898
F. W. Longee	1893-1894 1900-1901	John D. MacKenzie	1902-1903
		H. E. Leland	1902-1903

T. H. Rooney	1902-1903	C. E. Havens	1904-1914
H. F. Dugan	1902-1903	Samuel C. Irving	1906-1907
C. W. Gould	1902-1903	J. P. Berry	1908-1911
William Lyons	1904-1913	Walter Frear	1908-1911
A. C. Bane	1904-1913	E. M. Norton	1912-1914
William Thomas	1904-1905	Percy S. King	1914-1914

MEDICAL SUPERINTENDENTS.

Bedford T. Wood, M. D.	1885-1886	Wm. M. Lawlor, M. D.	1902-1904
A. E. Osborne, M. D.	1886-1902	Wm. J. G. Dawson, M. D.	1904-

APPENDIX A.

TABLE No. 1.

PERMANENT IMPROVEMENTS AND PURCHASE OF LAND.

	Legislative Appropriation.	Special Funds.	Contingent Fund.	Total.
Stockton	$1,231,065.00	$345,924.58	$204,076.75	$1,781,066.33
Napa	1,651,505.00	241,047.70	270,644.69	2,163,197.39
Agnew	2,378,449.86		203,868.91	2,581,318.77
Mendocino	389,724.38	365,728.73	85,914.01	841,367.12
So. California	1,248,081.41		227,439.47	1,475,520.88
Sonoma	895,410.66		51,038.05	946,448.71
Norwalk	250,000.00			250,000.00
Folsom	79,000.00			79,000.00
	[1] $8,123,236.31	$952,701.01	[2] $1,041,981.88	$10,117,919.20

TABLE No 2.

AMOUNT APPROPRIATED AND EXPENDED FOR MAINTENANCE (INCLUDING SALARIES).

	From Appropriations.	From Contingent.	Total.
Stockton	$11,735,695.83	$362,120.81	$12,097,816.64
Napa	8,347,960.69	435,035.19	8,782,995.88
Agnew	4,272,468.48	159,042.82	4,431,511.30
Mendocino	2,681,267.00	51,326.06	2,732,593.06
Southern California	3,637,258.11	197,377.62	3,834,635.73
Sonoma	2,921,932.68	62,679.07	2,984,611.75
	[3] $33,596,582.79	[4] $1,267,581.57	$34,864,164.36

[1] The above table shows expenditures and appropriations made available by the Legislature of 1913.

[2] Expended to July 1, 1914.

[3] The above table shows expenditures and appropriations made available by the Legislature to June 30, 1915.

[4] Expended to July 1, 1914.

TABLE No. 3.

	Permanent Improvements and Purchase of Land.	Salaries and Maintenance.	Total.
Stockton	$1,781,066.33	$12,097,816.64	$13,878,882.97
Napa	2,163,197.39	8,782,995.88	10,946,193.27
Agnew	2,581,318.77	4,431,511.30	7,012,830.07
Mendocino	841,367.12	2,732,593.06	3,573,960.18
Southern California	1,475,520.88	3,834,635.73	5,310,156.61
Sonoma	946,448.71	2,984,611.75	3,931,060.46
Norwalk	250,000.00		250,000.00
Folsom	79,000.00		79,000.00
	$10,117,919.20	$34,864,164.36	$44,982,083.56

THE LIVERMORE SANITARIUM.

LIVERMORE, CAL.

The Livermore Sanitarium was started in 1893 by Dr. John W. Robertson for the treatment of nervous and general diseases. Since 1894, however, it has been practically devoted to the treatment of mental diseases.

In 1912 Dr. V. H. Podstata, formerly superintendent of Elgin State Hospital, Illinois, and Dr. Willhite of Dunning, Chicago, became interested in the institution, since when it has been conducted under the joint names of Drs. Robertson, Podstata and Willhite.

There are no large buildings, but many isolated cottages, some for single individuals, and all without either window guards or enclosed restraints. All patients receive individual nursing and care.

The general hydropathic building was completed in 1906, and occupies grounds entirely separate from the cottages.

THE CARE OF THE INSANE IN COLORADO.

There is apparently no information available as to the care of the insane in Colorado prior to the establishment of the Colorado State Insane Asylum, at Pueblo, in 1879. No doubt a similar condition prevailed in Colorado as in other pioneer states, and the insane were cared for in jails, if dangerous to be at large, or allowed to roam at will, if harmless.

The Asylum at Pueblo was opened in 1883, and, remains to-day (1915) the only institution for the care of the insane of the state.

In 1909 the state established at Ridge, The State Home and Training School for Mental Defectives.

The investigation of the system of public charities and correctional institutions, and the inspection of charitable and correctional institutions and insane asylums receiving state, county, or municipal aid, is under the control of the State Board of Charities and Corrections, consisting of seven members, six appointed by the Governor for a term of six years, the Governor being an ex-officio member.

The State Insane Asylum is under the management of the State Board of Lunacy Commissioners, consisting of three members, appointed by the Governor for a term of six years. In addition, county institutions are under the control of individual boards consisting of six members, appointed for a term of three years.

The law allows the Board of Lunacy Commissioners to fix the capacity of the asylum at Pueblo. In consequence its management has not been obliged to contend with such crowded conditions as has been the experience of similar hospitals in other states.

All persons are entitled to admission to the Colorado State Insane Asylum.

Voluntary patients may also be received, but must not be detained more than three days after giving notice of their desire to go away. Voluntary patients must pay cost of maintenance.

Legal Proceedings in Commitment.—A person may be taken into custody upon a complaint filed by a reputable person that he is insane or so distracted in mind as to endanger his person and property or the person and property of others if at large.

Insane Persons Found at Large.—If a sheriff or constable find such person at large in his county he must apprehend him without order of the court. The person so arrested is taken before the county court and an inquest must be held without delay. He must be confined in a hospital or some suitable place until it is determined if he is insane. If found to be insane the county court must order his immediate transfer to the state hospital.

Inquest in Lunacy.—No inquest must be held until at least 10 days' previous notice has been given to the insane person and the guardian *ad litem* appointed by the court unless the guardian himself elects that the inquest be held sooner. If the guardian and the commissioner in lunacy endorse upon the citation that it is for the patient's best interest to hold an inquest at once or upon less than 10 days' notice, it may be held with the approval of the county judge.

Every inquest is brought in the name of the people of Colorado and prosecuted before a jury by the county attorney of the county or in his absence by a duly qualified attorney or other suitable person.

If the insane person has committed a criminal offense no proceedings can be held until notice has been given to the district attorney or other officer charged by law to prosecute him.

No insane person may be confined in any city or county jail unless he is violent and his absolute safety demands it and then upon order of the court. Under no condition may he be confined for more than 10 days.

Medical examiners in insanity are alone allowed to testify. They must be physicians of reputable character, graduates of an incorporated medical college and permanent residents of the state, in actual practice and not connected with any insane institution, and these qualifications must be certified to by a judge of a court of record.

Appeal from Commitment.—A person not committed or detained for any crime or supposed criminal act, who is restrained of his liberty, may apply for a writ of *habeas corpus* to the circuit or district court.

Costs of commitment are paid out of the estate of the insane person upon order of the county court; if there is no estate or the inquest results in his discharge the county commissioners of the county must allow them.

COLORADO STATE INSANE ASYLUM.

PUEBLO, COLO.

An act to establish the Colorado Insane Asylum and providing for its location was passed by the Legislature and approved February 8, 1879. Under the provision of this act, immediately after its passage the Governor appointed a superintendent of the proposed asylum and a board of three commissioners.

On the 11th day of June, 1879, the Board of Commissioners organized by electing Theodore Brown, president, and James McDonald, secretary.

Prior to this meeting the commissioners had given notice to the public when this meeting would be held, in order that donations of land might be made for a site, which, when selected, would be conveyed to the state. Several sites of 40 acres were presented to the board as a gift to the state for asylum purposes, and from among these a site of 40 acres, west of Pueblo, was accepted through George M. Chilcott.

This site contained a brick dwelling, which was remodelled, repaired and opened for the reception of patients in October, 1879; at the same time a one-story frame cottage was erected for women. These quarters were occupied until such time as new and more substantial buildings could be erected.

In 1880 the General Assembly appropriated $60,000 for the erection of buildings and the purchase of land—$55,000 for buildings and $5000 for additional land.

In April, 1881, plans for a new building were submitted to the commissioners and adopted by them. It had been understood and agreed that the cost of the building should not exceed the appropriation, but, owing to fluctuations in the prices of materials, it was found not sufficient to finish the work; an additional appropriation was, therefore, made by the General Assembly in 1882, after which the building was finished and occupied November 20, 1883. This building made room for 220 men patients and the quarters formerly occupied by men were utilized for women until such time as permanent buildings could be erected for their accommodation.

In 1888 money was appropriated for the erection of a wing of a permanent building for women, and in 1892 an appropriation was made for an administration building to be connected with the wing. The completion of one wing and an administration building gave accommodations for 185 women patients.

In 1904 the other wing, accommodating 100 more women, was added by means of an appropriation made for the purpose by the General Assembly. In 1894 a two story cottage for men, accommodating 70 patients, was completed at a cost of $40,000.

In 1893 a law was passed providing that all new or additional buildings erected upon the asylum grounds must be of moderate size and on the cottage plan; each building to accommodate not less than 50 and not more than 100 patients. In 1904 two cottages were completed, accommodating 200 men patients and costing $98,000. In 1908 one cottage, costing $50,000, was erected for the accommodation of 100 women patients. In 1909 three more cottages were erected for the accommodation of 300 patients, 200 men and 100 women. The cost was $150,000. Thus it will be observed that the property has undergone a steady increase from 1879, when it accommodated only 50 patients, up to the present time (1912), when it provides for 1200. All the cottages are modern in design and equipment, and one of the latest is fireproof.

Each succeeding year of the existence of the institution has shown improvement in the design of the buildings and in their management, the property at the present time being as good as the average institution of a similar character.

The institution has had three superintendents, Dr. P. R. Thombs, who was elected in 1879 and served until August 31, 1899, and Dr. A. P. Busey, who succeeded him on September 1, 1899. On January 1, 1913, Dr. Busey resigned, and was succeeded as superintendent by Dr. H. A. La Moure, who had been for two years assistant superintendent.

Three members constitute the Board of Commissioners, one member dropping out every two years. He is succeeded by a man elected for a term of six years.

BOARD OF TRUSTEES.

T. F. Brown	1879-1884	O. H. P. Baxter	1880-1887
Jose B. Romero	1879-1897	M. D. Currigan	1884-1889
James McDonald	1879-1879	A. Y. Hull	1887-1892
R. M. Stevenson	1879-1880	Dr. L. E. Lemen	1889-1895

L. W. Walker	1892-1897	M. Studzinkski	1905-1907
Dr. J. T. Eskridge	1895-1899	M. A. Vigil	1905-1908
Charles O. Unfug	1897-1899	J. W. Finkbiner (in office)	1907-
Fred. Warshauer	1897-1899	W. A. Hartman	1908-1909
Dr. W. W. Grant	1899-1905 1909-1911	G. F. Patrick	1909-1912
N. D. Owen	1899-1905	Dr. Louis Hough (in office)	1911-
J. D. Chamberlain	1899-1901	A. T. Stewart (in office)	1912-
E. G. Middlekamp	1901-1905		
Dr. Charles F. Andrew	1905-1909		

SUPERINTENDENTS.

Dr. P. R. Thombs	1879-1899	Dr. H. A. La Moure (in office)	1913-
Dr. A. P. Busey	1899-1913		

ASSISTANTS.

Dr. W. E. Cord	1899-1905	Dr. F. H. Kuegle	1910-1911
Dr. Annie W. Williams	1899-1900	Dr. Nellie Binford (in office)	1910-
Dr. Persis White	1901-1905	Dr. H. A. La Moure	1911-1913
Dr. B. T. Williams	1905-1906	Dr. Helena B. Pierson (in office)	1911-
Dr. Alice M. Lake	1905-1909	Dr. L. R. Bullick	1912-
Dr. E. H. Cahoon (a few months)	1907-	Dr. Evelyn B. Price	1913-
Dr. W. S. Osborne	1908-1910		
Dr. Emma J. Lucas (a few months)	1908-		

COLORADO STATE HOME AND TRAINING SCHOOL FOR MENTAL DEFECTIVES.[1]

RIDGE, COLO.

The Colorado State Home and Training School for Mental Defectives, located at Ridge, Colo., was created by an act approved May 5, 1909, and the building erected in 1910. It was opened for the reception of patients July 1, 1912.

The working capacity of the institution is 80 persons. This limit was reached some time ago, and there is now (Nov. 30, 1914), a waiting list of over 90 applicants. The age limit is

[1] Compiled from Second Biennial Report of the Board of Commissioners, November 30, 1914.

between 5 and 20 years. The work is custodial, educational and occupational.

In order to care for all the mental defectives in the state, the Board of Commissioners of the institution has asked the Twentieth General Assembly of Colorado for an appropriation of $318,000 for the biennial period beginning December 1, 1914. This includes, besides maintenance, repairs and furnishings, $110,000 for erecting and furnishing two cottages for 200 inmates, and $40,000 for erecting and equipping a hospital.

The site of the institution comprises 310 acres of land, valued at $31,000. The main building cost $115,000, and the power and laundry building, their furnishings, with the heating and lighting plants, water supply and sewerage disposal plants, an additional sum of $41,460. Besides the main buildings there are two frame cottages, cow barn and poultry house. The approximate value of the entire property on November 30, 1914, was $213,940.

The appropriation for support and maintenance for 1912-1914 was $60,000.

The population on November 30, 1914, was 80; 43 boys and 37 girls. A large number of the defectives are low-grade imbeciles and idiots.

The law of Colorado requires the legal commitment of all inmates to the State Home and Training School for Mental Defectives. This gives the management the control regarding the question of removal or discharge, and to a limited extent enables the institution to prevent this class of persons from coming under injurious influences.

The training school is giving special attention to the care, teaching and training of those who are susceptible of being benefited by such a course.

Many of the boys work on the farm and in the garden, in the laundry and in the kitchen. Girls and boys alike assist in making beds, sweeping, scrubbing floors, washing dishes and doing all kinds of housework.

At present there is no gymnasium, nor is there room for workshops.

While the law provides that all inmates of the institution shall pay board, if not all at least a part, they as a rule claim to be poor and pay but little, or nothing. There has been received from all sources since the opening of the institution but $770.

OFFICERS.

State Board of Commissioners.

Thomas F. Daly.................................President.
Benjamin F. Lowell.............................Secretary.
Charles D. Griffith.

Superintendent.
Dr. A. P. Busey.

Steward.
Robert H. Rubidge.

Assistant Physician.
Dr. H. C. Smiley.

Matron.
Mrs. Ida M. Connors.

WOODCROFT HOSPITAL.

Pueblo, Colo.

Woodcroft was founded by Hubert Work, M. D., its present superintendent and owner, in 1896, for the custodial care and treatment of female insane. The year following an additional building was opened for men.

In 1900 its location was changed from the center of the town to the present site, a farm of 60 acres in the suburbs of Pueblo, where a new modern building had been completed.

Four detached cottages for hospital purposes, having an aggregate capacity of 150 patients, were constructed as the population increased, and four brick cottages, now occupied by the assistant superintendent, night nurses and teachers, were added. In addition the equipment includes a modern laundry building, sanitary brick and concrete dairy barn with laboratory for milk testing, barns for cows and stabling for automobiles and horses.

The opening of Woodcroft marked the first attempt to operate a private hospital for the insane in Colorado.

In 1900 Woodcroft School for Feeble-Minded Children was opened on the same grounds, under the same management; this also was the pioneer in this branch of educational work in Colorado.

There have been admitted in the first 15 years of this hospital's history, 1775 adult insane, and to the school department 160 feeble-minded children.

THE CARE OF INSANE IN CONNECTICUT.

The first evidence of public relief for the insane in the State of Connecticut is to be found in the records of the colony of New Haven, in 1645. This record reads as follows:

"It was propounded to the court that Sister Lampson should be provided for at the town charge, so far forth as her husband is not able to do it."

In 1648 another record is made that Goodwife Lampson had been cared for in the house of the marshal for some time, with little amendment. The marshal, therefore, asked to be relieved from the burden and the court ordered her husband "to take her home or else get another place where she might be kept and looked to." No other allusion to the care of the insane is to be found before the year 1699.

The first real law of settlement for paupers, however, which was passed in 1656, undoubtedly included the insane, though they are not specified until later. In 1673 the general court ordered that each town should care for its own poor, but provided that the town might escape the responsibility in the care of strangers by warning them within six months of their arrival and transferring the warning to the court having proper jurisdiction. Unless so warned, a stranger became a lawful charge upon the town by a residence of two or three months in it.

In 1699 the General Court of Connecticut passed a law entitled "An Act for Relieving Idiots and Distracted Persons," which seems to have been copied verbatim from the Massachusetts law of 1694. This law, which made no distinction between idiots, the feeble-minded and the insane, provided that "whenever a person should be wanting of understanding so as to become incapable of providing for himself or herself, or should become insane, and no relatives appear that will undertake the care of providing for them, or that stand in so near a degree as that by law they may be compelled thereto; in every such case the selectmen or overseer of the poor of the town or peculiar where such person was born or is by law an inhabitant, be and thereby are empowered and enjoined to take effectual care and make necessary provision for the relief, support and safety of such impotent or distracted person at the charge of the town or place where he or she of right belongs; if the party hath no estate of his or her own the incomes whereof shall be sufficient to defray the same. And the justices of the peace within the same county at their county courts may order and dispose the estate of such impotent or distracted person to the best improvement and advantage toward his or her support, and also put the person to any proper work or service he or she may be capable to be employed in, at the discretion of the selectmen or overseers of the poor."

In 1711 a law was enacted entitled "An Act to Provide in Case of Sickness, Including Insanity, Feeble-mindedness, and Similar Conditions."

Capen remarks that the chief defects in the poor laws up to this time were due "to incompleteness or were inevitable at this early period." The laws of settlement made difficult a change of residence and may thus, in some instances, have contributed to pauperism. Had the population been larger, the lack of adequate provisions for the care of the poor, except in their homes or in service, would have become serious. The laws for the care of the insane were imperfect and, in fact, remained so for many generations. Yet, for a colony with a small population, supporting itself on farms, and desirous of keeping out those who would increase the disturbing elements already present in the colony, the poor law system of 1712 was very creditable. Its most serious defect was the lack of adequate methods for dealing with vagrants and tramps, who had already appeared.

In 1727 the number of disorderly persons in the colony became so great that it was decided to build a colony workhouse, to which, in addition to "rogues, vagabonds and idle persons," there might be committed "all common pipers, fiddlers, runaways, stubborn servants or children, common drunkards, common night-walkers, pilferèrs, wanton and lascivious persons (either in speech or behavior), common brawlers or railers, all such as neglect their callings, misspend what they earn, and do not provide for themselves or their families. In addition, the workhouse was to receive *"persons under distraction and unfit to go at large whose friends do not take care for their safe confinement."*

This measure, which was undoubtedly a step in advance in the care of the insane, divided those for whom the colony must make provision into four classes, namely, idlers, tramps, stubborn children or servants, and the insane; the poor were alone excluded from the workhouse.

In 1715 a law had been passed dealing with the support of the insane by their relatives, by which "those persons standing in the line or degree of parents, grandparents, children, and grandchildren" were required to relieve their insane relatives, if they were able, in such a manner as the county court where they dwelt should assess. Neglect to comply with this proviso was punishable by a fine of 20 shillings a week, to be levied by distress and sale of the offender's property. At the time the law was passed it applied only to cases of insanity, but in 1739 it was extended to all cases of need, while the fine for failure to comply with it was increased to 30 shillings. The proceeds of the fine, according to the provision of both laws, were assigned to the support of the needy or afflicted person.

In 1746 this law was changed so as to place the duty of enforcing the obligations of relatives upon the county court, the duty not having been previously so understood, and in 1750 the county court was empowered to take this action upon application "of the selectmen of the town or by one or more of the relatives."

It was further provided that the estate of any, who by "age, sickness or otherwise" had become "impotent and unable to support or provide for themselves," should be used for their support and they themselves might be put out to work or service." It was also provided that the court need not itself care for the estate, but might "appoint and empower some meet person as conservator to take care and oversee such . . . . persons and their estates for their support." In 1784 provision was made that where the property of an insane person was not sufficient to satisfy all debts, the court itself, without applying to the General Assembly, might order the sale of enough real estate to pay the same.

In the workhouse law of 1727, of which mention has just been made, an important clause had been included which provided for the confinement in the workhouse of any insane person who was unfit to go at large and whose friends did not care for him. It must be remembered that in those days there were no asylums and this was really a step taken in behalf of the insane. In 1756 a case arose which showed the need of a responsible person to see that the insane were placed under proper care. In that year the General Assembly ordered that the town of Wallingford should care for an insane woman whose settlement was unknown, but who was wandering through the town without clothing. Two years later it was again represented to the Assembly that an insane woman was permitted to wander from town to town and disturb people. Her relatives in Wallingford did not restrain her and the selectmen did nothing. The Assembly authorized any person who found her outside the town to apply to any justice for a warrant requiring him to take her to Wallingford and deliver her to the selectmen, who were ordered to pay the constable four pence for every mile he took her, together with his usual fees and allowances. An appropriation for the care of such persons was made in 1759 and 1761, but before the year 1750 the colony had helped to support several persons who had been made colony charges. In one case they had assisted a father to take care of an insane son who had become insane after military service.

In 1793, however, the unwillingness of the town to care for insane persons, who were thus permitted to wander without restraint, often to the danger of life and property, led to the passage of an act by which it was made the duty of the county authority or selectmen of the town of settlement or residence to order that such dangerous and insane persons be confined in a suitable place, if those responsible for their care did not obey the order requiring their restraint. If necessary, the authorities might have the insane persons committed to a county jail, to remain there during their insanity or commitment in accordance with the law; at the same time the authority to commit them to the workhouse was withdrawn. In 1797 the section regarding the confinement in jail was also repealed.

In the early years of the new century the question of caring for the insane was taken up by the medical profession in Connecticut and in 1812, at a meeting of the Connecticut Medical Society, a committee was appointed to secure information concerning the extent of insanity throughout the state. In 1814 this committee, which does not appear to have accomplished anything up to that time, enlisted the help of the General Association of the Congregational Clergy, an organization which extended into every town in the state, church and state not being as yet separated in Connecticut. From information thus obtained they reported that they had found " 146 persons who, in different degrees, are deprived of reason," but this estimate is certainly too small, since other authorities speak of 500 to 700. The condition of these persons was often very bad, as it was everywhere at that period, and the need of a hospital for the exclusive care of the insane became more and more evident to those who thought upon the subject.

The prime mover in securing such an institution was Dr. Eli Todd. He and Dr. Samuel Woodward had been much interested and pleased by the asylum for the insane established by the Society of Friends in Pennsylvania in 1817 at Frankford, and they were anxious to erect an institution of the same kind, at which the same methods could be put in practice, in Connecticut. Such an undertaking was very different at that time from what it is to-day. If a new hospital for the insane is needed at the present time the matter is laid before the Legislature and the necessary funds are provided by it, since the insane are now looked upon as wards of the state. Eighty to a hundred years ago, however, the state assumed no responsibility whatever and the money had to be raised by private subscription. The Medical Society appointed a committee to raise funds and itself contributed $200, a sum which was increased by another gift of $400 the next year. In the list of subscriptions it is noticeable that a large number of them are for very small amounts. Only three persons gave as much as $300, and the majority of them did not exceed $25, a number of subscriptions being for the sum of $1, while one is for 12 1-2 cents.

In this way, which was quite unique in this country, the necessary funds were raised and the Hartford Retreat was opened in 1824.[1] It was one of the earliest institutions of its kind, that is to say, for the exclusive care of the insane, in this country. Dr. Todd, who had been most active in the work of securing funds, was appointed superintendent and he began his work with convictions regarding the proper manner of treating the insane, which were radically different from those entertained up to this time. He

[1] See "History of the Hartford Retreat," in this volume.

was convinced that the system then employed of depletion by blood-letting, low diet, purges, blisters, etc., as well as the use of mechanical restraint and close confinement, was altogether wrong. The success of a different order of things, based upon the principle of liberal diet and strengthening medicine, with consistent kindness and as much freedom and liberty as possible, had recently been shown by Dr. Tuke of the York Retreat in England. But these ideas were as yet untried in America and it required considerable boldness as well as much tact and patience on Dr. Todd's part to make a place for them.

In 1837 a communication was received by the State Medical Society from the directors of the Retreat for the Insane, accompanying a copy of a "Memorial to the General Assembly," asking for an appropriation to provide an asylum for the insane poor of the state. The memorial was approved but nothing seems to have been done.

In 1839 the Society passed another resolution approving the establishment of a state institution and recommending that a committee of three be appointed to confer with the Legislature in the matter.

In 1851 a similar resolution was again passed and another committee was appointed. In 1853 another resolution was passed asking that an appropriation be made to the Retreat.

In 1855 the state began to help the towns to care for their insane poor. This involved the payment of a portion of the expenses of the patients in the Retreat by the state. In 1866 it was found that of the insane throughout the state, 147 were in the Retreat under state aid, 55 in the Retreat without state aid, 205 were supported and aided by the towns, and that there were 300 others, whose status was not known.

In 1866 the Connecticut Hospital for the Insane was finally created and located at Middletown, but it was not opened until 1868.

In 1903 the Norwich State Hospital for the Insane was established at the Town of Preston, Norwich; its capacity is 1030 beds.

There are two other state institutions for the care of the mentally infirm in Connecticut. One, the Connecticut School for

Imbeciles, was established at Lakeville, in 1858, as a private institution. It was taken over by the state on August 1, 1913.[1]

The Connecticut Colony for Epileptics, Mansfield Depot, Conn., was established by an act of the General Assembly, August 10, 1909. It was formally opened for the admission of patients May 15, 1914.

In 1838 a law was passed which committed persons acquitted of murder or manslaughter on the ground of insanity to a county jail, unless some one undertook to give bond of confinement under the direction of the court. In 1856 this law was amended to read, "the county jail or some other suitable place." Two years later a department for insane convicts was provided at Wethersfield, in connection with the penitentiary, but the building, though completed, was never occupied, and in 1859 was converted into a prison store house.

In 1860 insane criminals were to be sent to jail or "any other suitable place." In 1861 this law was made to apply to the person convicted of any crime, whether punishable by confinement or not. In 1865 the alternative "any other suitable place" was removed, and all insane criminals were sent to jail. In 1868 the trustees of the state hospital were directed to make provision at the hospital for insane criminals. In 1870 a law was passed providing for the confinement in the state hospital of criminals acquitted of crime because of insanity, as well as those who become insane after conviction.

All institutions in Connecticut where persons are held under compulsion are under the supervision of the State Board of Charities, which consists of five members, appointed by the Governor for a term of four years. The Connecticut Hospital for the Insane is controlled by a board of 13 members, of which the Governor is *ex-officio* a member; the members of this board are appointed by the Senate for a term of four years. The Norwich Hospital for the Insane is under the control of a similar board, but the term of its members is for six years.

All insane persons who are residents of the state are entitled to admission to the state hospitals.

[1] An act of the Legislature of January, 1915, provided for the removal of this institution to a site on property owned by the state in connection with the Connecticut Colony for Epileptics, Mansfield Depot, Conn.

Voluntary Patients.—Any asylum in the state may receive a voluntary patient who applies in writing, but such person must not be detained more than three days after he has given notice in writing of his desire to leave the asylum.

Legal Procedure.—The judge of the court of probate may commit patients, but only upon a written complaint, which may be made by any person. If the insane person is at large and dangerous to the community the selectmen of the town in which he resides or is at large must make complaint. No person may be committed without an order of the court of probate, except in case of one violently insane, when he may be detained for not more than 48 hours without special order of the court of probate, but the proceedings must forthwith be commenced.

Within 10 days after the complaint has been filed the probate court must appoint a hearing and give due notice to the person alleged to be insane and others concerned. The court may order the person to be brought before it and examine him if his condition or conduct renders it necessary; if not necessary or advisable he may state it in the final order.

While proceedings are pending the court may order the restraint of the alleged insane person.

In addition to oral testimony the court may require the sworn certificates of at least two reputable physicians, graduates of legally organized medical institutions and practitioners of medicine for at least three years within the state and not connected with any asylum nor related to the complainant nor to the person alleged to be insane.

One of the physicians must be selected by the court. Their certificates must state that they have personally examined the person within 10 days of the hearing and that he is insane and a fit subject for confinement in the hospital. If the court finds that he is insane and a fit subject for treatment it must order his commitment.

Admission of Pauper Patients.—When any pauper in any other town is insane a selectman may apply to the court of probate of the district for his commitment to a state hospital and the court must appoint two reputable physicians to investigate the facts and report. If they find him insane the court may order the selectman to take him to one of the state hospitals.

Admission of Indigent Patients.—When an indigent person not a pauper becomes insane application may be made by any person in his behalf to the probate court of that district and the court may appoint two reputable physicians and a selectman of the town to investigate the facts and report to the court. If the court of probate is satisfied that the person is indigent and insane and a resident of any town in its jurisdiction he must order him to be taken to one of the state hospitals. He must also state the town of which he is a resident and the amount of his estate. No probate court may commit a person who is not a resident of the town within its jurisdiction. When the court orders the admission of a pauper or indigent person it must record the order and give a certified copy of the procedings to be taken to the hospital and transmit a copy to the Governor.

Admission of Non-Resident Patients.—Insane patients not residents of any town may be committed by the Governor to any place of detention upon a sworn certificate signed by a reputable physician that he is found a pauper and insane.

Any person who becomes violently insane may be taken to a place of detention and held for not more than 48 hours without a special order of the court of probate on the certificate of one or more physicians, but the proceedings for his regular commitment must be commenced at once.

Appeal from Commitment.—Any person, relative or friend has the right of appeal from the order of the court finding any person insane. All insane persons confined in an asylum are entitled to the benefit of a writ of *habeas corpus.* Upon information that any person is unjustifiably confined in an asylum or in a neighboring hospital any judge of the Superior Court may appoint a commission to inquire into the case. If in the opinion of the commission the party is not legally detained or is cured and his confinement is no longer advisable, the judge may order his discharge, but no commission may be appointed with reference to the same person oftener than once in six months.

Costs of commitment must be paid out of the estate of the insane person if he has sufficient estate; if not, by his friends or relatives; if there are none, by the town to which he belongs; if found not to be insane, by the complainant.

THE HARTFORD RETREAT.

HARTFORD, CONN.

The Hartford Retreat was chartered in May, 1822, on petition and representations made by the Fellows of the Connecticut State Medical Society to the General Assembly. The subject of provision for the insane in the state had for several years previous received the attention of the society.

In 1812 Dr. Nathaniel Dwight, of Colchester, sent to the convention of the Medical Society held at New Haven, October 14 and 15, a communication upon the subject of a hospital for the insane, in consequence of which Mason F. Cogswell, John Barker, Samuel H. P. Lee, Gideon Beardsley, Thomas Hubbard, Elijah Lyman, Richard Ely, Jr., and John S. Peters were appointed a committee to collect information concerning the insane in their respective counties and report to the next convention.

At a meeting held October 20, 1813, this committee was continued. There is no record of any report having been made and probably little was accomplished by this committee, for at a meeting held October 19, 1814, it was voted that Mason F. Cogswell be appointed to obtain definite information from the General Association of the Congregational Ministers.

The investigation was evidently not very thorough, for "only 146 were reported as in different degrees deprived of reason"; and the matter seems to have rested until further action was taken by the Medical Society in 1821, when, at a meeting held in Hartford, May 9, Mason F. Cogswell presiding, the attention of the president and fellows was called to the helpless condition of the insane and their families by Dr. Eli Todd, relating his experiences of the difficulty of treating insane patients at their homes or in private dwellings. The subject, after some discussion, was referred to a committee, who recommended the establishment of an asylum for their relief. The proposition was approved by the convention and referred to a committee consisting of Drs. Eli Todd, Thomas Miner, William Tulley, Samuel B. Woodward and George Sumner.

The committee met every fortnight during the summer, most commonly at Rocky Hill, to suit the convenience of different members of the committee.

To obtain information they sent circulars into every town in the state, addressed to clergymen, physicians and other respectable gentlemen, requesting returns of the number of the insane, their ages, sex, cause of the disease, etc. The returns in answer to these circulars, although many of them were very imperfect, satisfied the committee that at least 1000 individuals within the limits of the state were mentally deranged, and that the condition of most of them was truly wretched.

The duties performed by this committee were arduous; they had obstacles to surmount requiring great perseverance. The field was untrodden; they had to learn the way as they proceeded; they had undertaken to accomplish an object which the indifferent asserted and the anxious feared would never be accomplished. The report made by them to the adjourned session in October, together with the annexed draft of a constitution, was the result of their labors.[1] The adjourned convention in October met for the express purpose of hearing and acting on the report of their committee. Every article of the proposed constitution was read separately and received a separate vote of acceptance, and finally, with little variation, the whole passed unanimously.

At the adjourned convention in Hartford on the 3d of October, 1821, it was "Voted, To accept and approve of the report of the committee appointed at the annual convention in May last on the subject of the establishment of an asylum for the insane in this state.

"Voted, To accept of the constitution for the organization of a society for their relief, reported by the same committee, as altered and amended by this convention.

"Voted, That Drs. Thomas Miner, Eli Todd, Samuel B. Woodward, William Tully, George Sumner, Jonathan Knight and Eli Ives be a Committee of Correspondence, to carry into immediate effect the plan laid down in the aforesaid constitution; and that the following persons be county committees to co-operate with them, viz.: M. F. Cogswell, M. D.; Rev. Thomas Robbins, Samuel Tudor, Hartford County; Rt. Rev. Dr. Brownell, Joseph Foot,

[1] See Appendix A, p. 93.

M. D., Simeon Baldwin, New Haven County; Elias Perkins, John O. Miner, M. D., Richard Adams, New London County; R. M. Sherman, Dr. Johathan Knight, Rev. M. R. Dutton, Fairfield County; Thomas Hubbard, M. D., Zephaniah Swift, Daniel Putnam, Windham County; Oliver Wolcott, Joseph Battell, William Buel, M. D., Litchfield County; S. T. Hosmer, Joshua Stow, J. R. Watkinson, Middletown County; John S. Peters, M. D.; Rev. A. Bassett, D. D., Benning Mann, Tolland County."

The Committee of Correspondence, whose duties were implied by the name, was instructed with great particularity. It was to keep in touch with the county committees, through whom it was to collect subscriptions in each town.

There was to be a joint meeting of the Correspondence and County Committees at the State House in New Haven on the Tuesday preceding the second Wednesday of May, 1822, for the purpose of adopting such measures as might conduce to the prosperity of the institution for the insane and for the transaction of any other business which might fall within the limits of their instructions.

The business of the Correspondence Committee appointed by the convention was to devise means of procuring funds for the establishment and maintenance of a retreat for the insane; to petition the General Assembly at their session in May for an act of incorporation or charter, and, if thought expedient, to request a grant of money from the treasury of the state to aid the benevolent object contemplated. The convention, also at this meeting, appropriated $200 of their funds to aid the Committee in prosecuting their plans. This grant, the first pecuniary aid which had been received, was very useful to the Committee. But for this they would have been obliged to make considerable advances of money from their own resources, or to have abandoned the undertaking in despair.

On the evening of the 7th of May, 1822, the general meeting of the Correspondence and County Committees was held by previous appointments at the State House in New Haven. Dr. Thomas Hubbard was elected chairman. The meeting ascertained that about $12,000 had already been subscribed to the funds. At this meeting it was resolved to present a petition to the General Assembly for an act of incorporation and for a grant of money. While the subject was before the Legislature many distinguished friends of the institution, both members and other gentlemen who were present, very generously offered their services to promote the interests of the cause in the Assembly. The act of incorporation and a grant of $5000 were both obtained, together with a brief permitting contributions in churches for five years. At the same time also the members of the Medical Society, then in session, showed their steady devotion to the cause by appropriating the remainder of their disposable funds, amounting to about $400, to the interests of this institution.

The act of incorporation was accepted and a Board of Directors was chosen at a meeting of the society held in Middletown on October 29, 1822. Supscriptions had been obtained in the several towns of the state for funds to aid in the establishment of the institution. The names of 2062 individuals appear as subscribers in the State of Connecticut, and 29 persons subscribed a little less than $400 in the other New England states. One subscription was for "$30 payable in medicine"; another for "one gross New London bilious pills, price $30"; and two for lottery tickets of the value of $5 each; one of these drew a blank and the other a prize, the net product being $17.

There were 224 subscribers in Hartford. The amount of individual subscriptions was declared to be not far from $14,000. The Connecticut Medical Society had appropriated $600, the state had granted $5000 upon certain conditions, and "in addition to the above sums the inhabitants of Hartford offered $4000, provided the institution should be established in that town."

At a meeting of the Society December 3, 1822, it was unanimously voted to establish the institution in Hartford, and on this date the directors appointed committees to fix upon a site and report a plan for a building. The committee, of which Bishop Brownell was chairman, reported on December 27 that they had examined nine different places and gave the prices at which each could be obtained and their several advantages and disadvantages. They gave the preference to Todd's place, 1 1-2 miles southwest from the State House, 15 acres of land, a house, two barns and cider house, price $2400. Advantages: excellent prospect, good building site, good grounds for walks, garden and meadow. The committee's report was accepted by the Directors and on January 27, 1823, the society unanimously resolved "that the land owned by Mr. Ira Todd be, and the same is, hereby fixed upon as the site of the buildings, etc., of a retreat for the insane, if the commissioners approve thereof."

The Society for the Relief of the Insane was organized by the election of the following officers for 1823: Nathaniel Terry, president; Right Rev. Thomas C. Brownell, vice-president; David Watkinson, treasurer; Samuel Tudor, auditor; and Jonathan Law, secretary.

The plan which was adopted for the building contemplated a center 50 feet square, three stories in height; and two wings, 50 x 30 feet each, of two stories, the whole not to exceed in cost the sum of $12,000. The building committee, consisting of Nathaniel Terry, David Porter and Henry L. Ellsworth, recommended that the buildings "be erected of Rocky Hill ironstone to be selected for that purpose; and to be covered with a white cement or rough cast similar to the Medical College at New Haven." They engaged as contractor "Mr. Scranton, of Derby, who had erected several buildings for Eli Whitney and was mentioned by him and several other gentlemen as a good mason." Mr. Scranton thought "that good walls for the building could not be made with Rocky Hill stone." The expediency of using the same appearing questionable, the directors resolved that the building of the retreat be constructed of Chatham freestone, or with that and other stone at the discretion of the committee; "and voted that $2 per day be allowed to the superintendent of the building when employed." As an illustration of the close economy and careful supervision of the committee, they reported January 28, 1824, "that the whole amount expended on the building, exclusive of the steps and iron sashes, falls a little short of $12,622."

The buildings were designed to accommodate 40 patients; and it was voted that they be opened for the reception of patients on April 1, 1824, and that they be "publicly consecrated to the blessing of Almighty God."

On January 7 the Board of Directors made choice of Eli Todd to be superintendent. Dr. Todd had been largely responsible for bringing to a successful issue plans that had been considered over a period of several years for the establishment of an institution for the insane. He had had unusual experience in the care of insane patients and it was most natural that he should be called to carry on the work. It is said that "long and perseveringly did he resist all entreaties—he wholly declined taking charge of an institution which he had so much agency in establishing. He could not bear for a moment that his zeal in this benevolent cause should by any be attributed to a selfish motive. He was, however, unanimously appointed by the committee whose duty it was to make the selection. He commenced the duties of his new station on April 1, 1824."

It is said that Dr. Todd had a great aversion to writing. Even his correspondence was too much neglected on account of his dread of taking up his pen. His reports were not full, and only a few short articles from his pen have been preserved.

Amongst these was found one in his own hand-writing, giving his plan of treatment of the insane, which was probably written soon after the Retreat was opened for the reception of patients. It may be assumed that he was actuated in his management of the institution by the feelings he expresses in this paper.[1]

[1] The great design of moral management is to bring those faculties which yet remain sound to bear upon those which are diseased, and by their operation to modify, to counteract or to suspend their morbid actions. This constitutes a process of self-control—the ground-work of cure, the grand tactical principle which is to decide the issue of the contest between reason and insanity. To effect all this successfully requires an art too refined and too difficult to be exercised in perfection; for who is there that possesses those rare endowments of head and heart, those sensibilities ever alive to the sufferings of the maniac, united with that exquisite tact of character by which at once is perceived, comprehended and felt the individualities of each case; who learns the secret avenues of approach to each several mind and with a masterly address and nice adaptation plies all the diversified modes of moral and mental influence? But fortunately there are certain plain and simple maxims in the moral treatment of the insane which are easily understood and of universal application. These are to treat them, in all cases, so far as possible as rational beings. To allow them all the liberty and indulgence compatible with their own safety and that of others. To cherish in them the sentiments of self-respect. To excite an ambition for the good-will and esteem of others. To draw out the latent sparks of natural and social affection. To occupy their attention, exercise their judgment and ingenuity, and to minister to their self-complacency by engaging them in useful employment alternating with amusement. . . . .

Under Dr. Todd's management the Retreat seems to have flourished and to have fully met the expectation of the large number of persons who were interested in and responsible for bringing it into existence. In the latter part of 1830 the Doctor's health became undermined, and, though he continued to direct the affairs of the institution for two years, he gradually failed and died November 17, 1833.

In Dr. Todd's third report to the Board of Managers he states that "37 cases have been admitted in the course of the year, to wit, 14 old cases and 23 recent cases. Of the recent cases 21 recovered, or 91.3 per cent." In the report for 1830, 14 old cases and 26 recent cases were admitted; two recent cases remained over from the previous year; 5 had been under treatment less than a fortnight when the report was made, "the remaining 23 have been the only subjects of treatment; of the latter 21 have recovered, being in the centesimal proportion of 91.6." It is further stated, "this institution reports a cure of 91 per cent of recent cases and an average of 51 per cent of all." The seventh report does not contain a report by the superintendent, but the medical visitors, Dr. Samuel B. Woodward, chairman, state, "during the last seven years, 147 recent cases of insanity have been admitted, of which number, 133, being more than nine-tenths, have been restored to reason. It is not an extravagant calculation that three-fourths of these would have continued under the influence of mental derangement if no establishment like the Retreat had been prepared for their reception."[1]

Soon after Dr. Todd's decease the position of superintendent was tendered by the committee of the Medical Society to Dr. George Sumner, but he refused the honor, "declining to take the office of physician on any terms." Dr. William H. Rockwell, Dr. Todd's first assistant and subsequently superintendent of the

[1] The Retreat was designed for those who could pay for treatment, but on May 19, 1830, the directors passed the following resolution:

"*Resolved,* That the managers of the Retreat be authorized to admit indigent lunatics being inhabitants of this state, whose disease has not exceeded six months, at two dollars per week, provided the number of such persons in the institution shall at no time exceed the number of ten; and, *provided, also,* That no individual shall remain in the institution upon the said terms over six months."

Brattleboro Retreat for many years, performed the duties of physician for about one year.

In a "Circular of the Directors of the Retreat for the Insane," issued in May 1834, it was reported "in accordance with the views of a committee of investigation appointed, the directors ordered the erection of rooms for the further accommodation of patients at the Retreat. At an expense of about $10,000, two pavilions three stories high and two wings connecting them with the original building, making an addition of 104 feet of front and comprising upwards of 50 separate apartments, were ready for the reception of patients in the spring of 1832."

In June, 1834, Dr. Silas Fuller, of Columbia, Conn., was appointed superintendent.

The late Gurdon W. Russell, for many years president of the Board of Directors of the Retreat, was authority for the statement that the arrangement with the superintendent permitted him to employ a portion of his time in practice outside the institution. Criticism and disagreement arose as a result of this plan, and it probably led to Dr. Fuller's resignation in 1840.

The position of superintendent was offered to Dr. Samuel B. Woodward, of Worcester, Mass., who declined it. Dr. Amariah Brigham was then nominated by the committee of the Medical Society, and was appointed superintendent in July, 1840. The following reference to Dr. Brigham occurs in the report for 1840: "At a late meeting of the directors of the Retreat, Dr. Brigham, of this city, was elected superintendent. His unblemished moral character, his professional industry, his acquirements and his manners pre-eminently fit him for the station for which he has been chosen."

After having served a little more than two years Dr. Brigham resigned in October, 1842, to accept the superintendency of the State Lunatic Asylum at Utica, New York (now Utica State Hospital).

Dr. Brigham stated in his first report: "It has been somewhat common to make a division of cases into chronic and recent; under the latter denomination, as was stated in the report of this institution for 1824, 'are comprehended all cases of insanity whose duration has not exceeded one year.' Entering upon the duties of superintendent in the middle of the year, it is impossible for me to say from personal inquiry how many of those discharged were recent cases, according to the above definition. I shall not, therefore, attempt such a classification, and I have grave doubts whether such can even be made with sufficient accuracy to be of any value . . . . ."

The two reports of the Retreat rendered by Dr. Brigham are among the most interesting and instructive of any that have been written. He investigated the admissions, discharges and recoveries in several institutions in England and France and all of those then in operation in this country, and gave at considerable length his views of the etiology of insanity and methods of treatment.

Dr. Gurdon W. Russell, for many years president of the Board of Directors of the Retreat, knew Dr. Brigham very well, and he has written of his administration: "Though it was short, yet he introduced many reforms, and by his untiring energy, ambition and close attention to his duties gave to the Retreat a reputation equal to any which it had ever possessed. He was required to give his whole service to it, this arrangement having become necessary on account of the number of patients. . . . . The ambition which was so prominent a point in his character led him to accept a more influential position for the development of his talents in a neighboring state."

In consequence of Dr. Brigham's resignation it became necessary for the Directors to provide for the temporary supervision of the patients. Dr. E. K. Hunt was selected for that purpose, and he discharged the duties assigned to him with great credit.

The number of patients in the Retreat at this time was 89—46 men and 43 women. The number of insane and idiots in the state was probably not less than 1000. The need of further accommodations had been brought to the attention of the General Assembly in May, 1838, and a committee was appointed to investigate the needs of the insane. Among other facts ascertained it was found that " 59 are caged or manacled, and a few others are in gaol or the state prison for safety."

In 1839 a committee of the General Assembly made a report recommending an appropriation of $20,000 by the state to erect a building for 150 patients. It passed the House of Representatives with only 12 dissenting votes; the Senate, however, proposed a substitute which was adopted by appointing a committee to prepare a plan with estimates, and likewise to select an eligible location, and make a report to the next General Assembly. This may have been the first attempt looking to the establishment of a state institution for the insane in Connecticut.

When the report was made in 1840 the subject was further postponed.

In 1841 a committee of the General Assembly recommended an appropriation of $20,000, and the appointment of a committee with power to select a site and erect a state asylum for the insane. The Directors of the Retreat "had presented a memorial to the same General Assembly offering some accommodation to the indigent insane at the Connecticut Retreat, and having in view the erection of additional buildings. No decisive action on the subject was taken until the session of 1842, when, by unanimous vote in both branches of the Legislature, $2000 a year for five years were appropriated for the support of insane poor persons at the Retreat."

"In May, 1843, the Board of Directors unanimously appointed Dr. John S. Butler superintendent, with a salary of $1400 per annum, with the use of a dwelling-house, garden and barn. They stipulated that his time be exclusively devoted to the interests of the Retreat, and only such other practice as "shall be offered him at the institution and his own dwelling-house." Dr. Butler was superintendent of the Boston Lunatic Hospital, and physician of the Public Institutions at South Boston from the autumn of 1839 to the autumn of 1842, when he was "not unwillingly superseded by a medical gentleman of opposite politics." In the annual report of the Directors for 1843 they said:

"The successor to Dr. Brigham, Dr. John S. Butler, of Boston, will assume the duties of his station in a few weeks. His experience in the treatment of the insane and the high encomiums which he brings from those who have been witnesses of his skill and humanity in another institution lead to the expectation of great good from his labors at the Retreat."

The lack of funds to provide for the needed increase in accommodations probably led the Directors of the Retreat to petition the Legislature to make available the amount that had been appropriated for the indigent insane before the appropriation fell due. At all events, the General Assembly, at the May session in 1843, passed this resolution:

WHEREAS, At the session of the General Assembly held in May, 1842, an appropriation of at least $2000 per annum was made in aid of the insane poor; and

WHEREAS, The Retreat for the Insane at Hartford has not at present suitable buildings for the accommodation of the insane poor, nor has said Retreat the present means of erecting such buildings; now, therefore, in order to encourage said Retreat to erect such buildings, it is hereby

Resolved, That the Governor of this state, as commissioner under said resolution of May, 1842, be, and he hereby is, authorized to *advance* to said Retreat said annual appropriation of $2000 per annum, for the ensuing five years; that is, to advance to said Retreat $10,000 instead and in lieu of the next five years' annual appropriation of $2000. And the Comptroller of Public Accounts is hereby authorized and directed to draw an order on the Treasurer of the state in favor of said commissioner for said sum of $10,000 in lieu of the annual sum of $2000 for the ensuing five years as now directed; *provided,* that said commissioner on advancing said sum of $10,000 shall take proper contracts on the part of said Retreat to support the insane poor at said Retreat on such terms as may be agreed upon between said commissioner and the officers of said Retreat; and *provided further,* that the relief to be furnished to the insane poor under this resolution should be extended through said period of the ensuing five years, and be as nearly equal in each year as can conveniently be made.

The Legislature made a further grant of $5000 at a subsequent session, payable half in 1845 and half in 1846. The Directors reported with reference to building operations:

"Upwards of $40,000, $5000 of which were granted by the state, payable half in 1845 and half in 1846, and the residue taken from a fund heretofore belonging to the corporation, and which is now nearly exhausted," were expended in the building of two wings, each 120 feet long and 36 feet wide, a house for the superintendent, and the rebuilding of the barns. The new buildings were constructed of Portland stone and stuccoed.

In the superintendent's report for 1846 Dr. Butler stated:

"The extensive additions and improvements which have been completed within the last 18 months have effected such a change, both in the external appearance and internal arrangements and accommodations of the Retreat, that it would hardly be recognized by those who have not watched from step to step their progress.

They in fact constitute a new era in the history of the institution. Its capacity for the accommodation of patients has been doubled, and the conveniences and appliances for successful treatment, as well as the arrangements for their more comfortable and pleasant classification, have increased in no less a ratio."

In 1853 the Legislature granted $8000, which became available on October 1 of that year, to be used toward the construction of a "lodge" for disturbed women patients. The building, a one-story structure, was completed in the fall of 1854. In 1858 a story was added, and the building is still used for the purpose for which it was originally designed. In 1855 another grant of $6000 was made for a building for disturbed male patients. The amounts appropriated by the Legislature up to this time were $5000 in 1822, $5000 in 1845, $8000 in 1853 and $6000 in 1855.

Under date of November 12, 1858, Miss Dorothea Dix, writing from Somerville, Mass., to Dr. Butler, said: "I cannot omit writing to express the sense I have of the value of the improvements you have made in and around the institution you direct." But she passes almost at once to say, "I must ask you to excuse me if I press on your consideration a few facts of the Retreat as seeming to me serious defects in an institution which must, in its nature, be to some extent custodial. First and most urgent of your wants, seems to me, means to arrest conflagration should it occur; a first prevention in your establishment should be adopted at once in common justice to yourself and your patients, as well as to the friends of those who are entrusted to your care, by adopting a safer method of warming your building, reducing your 28 or 30 fires to two or three at the most, and also by the introduction of gas to control the use of portable lights."

In 1862 Dr. Butler obtained $11,222 on an appeal for private subscriptions with which to provide "a conservatory for flowers, etc., a bowling alley for the exclusive use of ladies, and a building for a museum or reading-room for the gentlemen, and for the laying out and decoration of the grounds." The latter work was done in accordance with a design by Olmsted & Vaux, of New York, who gave their services to the Retreat. These improvements were carried out in 1861.

Steam heating was introduced in 1863.

In the superintendent's report for 1866 it is stated that "during the past year the wards of the institution have continued to be overcrowded. . . . . With a proper allowance of vacant rooms, with the necessity of changes and unexpected admissions, and the suitable limitation of numbers in our dormitories, 200 patients is the greatest number the Retreat should ever receive; 210 patients fill every proper accommodation in the institution . . . . our highest numbers for the last two years have averaged 241. . . . ."

In anticipation of the removal of the indigent insane to the State Hospital, which was opened in the spring of 1868, the Board of Directors, at a meeting held on March 5, 1868, appointed the Board of Managers a building committee to carry into execution the plans of Messrs. Vaux, Withers & Co., architects, for the alteration and improvement of the Retreat building. "These plans involved a radical and thorough reconstruction of the buildings, and embraced improvements in heating, ventilation, the enlargement of the halls and arrangement of a series of spacious single and also suites of other rooms, consisting of parlor, bed and bath rooms, all arranged and adapted for occupancy by patients whose habits and mode of life render these extra accommodations a sort of necessity." The improvements were completed in the spring of 1870, and the Managers said that "the result of the reconstruction is most satisfactory to the committee, the officers of the institution and others who have examined the alterations." The accommodations were reduced to about 140 beds.

On October 19, 1872, Dr. Butler presented to the Board of Directors his resignation as superintendent. He said therein: "I was elected to this office on the 13th of May, 1843, nearly 30 years ago. During this long period of service I have most earnestly and honestly and to the best of my ability endeavored to promote the highest interests of the institution. During my superintendency many important changes and improvements have been made in the Retreat; during the last four years the most important of all—its almost entire reconstruction. That this reconstruction has proved a success is evidenced by the universal approval of the external architecture, and of the home-like internal arrangements of the building, by its peculiar adaptedness, as shown by the decided increase of the percentage of recoveries, and by the decidedly favorable financial results . . . ."

When Dr. Butler became superintendent of the Retreat the accommodations were for about 90 patients. He witnessed its growth to provision for above 200 patients and an actual average occupation of almost 250 before the removal of the state beneficiaries; and, what is of more importance, he carried out the radical changes in the building whereby it was "remodelled and adapted to its new exigencies." Dr. Butler ever gave to the Retreat a deep, conscientious, abiding interest in its welfare and best good. He devoted himself without stint to the work and he expected of others the same loyal, conscientious service.

After Dr. Butler's retirement he lived in Hartford, where he died May 21, 1890.

Dr. James H. Denney was appointed acting superintendent October 27, 1872, and on the 25th of the following month was elected superintendent. Some disagreement with reference to the business management of the Retreat led to Dr. Denney's resignation in December, 1873. The question of a successor was one of grave concern to the Board of Directors, and the position was finally tendered to Dr. Henry P. Stearns, who at first declined the appointment; but on assurance that the circumstances that had led to Dr. Denney's retirement would be altered to accord with the methods of other institutions, he reconsidered and was unanimously chosen superintendent January 20, 1874. He did not, however, assume the duties of his office until May, having spent the intervening three months in the study of institutional practice and the methods of caring for the insane in England and Scotland.

Dr. Stearns' work comprehended the completion of the adaptation of the old buildings to the new needs and the construction of several new buildings; the chapel in 1876; a set of service buildings, including laundry, carpenter shop, stable and carriage house, in 1878; connecting corridors between the main buildings and the north and south lodges in 1880; the erection of Spencer cottage in 1881; of Hackmatack cottage in 1888; the north annex, the gate lodge and Warren cottage in 1893, and the south annex in 1894. The acquisition of the Barnard property and the construction of Belleview cottage in 1900 completed the addition of 21 rooms and 5 cottages.

During Dr. Stearns' term of service of more than 31 years, the Retreat maintained a high place among institutions and enjoyed an unusual degree of prosperity. The debts that had been incurred in rebuilding were in part left over to his administration, and these and other obligations incurred in acquiring land and erecting new buildings were met in the main from current income.

Impaired health led Dr. Stearns to tender his resignation in June, 1904, but subsequently, at the request of the Board of Directors, the resignation was withdrawn, and Dr. Whitefield N. Thompson, assistant physician at the Brattleboro Retreat, was selected assistant superintendent. He entered upon his duties October 28, 1904. At the annual meeting of the Board of Directors April 4, 1905, Dr. Stearns' resignation, which had been presented March 31, was accepted, and Dr. Thompson was chosen as his successor.

Dr. Stearns died May 27, 1905, in the house where he had lived as superintendent on the Retreat grounds.

In 1906 the average of attendants to nurses was 1 to 3. A course of instruction for nurses was instituted this year and lectures were given regularly by members of the staff, supplemented with lectures by the consulting physicians and surgeons.

Dr. Gurdon W. Russell, the president of the board, died February 3, 1909. He had served the Retreat in the dual capacity of medical visitor and director for more than half a century.

In 1911 the Retreat received a gift of $11,000, made by a gentleman in memory of his wife, "a patient lately deceased." The fund was given for the specific purpose of providing a home for the women nurses. This building was completed in 1912. It is of colonial architecture, and stands on Washington street, about 300 feet south of the west entrance. Each floor is provided with bath and toilet rooms, and spacious sitting rooms adjacent to the main hall and opening out on a wide veranda. The second floor has a suite for the head nurse. There are in all 20 sleeping rooms.

There were present at the beginning of the hospital year, April 1, 1912, 82 men and 89 women. There remained at the end of the year, March 31, 1913, 80 men and 84 women. The daily average for the year was 175 patients.

The Retreat is now receiving in two of the cottages acute borderline cases. The cottage service has heretofore been devoted to high-priced patients of the chronic class. The returns for the service that is now provided are fully up to those obtained under the old arrangement and the service is much more acceptable and useful to the public.[1]

OFFICERS OF THE HARTFORD RETREAT.

From the Opening in 1823.

PRESIDENTS.

Nathaniel Terry ....[2]	1823–1826	Gurdon W. Russell	1890-1909
Gideon Tomlinson	1827-1840	Jonathan B. Bunce	1909-1912
Thomas C. Brownell	1840-1865	John D. Brown	1912-1913
William A. Buckingham.	1868-1874	Charles P. Cooley	1913-
William R. Cone	1874-1890		

TREASURERS.

James Ward	1830-1840	Thomas Sisson	1865-1903
William T. Lee	1840-1865	J. M. Holcombe	1903-

MEDICAL VISITORS.

Mason F. Cogswell, M. D.	1823-1831	Edward P. Terry, M. D.	1827-1844
William Buel, M. D.	1823-1827	S. W. Brown, M. D.	1827-1830
Thomas Hubbard, M. D.	1823-1827	Horatio Gridley, M. D...	1830-1831
Eli Ives, M. D.	1823-1827	Chas. Woodward, M. D.	1831-1834
Thomas Miner, M. D.....	1823-1827 1831-1834 1840-1841	Amariah Brigham, M. D.	1834-1840
William Tully, M. D. ...	1823-1827	Archibald Welch, M. D.	1834-1843 1844-1849 1850-1859
S. B. Woodward, M. D..	1827-1834	Milo L. North, M. D. ...	1834-1840
George Sumner, M. D. ..	1827-1855	Eli Ives, M. D.	1840-1841
John L. Comstock, M. D.	1827-1840 1841-1843	William S. Pierson, M. D.	1840-1847
		Nathan B. Ives, M. D...	1841-1870

[1] In April, 1915, the directors of the Hartford Retreat purchased a tract of about 200 acres of land in Rocky Hill, with the purpose of establishing thereon a farm colony. The tract is situated on a plateau, overlooking the Connecticut Valley, with the Bolton Hills as a back ground; to the north the view opens as far as Mount Holyoke. It is planned to develop at Rocky Hill farming and other occupations, especially for men, and to build attractive cottages for wealthy patients who want rest and quiet and charming surroundings.

The site is accessible by trolley and by steam, and by a fine macadam highway, the latter of which brings it within half an hour's drive by motor from Hartford.

[2] The early records are incomplete and these dates may be only approximately correct.

Sam'l B. Beresford, M. D. 1843-1844
P. W. Ellsworth, M. D... 1843-1844
Benjamin Rogers, M. D. 1844-1853
E. K. Hunt, M. D. ...... {1844-1853, 1855-1890}
H. A. Grant, M. D....... 1847-1855
Richard Warner, M. D... 1849-1850
W. H. Cogswell, M. D... 1853-1860
J. G. Beckwith, M. D..... 1853-1860
Gurdon W. Russell, M. D. 1855-1909
M. W. Wilson, M. D. ... 1855-1856
P. M. Hastings, M. D. .. 1856-1898
Ashbel Woodward, M. D. 1860-1866
Rufus Blakeman, M. D.. 1860-1866
Isaac G. Porter, M. D... 1866-1870
Henry M. Knight, M. D. 1866-1880
Charles L. Ives, M. D.... 1870-1873
Lewis Williams, M. D... 1870-1882
Robert Hubbard, M. D... 1873-1875
Francis Bacon, M. D. .. 1875-1913
George L. Porter, M. D.. 1880-1913
E. C. Kinney, M. D. 1882-1893
W. A. M. Wainwright, M. D. 1890-1895
L. B. Almy, M. D. 1893-1907
Geo. R. Shepherd, M. D. 1898-1907
Harmon G. Howe, M. D. 1898-1913
William Porter, Jr., M. D. 1907-1913
Elias Pratt, M. D. 1907-1913
Edward K. Root, M. D... 1909-1913
Oliver T. Osborn, M. D.. 1913-

SUPERINTENDENTS.

Eli Todd, M. D. 1823-1833
Silas Fuller, M. D. 1834-1839
Amariah Brigham, M. D. 1840-1843
John S. Butler, M. D..... 1843-1872
James H. Denny, M. D.. 1872-1873
Henry P. Stearns, M. D. 1874-1905
W. N. Thompson, M. D. 1905-

ASSISTANT PHYSICIANS.[1]

William H. Rockwell, M. D.
T. G. Lee, M. D.
William H. Rockwell, M. D.
Daniel Brooks, M. D.
S. W. Hart, M. D.
William Porter, M. D.
James H. Denny, M. D.
Orville F. Rogers, M. D.
J. H. Whittemore, M. D.
Walter J. Norfold, M. D.
Charles W. Page, M. D.
Harmon G. Howe, M. D.
G. B. Packard, M. D.
George K. Welch, M. D.
Henry S. Noble, M. D.
F. H. Drury, M. D.
F. B. Thompson, M. D.
Joseph E. Root, M. D.
G. S. Wright, M. D.
F. H. Mayberry, M. D.
F. N. Barker, M. D.
R. C. White, M. D.
E. A. Down, M. D.
George S. Bidwell, M. D.
Edward Atkinson, M. D.
James R. Bolton, M. D.
H. O. Johnson, M. D.
H. M. Rauch, M. D.
William H. Walker, M. D.
Roy C. Jackson, M. D.
Harry G. Mellen, M. D.
Chester F. English, M. D.

[1] For several years, or until 1846, the superintendent's assistant was the apothecary, who seems not to have been a graduate in medicine.

RESIDENT OFFICERS FOR THE YEAR 1913.

Whitefield N. Thompson, M. D.....Physician and Superintendent.
William H. Walker, M. D..........First Assistant Physician.
Chester F. English, M. D...........Assistant Physician.
Rev. James W. Bradin.............Chaplain.
Henry J. Thompson...............Steward.
Harriet E. Bacon.................Matron.
Ella L. Carrier...................Assistant Matron.
Jean B. Glen......................Record Clerk and Stenographer.
George E. Moses.................Clerk.
O. S. Overlock...................Supervisor.

APPENDIX A.

Report of Committee, October 3, 1842.

The committee to whom was referred the subject of an asylum for the insane respectfully report that, in obedience to their instructions, they have framed a plan for its institution and government, an outline of which will be submitted to the convention. In detailing the course which has been pursued in relation to this subject, we claim your indulgence and need your cooperation; and, from the interest manifested in its behalf, we doubt not but we shall receive them both.

Our first object was to ascertain the *number and condition* of insane persons in this state. For this purpose circulars were distributed, soliciting information respecting their age, their employment, the duration of their malady and its supposed cause. The answers to these inquiries have been in many cases imperfect. Nor will they, except in those towns where the subject has been investigated with unusual care, furnish an adequate idea of the prevalence of mental derangement. In some instances it appears that *mania* has been the only object of inquiry; in others neither occasional nor partial insanity has been reported, while many have omitted to record cases which fell under their observation, from an apprehension that they would not immediately derive any benefit from the contemplated institution. We are therefore unable to determine with that precision which would have been desirable respecting the actual number of the insane; and we submit an abstract of the returns which have been received, confident that no member of the convention will hesitate to take into consideration the great proportion of cases which have not been noticed. And, however we may vary in our ideas relative to the extent of insanity, there is but one voice respecting a retreat for its cure. From our brethren we have assurances that in every part of the state the object of this meeting has been approved. From those with whom we have individually conversed we have received that encouragement which the humane are accustomed to give, and which an institution, so benevolent and so necessary, has a right to demand. An abstract of the returns which we have received will be presented to your view, from which it appears that in 70 towns there are somewhat more than 500 cases of insanity. Fifty-four towns remain to be heard from, and if the disorder should be found equally prevalent in them, the entire number will scarcely fall short of a thousand. How many escaped attention we presume not to say, but we have the strongest reason to believe that at least one-half have been overlooked. Their situation is wretched in the extreme. The victims of "moody melancholy" constitute a class of beings enslaved by the phantoms of their own imagination—phantoms which hover around their dwellings and pursue them in their customary rambles; as they enter a home endeared to them by many a fond recollection the anxious countenances of a family once lighted by the rays of cheerfulness and hope serve but to depress hearts already overloaded with sorrow. In their intercourse with society their spirits are wounded by a sneer or a jest, which would have fallen upon others equally innocent and harmless. The force of their disease is augmented from day to day, and at last suicide or confirmed insanity is the result of accumulated though imaginary sufferings. With them a retreat from the world is the only refuge from grief, and the *medicina mentis* with which that retreat should be stored is indispensable in the treatment of their disorder.

But the poor maniac, doomed to confinement in the lonely dungeon, and often to wear the chains which should be reserved for guilt alone, claims our intercession and our sympathy. In most cases he retains mind enough to see that he is an outcast from society or associated with its most infamous members. Thus situated and retaining a consciousness of his own innocence, he feels that he is injured and abused. But even the poor maniac does not, in most cases, require to be thus rigorously confined. Sometimes he wanders from place to place without food and without decent apparel; sometimes he occupies an apartment in the family mansion, at once the monument and the source of wretchedness, the victim, and in many cases the cause of insanity. With the utmost care on the part of his attendants, such a patient frequently suffers for the want of the ordinary comforts of life, and more especially for the want of that moral treatment which is almost incompatible with his situation. And hence it is that in the milder forms of insanity those cases become established which might have been readily cured by timely recourse to diversion and employment.

The wretchedness of those families upon whom devolve the care and maintenance of the insane can be estimated only by those who, from personal observation, have become acquainted with its extent. Their peace is interrupted, their cares are multiplied, their time is engrossed, and their fortunes reduced or entirely dissipated in attempting to retore to reason one unfortunate member. And when all their efforts have proved unavailing, when all their worldly goods are wasted, there is added to the preceding catalogue of afflictions the disappointment of high expectations and the anxiety which admits of no relief. The misery which they suffer is communicated to a large circle of friends and the whole neighborhood is indirectly disturbed by the malady of one. Less deplorable would it be if these sufferings were propagated only through the medium of friendly intercourse. But when the madman loses entirely his self-possession, especially if his unruly passions gain the ascendancy, he seems to delight in the waste of property and of life, and it may be literally said that "destruction and misery are in his paths."

From the returns which will be presented to the convention we infer that insanity is neither a rare nor a trivial disorder. Having no means of ascertaining the degree of its prevalence in former days, we cannot say whether it is a growing evil or not; but, from the little attention which it has hitherto excited among medical men, we are induced to believe that here, as in other countries, as the community has risen on the scale of refinement, it has been more and more exposed to the disease in question. Nor will it be difficult to assign a satisfactory reason for its prevalence in this section of the country. The people of New England inherit the constitution of their ancestors, and partake to a greater or less extent of their hereditary disorders. One of these, and by no means the least inconsiderable, is insanity. But other causes here operate with peculiar force. The easy transition from one rank of society to another and the facility with which wealth is accumulated serve to cherish even in humble life those hopes which in other countries are repressed or entirely subdued. Expectations high raised are the usual precursors of disappointment, and in the paper to which we have referred it will be found that numerous cases of insanity have been thus produced.

The residence of the insane with their respective families is perhaps a more productive source of their malady than the constitution we inherit, or the hopes we have unreasonably cherished. Many diseases become prevalent under circumstances which leave no doubt but sympathy is their exciting cause. The numerous cases of epilepsy which were at once cured by the ingenuity of the great Boerhaave all arose from sympathy with one unfortunate patient. It is so with insanity; and when an individual becomes insane, unless he is removed from his family and his associates, it is probable that some of them will become the subjects of the same disorder. In different sections of the state we find examples of insanity apparently produced in this manner, and hence it becomes endemic in particular villages and at particular seasons. In six towns adjoining each other on the banks of the Connecticut River there are, according to the returns which have been made, 172 cases of insanity. In six other towns, also contiguous to each other, but two cases have been noticed. Other facts in illustration of the same proposition have been communicated to us, but, instead of relating them at this time, we would refer each member of the convention to observations of his own in confirmation of its truth. In England the insane are sequestered from public view, and, being subjected to the most judicious treatment, they usually regain their reason. The incurable remain in asylums erected for their reception, secluded from society, and supported at a moderate expense by their families, or, in cases of necessity, by their respective parishes. Here they rove from house to house, alternately the objects of merriment and of dread; or, if confined in the family mansion, they awaken those sympathies which frequently lead to confirmed derangement.

From the preceding observations we infer that, while the causes which have been enumerated continue to operate, mental alienation will continue to prevail. And in private practice no disorder is more unmanageable. The patient suffers for the want of that steady course of discipline which is equally remote from cruelty and indulgence; for the want of attendants qualified for their task and faithful in its performance, and for the want of that medical skill which is rarely possessed by those whose attention is chiefly directed to other diseases. And, unfortunately, it often happens that the character and rank of the patient prohibit the use of those salutary measures which in a public institution might be pursued. Is he the master of a family? The recollection of his former ascendancy and the idea of his parental rights will cling to him until he is removed from the dwelling over which he claims control. Is he a child? Accustomed to indulgence, he brooks not restraint, but reproaches for their cruelty all who oppose his ungoverned passions. A madman in his own house has, of all situations, the worst. The same causes which produced his disorder in most cases continue to operate with their original force and oppose every exertion which is made to mitigate its symptoms or arrest its progress.

In the United States three public asylums, designed exclusively for the insane, have been established, and the munificence with which they are endowed is creditable to their respective benefactors. There can be no question but that these institutions are under good regulations and that they will attain the high rank they deserve among the public charities of the country. Situated, however, in the immediate vicinity of large towns, their expenditures and, of course, their charges, are very considerable; and, if we mistake not, none but the poor of the states in which they are located or of the societies by whom they were established are admitted on the most favorable terms. Hence it happens that the expense of supporting patients in either of these establishments prevents the people of this state from deriving much benefit from them. They are also too remote from us to admit of that easy communication with the residence of the insane which the friends are usually anxious to maintain. By these circumstances they are induced to delay for a time their application for relief; and often the only period which might have been employed in restoring to sanity the wandering and the shattered intellects is lost between hesitation and hope and fear. The disease becomes confirmed and the poor maniac is given up as finally and irrecoverably lost. We appeal to the physicians of the state and ask if this has not been the fate of their patients—to the connections, and inquire if this has not been the unhappy lot of their friends?

Painful indeed would have been the duty assigned us if, after investigating the extent of this evil, we had seen no prospect of its diminution. But when we turn our attention towards an asylum established on humane principles, and presenting to the unfortunate sufferers who enter its portals all that ingenuity can suggest or benevolence bestow for the cure of their disorder, that cheering prospect is ours. Such an asylum should be the reverse of everything which usually enters into our conceptions of a mad house. It should not be a jail, in which for individual and public security the unfortunate maniacs are confined. Nor should it be merely a hospital, where they may have the benefit of medical treatment; for without moral management the most judicious course of medication is rarely successful. Nor should it be merely a school, where the mind is subjected to discipline while the body continues to suffer in consequence of original or symptomatic disease.

At the present time it will not be expected that we do more than barely sketch the outline of a plan which may hereafter be modified by circumstances and matured by reflection. If the unanimous opinion of the committee receives the sanction of the convention, the first step will be to make the public acquainted with the value and the need of the contemplated asylum. And when that is once effected we doubt not but it will find an advocate and a patron in every friend of the public welfare. In this one object we shall all be united, and it would be strange indeed if, in its behalf, its future guardians should plead in vain. It seems desirable therefore that the generous and the wealthy in every part of the state should have an opportunity of expressing in terms never to be mistaken the interest they feel in its prosperity. Whenever its prospects will justify the measure, lands may be purchased and a building erected for the accommodation of the insane. The former should be divided, so as to furnish detached portions for walks, for a garden and for agricultural pursuits. The latter should be constructed of durable materials and so situated as to combine the advantages of health with a pleasant and variegated prospect. Its exterior should not exhibit the aspect nor even the faint resemblance of a prison; and at the same time, in its formation, the safety of its inmates should not be overlooked. The lunatic asylum at Wakefield, in England, is said to furnish an excellent model, worthy the attention of all engaged in the construction of similar buildings.

Much will depend upon the judicious choice of medical and domestic attendants, and much upon the economical expenditure of the funds. It has been our aim to guard against abuses in these several departments, and we call upon those to whom they are to be entrusted to act with deliberation and prudence. The friends of the unhappy patients must be assured that no effort will be wanting to correct the delusions and arouse the dormant energies of the mind diseased. They must be assured also that the inmates of this asylum will in all cases be treated with humanity, subjected to no unnecessary rigor of discipline and controlled by no force unless their personal safety requires it. The chains and the scourge which have too often been the implements of correction must be abolished, and every attendant dismissed from the institution who resorts to violence in the performance of his ordinary duties.

In ancient Egypt the insane were conducted to those temples in which were collected whatever seemed calculated to please the eye and rivet the attention. There, as they wandered from one magnificent object to another, the world and its vexations were forgotten, and amid the deep interest of the scene the gloomy images which haunted them were driven from their minds. In Greece, on the other hand, the followers of Hippocrates relied exclusively on the specific powers of hellebore and its adjuvants, medicines which at this day are rarely employed. Among the improvements of modern science, and we wish to impress it deeply on the minds of those who have the direction of the proposed asylum, must be ranked the co-operation of these two modes of practice.

The history and ceremony of the Retreat established by the Society of Friends in the neighborhood of York may be consulted with equal pleasure and advantage. It furnishes a lucid view of the effects of moral management and teaches how much may be effected by the perseverance and charity of a few. For many years that asylum excited little attention and received as little patronage, but it has now assumed that pre-eminent rank to which from its superior regulations it is justly entitled. Its managers appear, however, to have placed too little reliance upon the efficacy of medicine in the treatment of insanity, and hence their success is not equal to that of other asylums in which medicines are more freely employed.

It remains for us to notice some advantage which the community may expect to derive from the institution which we have recommended. *It will diminish the number of the insane.* At present no diseases are more dangerous and none more obstinate than those whose "seat and throne" are in the mind. The utmost skill is baffled in attempting to control them, and with faint hopes of success do the most intelligent of our professional brethren encounter an enemy by which they have so often been discomfited. In some instances, it is true that their efforts are successful, but the long catalogue of those who remain uncured and are deemed incurable will carry conviction wherever it is seen that such instances are comparatively unfrequent. In the contemplated asylum many whose cases are now deemed hopeless would regain their reason. We say this with confidence, for the experience of other institutions and the opinions of those physicians whom we have consulted all point to the same flattering conclusion. There are also many cases whose restoration to health is yet uncertain. To them a well governed asylum presents every prospect of immediate and permanent relief. Many a wandering maniac might have been restored to health if at the commencement of his disorder he had been placed in such an institution. He is now a burden to his family or to the state, increasing to a considerable extent their annual expenditures; he might have been a useful member of society. The injury which he has sustained cannot be repaired; but others, and we are all exposed to the same misfortune, may live to reap the benefit of our present exertions. On this subject, however, we wish no one to rely on the bare assertions of the committee, and appeal to statements, the truth of which cannot be doubted, to prove the justness of these observations. It was long since stated by Dr. Willis, in his evidence before the Parliament of England, that nine out of ten cases recovered if placed under his care within three months of the attack. The records of the great French hospital over which Pinel so ably presides present the same flattering result; and in the extensive practice of Dr. Burrows the proportion of cures has been still greater. By the latter it is announced that of 100 recent cases, 91 have been cured; that 35 of 100 old cases, such as are generally deemed hopeless, have recovered, and that the aggregate proportion of cases has been 81 in 100.

What has been the experience of physicians in this state we leave for others to decide; but excepting cases of *delirium* which occur in febrile and other disorders, it is feared that a large proportion of the insane never regain their reason. The above statement, while it refutes the popular opinion that insanity is incurable, exhibits in its true light the importance of directing the energy of a few minds to those diseases which baffle the ordinary resources of our art.

Having already referred to sympathy and grief resulting from the promiscuous residence of the insane with their respective families as frequent causes of the malady in question, it is perhaps unnecessary to state that by their seclusion from society these causes will be removed, and the disease whose frequency has become alarming will be less frequent and more easily subdued. We conclude, therefore, that by removing some of the exciting causes of insanity and subjecting it more completely under the control of medicine, the proposed asylum will materially diminish the number of its unhappy subjects. *It will also diminish the expense of their maintenance.* Knowing how much the peace of a neighborhood is often disturbed by a single maniac, that two or three constant attendants are necessary to secure him, and that medical advice can be obtained only at distant intervals or at considerable expense, we believe that in cases of *mania* no one will refuse assent to the above proposition. And in milder forms of insanity, where restraint is unnecessary, we have usually observed a gradual waste of property, making poor those families who once possessed a respectable fortune, and reducing to penury those whose possessions were originally small. We doubt not but others have made the same observation and will conclude with us that the present mode of treating the insane is as ruinous as it is ineffectual. In an asylum they might be supported at a moderate expense and their friends enabled to pursue their customary avocations without molestation and without fear. They and the public would be secure from the depredations of these unhappy beings, many of whom annually destroy more property than would be necessary to maintain them. And the admittance of the insane into an asylum would add very materially to their own comfort. There they would be treated with humanity and allowed every indulgence compatible with their recovery; and there they would experience the benefit of judicious medical treatment, associated with the experience of benevolent and faithful attendants. There, too, they would find neither solitude to depress nor unwelcome society to estrange the diseased mind; and, with these advantages, it is reasonable to expect that the subject of melancholy will become cheerful and the wild maniac regain his composure.

As Christians, and as men, it is our duty to alleviate the sufferings of others; as physicians, it is also our imperative duty to use every exertion for the improvement of medicine. No one conversant with the records of our profession can hesitate for a moment to believe that its interests would be greatly promoted by adopting the plan which we have suggested. When, we ask, did Crowther, Haslam and Coxe become familiar with the diseases of the mind? Bethlem Hospital was the great school in which they were instructed. To what source do we owe the masterly sketches of Pinel and Rush? The public charities of Paris and Philadelphia, which furnished the subjects of their observations, have been, perhaps, of more utility to the world at large than to their respective patients. They served to accumulate observations, and that information which is lost by diffusion becomes of immense value when concentrated in the mind of one. Such a mind is not merely illumined, it is *luminous,* and there is not a member of our profession so remote but he may occasionally be guided by its rays.

With this view of the subject we conclude, believing that the convention will take immediate measures for the formation of a society for the relief of the insane. The principles upon which such a society should be formed are embraced in the annexed constitution.[1]

T. Miner,
Eli Todd,
S. B. Woodward,
W. Tully,
G. Sumner.

[1] The constitution of the Society for the Relief of the Insane is embodied in the original charter.

CONNECTICUT HOSPITAL FOR THE INSANE.[1]

MIDDLETOWN, CONN.

In 1866 an act to create a hospital for the insane in the State of Connecticut was passed, but the birthday of the Connecticut Hospital for the Insane cannot truly be said to have occurred until it was delivered to the public April 30, 1868.

The report of the commission appointed by the Assembly in the year 1865 showed that there were 706 insane persons in the State of Connecticut, of whom 202 were in the Retreat at Hartford; 204 in the almshouses; and 300 outside of both; that it was impossible to secure suitable care and medical attention for this large and deeply afflicted class, either in the Retreat or in the almshouses, or in private houses; and that considerations of humanity and of true economy, as well as public welfare, demanded that these persons should liberally be provided for by the state.

The act, modified and supplemented by other acts, appears in the revision of the General Statutes, 1888. It provided that "The land of the state and its appurtenances in Middletown shall be and remain the Connecticut Hospital for the Insane." Further, "That the government shall be vested in a board consisting of the Governor and 12 trustees to be appointed by the Senate, one from each county and four from the vicinity of the institution. During the regular session of the General Assembly of 1889 the Senate shall appoint six of said trustees, of whom three shall hold office for four years from the first day of July, 1889, and three for three years from the first day of July, 1890. During the regular session of the General Assembly of 1891, and biennially thereafter, the Senate shall appoint six trustees, who shall hold office for four years from the first day of July following their appointment. The Governor may fill any vacancy which occurs during the recess of the General Assembly until its regular session. No trustee shall receive compensation for his services.

[1] This history was prepared by the late Dr. Henry S. Noble.

"The trustees shall have charge of the general interests of the institution, make and execute its by-laws, appoint and remove its officers and attendants, fix their compensation, exercise a strict supervision over all its expenditures, and may receive by bequest, devise or gift property for the use of the hospital.

"They shall appoint a superintendent, not of their own number, who shall be a competent physician and reside in or near the hospital.

"They shall appoint a treasurer, with a salary not exceeding $400 a year, who shall give a bond to the state of $10,000 and whose accounts, with the vouchers, shall be submitted quarterly, and oftener if required, to the trustees, with a written statement of his disbursements and funds in hand; and his books shall be at all times open to the trustees."

From 1866 the successive Governors of Connecticut have been ex-officio members of the Board of Trustees.

Middletown, which is situated on a bend of the Connecticut River, nearly at the center of the state and easily reached from all points, was chosen as the location for the Hospital, not only because it was central, but also because here it was possible to obtain abundance of water from a reservoir by gravity, and to dispose of sewage by the simple method of surface irrigation on the farm; moreover the river was conveniently near for the delivery of coal and other freight. The people of Middletown granted a suitable farm and valuable water privileges.

Besides the land given by the town of Middletown, 80 acres adjoining it were purchased. From time to time other purchases of land have been required by the growth of the Hospital until in 1912 the total amounted to 650 acres.

In 1867 connection was made with the first reservoir by a cast-iron pipe six inches in diameter. In 1887 a companion water main eight inches in diameter was laid.

After the site was chosen building operations progressed sufficiently to permit the corner-stone of the Hospital to be laid June 20, 1867. On May-day, 1868, the center and one wing of the main building were ready for the accommodation of patients. During the succeeding six years the other three wings were added, and in 1874 the Hospital was considered to be complete, having beds for 450 patients.

This stone structure, four stories high, was built on the so-called "linear" plan, with eight wards for patients on either side of the central portion, in which were the kitchens and offices. Back of the center and connected by an underground tramway were the laundry, bakery, sewing room, engine room and the boilers. Still further back was the "annex," at first used as a joiners' and painters' shop, although erected "with the ulterior view" of being devoted to the isolation of insane convicts.

Already the utility of the "cottage system" had been demonstrated by lodging certain demented patients in two old dwelling houses left standing on the hospital grounds. By the river, a third of a mile away, was the hospital dock, and near it the coal house. A large barn and a piggery completed the list of structures at that time. The total appropriations for land and construction, 1866-1876, amounted to $640,043.

These provisions did not long suffice, for the trustees state in their report to the Legislature of 1877, that as they "do not deem it desirable to enlarge this hospital, they earnestly urge the importance of immediate provision for the erection of a new hospital"; and to the Legislature of 1878 they mention the urgent need of "another hospital of similar grade." The next year the board repeated this advice, as the Hospital was overcrowded and insane persons were obliged to wait for weeks to be admitted, or else be cared for in other institutions.

It was also in 1879 that a commission, consisting of Gurdon W. Russell, M. D., Henry W. Buel, M. D., and Ephraim Williams, appointed by the Governor to investigate the need of further accommodations for the insane poor of the state and to report upon a location and plans for such hospital buildings if needed, reported to the General Assembly that further accommodations were necessary, there being about 400 insane poor for whom the state had made no hospital provision, and they recommended erecting in the immediate vicinity of the existing hospital plain buildings of brick, containing 250 beds.

Nevertheless, no legislative action was taken until the following year, when it was resolved by the General Assembly and approved by the Governor, March 24, 1880, "that a committee of three be appointed by the Governor, who shall cause to be built within one year additional buildings for the accommodation of the insane, adjacent to the present hospital at Middletown, according to the plans and estimates of the commission presented to this General Assembly; and that there be appropriated from any moneys now in the treasury of this state a sum not exceeding $130,000 for the erection and furnishing of said buildings. Said committee shall make report to the next session of the General Assembly; provided, that of the sum hereby appropriated not less than $5000 shall be reserved for the construction of suitable buildings or apartments upon the grounds of said Connecticut Hospital for the Insane wherein insane convicts shall be placed and cared for separate from the other inmates of said hospital."

In accordance with this act the Governor appointed as a building committee Melancthon Storrs, M. D., William J. Atwater and Charles G. R. Vinal, who immediately entered upon their duties.

It was found that the inclination of the ground at the south end of the proposed building favored the construction of a small ward in the basement, and the required separate apartments for insane female convicts were there provided, the trustees having already devoted the "annex" to the use of male convicts.

To the Legislature of 1881 the committee was able to report satisfactory progress, and July 20 the building, finished and furnished at an expense of $130,000 with 262 beds for patients, was formally transferred by the committee to the Board of Trustees. This was made the occasion of a memorial gathering of many friends of the hospital.

The pressing need of more room may be inferred from the fact that the new building was soon filled to excess, and that the Legislature in 1884 and 1885 made appropriations for the erection, on land purchased by special appropriations in 1882, of an additional building "for the care of the insane of this state, and particularly to furnish one or more wards for the better classification and accommodation of the epileptic insane."

This building, completed early in 1886 and furnished with 300 beds, stands about 175 feet south of the building erected in 1881; both front westward, and resemble one another in their essential features. Each is of brick, three stories high; has six wards containing 50 beds, more or less, in rooms on either side of a long corridor, broken in the center by a bay which serves as a day room; has two large dining rooms, where the patients congregate for their meals. In this particular these two buildings differ markedly from the old main building, in which every ward has its separate dining room.

The total number of patients was now above 1000, and the revenue began to exceed the cost of maintenance.[1] The resulting surplus of cash enabled the trustees to make several improvements rendered necessary by the growth of the hospital.

An addition to the annex provided a workshop for convicts. A reception room and a medical office were added to the middle hospital. A supplemental water main was laid; a green house and bowling alley were built; a brick cottage, accommodating 70 patients, chiefly those working out of doors; a horse barn, coal house, an ice house and a cottage for employees were also erected.

The Legislature bestowed more than tacit approval upon these expenditures, for in 1889, the Hospital then having 1300 patients,

[1] The trustees of the hospital are the custodians of a certain fund known as the Atwater fund, created by the following clause in the will of the late George Atwater, of the town of Hamden, dated October 2, 1867:

"I direct and require that the said assistant trustees of my estate shall within two years after the death of my said wife Maria, if she shall survive my said daughter Eunice, or within two years after the death of my said daughter Eunice, if she shall survive her mother, convey to the persons who shall at that time constitute the Board of Trustees of 'The General Hospital for the Insane of the State of Connecticut,' located in Middletown, to them and their successors in office, all the remainder of my estate, both real and personal, to have and to hold the same in trust for the uses, intents and purposes hereinafter mentioned and declared concerning the same, viz.:

"The said trustees of the General Hospital for the Insane of the State of Connecticut shall reserve the whole amount received from my estate as a separate fund (to be known as the Atwater fund) for the benefit of the insane poor of the State of Connecticut, and shall have the right to appropriate and expend the annual income of the fund for the support of indigent insane persons, giving preference to indigent insane persons, if any such there may be, belonging to and having legal residence in my native town of Hamden; but the said trustees shall not appropriate or expend the principal of the fund."

This trust fund was accepted by a vote of the trustees of the hospital January 14, 1886.

it was resolved by the General Assembly that the Board of Trustees be authorized and instructed to expend from the funds of the Hospital an amount necessary to erect a building furnishing accommodations for at least 120 persons. By an addition to each wing of the south hospital, and by the completion of the unpretentious, but very comfortable and convenient, cottage, of which one-third was built the year before, 150 patients were accommodated.

Other items of construction followed, of which the most costly was an assembly room, seating over 600 persons, the original chapel and amusement hall being no longer adequate.

As the number of patients again exceeded the capacity of the institution and a disposition to enlarge it still further was manifested by the Legislature, it was voted at a special meeting of the Board of Trustees, April, 1889, that "in the opinion of this board the economic and humane interests of the state require that additional accommodations for its insane be provided in some other locality."

In 1893 the General Assembly resolved "that a building committee of five members, three of whom shall be elected by the Trustees of the Connecticut Hospital for the Insane, and two of whom shall be elected by the Senate, be authorized and directed to cause the erection in the town of Middletown of a suitable building sufficient for the accommodation of 250 insane persons of the class known as incurable insane; and to expend for said purpose a sum of money not to exceed $70,000. A further sum of $30,000, or so much thereof as shall be necessary, is hereby appropriated from the State Treasury to furnish and complete said building."

This act was approved June 30, 1893, and the Trustees elected from their number Henry Woodward, Andrew C. Smith and Samuel Russell to be members of the building committee.

Already the Trustees, finding the water supply insufficient in the time of drought, had availed themselves of the privileges guaranteed to them by the town of Middletown, "the full and complete use and enjoyment of the water of Butler's Creek and Silver Creek," by purchasing the requisite land and constructing a reservoir on Silver Creek. Fortunately, too, just at this time, a farm extending from the northern limit of the hospital grounds to the Connecticut River was for sale, and its purchase provided a most admirable site for the future buildings. As from time to time the water supply has threatened to be inadequate, other reservoirs have been added to the first one built in 1867. The water is all delivered to the hospital by gravity, and efficient fire protection is maintained by the pressure afforded by the 160-175 feet elevation of the principal reservoirs, but this has been supplemented by the installation of a powerful fire pump.

Section 7, Chapter 102, of the Public Acts, 1867, provides that "the trustees are hereby authorized and empowered to make and establish such by-laws as they may deem necessary and expedient."

Accordingly, the Board of Trustees adopted certain by-laws and regulations and revised them in 1887 and again in 1902, designating the duties of the persons employed in the Hospital, viz.:

1. The superintendent is required to exercise "entire official control over all subordinate officers" and over the treatment of all patients; to conduct the correspondence and to see that due care is taken of all hospital property.

2. The assistant physicians, each has under his special care a certain number of patients for individual study and treatment.

3. The business manager and assistant keep all the accounts of the hospital, except those in the hands of the treasurer, and purchase the groceries, provisions and supplies for the institution.

4. The farmer has charge of the agricultural operations, the butchering, preservation and distribution of meats and the delivery of freight.

5. The matron has charge of all work done in the laundry and the sewing rooms.

6. The housekeepers have charge of the ordinary domestic matters in their respective households and attend particularly to the preparation of food for the patients.

7. The supervisors have the immediate direction of the ward attendants and instruct them in their duties, such as the management of patients, the nursing of the sick, the prevention of escapes, the care of patients' clothing and the cleanliness of the wards.

8. The storekeeper, under the instruction of the business manager, takes care of the stock in store and issues supplies on requisition of housekeepers, supervisors and others, keeping due account of the same.

9. The mechanics, comprising the engineer and electrician, have charge of the heating apparatus, plumbing and gas-piping, and all electrical power and machinery.

By 1893 the Hospital buildings had increased from one to five, with capacity ranging from 250 to 675, aside from cottages, and the population of the institution had risen to 1535.

The Legislature of that year having decided to provide additional accommodations for the insane, the work of building what is now known as the north hospital was at once commenced, and about 52 acres of land were purchased from the heirs of Elisha S. Hubbard. This tract included a substantial farm house, which has since afforded accommodations for about 36 male patients. The farm extended from the northern boundary of the hospital grounds across the Valley Railway to the Connecticut River, and afforded a site for the present wharf, coal pocket, spur tracks, coal and merchandise hoisting apparatus, and shuttle railway operated by electricity, by which all coal and heavy merchandise are delivered to the hospital buildings.

The north hospital, with accommodations for 250 patients of the chronic class, was completed within the appropriation of $100,000, $70,000 of which was taken from funds in the hands of the Trustees, and $30,000 was appropriated by the Legislature. This building was scarcely complete when the urgent necessity of additional accommodations was apparent. To meet this demand the Trustees proceeded to erect an additional wing to the north hospital for the accommodation of 50 female patients, at a cost of $20,250, which was taken from Hospital funds.

This wing was no sooner completed than an equally urgent demand arose for further accommodations for male patients. This was met by the erection of a wing at the north end of the north hospital, corresponding to that erected for female patients at the south end, and contained accommodations for 50 male patients. The cost was $17,623. At the close of the fiscal year ending September 30, 1898, the census of the Hospital had risen to 1895.

In 1896 the training school for nurses and attendants was inaugurated and has continued ever since, with the exception of an interval from 1896 to 1901.

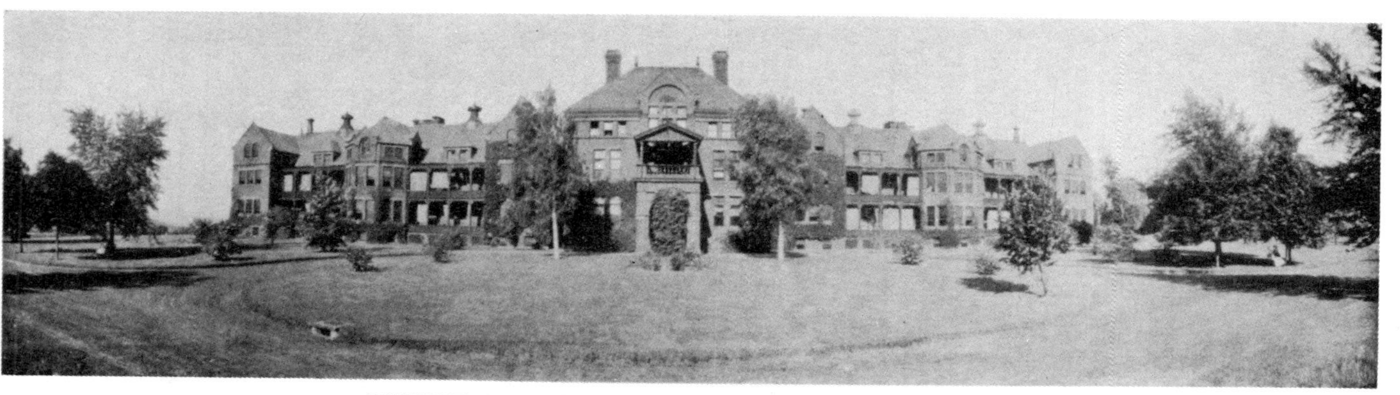

CONNECTICUT HOSPITAL FOR THE INSANE, BUILDING A.

During the biennial period ending September 30, 1898, several buildings of importance were added to the equipment. A mortuary building of stone and brick, with tiled roof, was erected at a cost of $6524.54. A substantial iron fence was built on the north and south sides of Silver Street in front of the main grounds. Iron verandas and fire escapes for three stories were added to the south hospital, which afford airing facilities for such patients as are unable to avail themselves of out-of-door exercise. A brick, iron, cement and glass cow barn was erected, with stabling for 100 cows, at a cost of $16,902.10.

During the following biennial period, ending with September 30, 1900, two infirmary wards, with accommodations for 70 patients each, were added to the north hospital at a cost of $6471.53. The laboratory for clinical and pathological work was established and equipped in the south end of this building, and has since proved a valuable adjunct to the scientific work of the institution. Day balconies and fire escapes, which during the winter months are enclosed in glass, were added to the main hospital at a cost of $3840.

The unprecedented drought of 1899 aroused the Trustees to the necessity of providing an additional water supply, which resulted in the building of No. 4 reservoir. This was completed in the summer of 1900 at a cost of $15,813.19, and has a capacity of 33,000,000 gallons.

During the following period from 1900 to 1902 the heating system was thoroughly reorganized, and the several detached heating plants were consolidated into one central one. The congregate building was built, comprising a congregate dining room with a capacity of 1500 persons, with kitchens, serving room, bakery, store, meat market, cold storage plant, laundry, sewing and ironing rooms, and hydrotherapeutic establishment, with a dining room for employees, at a total cost of $272,530. With the reorganization of the boiler and heating plant steam as a motive power was dispensed with, and electricity substituted. Lighting the entire institution with electricity was commenced and carried forward as rapidly as possible. Electrical power was provided for the carpenter shop, laundry, and ensilage cutters. Electric irons were provided in the ironing room. Electric elevators provided with

9

automatic safety devices were installed in the congregate building. The steam mains for heating the south and middle hospitals and main cottage, as well as the barns and carpenter shop, were carefully insulated in earthen conduits, so as to prevent condensation. The new chimney, 141 feet in height, afforded ample draught, and the economizer and hot water heaters gave the highest percentage of return for the coal consumed. The cold storage plant, with auxiliary ice-making facilities, did excellent service, and the latter during one whole season since has supplied the Hospital with all the ice required.

During the season of 1912 the local telephone system was thoroughly overhauled and enlarged. Fifty-six stations were installed and the service handled by three operators on duty eight hours each.

During the biennial period the capacity of the south hospital was again increased to meet the ever recurring demands for more accommodations, by the erection of a three-story brick and iron addition to the north wing, 60 feet by 40 feet, containing 80 beds. The framework is of iron and the floors granolithic, covered with linoleum. These wards contain bath and toilet accommodations and communicate with the main wards of the building on the same levels through fireproof iron doors. The second and third floors are each provided with an iron veranda having an eastern exposure. These verandas serve the purpose of fire escapes, and in winter are enclosed with glass and make desirable infirmaries. The entire cost was $14,221.

The old laundry building was repaired and altered for the accommodation of female patients at a cost of $6000. Excellent accommodations were thus secured for over 100 female patients, at a cost of $68.97 per bed in addition to the value of the building prior to making the repairs.

On June 21, 1906, the most destructive fire in the history of the institution occurred, during which the amusement hall, chapel, dynamo, engine and tool rooms were destroyed, and for a time the center portion of the main building was in danger. Fortunately, there was no loss of life to either patients or employees.

Plans were at once completed for the erection of a thoroughly fireproof structure for engines, electrical apparatus, cold storage

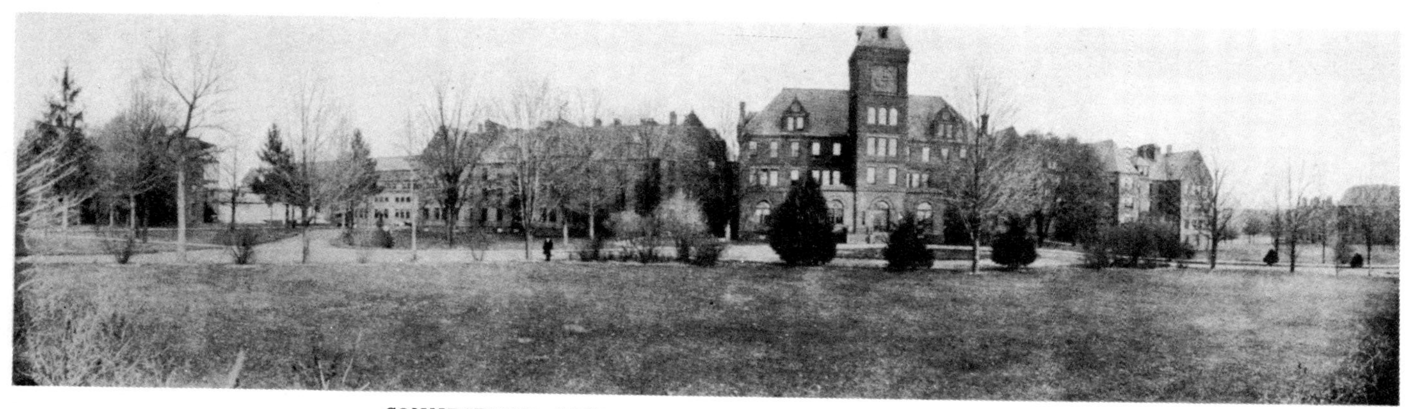

CONNECTICUT HOSPITAL FOR THE INSANE, BUILDING B.

machinery, etc. The insurance, amounting to $30,499.04, was immediately adjusted and paid.

A municipal fire system was inaugurated, covering the entire premises by means of 24 stations, by which a repeating signal is sent to the central station, where an organized fire department is always on duty. The more hazardous localities on the premises are protected by automatic sprinklers.

Electric lighting has been gradually extended, until it now covers the entire institution.

During the biennial period ending with September 30, 1906, a new underground root and vegetable cellar was constructed, at a cost of $5983, for which no legislative appropriation was called for.

In addition the Legislature granted an appropriation of $20,000 for an isolation hospital, and the building was completed within the appropriation. It is located apart from the other hospital buildings, is thoroughly fireproof and built according to modern conceptions. It affords accommodation for 30 patients of each sex and the requisite number of nurses. It is lighted by electricity, heated by steam and provided with gas ranges for the preparation of food. To complete the equipment a large Kinyoun-Francis sterilization chamber was installed, at a cost of $1350.

The Legislature of 1906 granted an appropriation of $75,000 with which to provide a chapel or assembly room. The result was a thoroughly fireproof structure, the auditorium of which has a seating capacity of about 1400. It is connected with the main hospital, congregate dining room, middle hospital and main cottage by overhead bridges. The main floor consists of an auditorium, gallery, lobby and stage, the first two of which are provided with set opera chairs. Toilet and dressing rooms are placed at convenient points. The stage is protected from fire by automatic sprinklers and an asbestos curtain; and is furnished with ample scenery, several drop curtains, and various electrical appliances. In the basement a room has been provided for dancing. Scarcely anything other than brick, steel and concrete enters into the construction of the building. It is heated by steam and lighted by electricity, with an additional gas equipment in case of emergency.

A drop curtain, pulpit and chairs effect a transformation of the stage and make it appropriate for chapel services.

The same Legislature which rendered the assembly room possible granted an appropriation of $45,000 for the purpose of building a new wharf, coal hoisting works and pocket, with an electric industrial railway for the transportation of coal and heavy merchandise from the wharf and railroad to the Hospital. A siding has been built on the Valley Division of the N. Y., N. H. & H. R. R., upon which car-load lots of merchandise are delivered and transported to the Hospital.

During the biennial period ending September 30, 1908, a mechanical filter was installed, with a capacity of 100 gallons per minute, to obviate any risk of illness from possible contamination of the water from reservoirs No. 2 and No. 5. All water supplying the institution is analyzed at regular intervals and has invariably been found free from pathogenic bacteria.

The last building to be added to the hospital equipment was the nurses' home, erected in 1909-10, for which the Legislature appropriated the sum of $75,000. This building is also fireproof, and contains comfortable quarters for over 90 employees. Twelve of the rooms in the central portion of the building are designed for married couples. Each wing provides accommodations for 35 nurses and attendants of each sex. The basement under the east, or male, wing, has been fitted up as a recreation and reading room, with billiard and card tables, magazines, periodicals, etc.

During this same biennial period the last and largest water main connecting the system of reservoirs with the Hospital buildings was laid, at a cost of $18,000, which was covered by a legislative appropriation of that amount. This main is sixteen inches in diameter and affords not only an ample supply of water for all ordinary purposes, but likewise provides increased pressure and supply in the event of fire.

The buildings constituting the institution have increased during the progress of years from one or two up to 34. The aggregate of legislative appropriations amounts to the sum of $1,470,573. Various improvements have been made from time to time, which have been paid for from the earnings of the Hospital over and above running expenses; the cost of these improvements amounts to nearly half the above mentioned sum.

Insurance is carried on the Hospital property, including buildings and contents, to the amount of $1,200,000.

The institution is now (1912) caring for 2535 patients, and has for the past two or three years been overcrowded, notwithstanding the existence of the Norwich State Hospital, with a census of about 800. Whether there will be any further expansion of the Connecticut Hospital for the Insane is problematical. It would seem to be much the wiser policy to organize a third institution in the southwest quarter of the state, rather than to continue overcrowding those already in operation.

SUPERINTENDENTS.

Abram Marvin Shew, M. D.[1] 1867-1886
James Olmstead, M. D.[1] 1886-1898
Charles W. Page, M. D. 1898-1901
Henry S. Noble, M. D.[1] 1901-1915
C Floyd Haviland, M. D. 1915-

ASSISTANT SUPERINTENDENTS.

Henry S. Noble, M. D.[1] 1898-1901
William E. Fisher, M. D. 1902-

ASSISTANT PHYSICIANS.

Winthrop B. Hallock, M. D.[1] 1868
Calvin S. May, M. D. .. 1873
James Olmstead, M. D.[1]. 1877-1886
William E. Fisher, M. D. 1877-1902
Charles E. Stanley, M. D. 1878-
Henry S. Noble, M. D.[1].. 1881-1898
James M. Keniston, M. D. 1882-
Edwin A. Down, M. D... 1887
A. B. Coleburn, M. D.... 1890-
A. Josephine Sherman, M. D. 1890
L. Pierce Clark, M. D... 1894
Mary Harley, M. D. ....
Jessie W. Fisher (neé Weston), M. D. 1894-1908
John W. Duke, M. D.... 1895
Ross E. Savage, M. D... 1897
John H. Mountain, M. D. 1899
Albert C. Thomas, M. D. 1901
Walter S. Lay, M. D..... 1902
George Streit, M. D..... 1902
E. A. Ehlers, M. D....... 1903
Leon F. LaPierre, M. D. 1904
C. W. Glover, M. D..... 1905
Edmund S. Sugg, M. D.. 1906
F. Frank Morrison, M. D. 1906
Louis R. Brown, M. D.. 1908-
Hamilton Rinde, M. D... 1908
William M. Kenna, M. D. 1912

PATHOLOGISTS.

Edward C. Seguin, M. D.[1] 1870
A. R. Diefendorf, M. D. 1899
Jessie W. Fisher, M. D. (Assistant 1900) 1908-

[1] Deceased.

THE NORWICH STATE HOSPITAL FOR THE INSANE.[1]

NORWICH, CONN.

The plan to erect a second state hospital in Connecticut had its origin in 1890, when a special committee appointed by the General Assembly to inquire into the necessity of providing further accommodations for the insane at the Connecticut Hospital for the Insane, or elsewhere in the state, reported "that for the good of the patients themselves and as a matter of economy in the end to the state such accommodations should be provided in some other locality."

Although the matter was from time to time discussed by various medical societies and others interested, and although certain towns in the state had made plans to secure the proposed institution should it finally be established, little was actually accomplished until the legislative session of 1897, when the following resolution was passed:

> That Lucius Brown, of Norwich; O. Vincent Coffin, of Middletown; Dr. Amos J. Givens, of Stamford; Dr. Clifford B. Adams, of New Haven; Dr. Clinton E. Stark, of Norwich; Dr. Patrick Cassidy, of Norwich, and Dr. Edward B. Hooker, of Hartford, be, and they are hereby appointed a commission that shall serve without compensation and whose duty it shall be to investigate the necessity of additional accommodations for the insane of this state, to consider the expediency of erecting new buildings for this purpose, to inquire into the desirability of the site which the people of Norwich have offered to give to the state for an asylum for the insane, to inquire into the desirability of any other site which any other town may propose to donate and report the results of their investigations to the next Legislature at the beginning of the session.

Dr. Clifford B. Adams died shortly subsequent to his appointment and was never able to meet with the committee, but the remaining members had frequent conferences and after an unusually careful study of the question in accordance with the creating act submitted its report to the General Assembly of 1899. The committee, while agreeing that additional accommodations should be provided, and that Norwich had offered an ideal site, was not unanimously in favor of establishing a second state hospital. The investigations of the committee had disclosed that

[1] By Henry M. Pollock, M. D., superintendent.

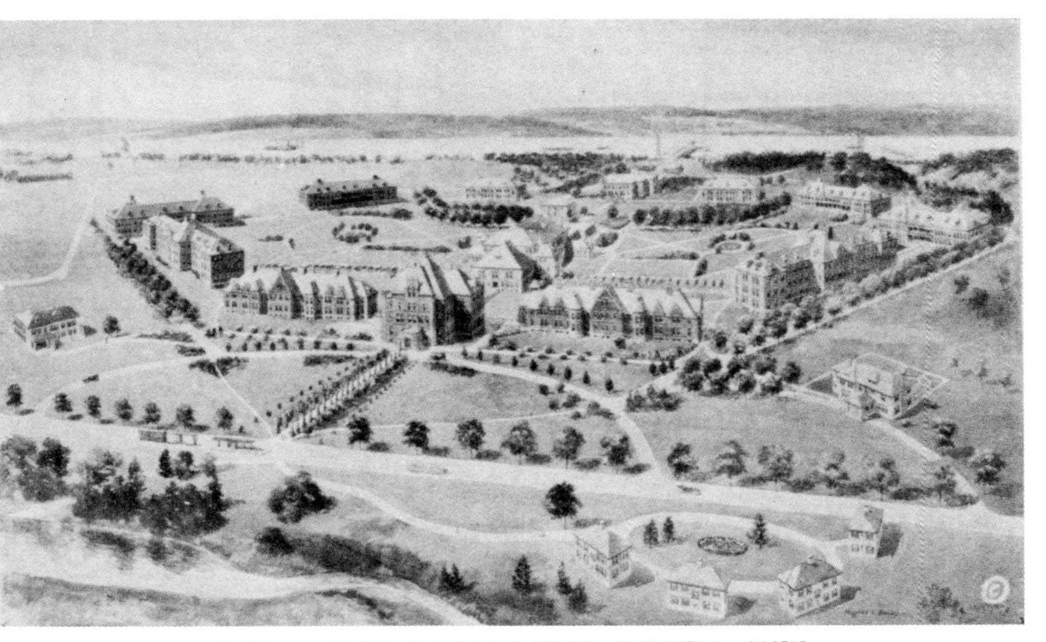

GENERAL VIEW, NORWICH STATE HOSPITAL, CONN.

there were 120 patients at the Connecticut Hospital for the Insane in excess of its normal capacity; that 336 insane were being improperly cared for outside of the state hospital and that the average yearly increase of the insane in the state was 64. The committee also found that the trustees of the Connecticut Hospital for the Insane and the newly elected superintendent, Dr. Page, were planning to add to the capacity of that hospital by the conversion of the ward dining-rooms into dormitories through the construction of a congregate dining-room, where, using the phraseology of the majority report, "1500 or more patients could be massed together for their meals." Mr. O. Vincent Coffin, who presented the minority report, felt that the erection of such a building would greatly enhance the welfare of the patients, would in all probability meet the needs of the state for the ensuing five years and would be a more economical solution of the problem than the establishment of a second state hospital. The remainder of the committee submitted a majority report which closed as follows:

> Your committee therefore concludes that there is an immediate necessity that additional accommodations for the insane of the state be provided by the erection of a suitable building to accommodate at least 1000 patients; that such hospital should be established at a place other than Middletown, and that the Norwich site should be accepted for that purpose and the construction of the building begun at once under such wise plans as will necessitate no extravagance, but shall give the best results with the least possible expense.

In accordance with the majority report of the committee, a bill establishing a second state hospital at Norwich was prepared and presented during the 1899 session of the General Assembly, but the committee to which it was referred reported unfavorably. A similar bill introduced during the legislative session of 1901 also met with a like fate. Dr. Clinton E. Stark, of Norwich, notwithstanding these discouragements, continued to keep the question before the public and it was largely due to his efforts that the act establishing a second state hospital for the insane in or near the town of Norwich was finally passed by both houses of the General Assembly and received the approval of Governor Abiram Chamberlain on June 12, 1903. The location and the granting of the initial appropriation of $100,000 were, however, made contingent upon the town of Norwich donating the necessary site, the town having voted at a regularly called town meeting in 1898 that if a state hospital for the insane was established in Norwich a suitable site would be given. The citizens of Norwich carried out their agreement and deeded to the state a level tract of some 60 acres in the town of Preston, adjacent to the division line of the two towns. This site, two and one-half miles distant from the City of Norwich, some 60 feet above and on the east bank of the Thames River, may be regarded as almost ideal for the erection of a public institution. The situation upon the Thames River, with the tracks of the New York, New Haven and Hartford Railroad upon its banks, provided an economical disposition of the sewerage at tidewater and every facility for the reception of freight, while the Norwich and Westerly Trolley, passing through the hospital grounds on the east and the station of the railroad distant some five minutes walk from the proposed administration building, secured easy accessibility. A brook which wound its way down through the valley on the east of the property with its square mile of watershed ensured, with the construction of the necessary storage reservoirs, an abundant water supply, and the character of the soil—a sandy loam with a subsoil of sand and gravel, a depth of three or four feet—furnished not only excellent drainage and a firm foundation, but much of the material for the construction of the future buildings.

The first Board of Trustees as appointed by the State Senate was composed of Governor Chamberlain, ex-officio chairman, Costello Lippitt, Clinton E. Stark, M. D., Calvin L. Harwood, Frank T. Maples and Henry H. Gallup, of Norwich; George C. Waldo, of Fairfield County; Franklin H. Mayberry, M. D., of Hartford County; Eugene H. Burr, of Middlesex County; Edwin S. Greeley, of New Haven County; J. Deming Perkins, of Litchfield County; Edwin C. Pinney, of Tolland County, and Frederick E. Wilcox, M. D., of Windham County.

The trustees organized by selecting Costello Lippitt as president and Frank T. Maples as secretary, and made plans for the active prosecution of the work. Dr. N. Emmons Paine, of Boston, who had appeared before the several committees and advocated the passage of the act, was retained to advise with the architects in the designing of the first buildings. Cudworth & Woodworth, of Norwich, were selected as architects, the R. D. Kimball Company, of Boston, as heating engineers, and Chandler & Palmer, of Norwich, as civil engineers. These firms continued in their several capacities throughout the construction of the hospital. Plans were rapidly prepared for the construction of two ward buildings, each with accommodations for 50 patients; the various contracts were let and the work of construction was begun on October 28, 1903. The limited appropriation granted made temporary arrangements necessary for the power station, kitchen and laundry. The location of two farm houses, acquired with the property and since razed, adjacent to the ward buildings and to one another made it practicable to remodel one into a kitchen and the other into a laundry and to provide a temporary power house at a minimum expense by erecting a roof between them. A sewer of sufficient size to care for the future growth of the hospital was laid and a temporary water supply was installed. A third farm house, situated a short distance from the ward buildings, small in size and of unusually cheap construction, served not only as a residence for the superintendent and his family, but also as a temporary administration building. It was the constant aim of the trustees to install all temporary work at a minimum of cost and as far as possible to make the apparatus purchased available for the future needs of the institution; in reviewing the constructive work of the hospital it is surprising to observe the meagerness of the expenditures for this purpose. The entire work was pursued with the utmost diligence and on October 10, 1904, less than one year subsequent to starting construction, the buildings were completed and furnished and ready for the reception of patients.

The act establishing the hospital failed to provide for the direct commitment of pauper and indigent insane, and until the convening of the General Assembly in 1905 and the approval of an act on May 19 of that year, providing that all of the provisions of the general statutes relating to the commitment of insane persons to the Connecticut Hospital for the Insane at Middletown should apply to and authorize commitment to the Norwich Hospital for the Insane, or to any other state hospital for the insane that might thereafter be established, it was possible for commitments to be made to the Norwich Hospital only after the committing court had found that the Connecticut Hospital for the Insane was unable, because of an excess of patients, to accommodate the person to be committed.

The hospital also found itself in an embarrassing position through the fact that no maintenance appropriation had been made and in consequence the only fund applicable for support was the allowable weekly charge per patient of $3.50 due and payable quarterly. However, the hospital, through the use of a small sum remaining from the original appropriation and the exercise of the strictest economy, managed to meet its obligations until the convening of the Legislature in 1905, when an appropriation for current expenses was granted.

The opposition to the establishment of the hospital was again manifested during the General Assembly of 1905, when two bills were introduced, evidently with the object of hampering its development. The one provided that the Board of Trustees of the two hospitals should be consolidated and that the new board should be composed of eight of the trustees from the Connecticut Hospital for the Insane and four from the Norwich board; the other provided that commitments to the Norwich hospital should only be made from New London County, one of the smallest and least populated of the eight counties of the state, and that the insane from all the remaining counties should be sent to the Connecticut Hospital for the Insane. The former of these bills was defeated and the latter so modified as to give the Norwich institution three counties and to permit the friends or relatives of indigent patients (those paying a portion of the cost of their support), no matter where they resided, to elect to which of the two institutions commitment should be made. Certain of the influential members of the General Assembly of 1907 advanced the opinion that chronic custodial patients could be as well and more economically cared for in an institution that might be designated as a state almshouse and that further provision for the care of the insane should be made at such an institution rather than at the state hospitals. The Board of Trustees of the Norwich State Hospital answered this argument by pointing out that it would be more economical to establish colonies in connection with the existing hospitals than to establish a separate and distinct institution, and this led to an appropriation of $50,000 to the Norwich State Hospital for a colony and colony development.

With this appropriation the Board of Trustees erected a fireproof building a mile distant from the parent hospital with accommodations for 100 male patients. Although the erection of the colony building may be regarded as illogical at the time of its construction, owing to the small size of the hospital and the consequent limited number of patients capable of colonization, its building in all probability served to prevent a certain class of the insane being cared for in a state almshouse. The colony with the growth of the hospital has since proved its utility and the wisdom of the course adopted.

Since 1907, and indeed since 1905, legislative opposition to the hospital has disappeared and its development has been comparatively rapid. Additions have been made to the original site until it now comprises more than 500 acres and there have been expended for buildings, land and permanent improvements more than $1,500,000.

The several completed buildings are arranged as follows: In the center, in the order mentioned, from front to rear are located the administration building, amusement hall and dining-room building, kitchen and store rooms, central fire station and garage, laundry, shop building, laboratory and club house for employees. Below the general level of the plateau and adjacent to the Thames River, the tracks of the New York, New Haven and Hartford Railroad and a freight track of the Norwich and Westerly Trolley, is situated the power house and central heating plant. The power house is connected with the main group of buildings by a head house and covered bridge of concrete. Extending from this concrete bridge is a subway, also of reinforced concrete, eight feet in height and width, which, in conjunction with the basements of the several buildings, and connecting subways and basement corridors, makes a continuous passageway 977 feet long, terminating at the administration building in front. This central passage serves for the conveyance of the steam, water and electric mains, gives ready communication between the several buildings in inclement weather without exposure to the elements, and provides with the freight elevator at the power house an easy and economical means for the distribution of supplies received in carload quantities.

Lateral subways and basement corridors equally well lighted and ventilated connect the several ward buildings with one another and the central group.

The ward buildings separated in each instance from the nearest building by a distance of not less than 100 feet are arranged on either side of the central group in the form of a hollow square. On each side there is a convalescent building (the original ward building) for convalescents, a building for quiet chronic patients, a building for the semi-disturbed and epileptic and a building for acute and chronic disturbed patients. These ward buildings and the colony provide normal accommodations for 1230 patients.

Comfortable houses have been built for the superintendent and medical staff in front and on either side of the administration building and across the highway and approximately an equal distance from the administration building are cottages for nurses. All of the buildings comprising the main group, including the staff house, superintendent's house and nurses' cottages are heated from the central power house and, with the exception of the outlying buildings and the ward buildings, constructed out of the first appropriation, are practically fireproof.

The farm buildings are situated approximately one-half mile distant from the main group of buildings, midway between them and the colony, and are constructed largely of reinforced concrete. They comprise a horse barn, large dairy barn and piggeries. The poultry plant is located at the colony.

The daily average number of patients and the weekly per capita cost during the several years since the opening of the hospital have been as follows:

Year ending Sept. 30	Average No. of patients	Weekly per capita cost
1905	77	$6.58
1906	150	4.76
1907	208	5.38
1908	373	4.01
1909	524	3.63
1910	660	3.51
1911	728	3.50
1912	813	3.61
1913	918	3.53
1914	998	3.64
1915	1109	3.51

Early in the history of the institution the practice was adopted, which has since been continuously followed, of purchasing practically all supplies upon monthly competitive bids, the estimates being sent to any firm either within or without the state that had signified a desire to compete. A system of internal accounting, giving the net cost of the various departments, was installed in the hospital in 1905 and each month a statement is sent to the department head giving the net cost of his department for the previous month. Credit is given to the various mechanical departments for construction or repair work performed for other departments.

An industrial teacher, who has devoted her entire time to the instruction of the patients, has been continuously in the employ of the hospital since March 1, 1909. Sales of the various articles manufactured are daily made and after the cost of the materials is deducted half is retained by the hospital to carry on the work and half is placed to the credit of the individual patient. Certain of the patients, however, who devote their entire time to industrial work are not credited with their full earnings, a deduction being made and placed to the credit of patients employed in the kitchen, laundry or other departments, whose opportunities to perform remunerative work are limited.

A training school for nurses offering a two-years' course was established in 1907. All instruction is given with special reference to the intelligent nursing of mental and nervous diseases and to prepare for post-graduate work those desiring to become proficient in general nursing. Since 1908 the course in the hospital has been supplemented by supplying from the senior class a district visiting nurse to the indigent poor of Norwich and vicinity. Each pupil-nurse is required to serve four weeks in the diet kitchen and six weeks in the surgical dressing room.

Since September 12, 1912, a general head nurse has been employed, who has devoted her entire time to the supervision of the nursing on all the male and female wards and the instruction of the nurses in the care of patients, both at the bedside and in the training school.

On September 3, 1913, with the purpose of giving positive rather than negative instruction to the new ward employees and more rapidly acquainting them with their duties and the customs of the hospital, a three-months' attendants' course, repeated four times during the year, was inaugurated. It was intended that the course should supplement rather than supplant the regular two-years' course of the training school. The instruction consists of 12 talks by the various members of the medical staff and ward demonstrations by the general head nurse and supervisors.

On October 1, 1912, with a view of obtaining helpful suggestions and criticisms from the relatives and friends of patients, and also with the purpose of giving visitors a better knowledge of the hospital, the following was printed on the reserve side of the visiting cards, of which a supply is always on hand in the reception rooms:

The Norwich State Hospital for the Insane is not an endowed institution, but has as its only source of income the $3.50 per week received for the care and treatment of each patient. Of this amount $1.50 per week is paid by the state and the balance by the relatives and towns. No distinction is made in the treatment of patients, and, though it is impossible to provide certain luxuries, it is the constant endeavor of the superintendent and staff to supply everything that will contribute either to increased happiness or recovery.

Often a desire might have been gratified had it been known, or the relatives or friends may have a valuable criticism or suggestion. The desired success of the hospital can only be attained through the co-operation of the friends and relatives of each patient. If you have a suggestion or criticism, if you are dissatisfied with the treatment, or if a patient expresses to you a reasonable desire, communicate it at once to a member of the staff or write a note to the superintendent. Writing materials for this purpose may be obtained of the usher.

This plan proved to be so helpful in the administration of the hospital that on October 1, 1912, the following was printed and posted on each of the hospital wards:

Each patient at the Norwich State Hospital for the Insane should know:

1. That any patient committed by a probate court is not sent to the hospital for a definite period. Commitment is made until such a time as, in the opinion of the superintendent and the medical staff, the patient has sufficiently recovered. He or she is then entitled to be released from the hospital under such arrangements as the superintendent shall deem advisable.

2. That any patient committed by a probate or other court may write to any proper person without the hospital (the Governor of the state, the State Board of Charities, a member of the Board of Trustees of the hospital, his attorney-at-law, a conservator or guardian, a relative or intimate friend) and that writing materials and stamps will be furnished by the hospital. Letters may be sealed or unsealed, must be free from obscenity or vulgarity and handed for mailing to a physician or supervisor.

3. That any patient may be visited by his or her family physician, an attorney-at-law, a relative or intimate friend on any week-day between 10 to 11 a. m. and 2 to 4 p. m. and by relatives on Sunday during the same hours.

4. That any patient may inquire of a visitor, if he be a member of the Board of Charities or a trustee of the hospital, and if so may engage him

in conversation; that otherwise patients should not talk to visitors who come to see the hospital or other patients.

5. That any patient is entitled to make reasonable requests of all nurses and attendants.

6. That any patient is entitled to the best treatment the hospital affords and that abuse and ill treatment of any kind is prohibited and should be at once reported to the superintendent, a physician or a supervisor.

7. That any patient is urged to call the attention of the superintendent or a member of the medical staff to anything which he or she believes will add to his or her comfort or happiness or to the comfort or happiness of others.

The General Assembly of 1911 made an appropriation of $10,000 for the building and equipment of a club house for employees. The building, especially designed for the purpose, was formally opened with appropriate ceremonies on the evening of November 26, 1913. As far as can be ascertained this is the first building of its kind erected at a state hospital for the insane with a specific appropriation granted by a state legislature.

The club, which is entirely under the management of the club directors chosen by the nurses and other employees from among their number, has had a decided influence toward promoting a feeling of loyalty and good fellowship and has been a material aid in obtaining and retaining the services of desirable employees.

The 1915 session of the General Assembly granted an appropriation for providing additional accommodations for patients.

The trustees have decided to employ a portion of the money appropriated in building a psychopathic or reception hospital, somewhat apart from the main group. The psychopathic department will be composed of a central or administration portion, with the requisite offices and quarters for nurses and two wings giving accommodation to 50 patients of each sex.

The General Assembly during the 1915 session established a state farm for inebriates as a department of the Norwich State Hospital. For several years a persistent effort had been made by the various heads of the several state institutions, various civic organizations and certain individuals to have a state farm for inebriates established as a separate institution. In 1913 a bill establishing a state farm passed both houses, but received the veto of the executive. When it became apparent that no appropriation for this purpose would be granted by the 1915 session of the

General Assembly it was proposed that a state farm for inebriates be established as a department of the Norwich State Hospital and that a farm house and out-buildings situated some two and one-half miles distant from the main hospital, on land already owned by the state, be taken for this purpose. The suggestion was adopted, an act passed placing the management of this department under the hospital's Board of Trustees and providing for the commitment of inebriates and dipsomaniacs by the various criminal and probate courts of the state to the state farm for a period of not less than six months nor more than three years.

The trustees expect to provide for 50 inmates and to demonstrate in this small way that an institution of this character may be made practically self-supporting and that much greater good will accrue to the individuals than under the present methods of jail commitments.

TRUSTEES.

Costello Lippitt	1903-	Frederick E. Wilcox, M. D.	1903-1913
Edwin S. Greeley	1903-	Edward P. Hollowell	1907-1913
George C. Waldo	1903-1915	P. LeRoy Harwood	1907-1913
Clinton E. Stark, M. D.	1903-	James A. Doughty	1911-
Henry H. Gallup	1903-	L. Lester Watrous	1913-
J. Deming Perkins	1903-1911	Kirk W. Dyer	1915-
Edwin C. Pinney	1903-	James J. Donahue, M. D.	1913-
Eugene H. Burr	1903-1915	Charles A. Jenkins, M. D.	1913-
Franklin H. Mayberry, M. D.	1903-1913	James H. Naylor, M. D.	1913-
Calvin L. Harwood	1903-1907	E. Everett Rowell, M. D.	1915-
Frank T. Maples	1903-1907		

In January, 1904, Dr. Henry M. Pollock, then assistant superintendent at the Fergus Falls State Hospital, was appointed superintendent, and Dr. Harry O. Spalding, formerly of the Newton Nervine, assistant superintendent. Dr. Pollock assumed his active duties on May 1, 1904, and has since continued as superintendent of the hospital. Dr. Spalding, who assumed his duties on October 1, 1904, resigned March 22, 1912, to accept the superintendency of the Westborough State Hospital. The other medical officers who have held positions at the hospital are:

ASSISTANT PHYSICIANS.

Dr. J. Evan Shuttleworth	1906-1907
Dr. Thomas F. Erdman..	1907-1912
Dr. Jennie G. Purmort..	1907-1912
Dr. Harry F. Hoffman..	1910-1912
Dr. Julius S. Kohn.....	1910-1910
Dr. Gaius E. Harmon (pathologist)	1910-1912
Dr. Frederick H. Lovell.	1911-1912
Dr. Esther S. B. Woodward	1912-1915
Dr. D. T. Brewster......	1912-1912
Dr. C. Fletcher Souder..	1912-
Dr. Mark S. Bringman..	1912-1914
Dr. John F. Lovell (pathologist)	1912-1913
Dr. Franklin B. Pedrick	1913-1914
Dr. James B. Quinn (pathologist)	1913-1914
Dr. Dana F. Downing..	1914-1914
Dr. Edward A. Everett..	1914-
Dr. Frederick N. Beardslee	1914-1915
Dr. Simon R. Klein (acting pathologist)	1914-1915
Dr. William W. Gleason	1915-1915
Dr. Elizabeth E. Enz....	1915-
Dr. Richard Blackmore.	1915-
Dr. W. Franklin Wood..	1915-

INTERNES.

Dr. Harry F. Hoffman..	1909-1909
Dr. Harry Millspaugh...	1910-1910
Dr. John W. Callahan..	1910-1910
Dr. John J. Bendick.....	1912-1912
Dr. James B. Quinn.....	1912-1912
Dr. Bruce Greenway....	1914-1914
Dr. Helen B. Todd	1914-1915
Dr. J. Lewis McAuslan.	1915-
Dr. Hartwell J. Thompson	1915-1915

CONNECTICUT SCHOOL FOR IMBECILES.

Lakeville, Conn.

As no records were kept of the early history of the Connecticut School for Imbeciles, it is impossible to give more than a brief sketch of its inception.

In 1858 Dr. Henry Knight began to take a few imbecile cases into his own home for treatment and care. The School was conducted as a private institution until Dr. Knight's death in 1861, when a charter was secured and a corporation formed under the control of a board of directors and continued by a second Dr. Henry Knight until his death in 1885. His son, Dr. George H. Knight, then assumed control, and conducted the institution until his death October 4, 1912. He was succeeded by Mrs. George H. Knight, who remained in charge until the state assumed control on August 1, 1913.

The first superintendent appointed by the state was Dr. Robert Knight, of Sharon, a brother of Dr. George H. Knight. He remained in charge until February 1, 1914, when Dr. Charles T. La Moure was appointed to succeed him.

As there was no other institution in the state for the care of the feeble-minded, many state cases were received at this institution from its inception, and the School received state aid for their care.

In 1914 the institution consisted of a group of three-story, cheaply constructed wooden buildings, connected by corridors, a small two-story wooden hospital building, and a three-story wooden building for custodial care, with a laundry in the basement. In the last six months of 1914 there were two fires in this laundry.

The site of the institution comprises six acres of ground, and there are 300 cases under care. The institution has always been lighted by kerosene lamps.

The General Assembly of Connecticut in January, 1915, enacted a law changing the name of the "Connecticut School for Imbeciles" to "The Connecticut Training School for the Feeble-minded," and providing for its transfer to a new institution constructed on the property of the state in the town of Mansfield.

Provision was made in the act for the selection of a site in the town of Mansfield by a commission consisting of three members of the Board of Trustees of the Connecticut Colony for Epileptics and three members of the board of the Connecticut Training School for Feeble-minded. In case of the failure of this commission to locate a site on or before August 15, then the Governor was empowered to select such a site. The act further provided that the site selected should be so situated that one heating, power, lighting and sewage plant could serve both the new institution and the Connecticut Colony for Epileptics.

The trustees of the Connecticut School for Feeble-minded were authorized by the act to sell the property in the town of Salisbury for a sum not less than $25,000. This, together with $200,000 appropriated by the act, was to provide at the new location at Mansfield such buildings, etc., as might be necessary for the conduct of such school.

THE CONNECTICUT COLONY FOR EPILEPTICS.[1]

MANSFIELD DEPOT, CONN.

In 1905, after investigations made by the Connecticut State Medical Society, extending over a period of several years, the results of which were brought before the General Assembly, a resolution was passed by that body as follows:

Resolved by this Assembly, That there shall be appointed by the Governor in July, 1905, a committee of three persons, who shall investigate methods for the care and treatment of persons resident in this state who are affected with epilepsy in any of its forms and conditions, and report to the General Assembly at its January session, 1907, the result of such investigation, together with what is deemed by said committee to be the most practical plan to be adopted for such care and treatment by the state as shall secure the most humane and curative results.

A committee, consisting of Drs. Max Mailhouse, Frank K. Hallock and Edwin A. Down, was accordingly appointed by the Governor. This committee, after making extensive investigations, reported to the General Assembly in January, 1907. No definite action was taken by this Assembly, but the next Assembly passed an act providing for the establishment of a colony for epileptics. This act became effective from August 10, 1909. Section 1 of this act reads as follows:

There shall be established within this state a colony for epileptics, the object of which shall be the scientific treatment, education, employment and custody of epileptics, and which shall be known as the Connecticut Colony for Epileptics.

The act empowered the Governor to appoint a commission of three persons to secure a suitable location for the institution, consisting of not less than 200 acres, and also empowered him to appoint a board of trustees for the government and control of said institution. The trustees were authorized to admit patients to the said institution under special agreements, provided, however, that hopeful cases should have preference as to admission, and in no instance shall a hopelessly or violently insane person be admitted.

In August, 1910, the Commission appointed by the Governor

[1] Prepared by Donald L. Ross, M. D., superintendent.

purchased a site of about 222 acres half a mile from Mansfield Depot, County of Tolland, on the Central Vermont Railroad.

In September, 1910, the first Board of Trustees, consisting of eight members, one from each county in the state, was appointed.

The site purchased contained no buildings suitable for the care of patients, and the Board of Trustees proceeded at once to prepare plans for building the institution.

Upon January 10, 1911, Donald L. Ross, M. D., assistant physician at Kings Park State Hospital, Kings Park, N. Y., and formerly first assistant physician at Craig Colony for Epileptics, Sonyea, N. Y., was appointed superintendent by the Board of Trustees.

The General Assembly of 1911 appropriated as follows for the development of the institution:

For current expenses	$25,000.00
For two ward buildings, 40 patients each	60,000.00
For dining hall and kitchen building	15,000.00
For central heating plant	35,550.00
For development and construction of sewage disposal plant	10,000.00
For construction of a spur track to connect with the Central Vermont Railway	12,000.00
For fees of architects and engineers	5,000.00
Total	$162,550.00

Following the above appropriations, the Board of Trustees set to work to carry out the different objects for which the money had been appropriated.

In June, 1911, more land was purchased in order to obtain the right of way for a spur track and to secure better building sites, thus increasing the amount of land to 354 acres.

The general plan of the institution provides for a centrally located building to be used for administration purposes and as quarters for officers. Other special buildings planned are as follows: A central heating and power plant, laundry, store room, bakery, assembly hall, industrial building, school and hospital. The buildings for patients are to consist chiefly of cottages accommodating from 20 to 40 patients, the smallest to contain the better class, mentally, and to have their own dining rooms and kitchens. For the lowest class, mentally, a cottage for each sex is planned, these to accommodate not more than 100 patients. A congregate dining room is planned for each sex, excepting for those in the smallest cottages. The buildings for males are to be separated as thoroughly as the contour of the site will permit, excepting the two largest buildings, which will be located closer together as the inmates in these will be under stricter supervision. It is expected to employ female nurses in both. It is also planned to employ the patients as much as possible in assisting in the work of the different departments. Male patients especially will be employed at farm work.

The institution will open for the admission of patients, May 15, 1914.

ELM CROFT

Enfield, Conn.

Elm Croft, situated in Enfield, Conn., was established in 1890, by Dr. Edward Smith Vail, for the treatment of persons suffering from nervous diseases.

The houses are of modern design, heated by steam and lighted by electricity. They have open fireplaces and hardwood finish. There are 50 acres of grounds, and the farm furnishes cream, milk, butter, eggs, vegetables, etc., for the institution.

Dr. E. S. Vail is now assisted by his son, Dr. T. E. Vail, both of whom reside on the grounds of the institution.

DR. BARNES' SANITARIUM.

Stamford, Conn.

This Sanitarium was organized in 1894 by an act of the Legislature. Subsequently in 1898, when it became The Dr. Barnes Sanitarium, it was licensed under a new act which applied to all the institutions of the state.

The sanitarium is situated in a park of 50 acres on high ground overlooking Long Island Sound. The buildings are six in number. They are so arranged that patients can be classified in a thorough manner. A farm is connected which gives an abundant supply of vegetables and fruit. It also gives an opportunity for out-of-door work by the patients.

Among the special features of treatment are freedom from bars and bolts, and the insistence on proper physical exercise in the open air.

The medical superintendent is Dr. F. H. Barnes, who for the past five years has been connected with the neurological department of the New York Post-Graduate Hospital, and is neurologist to the Stamford Hospital.

THE CARE OF THE INSANE IN DELAWARE.

No reference to the care of the insane in Delaware can be found prior to 1793. Before that date the colony was so sparsely settled and the population so scattered that each family cared for its own insane, unless they became unmanageable and therefore a source of danger to the community in general, in which case they were sent to the nearest county jail.

The earliest legislation on the subject was an act passed on February 2d, 1793,[1] to vest in the Court of Chancery the care of all idiots and insane over the age of 21, so far as to appoint a trustee or trustees to take charge of their persons and assume the management of their property, both real and personal. This act had to do principally with the property of the insane. Nearly 20 years later in 1812 a further act was passed giving the Levy Court in each county the power to remove all idiots and insane from the county jail to their respective poorhouses.

No state care was provided for the mentally defective until 1889, the only provision for them up to that time being made by the counties, of which there were three, New Castle, Kent and Sussex. New Castle had established a four-story brick building at Farnhurst for the accommodation of the chronic insane of that county, while Sussex, about the same time, erected a two-story wooden building for the same purpose. Prior to this the insane were housed in poorhouses and jails and received but scant care and attention.

The condition of the insane in these county establishments was deplorable and the history of the state shows that from time to time public-spirited citizens made many attempts to induce the General Assembly to take steps to ameliorate the existing state of things.

It was not until 1889, however, that the Legislature was prevailed upon to make the necessary provisions for state care. Even then New Castle and Sussex refused to sanction the passage of the act for a state asylum unless the state would agree to purchase the buildings already erected by them. A proviso was accordingly added to the bill by which the state bought the New Castle building for $75,000 and that belonging to Sussex for $8000. It was also

[1] Vol. I, Delaware Laws.

provided that the New Castle Asylum should be used as a nucleus for the new institution to be erected by the state. With these amendments the act was passed by the Legislature on April 25, 1889.

This act provided that the hospital should be under the control of a board of nine trustees, distributed regularly between the three counties, and one of them a physician; it was further provided that they should not all be of the same political faith.

By the passage of this act Delaware became the first state to accept all the indigent insane as her wards and to make state provision for them. During the session of 1889 and 1890 New York, it is true, by act of assembly, provided for the treatment of all her insane in state hospitals. While the Legislature of New York was discussing the propriety of such provision, Delaware had its insane already housed, and, though hampered by limited means, was endeavoring to institute a new era of care for her dependent defectives.

Classes Committed.—All indigent insane persons and also insane persons from Delaware and other states who are able to pay for their maintenance and support.

Legal Procedure.—Certificates must be filed with the superintendent of the hospital, signed by two physicians residents of the state who have been actively in practice, stating, after separate examinations, that they believe the patient's disease requires hospital care and treatment and that they are in no way related to the patient by blood or marriage or connected with any hospital.

Commitment.—Patients coming from the New Castle County almshouse must be accompanied with certificates signed by at least one of the physicians required by law to examine the patient and made within one week after the examination and within two weeks of the time of application for admission to the hospital. In all cases certificates must be accompanied by an order of admission signed by one or more of the trustees of the hospital.

These provisions do not apply to commitments to the hospital made by the Chancellor or in any court of the state as provided by law. In the City of Wilmington the State Board of Trustees is required to appoint as examiners two physicians of different schools of medicine residing in Wilmington for a term of three years.

No person may be admitted to the state hospital from the City of Wilmington unless the certificate is signed by at least one of the physicians appointed by the State Board of Trustees.

In the case of indigent patients, if the relatives or friends or a citizen apply to the Chancellor personally or by petition presenting certificates of two practising physicians, one of whom must be the regular physician of the almshouse, stating that the person is insane and in need of medical treatment, the Chancellor, if satisfied, must refer the application to the trustees of the poor of the county for information, and if their report is satisfactory he must recommend in writing to the Governor that the indigent insane person be removed to the insane department of the New Castle Almshouse.

Appeal from Commitment.—Any person committed to the state hospital or any person related to the person committed within the third degree of consanguinity or any other three persons may make a sworn petition to the Chancellor at any time for a warrant to the sheriff to determine whether the patient is sane or insane; the Chancellor must then issue a writ committing him and summon a jury within five days to determine the case and to return the findings by the jury to the Chancellor within two days. If the jury finds that the person is sane the patient must be released.

Costs of Commitment.—These must be paid by the county of his residence.

DELAWARE STATE HOSPITAL AT FARNHURST.

Under the act of April 25, 1889, Chapter 553, Vol. XVIII, Laws of Delaware, Lewis Thompson, John J. Black, M. D., Nathaniel Williams, Zebulon Hopkins, John B. Cooper, James H. Wilson, M. D., Alfred P. Robinson, Eli R. Sharp and Hiram R. Burton were appointed as members of the State Board of Trustees of the Delaware State Hospital at Farnhurst. They were empowered to take over the insane department erected by "The Trustees of the Poor of New Castle County" for the sum of $75,000, and also the building in Sussex County known as "The Insane Department" for the sum of $8000.

As the bill provided that the building erected by New Castle County should be the nucleus of the new state hospital, the board held its first meeting at that place July 10, 1889.

Upon assuming charge of the institution the trustees received from New Castle County ten acres of ground and a large building, scantily furnished and in need of repairs and a general overhauling—a plant absolutely unfit in its then condition for a modern hospital of any kind—with $28,000 in money to carry on the institution in every department until April 25, 1891. They recognized the fact, however, that the whole act in relation to the State Hospital for Insane, as passed by the Legislature of 1889, was tentative and that vigorous action would be taken by the Legislature of 1891 to place the institution upon a solid and creditable footing.

The Board organized at its meeting July 10, 1889. Dr. John J. Black, of New Castle, was elected president and Dr. James H. Wilson, of Dover, secretary on July 31. At its second meeting the Board elected Dr. D. D. Richardson, of Philadelphia, as superintendent.

Dr. Richardson was well qualified for the position for which he had been chosen. He had for years devoted his time and talents to the welfare of the insane, having been superintendent of the insane department of the Philadelphia Hospital and later having organized and opened the State Hospital at Warren, Pa.

On August 1, 1889, which was practically the initial hospital day, 99 patients, all accredited to New Castle County, were admitted. On the 3d of September 12 patients were admitted from Sussex County, and on the 11th 18 patients from Kent County entered the institution. There were 138 subsequent admissions from the three counties.

During the legislative session of 1891 the official name of the hospital was changed from the Delaware State Hospital to the Delaware State Hospital at Farnhurst. A joint resolution was also passed empowering the Board of Trustees to make contracts in relation to the board and maintenance of any insane person and to collect from the relatives of the same any compensation agreed upon at the time of admission of said insane person. This session of the Legislature also passed an act appropriating $30,000 for the improvement of the grounds and buildings. With the money thus appropriated the superintendent's residence was built and a new laundry and amusement hall; several fire escapes were placed in position; new furniture, beds and bedding were added to the equipment, and the entire building was painted and renovated.

Dr. D. D. Richardson, the superintendent, resigned his position in September, 1893, to accept the position of superintendent of the Norristown State Hospital, Pennsylvania. Dr. Richardson's resignation was a great loss to the institution, as he had labored unceasingly to place the institution upon a firm basis.

The Board of Trustees at its meeting in October, 1893, elected Dr. Wm. H. Hancker, who had been Dr. Richardson's assistant for the previous year, as the new superintendent. Dr. Hancker had formerly been assistant superintendent of the Northern Hospital at Oshkosh, Wis., for a period of 18 years.

On June 22, 1894, the Board purchased 13 acres of land adjoining the hospital grounds on the north. The property was unimproved, about one-half consisting of low and marshy land. This was converted into a pond, fed by numerous springs, and the ground surrounding it was sodded and otherwise improved and beautified.

At the close of the year 1894 the population of the hospital had increased to 232. As the capacity of the building was 150, the Board decided to ask the incoming Legislature to appropriate $35,000 for a new building to join the existing structure. In January, 1895, in accordance with the above request, the Legislature passed an act authorizing the issuing of state bonds for the sum of $35,000. The bonds were sold for $36,568; a bonus of $1568. The building was finished and occupied in June, 1897.

It is immediately in the rear of the original building and at right angles with the same, being connected with it by means of a covered passage-way 25 feet in length. The building is 186 feet in length, three stories in height, and built of hard and stretcher brick with red stone trimmings, the inside being of hollow brick to prevent dampness.

In 1898 a well-organized laboratory was established, thoroughly equipped with instruments of precision and all necessary paraphernalia to carry on the work required. As there was no public laboratory in the state for the examination of sputa, blood work, etc., the Board of Trustees passed a resolution that the practitioners of the state should have the privilege of sending specimens to the institution for examination free of charge. It goes without saying that they fully appreciated the benefits to be derived from an offer of this kind and fully availed themselves of the privilege. Naturally the work of the pathologist and bacteriologist was greatly augmented, so much so that it was deemed advisable to ask the next Legislature for a sufficient sum to build a state laboratory on the grounds of the present hospital. The bill was introduced and was ably supported by the medical fraternity of the state. Although it was defeated, it was the means of establishing a state laboratory on the grounds of the Delaware College at Newark, under the supervision of the State Board of Health.

In May of 1900, Elza Wade, an honest old employee of the hospital, died. Having no relations, he left all of his savings, amounting to $1300, to the superintendent, with the injunction that he be decently buried and that the residue be applied to the best use of the hospital. With the consent of the Board, the superintendent applied the money to the establishment of a modern surgery, equipped will all necessary appliances. This is now known as the Elza Wade Surgery.

On April 14, 1902, smallpox was discovered in one of the female wards. The president of the Board of Trustees and the secretary of the State Board of Health were immediately notified. A consultation was held at the hospital at once. The hospital was quarantined and the line of work necessary to suppress the epidemic was outlined.

Immune nurses from Philadelphia were immediately employed and four of the employees of this institution, two males and two females, volunteered their services. They had never seen a case of this loathsome disease, nor were they in a strict sense immune. Too much honor or praise cannot be given this little band of workers for the amount and character of the work they accomplished. One of the males was taken with the disease; was in bed but a few days and was again up and doing. The upper ward of the annex was emptied of male patients and a systematic fumigation of all wards and corridors begun. In spite of all efforts the disease rapidly spread until there were 22 cases. The number of deaths were seven. The supervisor, Samuel McMullen, and the painter, John M. Cheffins, were among those who succumbed. All who died were over 73 years of age and the average was 76½ years.

In 1902 the new tuberculosis hospital was opened, capable of accommodating 20 patients, complete in every detail, with all modern appliances necessary. This building was built entirely from the receipts of pay patients and no appropriation of any kind was made by the state.

The population of the hospital steadily increased and in 1907 there were 423 patients being cared for, while the capacity of the institution was only 250.

The Legislature of 1907 appropriated $40,000 to erect and equip a building to accommodate the overflow. In 1908 the building was opened for the reception of patients. At a meeting of the Board of Trustees December 5, 1907, it was moved and carried that the new building be known as the John J. Black Cottage. This action was in recognition of the active interest Dr. Black had taken in the affairs of the institution since its opening in 1889. At the first meeting of the Board of Trustees in May, 1889, he was elected president of the board, and was yearly re-elected to the chairmanship without opposition. His untiring devotion to the best interests of the hospital, his advanced ideas, and the aptitude with which he grasped the intricate problems that constantly arise in the management of an institution of this size were thus acknowledged by the board.

On September 27, 1909, Dr. John J. Black died after a brief illness. Dr. Black had ever been the friend of the afflicted. His interest in the welfare of this institution and its inmates never flagged. His frequent visits made him thoroughly familiar with the patients and with the general administration of the hospital. His genial nature, affability and ready desire to hear all sides of a disputed question before judging its merits were some of his predominant virtues. His loss was a severe one to the institution. His interest and his fight for state aid for those suffering from tuberculosis dates back for years and he was always in the vanguard of those who persisted that this so-called fatal disease could, under advantageous circumstances, be classed in the category of disease amenable to treatment.

The Trustees of the Delaware State Hospital at Farnhurst for the year 1913 are as follows:

William H. Swift ....President.
James H. Wilson, M. D. ....Secretary

George S. Capelle.	William P. Orr, M. D.
George H. Murray.	Thomas C. Frame, M. D.
Rowland G. Paynter, M. D.	Walter H. Steele, M. D.

Philip L. Cannon.

The resident officers since the founding of the Delaware State Hospital at Farnhurst have been as follows:

Dr. David D. Richardson	1889-1892	Dr. William E. Curtin..	1902-1902
Dr. William H. Hancker	1892-	Dr. Charles G. Brown...	1903-1903
Dr. John H. Hammond..	1893-1901	Dr. Taleasin H. Davies..	1903-
Dr. Edith A. Barker	1898-1899	Dr. Blanche Dennes.....	1904-1908
Dr. Jean M. Wilson.....	1899-1901	Dr. Edith Clime Weber..	1909-1909
Dr. Florence Hull Watson	1901-1902	Dr. Elizabeth W. Allison	1910-1910
Dr. Clarence Van Epps..	1901-1902	Dr. Anna J. Gardner....	1911-1912
		Dr. Hannah Morris	1913-

THE CARE OF THE INSANE IN THE DISTRICT OF COLUMBIA.

In the *Journal of Insanity* for July, 1844,[1] the following note is found:

"The subject of a lunatic asylum in the District of Columbia has several times engaged the attention of Congress. In 1841 an act was passed providing for the accommodation of patients at the Maryland Hospital, at an expense not exceeding $300 a year. This was deemed too expensive and it was proposed to fit up a building in Washington for the reception of patients. During the last session an act was passed appropriating $4000 for the support of the lunatics of the District, about 20 in number, at the Baltimore or some other suitable lunatic asylum for the ensuing year at a price not exceeding $4 per week for each patient."

The institution chosen for the care of the "lunatics of the District" was the Maryland Hospital for the Insane,[2] then located on North Broadway, Baltimore, on a site now occupied by the present Johns Hopkins Hospital. There the insane of the District were cared for until January 15, 1855, on which date they were transferred to the Government Hospital for the Insane, which had been provided for by an act of Congress in 1852.

At present the Government Hospital for the Insane receives patients from the military organizations stationed throughout the United States, from our island possessions, and from the District of Columbia.

The supervision of charitable, correctional and reformatory institutions and associations which receive appropriations from Congress for care or treatment of residents of the District of Columbia is in the hands of a board of charities, consisting of five members, appointed by the President of the United States, for a term of three years. In addition there is a board of visitors for the Government Hospital, consisting of nine members, appointed by the President of the United States, for a term of six years. The members of both these boards serve without compensation.

[1] Volume I.

[2] Now Spring Grove State Hospital, Catonsville, Md.

The Government Hospital is under the direct charge of the Department of the Interior; and the superintendent, who must be a well-educated physician, experienced in the treatment of the insane, is an appointee of the Secretary of that department.

The cost of maintenance of indigent patients of the District of Columbia is paid one-half by the District and the remainder by the United States. Other patients are supported directly by the federal government or by their pensions, or by the individuals themselves, when able.

Legal Procedure.[1]—Proceedings in cases of indigent insane residents and insane persons having dangerous tendencies are instituted upon petition of Commissioners of the District of Columbia. All writs *de lunatico inquirendo* issue from the Equity Court and the justice holding it presides at all inquisitions and may call a jury or may summon a special jury.

Detention of Insane Persons.—An insane person within the District may be apprehended and restrained without warrant by any member of the police or any other official authorized to make arrests.

The superintendent of the metropolitan police is authorized to order the apprehension and detention without warrant of any indigent person alleged to be insane or who has homicidal or dangerous tendencies and found elsewhere than in public places, upon the affidavits of two or more responsible persons that they believe the person to be insane. But before apprehension the superintendent must require the certificates of at least two physicians, who shall certify that they have examined the person alleged to be insane and that he should not be allowed to remain at liberty, and that he is a fit subject for treatment.

The Commissioners of the District of Columbia are authorized to place in the Government Hospital for the Insane for a period not exceeding 30 days indigent persons alleged to be insane, residents of or found within the District of Columbia and alleged insane persons of homicidal or otherwise dangerous tendencies, apprehended and restrained, pending their formal commitment to the

[1] Provisions relate to residents of the District of Columbia who are indigent or dangerously insane. Persons from the army, navy or marine corps and other government services are admitted by the superintendent upon the order of the Secretary of War, Secretary of the Navy, or Secretary of the Treasury, as the case may be.

hospital or their transportation to the homes when their places of residence are ascertained.

The Commissioners may authorize the temporary commitment of insane persons for periods not exceeding 30 days in any other hospital which is properly equipped, pending the temporary commitment or formal commitment to the Government Hospital for the Insane or to any other hospital or asylum. Such a person may be detained in a police station or house of detention pending arrangements for his temporary detention in the government hospital or other institution; or they may be detained there until formally committed, in case no other provisions are feasible. If the superintendent of the hospital for the insane certifies in writing to the physicians of the hospitals in the District of Columbia that he is not insane or has recovered his reason, the officials must at once discharge the insane person and report their action to the Commissioners. No certificate is valid if made by a physician not regularly licensed to practice medicine in the District of Columbia, unless a commissioned surgeon of the United States Army or Public Health and Marine Hospital Service; or a physician not a permanent resident of the District of Columbia; or by a physician not actually engaged in practice for at least three years; or by a physician related by blood or marriage to the person whose mental condition is questioned. No certificate is valid if made by a physician financially interested in the hospital or asylum in which the alleged insane person is to be confined or who is officially connected with it.

Appointment of Guardian.—In case any person adjudged to be of unsound mind has property, the Equity Court has full power to appoint a committee or trustee of the person and estate, who must reimburse out of the funds the District of Columbia for all costs expended or incurred by it and the Equity Court has full power to superintend and direct the affairs of persons *non compos mentis*, and to appoint a committee or trustees for such persons.

Non-resident insane to be returned to their place of residence. All necessary expenses are paid by the District.

Appeal.—Any person restrained of his lawful liberty may apply by petition to the Circuit Court of the District for a writ of *habeas corpus*.

Costs of commitment are chargeable to the District of Columbia unless the person has an estate, in which case he is liable.

GOVERNMENT HOSPITAL FOR THE INSANE.[1]

WASHINGTON, D. C.

The first appropriation towards building the Government Hospital for the Insane was of $100,000, and was made by Congress in 1852 for the purchase of land. The organic act creating the institution and outlining the duties of its officers and providing for the admission of various classes of insane patients was not approved until March 3, 1855. The hospital, however, had been opened for the reception of patients on January 15, 1855.

The creation of the hospital was due very largely to the activity of Dorothea L. Dix. She drew up with her own pen the outlines of the organic act establishing the institution, and virtually named its first superintendent, Dr. C. H. Nichols. During the latter part of her life Miss Dix spent much of her time at the hospital, where quarters were always reserved for her, and the little desk upon which she drew up the original act creating the hospital stands in the board room in the main building.

On the first of July, 1855, the President named a board of visitors, as follows: Benjamin F. Bohrer, M. D., president; William W. Corcoran, Jacob Gideon, Professor Grafton Tyler, M. D., Daniel Ratcliff, Professor Thomas Miller, M. D., William Whelan, M. D., U. S. N., Robert C. Wood, M. D., U. S. A., and Rev. P. D. Gurley, D. D. The make-up of the board has, in the main, followed the plan of the first board, namely, to name as members of the board one representative of each of the classes cared for in the hospital; thus a representative from the Army, the Navy and the Public Health and Marine Hospital Service, usually the acting or the retired surgeon-general of these several services, a lay physician, a lawyer, a clergyman, a layman, and in recent years two women.

The original main building was built from bricks made on the place, and in architectural style is a modification of the Kirkbride plan, each wing receding from the center, in echelon. The building itself is in the collegiate Gothic style. This main building was several years in building and wings were added to it from time to

[1] Prepared by William A. White, M. D., superintendent.

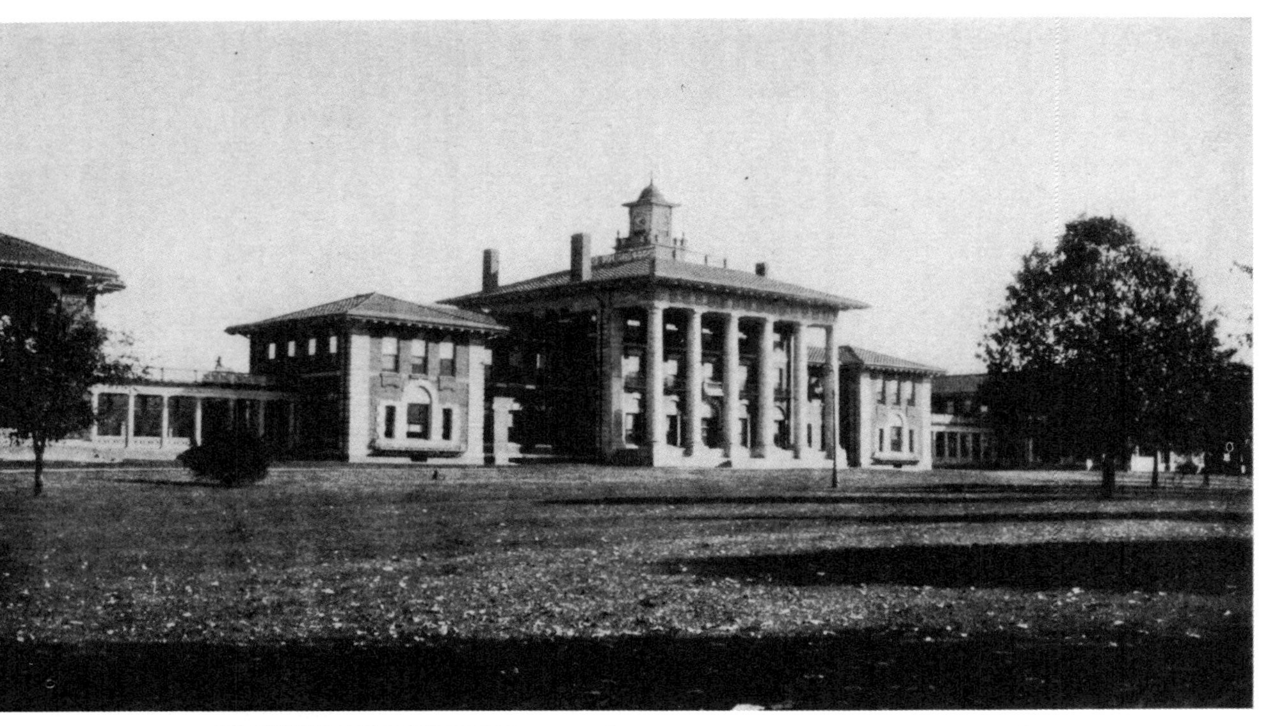

ADMINISTRATION BUILDING, GOVERNMENT HOSPITAL, WASHINGTON, D. C.

time. Other construction, however, was undertaken in the meantime, and shortly after the opening of the hospital, during the fiscal year 1855-6, a building was opened for the colored insane, which the superintendent stated in his report he believed to be the "first and only special provision for the suitable care of the African when afflicted with insanity which has yet been made in any part of the world."[1]

While it was undoubtedly very largely in Miss Dix's mind that the Government Hospital for the Insane should be essentially a military institution, still the organic act provided also for the admission of patients from the District of Columbia. The District of Columbia in those years, however, was a rather small affair and so the number admitted to the hospital was not very great. The total number of patients admitted from all sources during the first year was only 63. During the Civil War, however, the hospital was conveniently located for utilization by the army and navy, and in 1861 one of its buildings, the West Lodge, was set aside for the wounded seamen of the Chesapeake and Potomac fleets, and a little later a couple of wards in the main building were prepared for the reception of sick and wounded soldiers. The following year the annual report shows that the General and Quarantine Naval Hospitals, with 70 beds, in charge of Surgeon N. Pinkney, of the Navy, and the General Army Hospital, with 250 beds, in charge of the medical officers of the Government Hospital for the Insane, "have been in successful operation during all of the past year"; while in the following year it is again noted that the General Hospital, with 250 beds, known as the St. Elizabeth Hospital, and the separate General and Quarantine Naval Hospitals, with 60 beds in both, "all free tenants of the institution, under our supervision, are maintained in full activity and usefulness."

Here is the first mention of the name of St. Elizabeth as applied to the hospital. It was taken from the name of the tract of land upon which the hospital stood, which has been known ever since the settlement of the country as the St. Elizabeth tract. The application of the name St. Elizabeth to the hospital was the result of the disinclination of many of the soldiers who were not insane to have the institution in which they were temporarily resident

[1] This was incorrect, Williamsburg, Va., having made separate provision for colored insane prior to 1850.

called the Government Hospital for the Insane. In January of 1863, at the request of the Surgeon-General of the army, certain rooms of the hospital were set aside for the convenience of one of the manufacturers of artificial legs, and soldiers who had lost a limb by amputation in any one of the district or neighboring hospitals might, if they wished, be transferred to the St. Elizabeth Hospital as soon as the stump was healed, to be fitted with an artificial leg. These were the men who, while resident in the hospital and getting their artificial limbs adjusted, did not wish to be considered patients in an institution for the insane, and so St. Elizabeth Hospital came to be a name applied to the institution. The St. Elizabeth referred to is the Hungarian saint about whom many legends of kindness to the sick and afflicted folks were written, and so the name came to be retained because of its singular appropriateness.

The first superintendent, Dr. Nichols, resigned in 1877 to take charge of the Bloomingdale Hospital for the Insane in New York City. He had served the institution for practically 25 years, having been called to the superintendency in October of 1852, after the passage of the first appropriation act; from that time until the opening of the hospital in January, 1855, he selected the sites of the buildings and planned and supervised the construction of the original edifice and its successive additions down to the time of his resignation. Dr. Nichols was a Quaker and brought to his work the humanitarian principles of that sect, which has been closely identified with the care of the insane in this country. Dr. Pliny Earle was a close friend of Dr. Nichols and a frequent visitor at the hospital, as was also Miss Dorothea L. Dix. Dr. Nichols was succeeded by Dr. W. W. Godding, who took charge of the institution in 1877.

Dr. Godding had been appointed upon the hospital staff some time in 1863. He came from Fitchburg, Mass., and previous to his connection with the Government Hospital for the Insane had been connected with the New Hampshire Hospital for the Insane at Concord. Later he had been superintendent of the Taunton State Hospital for a number of years and resigned the position to return to Washington.

During Dr. Godding's incumbency of 22 years the institution grew rapidly. When he took charge of the hospital in 1877 he found only six buildings. During his superintendency he erected 22 buildings and various extensions and additions. The larger buildings erected were the Relief Building, the Home Building, Howard Hall for the criminal insane, the Toner Building and Infirmary, a large refectory, the Oaks Building for the epileptic insane, with its large kitchen, a power house with electrical installation, and the Allison Building. When he took charge there were 765 patients; when he died he left a population of 1967 patients. He found, in 1877, 227 employees. He left an organization of 540 employees, or a total of over 2500 patients and attendants. Besides the erection of these buildings he added over 500 acres to the hospital grounds and established a farm colony at Godding Croft. During this period of growth the appropriations for the support of the institution trebled, and at the time of his death he was annually disbursing over $500,000.

The Government Hospital for the Insane was one of the early institutions in the country to recognize the value of scientific work and one of the first to appoint a pathologist. Dr. I. W. Blackburn, who had been associated with Professor Formad of Philadelphia, was appointed special pathologist in the fiscal year 1883-4. In after years his work became well known, and at the time of his death—June 18, 1911—he had established for himself a national reputation among workers in this field.

The Government Hospital for the Insane was also one of the first to take up the systematic application of hydrotherapeutic measures to the treatment of the insane. The active man on the staff in this work was Dr. G. W. Foster, who had charge of the Toner infirmary. The report for 1895-6 shows that during the previous two years he had been actively engaged in using hydrotherapeutic measures and had made special application of this form of treatment to general paresis. Subsequent reports made considerable mention of this treatment, describing both Dr. Foster's methods and his conclusions. During the first three years no special hydrotherapeutic apparatus was installed, the treatment consisting mostly of the application of the cold pack accompanied by cold to the head in the form of a wet towel or ice pack. During the fiscal year 1897-8 a complete hydrotherapeutic outfit was installed, the form of apparatus being that designed by Dr. S. Baruch, of New York City. Dr. Godding died in office on the 6th of May, 1899.

During the interval between Dr. Godding's death and the appointment of his successor, Dr. A. H. Whitmer became acting superintendent. During his short period of service the school of instruction in nursing, which had been begun in 1894, was reorganized and extended, and arrangements were made to give a certificate after the completion of a two years' course, with promotion and increase in pay.

Dr. Witmer died January 18, 1900.

On October 17, 1899, Dr. A. B. Richardson was appointed superintendent as Dr. Godding's successor. He came from Ohio, where he had much experience as administrator and had recently built the Massillon State Hospital.

When Dr. Richardson took charge of the hospital his survey of the situation showed that the buildings were calculated to accommodate properly and care for a population not to exceed 1600 patients, while the population on June 30, 1900, was 2076, an excess of almost 500 beyond the capacity of the institution. The superintendent reported that in some of the male wards which were intended for 18 patients there were 43 and 44 patients, and in other wards from 16 to 18 beds were made on the floor each night along the corridors, while in the most disturbed female wards, with a normal capacity of 36 each, there were 58 to 60 patients. This condition of affairs was reported to Congress, which authorized an extension of the hospital for 1000 patients, and limited the total cost of said extension to $975,000. Arrangements were immediately made for securing plans and entering upon the work of extension. After the preliminaries were finally completed a contract was let for the construction of 12 buildings. The original contract for 12 buildings included two psychopathic reception buildings, one building each for disturbed men and women, an infirmary and six cottages. Five larger buildings were built to accommodate from 104 to 120 patients each, and the six cottages from 40 to 60 patients each. The twelfth building was the nurses' home. In addition to these buildings, a cold storage building and storehouse, a kitchen for the detached group of buildings, and a new stable were constructed, artesian wells were bored for supplying the hospital with water, and a railroad switch constructed extending from the Baltimore & Ohio Railroad to the power house. During the following session, in 1902, Congress provided for an

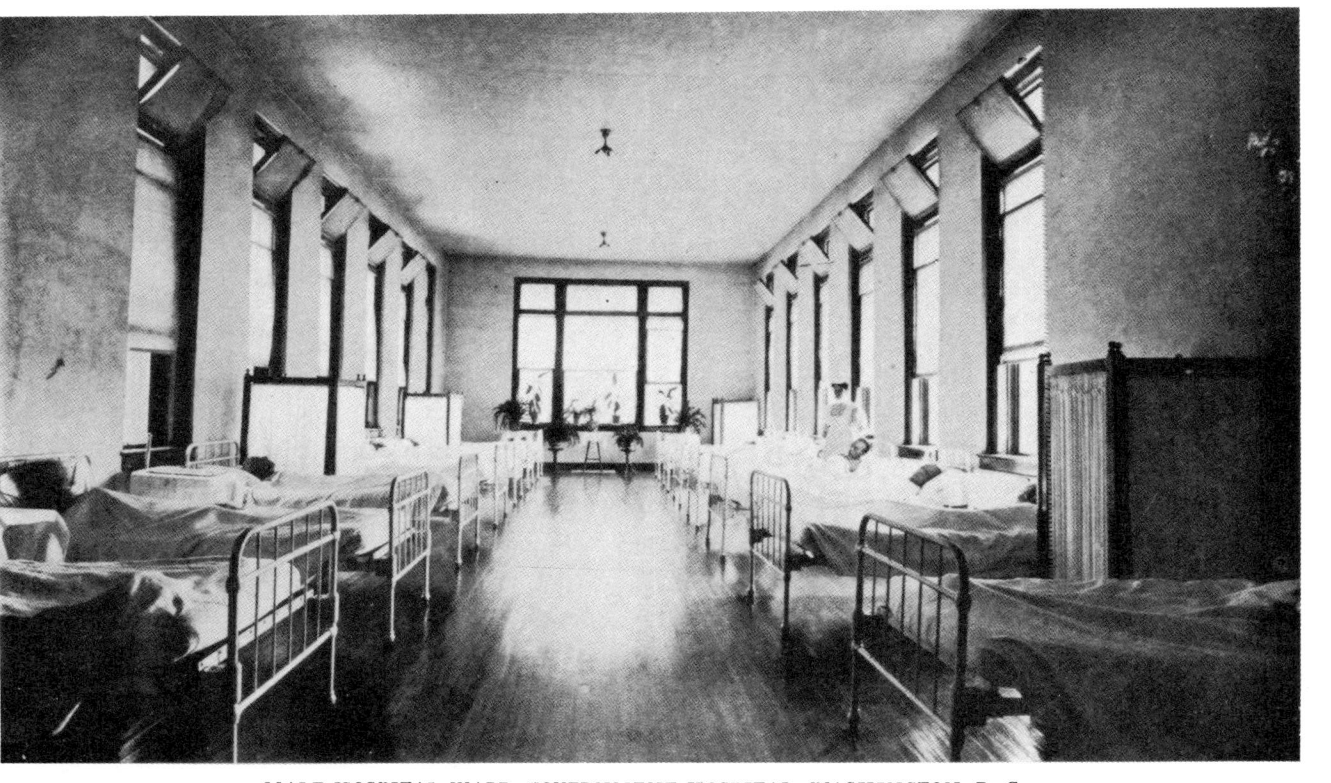

MALE HOSPITAL WARD, GOVERNMENT HOSPITAL, WASHINGTON, D. C.

additional administration building, a kitchen building, and a central power, heat and lighting plant by an appropriation of $425,000, making a total appropriation for the hospital extension of $1,400,000, to which was added afterwards a little over $100,000 for furnishing, etc., completing the sum of $1,500,000 expended for the accommodation of 1000 patients; for centralizing the power, heat and lighting, and for centralized administration, making a per capita cost per patient of somewhere between $1000 and $1500.

In the midst of this work and before any of the buildings of the hospital extension had been completed and occupied, Dr. Richardson, who was apparently in good health, suffered a stroke of apoplexy and died suddenly on the 27th of June, 1903.

He was succeeded by the present incumbent, Dr. William A. White, who took charge of the hospital on October 3, 1903. During the intervening three months between Dr. Richardson's death and the appointment of the new superintendent, Dr. Maurice J. Stack, first assistant physician, was in charge.

On the first of October, 1903, there were 2293 patients in the hospital, and the 15 buildings of the hospital extension were under construction, but no one of them had been finished. The work of building this large addition to the institution, reclassifying the population, occupying new buildings, shifting the center of administration and getting the new power, heat and lighting plant in operation immediately devolved upon the incoming superintendent. The first of the new buildings was placed in commission and occupied on August 12, 1904, and from that time forth various buildings were gradually occupied. The officers were changed to the new administration building and the central power plant started in operation.

During the last few years of Dr. Godding's life and during the short period of Dr. Richardson's superintendency the hospital had rapidly grown; when the large extension for 1000 beds had been completed and was ready for occupancy the problem of the reclassification of patients to meet the new possibilities of housing required to be solved, and it was suddenly borne in upon the management that the hospital had in some way suddenly expanded from an institution of medium size to a tremendous plant. Dr. Godding had been many years connected with the institution and knew all of its ramifications so intimately that he had not felt keenly the need for newer administrative methods. Dr. Richardson was so completely occupied with the great problem of building that he had not time and energy to devote to a revision of administrative methods, and when therefore the new buildings were to be occupied it became apparent that the whole institution required to be placed upon a new administrative basis, and that the psychological moment had arrived for undertaking this extensive work.

With the occupation of the new buildings the population was redistributed and reclassified. Tubercular patients were segregated from the others, porches and sun parlors being built for their accommodation; epileptic patients were separately housed; and the problem of classification generally was carefully worked out as best it could be under all the circumstances.

The administrative department of the hospital, so far as its outside work and the business office were concerned, was also entirely reorganized. The different groups of mechanics were collected under heads and sub-heads, and the whole scheme arranged in such a manner as to concentrate it in the office of the superintendent. The financial department in the same way was entirely revised; a new system of accounting was adopted, and the whole scheme was placed in better relations with the financial offices of the government.

The medical service was similarly reclassified. The position of clinical director was created. The clinical director is the personal representative of the superintendent in the wards, and it is his primary business to look after the medical work of the hospital and, to a certain extent, to relieve the superintendent on the one hand and the first assistant physician on the other, who must be prepared to take the superintendent's place in his absence.

A scientific department was also organized. The nucleus of this department previously consisted of a pathologist and a clinical pathologist only. There were added a psychologist, histopathologist, and various assistants from time to time, and the whole work was organized under a scientific director. During the past four years the research work of this department has been published annually as a bulletin from the hospital.

In addition to the work of reorganizing the institution, the hospital sought to extend its usefulness into many other channels.

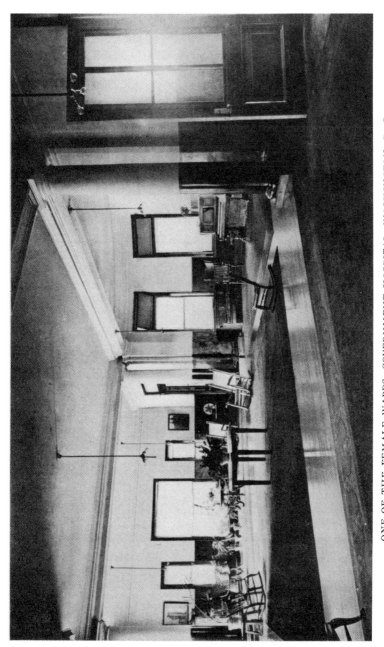

ONE OF THE FEMALE WARDS, GOVERNMENT HOSPITAL, WASHINGTON, D. C.

Accordingly it took surgeons from the Public Health and Marine Hospital Service for training for work on Ellis Island in discovering insane immigrants. The hospital also brought the subject of military psychiatry to the attention of the Army and Navy, and has had for some years surgeons from the army and navy stationed at the institution to study psychiatry in order to apply its results for the betterment of their respective services.

The institution also has gone on growing, increasing at the rate of nearly 100 patients per annum, until to-day there are 2946 patients. The hospital spends approximately $750,000 per annum. From being an institution of only local reputation, its influence now has wide ramifications. It receives patients from the military organizations stationed throughout the United States and, since the war with Spain, from our island possessions. The growth of scientific work has had much to do with the modifications of opinion regarding the insane in the District of Columbia and the practice among the local authorities in dealing with this class in the community. The staff of the institution has been very active in a medical and scientific way, and their numerous writings are scattered throughout the literature of the medical world, original publications from this institution appearing not only in the United States, but in Spain, Italy, Germany and France.

During the nearly 60 years of the hospital's existence many men prominent in public life and eminent in civil and military circles have been connected with the Board of Visitors as a result of its military functions and its location in Washington.

LIST OF THE MEDICAL OFFICERS OF THE INSTITUTION FROM THE BEGINNING.

C. H. Nichols, superintendent, 1855-77; William P. Young, 1855-58; S. Preston Jones, 1858-59; Bela N. Stephens, 1859-65; W. W. Godding, assistant physician, 1863-70; superintendent, 1877-99; Bernard D. Eastman, 1865-73; Thomas M. Franklin, 1865-72; Warren G. Hutchins, 1871-72; William H. Morrell, 1872-77; Francis M. Hamlin, 1873-76; Robert H. Chase, 1872-80; A. H. Witmer, 1876-1900; Maurice J. Stack, 1876-1909; George W. Foster, 1880-82, 1893-1900; Samuel B. Lyon, 1880-86; A. C. Paterson, 1881-97; J. C. Simpson, 1883-1904; J. E. Kenney, 1884-88; I. W. Blackburn, 1884-1911; J. V. Calver, D. D. S., 1886-97; Charles H. Latimer, 1888-1900; Samuel R. Means, 1889-90; Charles A. Drew, 1890-93; J. A. Barry, 1891-96; J. E. Toner, 1896-1904; A. D. Weakley, D. D. S., 1897 to the present; George H. Schwinn, 1898 to the present; Thomas Dowling, Jr., 1898-99; A. B. Richardson, superintendent, 1899-1903; C. H. Clark, 1900-07; Harry R.

Hummer, 1900-08; Patrick McGrath, 1900-01; Benjamin R. Logie, 1901-10; Cornelius Deweese, 1901-05; John M. Pulliam, 1901-03; Orrville G. Brown, 1901-03; Arthur H. Wise, 1902-03; William A. White, superintendent, 1903 to the present; Paul L. Freeman, 1903-05; Frank R. Webb, 1903-05; Alfred Glascock, 1903 to the present; William W. Richardson, 1904-05; W. H. Hough, 1904 to the present; L. H. Taylor, 1904-05; W. F. Hemler, 1904-07; Arthur H. Kimball, ophthalmologist, 1904 to the present; John P. Turner, V. M. D., 1904 to the present; A. C. Fitch, 1904-09; Mary O'Malley, 1905 to the present; H. R. Nichols, 1905-06; Heber Butts, 1906-07; George Peterson, 1906-06; Edith Conser, 1905-06, 1907-12; Nicholas J. Dynan, 1907-13; William N. Mebane, 1907-07; Wm. L. Sheep, 1907-09; Shepherd I. Franz, scientific director, 1907 to the present; C. R. Bell, 1907-08; M. H. Darnell, 1907-08; David G. Willetts, 1907-07; Erwin E. Downing, D. D. S., 1908-09; Harry Sicherman, 1908-10; George M. Gehringer, 1908-09; Eva C. Reid, 1908-13; Larry B. McAfee, 1909-09; Henry W. Miller, 1908-10; Nicholas Achucarro, 1908-10; Lucien C. Smith, 1908-08; Lawrence M. Drennan, 1907-09; A. H. Sutherland, 1909-10, assistant in psychology; George L. Echols, 1909-10; William H. Braithwaite, 1909-10; Charles R. Irby, D. D. S., 1909-13; Gonzalo R. Lafora, 1910-12; Francis M. Barnes, Jr., 1910-13; Rose Alexander, 1909-11; Paul E. Bowers, 1909-11; Myer Solomon, 1910-12; Bernard Glueck, 1909-12, 1913-14; Isaac N. Kelly, 1910-11; John H. Thorne, 1910-12; Josephine M. Stransky, 1910-12; James J. Loughran, 1910-13; Halbert Robinson, 1911-12; Hyman Laveson, 1911-11; Grace H. Kent, assistant in phychology, 1910-11; Oliver C. Cox, 1911-11; Helen A. Binnie, 1911-12; John A. F. Pfeiffer, 1912 to the present; Samuel McEwan, 1911-12; Grace DeWitt, 1912-14; Edwin G. Boring, assistant in psychology, 1912-12; Orlando J. Posey, 1912-13; Hagop Davidian, 1912 to the present; Arrah B. Evarts, 1912 to the present; John B. Anderson, 1912-13; Dennis J. Murphy, 1912 to the present; Frank H. Dixon, 1912 to the present; James C. Hassall, 1912 to the present; Raymond Apgar, 1913-13; J. P. H. Murphy, 1913 to the present; William E. Coyle, 1913-13; D. G. O'Neil, 1913 to the present; John E. Lind, 1913 to the present; William E. Detweiller, D. D. S., 1913-13; Edith A. MacDowell, 1913-13; Francis M. Shockley, 1913 to the present; Louis Wender, 1913 to the present; John R. Ernest, 1914 to the present; Wm. J. Lanahan, D. D. S., 1913-14.

VISITORS.

TAKEN FROM THE FIRST ANNUAL REPORT OF THE HOSPITAL, 1857.

Jacob Gideon, Esq., President of the Board.
Dr. Benjamin S. Bohrer.
Daniel Ratcliff.
Professor Thomas Miller, M. D.
Dr. William Whelan, U. S. N.
Dr. Robert C. Wood, U. S. A.
Rev. P. D. Gurley, D. D.
W. W. Corcoran.
Professor Grafton Tyler, M. D.

OFFICERS OF THE HOSPITAL FOR 1914.

Board of Visitors.

Brig.-General Geo. M. Sternberg, U. S. A., President of the Board.
Mrs. Henry G. Sharpe.
Mr. John W. Yerkes.
Walter S. Harban, D. D. S.
Rupert Blue, M. D., Surgeon-General, P. H. S.
Lewis E. Smoot.
Mrs. Archibald Hopkins.
Wm. C. Braisted, M. D., Surgeon-General, U. S. N.
Wm. C. Gorgas, M. D., Surgeon-General, U. S. A.

CHAPLAINS.

Rev. C. H. Butler.
Rev W. G. Davenport.
Rev. C. M. Bart.
Rev. Hugh T. Stevenson.
Rev. Geo. M. Cummings.

MEDICAL STAFF, 1914.

William A. White, M. D. ....Superintendent.
George H. Schwinn, M. D. ....First Assistant Physician.

SCIENTIFIC DIRECTOR.

S. I. Franz, A. B., Ph. D.

SENIOR ASSISTANT PHYSICIANS.

Mary O'Malley, M. D.
Alfred Glascock, M. D.

ASSISTANT PHYSICIANS.

William H. Hough, M. D.
John A. Pfeiffer, M. D.

JUNIOR ASSISTANT PHYSICIANS.

Arrah B. Evarts, M. D.
Hagop Davidian, M. D.
Frank H. Dixon, M. D.
John E. Lind, M. D.
John P. H. Murphy, M. D.
Anita A. Wilson, M. D.
James C. Hassall, M. D.
Dennis J. Murphy, M. D.
D. G. O'Neil, M. D.
Francis M. Shockley, M. D.
Louis Winder, M. D.
John R. Ernest, M. D.

VISITING DENTIST.

A. D. Weakley, D. D. S.

STEWARD.

Monie Sanger.

CHIEF CLERK.

Frank M. Fenotti.

PURCHASING AGENT.

A. E. Offutt.

MATRON.

H. O'Brien.

CHIEF OF TRAINING SCHOOL.

Miss Cornelia Allen, R. N.

THE CARE OF THE INSANE IN FLORIDA.

The insane of Florida were cared for in the asylums of other neighboring states—Georgia, South Carolina and Alabama—at the expense of the State of Florida until 1877. The larger number of the patients had been cared for at the Georgia State Sanitarium at Milledgeville, but the Legislature of that state, having ordered the return of all patients not resident citizens on account of the crowded condition of the Georgia Asylum, Florida decided to establish an institution of its own. The result was the establishment of the Florida Hospital for the Insane, located at Chattahoochee, in the western part of the state. This is the only state institution for the care of the insane in Florida. The institution is under the management of a Board of Commissioners of State Institutions, which consists of the Governor and the administrative officers of executive departments, *ex-officio*.

The hospital is under the direct charge of a superintendent, who is a layman. The medical service is in charge of a chief physician and three assistant physicians.

The cost of maintenance of patients is paid by the state.

There is no provision for the admission of voluntary patients; but pay patients, other than voluntary patients, not committed by judicial proceedings, may be admitted.

Classes Committed.—Destitute insane other than the incurable and harmless are admitted to the State Hospital.

Legal Procedure.—Residents of the state supposed to be insane, either *non compos mentis* or sufficiently devoid of reason to be incapable of self-control, are committed by a petition signed by five reputable citizens stating their belief that a patient is insane and asking that legal examination be made, presented to the county judge or judge of the circuit court having jurisdiction. The judge must, without delay, appoint an examination committee of one intelligent citizen, not a petitioner in the case, and two practicing physicians of good professional standing, graduates of a school of medicine recognized by the American Medical Association and residents of the county. The committee must examine the person to ascertain his mental and physical condition, and, if insane, whether the insanity is acute or chronic, its apparent cause, the hallucination, if any, his age and his propensities; also, whether he is indigent or has available means for his support.

If a contest is made the court must appoint a hearing. If the accused is indigent and unable to procure witnesses, the court must summon them at the expense of the county.

The examining committee must report its findings to the county judge, each member of the committee signing the report.

On receiving the report of the committee the judge must order the sheriff of the county from which the report is submitted to deliver the insane person to the superintendent of the hospital. The order of commitment must include a copy of the information and report of the committee.

If the report of the committee is that the alleged insanity is chronic or produced by epilepsy or senility and confinement or restraint are not necessary to prevent self-injury or violence, the judge must find him incurable, harmless and indigent and order the sheriff to deliver him to the county commissioners of the county of his residence.

FLORIDA HOSPITAL FOR THE INSANE.

CHATTAHOOCHEE, FLA.

The Florida Hospital for the Insane at Chattahoochee was established by the Legislature of Florida in 1876. The building was erected in 1834 as a government arsenal, at great cost and from the best material. After the Civil War it was sold to the state authorities to be used as a state prison. In March, 1877, the Legislature abolished the state prison, and the building was then converted into a lunatic asylum and was opened as such in May, 1877. The institution is located about a mile from the Apalachicola River, near its head and within a few hundred yards of the Georgia line. The country is undulating and beautiful, one of the most elevated portions of the state and well watered with springs, but its proximity to the river and swamps subjects its inhabitants to malarial fevers.

At present (1914) the institution has a population of 332 white men, 325 white women, 296 colored men and 257 colored women. The sexes and colored are separated and cared for in special buildings.

In general, the operation of the institution is divided into two departments, one for the care of chronic cases and one for the care of acute cases. For the chronic cases industrial re-educational pursuits are carried out as far as practicable. The industries consist of farming, sewing, mattress making, labor in a planing and saw mill, carpenter shop, ice and power plant, gardening and dairy department. Weekly dances, occasional theatrical performances, music, games and reading matter are provided for all classes.

The dormitory plan of treatment has been adopted, the isolation room has been abolished, and segregation of classes has been carried out with satisfactory results. Ward dining halls have been replaced by a large congregate dining hall.

Mechanical restraint, while not entirely abolished, has been reduced to a minimum. Iron bars and other devices that tend to give the place a prison atmosphere have been replaced in the newer buildings by light porch screens, and the windows have been left unobstructed as far as safety will permit.

Owing to the mild climate practically the entire population of the hospital is kept in the open air nearly all the year. Even during rainy weather the large and spacious porches eliminate the necessity of keeping the patients indoors.

It is the aim and endeavor of the hospital to provide at least one nurse for each ten patients, and the ward reports are so arranged as to give an accurate report of the conduct and general conditions of each patient during the entire 24 hours.

A new receiving hospital has recently been erected, and has four departments; two for the care of acute medical and surgical cases and two for the care of acute mental cases. A modern operating room equipment has been installed. A diet kitchen enters into the general operation of this department. The hydrotherapeutic equipment consists of continuous bathing devices, steam vapor cabinets, and large porcelain tubs for ordinary hydrotherapeutic uses.

The institution sends a nurse for patients that have been committed from the different portions of the state. By this method tactful nurses bring patients into the hospital without difficulty, whereas, previously, harsh restraint and methods of deceit were often practiced.

The erection of a tuberculosis colony is contemplated in the near future, and this department will probably be constructed along the lines of a tent colony.

RESIDENT OFFICERS (1914).

Worth W. Trammel........................Superintendent.
Dr. Ralph N. Green........................Chief Physician.
Dr. N. F. Barnes..........................Assistant Physician.
Dr. A. E. Conter..........................Assistant Physician.
Dr. H. S. Holloway........................Pathologist.
Dr. J. G. Wilson..........................Dentist.
Rev. R. A. Lowell.........................Chaplain.

THE CARE OF THE INSANE IN GEORGIA.

The first reference of any kind to the necessity of establishing an institution for the care of the insane in Georgia is to be found in the annual message of Governor Wilson Lumpkin, addressed to the Senate and House of Representatives of the Georgia Legislature November 4, 1834, as follows:

"While our thoughts are turned to the abodes of the unfortunate, I would avail myself of the occasion most earnestly to invite the serious attention of the Georgia Assembly to another class of individuals who are to be found in every community and who deserve to be among the first objects of legislative care and attention. I allude to idiots, lunatics and insane persons of every description. Every government possessing the means should, without hesitancy or procrastination, provide suitable asylums for these most distressed and unfortunate of human beings." There is no record of any action following this recommendation.

According to Powell, Georgia made no provision for the care of the insane prior to 1837. He states[1] "that year there came to Milledgeville a Northern philanthropist, whose object was to petition the Legislature to do something for them.

"No blaring trumpet sounded out his fame;
He lived, he died—I do not know his name!"

Milledgeville, the town in which the Legislature met, had a small faculty of distinguished physicians, Drs. White, Fort, Case and Green, and he solicited and received their hearty co-operation in his worthy effort. These physicians, aided by Drs. Philips and Arnold and Judge Harris, who were members of the Legislature, appealed to that body for assistance. The Legislature yielded somewhat reluctantly to their entreaty, made an appropriation, and appointed a commission.

The commission purchased a site, and work on buildings was begun, but owing to great financial depression the institution was

[1] "A Sketch of Psychiatry in the Southern States." Transactions of the American Medico-Psychological Association, Vol. IV, 1897.

not completed for the reception of patients until December, 1842. This institution is now known as the Georgia State Sanitarium, Milledgeville, Ga., and is the only state institution for the care of the mentally defective in Georgia. Its capacity in 1914 was 3400 beds.

Originally the counties were to pay for their pauper insane, but in 1846 they were transferred to state care. Up to 1877 patients were received from other states. At first the institution was in charge of a layman, a physician being employed only when his services were demanded. In 1843 this system was changed and a physician was appointed as superintendent.

It is of interest to note that in 1852 Miss Dix lent her assistance to the then superintendent, Dr. Green, in securing legislative appropriations for added improvements.

At present the institution is under the control of a board of ten trustees, who are appointed by the Governor for a term of two years.

Legal Procedure.—A pay patient in the state may not be admitted unless accompanied by authentic evidence of insanity, or a certificate of three reputable practicing physicians, or from one physician and two respectable citizens. A pay patient not resident may not be admitted, unless record of conviction or certificates of physicians endorsed by the judge having jurisdiction are presented.

A pay patient, resident or non-resident, alleged to be a lunatic may demand a trial by jury. The certificate of the ordinary of the county where an insane negro resides, of his condition, mental and pecuniary, is sufficient to grant his admission to the hospital.

On the sworn petition the ordinary, after notice to the three nearest adult relatives, must issue a commission to 18 discreet persons, requiring any 12 of them, including the physician, to examine the person for whom commitment to the sanitarium is sought. In lunacy cases the number of jurors may be six, one of whom must be a physician, unless 12 are demanded by the person tried, or by his relatives or friends. The commission must find whether the person is to have a guardian or to be committed to the state sanitarium and make return to the ordinary.

Guardians of insane persons may place them in the Georgia State Sanitarium. When there is no guardian for an insane person or the guardian refuses or fails to confine his ward, if any person makes oath that the insane person should not longer be left at large, the ordinary or judge of the Superior Court must issue a warrant, as in criminal cases, for the arrest of the insane person, and, after an investigation of the facts, may commit him to the state sanitarium.

Furlough.—No provision exists for furlough.

Temporary Disposition of Patients.—The superintendent of the sanitarium may receive and provide for persons for a reasonable time.

Appeal from Commitment.—Trial by jury may be had by patients convicted of lunacy if a relative or friend makes affidavit that he believes the alleged cause of commitment did not and does not exist and that the conviction was obtained by fraud, collusion or mistake.

Costs of commitment must be paid by the estate of the insane person; if he has none, out of the county funds; also the cost of conveying the person to the state sanitarium.

GEORGIA STATE SANITARIUM.[1]

MILLEDGEVILLE, GA.

The Georgia State Sanitarium, Milledgeville, Ga., was established by an act of the Legislature of 1837, which made an appropriation and appointed a commission to purchase a site and erect a building.

The commission bought for a small price 40 acres of sterile pine land located on a high hill, about two miles distant from and overlooking the town of Milledgeville. Plans for buildings were secured and work was begun, but, as it was a time of great financial depression and the state was burdened with debt, the Legislature ordered all work to be confined to one building. This was made ready to receive patients, and in December, 1842, the first patient was admitted. The plan of self-support was adopted. The counties were to pay the expenses of their pauper patients and the friends of patients who were able to pay were to provide for their dependents. About 1846 this plan was changed to state care of the pauper insane. Up to 1877 patients were received from other states, but at that time the General Assembly passed an act sending all non-resident patients to their respective states, on account of the overcrowded condition of the institution. During the same year an act was passed making the institution free to all *bona fide* citizens of the state. This act also provided that relatives of patients could deposit with the steward funds for extras to be used by the patients individually, but no part of this was to go to the support of the institution.

When this institution was first opened it was in charge of a layman, and a physician was employed only when his services were needed. These methods were gradually changed. In 1843 Dr. David Cooper was elected superintendent. He was a man of ability, but of great eccentricity, and was entirely unacquainted with the real demands of his work. He retained his position three years,

[1] The material for this history, prior to 1897, has been taken from "A Sketch of Psychiatry in the Southern States" by T. O. Powell, M. D., Transactions of the American Medico-Psychological Association, Vol. IV, pp. 108-112. The history of the institution subsequent to 1897 has been furnished by L. M. Jones, M. D., superintendent.

and during that time had but few patients. The attention of the trustees had been directed to Dr. Thomas F. Green as one who was likely to succeed with a very unpromising enterprise, and he was persuaded to accept the superintendency. Dr. Green was the son of an Irish exile who was in the rebellion of 1798. His father was a physician, a man of high culture, and was professor in the State University. Dr. Green was born in Beaufort, S. C., in 1803. He received his general education at the State University of Georgia and his medical education at Charleston, S. C. He settled in Milledgeville as a physician and was a successful and popular practitioner when he was chosen superintendent of the asylum. The patients he found in the asylum were of the worst possible description. Only those who were a burden at home and for whose recovery there was no hope were sent to the asylum, which, being regarded as a mad-house, inspired the people with terror.

Dr. Green was admirably adapted to perform the difficult task before him. He was a man of kindest heart, most genial manner, and of great enterprise and energy. He soon secured the confidence, not only of the patients, but of the people of the state as well. Year after year he succeeded in obtaining appropriations, in making improvements, in securing a suitable corps of attendants, and in every way providing for the treatment of the insane. Being himself a man of great intelligence, his own measures were eminently wise and he had assistance in the visit of Miss Dix in 1852. He remained in charge of the asylum from 1847 to 1879, when, in the beauty of a serene old age, he suddenly passed away. His monument was the magnificent institution which he had watched over almost from its foundation. For 20 years Dr. Green and Dr. T. O. Powell had been associated as colleagues in the management of the asylum, and when he died Dr. Powell was selected to take charge of it. He remained in charge for nearly 20 years and in connecttion with the institution for 35 years.

In none of the exciting political campaigns of the state was there at any time any decided interference with this institution, and the Legislatures have as a rule generously granted all the requests made by those in charge.

The asylum is charmingly located. A magnificent view is had from every direction, and perhaps in no part of the land is there a better health record. The completion of the second building in

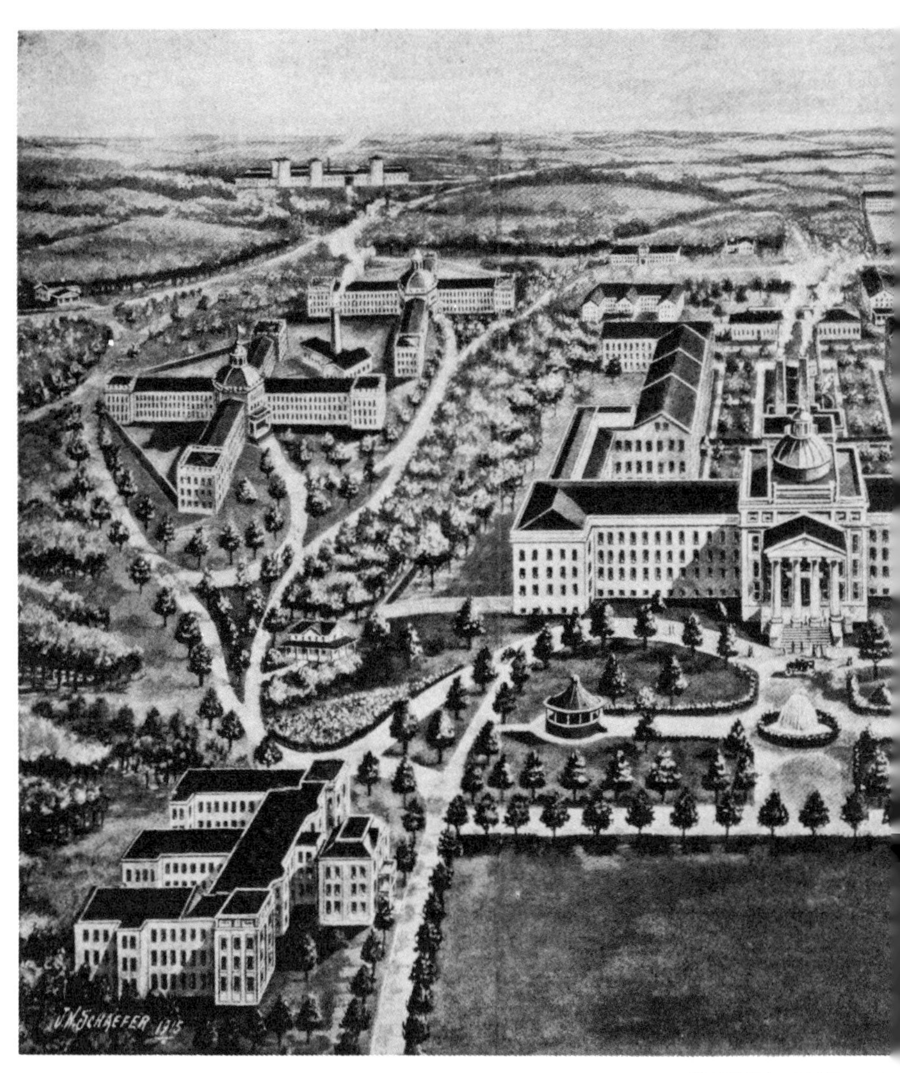

GEORGIA STATE SA

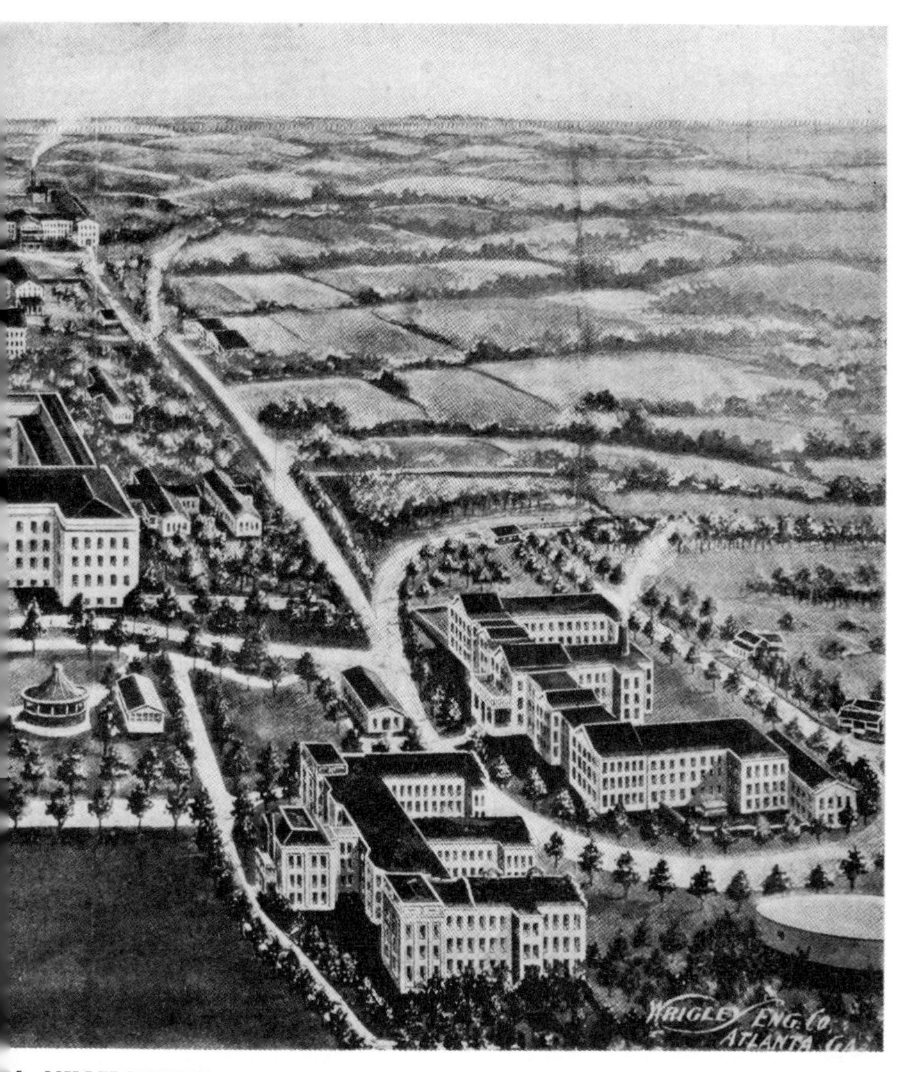

M, MILLEDGEVILLE.

1847 enabled the trustees to make markedly beneficial changes in the asylum. The female patients were placed in the new building, thus entirely separating them from the males. This enlargement also offered greater facilities, and the increased appropriations of money for maintenance enabled the authorities to make many improvements; the substitution of white attendants for negroes who had formerly discharged this duty being one of them. In 1849 it was found urgently necessary to make additional provision for the insane of the state. Plans and estimates were submitted to the Legislature for enlarging the asylum accommodations. The plan contemplated was the Kirkbride plan, consisting of a large, showy building to be erected in front of the existing wings, and additions to the latter which would make the structure in the shape of the capital "E." The Legislature appropriated $10,500 for the enlargement of the institution and in 1851 $24,500 additional. Every dollar of this approriation was expended upon the foundation of the present center building before the walls had reached the surface of the site. Supplemental appropriations were made as follows: In 1853, $56,500; 1855, $110,000; 1857, $63,500; 1858, $30,000.

The building was completed in 1858. It provides accommodations for asylum officials and necessary offices, and for a large number of patients; each patient occupying a separate room 10 by 12 feet. This building, as well as all others attached to it, is divided into sections or wards, each provided with a dining-room, parlor, etc., and all modern improvements. In 1870 and 1871 an appropriation amounting to $105,855 was voted for the enlargement of the asylum. This sum was expended in enlarging the main building. In 1881, at the urgent solicitation of the Board of Trustees, the Legislature decided to erect two separate buildings for white convalescents, one for males and the other for females, and appropriated $165,000 for this purpose. In 1883 a supplemental appropriation amounting to $92,875 was voted by the Legislature. In 1893 the Legislature, after an urgent appeal from the Board of Trustees, voted $100,000 for the erection of additional buildings for white and colored insane. The building for whites has a capacity for 600 patients, and the two annexes to the building for negroes will afford accommodations for about 300 patients.

The emancipation of the negro population in 1865 necessitated asylum accommodations for the insane of this race. In 1866 the Legislature appropriated $11,000 for an insane asylum for negroes. The building was located on the grounds of the asylum for the whites. In 1870, additional accommodations for this class being deemed necessary, the Legislature appropriated $18,000 for enlargement of the building for negroes. In 1879 the Legislature appropriated $25,000 for the same purpose, and in 1881 an appropriation of $82,166 for a new building and heating apparatus for the same was made for the colored insane. These several enlargements provided for 541 negroes. The overcrowded condition of the negro building and the urgent demand for care of a number of negro insane who could not be admitted for want of room caused the Board of Trustees to add two annexes, 128 x 31 feet each, four stories high, to the existing negro asylum. These additional buildings provide accommodations for about 300 patients in the negro institution.

There have been made from time to time large purchases of land adjoining the asylum until the institution now owns over 3000 acres. The institution has its own water works, the water being furnished from a bold stream on its own grounds, and has, besides, a well 960 feet deep, much of it through solid rock.

There is a training school for nurses, and a well equipped laboratory under an efficient neuropathologist. The non-restraint system has prevailed for many years. In 1912 there were over 2100 patients in the institution. The asylum comprises a number of buildings as follows: First, the main building. The front presents a handsome, showy brick structure, three stories high, of Grecian architecture. With the exception of the capitol building in Atlanta, the center asylum building is the handsomest edifice in the State of Georgia. Besides the superintendent's apartments, rooms for visitors and officers, the building accommodates about 500 patients, with necessary nurses, etc. Second, two brick buildings for convalescents, three stories high, accommodating 140 patients and nurses each. These are located on each side of the front of the center building, about 500 feet from the latter, and about 1000 feet apart. Third, in the rear of the center edifice, two brick detached buildings, three stories high, accommodating about 100 patients each. Fourth, two one-story wooden detached buildings for patients too feeble to ascend to the higher floors, accommodating 40 patients each. Fifth, the building for negroes located a quarter of a mile in the rear of the building for whites. This is also of brick, three stories high, and, like the building for whites, is provided with all modern conveniences. It provides for 650 insane negroes, besides the supervisor and attendants. About a mile distant from the asylum proper is located the contagious diseases hospital, which is reserved for treatment of any contagious disease that may be brought into the institution. It accommodates 60 patients and attendants. In addition to the above-described buildings, the new building for whites accommodates 600 patients. The total cost of the land and buildings is more than $1,000,000.

The advisability of establishing a colony for patients who were able to do farm work was agitated for several years, until finally, during the summer of 1898, three frame buildings were erected on a portion of the sanitarium land about three miles from the central plant. One of them, having a capacity for 40 patients, was used as a dormitory, one as a dining hall and kitchen, while the remaining cottage was occupied by the farm supervisor. It was proposed that these buildings should form a nucleus for a larger group to be known as the Farm Colony. In the fall of 1898 about 40 harmless, able-bodied negro men were sent to the colony, and the wisdom of this policy of colonizing them was soon apparent.

In 1900 the overcrowded condition of the institution led the Board of Trustees to ask for an appropriation large enough to warrant the erection of "a building capable of caring for 900 inmates." During the following year the Legislature acted favorably upon this recommendation and appropriated the sum of $150,000 for the erection and equipment of such a building, stipulating, however, that it should be large enough to accommodate 1200 patients. With this fund in hand, two buildings were determined upon, each structure consisting of a central octagon, four stories high, with four wings three stories high radiating therefrom. Between the two buildings and communicating with them by a covered passageway were located two congregate dining halls, with kitchen and boiler room attached.

These buildings were located one-half mile from the central group and were occupied by white male patients in November, 1903.

During the year 1901 a suite of rooms for surgical operations was built as an annex to the infirmary for white females; both operating and sterilizing rooms were equipped with all modern conveniences.

In 1903 three additional frame buildings, each having a capacity for 40 patients, were erected at the colony. A cottage was built for employees and two large barns for the stock. These buildings were lighted by acetylene gas, while two hydraulic engines forced an abundant supply of water into a large steel tank situated near the buildings. About 100 negro males are employed at this colony, and more than 1000 acres of land are cultivated by them, while two large peach orchards and a vineyard bountifully supply all the patients with fruit in season.

The General Assembly in 1905 made a further appropriation of $75,000 for the installment of an improved system of water works and an electric plant. This system was completed in 1907 and the institution has since that date been furnished with an unlimited supply of pure, filtered water from the Oconee River.

On August 18, 1907, the institution suffered an irreparable loss in the death of its venerable superintendent, Dr. T. O. Powell, who had served it in the capacity of assistant physician and later as superintendent for 45 years.

The vacancy caused by the death of Dr. Powell was filled on August 22, 1907, by the election of Dr. L. M. Jones, who had been connected with the institution as assistant physician for 24 years.

During the year 1908 four frame buildings were erected for the use of those suffering from tuberculosis, each having a capacity for 20 patients. On completion, these buildings were immediately filled, and a larger building for white females of the same class is now in process of erection.

In 1909 the Board of Trustees created the office of clinical director. "Two objects were thus sought; one to increase the medical efficiency of the sanitarium; the other to grant the superintendent needed assistance in this important branch of the work and give him more time for the administrative duties of his office."

This action of the board resulted in the establishment of uniform and systematic methods of conducting the medical work of each department of the sanitarium, the institution of daily staff meetings and an increase of interest and efficiency on the part of every member of the staff.

Although the attendants had received instruction in nursing for some years, it was not until the year 1911 that a chartered training school was established, which school is now in successful operation.

From time to time, as the number of patients increased, it has been found necessary to enlarge the medical staff until it is now composed of 16 physicians, the superintendent included.

The scientific department has made steady progression and its standard at the present time is higher than at any former period in the history of the institution.

SUPERINTENDENT AND RESIDENT PHYSICIANS.

David Cooper, M. D. 1843-1846
Thomas F. Green, M. D. 1847-1879
Theophilus O. Powell, M. D. 1879-1907
L. M. Jones, M. D....... 1907-

CLINICAL DIRECTOR.

E. M. Greene, Jr., M. D. 1909-

ASSISTANT PHYSICIANS.

Theophilus O. Powell, M. D. 1863-1879
George M. Lucus, M. D. 1868-1870
Charles H. Bass, M. D... 1870-1872
Thomas H. Kenan, M. D. 1870-1882
W. W. Flewellen, M. D... 1879-1879
J. M. Whitaker, M. D... 1879-1911
Harris Hall, M. D....... 1880-1890
L. M. Jones, M. D....... 1882-1907
W. A. O'Daniel, M. D... 1882-1900
J. C. Patterson, M. D..... 1890 1901
E. M. Greene, Jr., M. D.. 1901-1908
N. P. Walker, M. D..... 1901-1909
R. C. Swint, M. D. 1901-
J. W. Mobley, M. D. 1903-
R. V. Lamar, M. D. 1904-
J. E. Hunt, M. D. 1904-
Y. A. Little, M. D........ 1906-
L. P. Longino, M. D..... 1907-
Y. H. Yarborough, M. D. 1908-
W. J. Cranston, M. D.... 1909-
B. McH. Cline, M. D. ... 1910-
George L. Echols, M. D.. 1910-
J. I. Garrard, M. D...... 1911-
W. F. Tanner, M. D..... 1911-

PATHOLOGISTS.

T. E. Oertel, M. D....... 1895-1899
M. L. Perry, M. D. 1899-1903
W. C. Pumpelly, M. D... 1903-1905
R. V. Lamar, M. D. 1905-1908
D. G. Willets, M. D...... 1908-1910
S. S. Hindman, M. D.... 1912-

ASSISTANT PATHOLOGIST.

J. W. Mobley, M. D...... 1896-1902

ALLEN'S INVALID HOME.

MILLEDGEVILLE, GA.

This institution was opened by Dr. H. D. Allen in 1890, on the site of the old Oglethorpe University, which comprised 40 acres of land and a three-story brick building with 17 rooms and a large hall on the third floor. In 1891 a large house and 46 acres of land, about 150 yards distant from the original building, were purchased by Dr. Allen. This gave the institution two separate buildings, one for men and one for women, and this complete separation of the sexes has continued to the present time.

There have been built since 1891 an additional cottage for men and two buildings for women. Two hundred and fifty-three acres of land have been added to the original holdings, on which are grown a great variety of vegetables, etc., for the use of the institution.

At first only chronic incurable cases were received; the first two patients, received in the early part of 1891, being still in the institution (1915). Afterwards acute cases were accepted, and this practice continues to the present time. It is the endeavor of the Home to have a nurse with every acute case, and to give such cases every possible diversion that their physical condition warrants. There is no attempt made to employ patients other than what they themselves are inclined to do for their own occupation and amusement.

A training school under a charter was started in 1908, and three years later the first class was graduated. Every year since then a similar class has graduated, and, with the exception of one nurse, all those graduated have continued in the service of the institution.

The men nurses have never taken an interest in the training school. The men patients are attended by men nurses exclusively, and the women patients by women nurses. There are no women in the men's building.

The average population is 50 patients, although as many as 65 have been in residence.

Dr. H. D. Allen is superintendent and the assistant physician is Dr. W. A. Ellison.

DR. BRAWNER'S SANITARIUM.

SMYRNA, GA.

This institution was established by Dr. James N. Brawner as a private sanitarium in 1910. It is located at Smyrna, 16 miles from Atlanta, and consists of a 40-room building, erected at a cost of $50,000. There is a truck farm in connection with the sanitarium and a training school for nurses, with eight pupil nurses in attendance.

Dr. James N. Brawner has associated with him, Dr. Hansell Crenshaw.

AFTON VILLA SANITARIUM.

ATLANTA, GA.

Afton Villa Sanitarium, which was opened June 1, 1915, is the successor to Howell Park Sanitarium, which was organized by Dr. J. Chester King in October, 1905, as a private institution for the treatment of nervous and mild mental cases, alcoholic and drug addictions and general invalidism.

The original building was located in a suburb of Atlanta, and consisted of a three-story brick and stone structure, with slate roof.

The new institution is located on a tract of 25 acres on Peachtree Road, Atlanta. The building is of concrete and pressed brick, with tile roof, and has a capacity of 125 rooms. It is modern in every respect, being modelled on the best of European and American institutions of like character. The value of the entire plant is estimated at $150,000.

The sanitarium possesses a complete equipment, such as is found in a first-class clinical establishment.

The nursing is entrusted to carefully trained nurses and a staff of skilled persons is in attendance for the various forms of treatment.

Dr. J. Chester King, who was the founder and medical director of Howell Park Sanitarium since its organization in 1905, is the medical director and proprietor of Afton Villa Sanitarium. Dr. W. A. Gardner is assistant medical director.

THE CARE OF THE INSANE IN IDAHO.[1]

Prior to 1881 no provision was made for the care of the insane in Idaho beyond what could be procured by county commissioners in private families. In 1881 the Legislature of the state authorized the Governor and the president of the legislative council to make a contract with the owners or managers of some institution, either in Oregon or California, for the care of the insane of Idaho who were public charges. A contract was finally made with a private asylum, conducted by Drs. Loryea and Hawthorne, in East Portland, Ore., which continued in force until October, 1883, when Oregon established a state asylum at Salem. The authorities of Idaho thereupon made a contract with the authorities of Oregon to care for her insane. This arrangement continued until 1886, when the State of Idaho established an asylum about one mile east of the village of Blackfoot. This institution is now known as the Idaho Insane Asylum, Blackfoot, and has a capacity of 300 beds.

In March, 1905, the Idaho State Legislature appropriated $30,000 for the erection of a second state asylum for the care of the insane. The new institution was located at Orofino, in the northern part of the state, and was opened in April, 1906. It is now known as the Northern Idaho Sanitarium, Orofino, and has a capacity of 250 beds.

A third institution, the Idaho Sanitarium for the Feeble-minded and Epileptic, was established in 1912 and located in Boise Valley; it is still in process of construction.

The state institutions are under the direction of separate boards of directors, which consist of three persons, appointed by the Governor, for a term of two years. The superintendent of each individual hospital is required to be a graduate in medicine with at least five years' practice.

No non-resident insane person must be received in the asylums unless he becomes insane within the state. Indigent insane must have preference.

[1] The material for this chapter has been furnished by John W. Givens, M. D., superintendent of the Northern Idaho Sanitarium, Orofino, Ida.

Legal Procedure.—If affidavits satisfactory to the magistrate of the county that a person is so far disordered as to endanger health, person or property are presented, he must cause him to be arrested and taken before any judge of a court of record for examination. Two or more witnesses acquainted with such insane person and at least one graduate physician must testify at such examination. If the physician, after hearing the testimony and making the examination, believes him to be dangerously insane, he must make a certificate as to the fact. The judge, after such examination and certificates, must order that he be confined in the insane hospital.

Appeal.—Upon petition a writ of *habeas corpus* must be granted by the circuit court or by the district court.

Costs of commitment are paid by the hospital; the physician by the treasurer of the county.

The judge must inquire into the ability of the insane person to pay for his transportation to the asylum, the expense of the examination and the actual charges and expenses for the time that such person may remain in the asylum. In case an insane person committed to the asylum is possessed of real or personal property sufficient to pay such charges and expenses, the judge must appoint a guardian for him, who must pay to the Board of Directors the sum for the maintenance and clothing of such ward.

The cost of maintenance of indigent patients is a charge against the state.

IDAHO INSANE ASYLUM.

Blackfoot, Ida.

The Idaho Insane Asylum, the first asylum to be erected in the state for the care of the insane, was established in 1886 upon a tract of seven acres of land about one mile east of the village of Blackfoot. This location was in a section of the country which had always been known as a part of the Great American Desert. Two trunk railway lines crossed the state from east to west, the Oregon Short Line through the south and the Northern Pacific Railway through the north. These railways were connected by the Utah Northern Railroad, extending north and south through Idaho. The village of Blackfoot being located upon this railway, was fairly central for transportation.

The asylum when erected was a three-story building, with a basement 60 x 70 feet. The basement was of stone and the outside walls of the first and second stories were of brick, but the inside walls of the first, second and third stories and the outside walls of the third story were of wood. The cost of construction and furnishing was only $30,000.

In July, 1886, the directors appointed Dr. T. T. Cabiness, of California, medical superintendent; he served until November, 1886, when he was succeeded by Dr. John W. Givens, who had formerly been an assistant physician of the Oregon State Insane Asylum.

In 1886 a kitchen, built of corrugated iron, one story in height and 26 by 28 feet in dimensions, was added. A water supply was procured from a well connected with a water tank of the capacity of 10,000 gallons, placed upon a wooden water tower, supplied by a wind mill attached to the well. From this tank water was pumped to the asylum buildings.

During the summer 73 acres of land surrounding the buildings were purchased and fenced in and 15 acres were put in cultivation. A ditch six feet in width and three-fourths of a mile long was constructed to convey water from an irrigating ditch to the asylum land. The following year a second irrigating ditch, seven miles long, 12 feet wide and three feet deep was constructed from the Snake River to irrigate the asylum farm, as the former irrigating ditch from Blackfoot River had proved insufficient. In the same year an appropriation of $15,000 was received from the Legislature to erect an additional building.

During the night of November 24, 1889, a disastrous fire of unknown origin occurred in the asylum, which resulted in the loss of the lives of two patients and the destruction of the main building and its contents. Fortunately the new building for which provision had been made during the previous year and which was nearly ready for occupancy was not injured to any extent. Of the 67 patients at the time in the asylum, one man and one woman are known to have perished in the fire, their charred remains being found in the ruins. Four men and one woman were missing and it was never known whether they escaped or were burned to death. The loss of property was about $25,000. The lesson taught by the fire was that an asylum population is most helpless at such a time, and the directors decided that all future buildings for patients must be fireproof. Unfortunately, all the records of the asylum were destroyed at this time.

In 1889 the building previously referred to was finished; it was 117 feet long and 30 feet wide and two stories in height. It contained 21 sleeping rooms, four dining rooms, three bath rooms and lavatories. A wooden building 30 x 60 feet for a laundry was also built. Brickmaking as an industry was introduced during the year, 75,000 bricks being made and burned.

In 1891 a new building, situated about 700 feet above the old one, overlooking the village of Blackfoot and commanding a good view of the Snake River Valley, was constructed.

In 1892 a ward building 30 x 50 feet, two stories high, was added; also an orchard of 1500 trees was planted, and a farm of 40 acres of choice land adjoining the asylum was purchased. In 1894 an electric light plant was installed, 360 acres of land adjoining the asylum were purchased and 1480 acres near the asylum were procured through "relinquishment." This gave the asylum 2100 acres of land.

The law was changed so that all patients were brought to the asylum by attendants sent out by the institution; men by men attendants, women by women attendants. This law did away with the manifest impropriety of insane women being brought at times a distance of 800 miles under the care of a sheriff only.

In this year an additional building 24 x 25 feet was erected and a well 50 feet deep and eight feet in diameter was dug; a new ward was also built and 2000 bricks were made by the labor of the patients.

In 1898 an additional ward building was constructed mainly of bricks manufactured on the premises, and 100 acres of land were put under cultivation. In 1899 the whole of the 2000 acres of land belonging to the asylum were fenced in, and a pump was put in the well for domestic purposes, operated by electric power from the American Falls, 50 miles distant.

MEDICAL SUPERINTENDENTS.

Dr. T. T. Cabiness...... 1886-1886
Dr. John W. Givens..... 1886-1895
Dr. I. N. Moore......... 1895-1896
Dr. John W. Givens..... 1896-1905
Dr. C. H. Hoover....... 1905-1911
Dr. Francis Poole....... 1911-1913
Dr. George Hyde........ 1913-

THE NORTHERN IDAHO SANITARIUM.

OROFINO, IDA.

In March, 1905, the Idaho State Legislature made an appropriation of $30,000 to buy a site for the erection of a second state asylum for the care of the insane in one of the northern counties, and in addition gave $20,000 to maintain it for two years. The law further authorized the Governor to appoint a commission of five persons, of which he was to be one, to select the site.

The commissioners appointed were Governor Frank R. Gooding, John W. Givens, medical superintendent of the State Asylum at Blackfoot; James Stephenson, State Engineer; Robert Hays, an attorney, and Robert Aikman, a prominent business man. They selected a site near Orofino, in a pine grove overlooking the Clearwater River, and on a branch line of the Northern Pacific Railroad. The site was fairly central for Northern Idaho; it had an agreeable climate, a long growing season, and short, mild winters. All crops of the temperate section and also most fruits grow well in the region.

The Governor appointed J. K. Bell, J. G. Rowton and T. J. Taylor a board of directors to manage the asylum, who in turn appointed Dr. John W. Givens, medical superintendent in July, 1905.

The medical superintendent took 20 male and 5 female patients from the State Asylum at Blackfoot, together with a few attendants, to the new site, made them reasonably comfortable in tents and temporary wooden buildings and commenced the work of building the new institution.

Four hundred thousand bricks were made at the building site. Masons and carpenters were employed, and a four-story brick and stone building 55 x 60 was ready for occupancy by the following April, since which time all insane persons from Northern Idaho have been received into this asylum.

In addition to the 30 patients already brought from the State Asylum at Blackfoot on June 27, 1906, 18 other female patients were transferred from the same institution. These patients had been committed originally from the counties of Northern Idaho.

During the first year $29,218.68 were expended from the fund of $30,000 for 235 acres of land and for clearing and cultivating about 20 acres of it, planting 1500 fruit trees, piping water from springs in the adjoining hills to the asylum for domestic use, and for the construction of a central building, barns and other farm buildings.

From the maintenance appropriations of $20,000 there were expended $15,633 for furniture, household furnishing supplies, provisions, clothing, fuel and the pay of employees.

Many improvements of wards and grounds were made during the year 1906. Twenty acres of asylum lands were cleared of brush and stumps and put under cultivation, and a kiln of 250,000 bricks was made ready for burning in anticipation of additional buildings.

On July 1, 1907, there were in the asylum 71 patients, of whom 44 were males and 27 females. During the year 65 patients were admitted—50 males and 15 females.

The total number treated in the asylum during the year was 136—94 males and 42 females.

The bricks made by the employees and patients during the previous season were used in the construction of a ward building 33 x 70 feet, of two stories, and a laundry building 25 x 50 feet, of one story.

An additional orchard of 1000 trees was planted during the year; and a silo of 100 tons capacity was constructed and filled with corn grown on the asylum farm.

July 1, 1908, there were in the asylum 67 males and 34 females; total 101. Fifty males and 24 females were admitted during the year.

The whole number under treatment during the year was 118 males and 56 females.

A ward building three stories high, from 30 to 50 feet wide and 150 feet long, was erected during the year. This building was of stone, cement and brick throughout, and of fireproof construction except the floors and doors. Electric wires and lights were installed in all the occupied buildings.

An irrigating ditch one and one-half miles long from Orofino Creek across the asylum grounds was dug, and afforded water to irrigate 25 acres of garden and orchard. Roads were widened and improved and a board side-walk four feet wide was completed from the asylum buildings to the Northern Pacific Railway.

July 1, 1909, there were in the asylum 81 males and 40 females; total 121. Seventy-nine males and 21 females were admitted during the year. The whole number under treatment during the year was 160 males and 61 females.

A hot water heating apparatus was put in the ward built the previous year, which comfortably warms it. The new ward is now occupied, although not entirely finished. The laundry was equipped with a steam boiler, a metal steam dry-room, an extractor, an electric motor and electric hand irons, and the hand washing machines have been fitted with power attachments, so that all laundry work is now done by machinery except such portion of the ironing as requires a power mangle.

Two additional water tanks, each 16 feet in diameter and 16 feet high, were placed on the side hill 150 feet higher than the asylum buildings and a three-inch pipe was laid from the tanks to the building, a distance of 100 feet. A three-inch steel water pipe has been laid from Rock Creek, a distance of 2600 feet, to supply these tanks. Three hydraulic rams were installed to supplement the domestic water supply. Rams supplied with water from the irrigating ditch lift the water 300 feet to the reservoir tanks above the buildings. The water thus procured by gravity from Rock Creek and by hydraulic ram from the irrigating ditch is for the present sufficient for domestic use.

July 1, 1910, there were in the asylum 179 patients, of whom 126 were males and 53 females. During the year 66 patients were admitted—47 males and 19 females. The total number treated in the asylum during the year was 249—175 males and 74 females.

In February, 1912, the total number of patients was 217—148 males and 69 females.

There are 365 acres of land in the asylum plant, and the total value of the asylum property is estimated at $165,000. In 1913 the Legislature of Idaho changed the name of the institution to the Northern Idaho Sanitarium.

MEDICAL SUPERINTENDENT.

Dr. John W. Givens..... 1905-

THE IDAHO SANITARIUM FOR THE FEEBLE-MINDED AND EPILEPTIC.

BOISE, IDA.

This institution was established in 1912 and is still in process of construction. It has been located on a tract of 2000 acres of raw sage brush land, in Boise Valley.

The institution is to be developed on the cottage plan with cut stone two-story buildings of the colonial type. The buildings are to be placed in a circle around the crest of the site, which is on a knoll.

Much of the preliminary work has been done by the prisoners from the state penitentiary.

The establishment of the institution has been under the direction of Dr. John W. Givens, superintendent of the Northern Idaho Sanitarium, but, owing to the parsimony of the Legislature, but little has been accomplished. The legislative appropriation for 1913 was for $17,000 only. In consequence the center building, 120 feet by 40 feet, two stories in height, of cut stone, has remained unfinished, and, as a result, no patients have been received. It is doubtful if the institution will be opened for some years, as the state is passing through a period of extreme economy.

THE CARE OF THE INSANE IN ILLINOIS.

Prior to the establishment of the Illinois State Hospital for the Insane, now the Jacksonville State Hospital, the insane of the state were cared for in jails and almshouses, and, according to Miss Dix, "in even more dismal abodes—noisome pens and cages unfit for human habitation." No doubt many unfortunates wandered at large, a prey to ill treatment and wretchedness, and that, as regards the neglect of the insane, the State of Illinois but repeated the history of nearly every other state in the Union.

In the summer of 1846 Dorothea Dix travelled through the northern, central and southern districts of the state for the purpose of investigating conditions then prevailing. In December of the same year she returned to Illinois and, when the Legislature assembled in January, 1847, presented an eloquent and effective memorial at a special hearing given for the purpose before the House and Senate. Her labors resulted in the passage of an act creating the Illinois State Hospital for the Insane, which was signed by the Governor in March, 1847.

The "hospital" was located within four miles of Jacksonville, in Morgan County, and the act of incorporation provided that in the admission of cases preference should be given to "recent cases," and also that "indigent insane in this state shall always have precedence."

Work was begun on the hospital in the fall of 1847, but it was not until November, 1851, that patients could be received. The legal name of the institution was changed to Illinois Central Hospital for the Insane, in 1875, and to Jacksonville State Hospital, in 1910.

Since the establishment of this hospital the State of Illinois has at different times made appropriations for additional hospitals for the care of the insane. In the order of their establishment they are as follows:

The Northern Illinois Hospital and Asylum for the Insane, established in 1869 and opened for the reception of patients on April 3, 1872. In 1875 the name of the institution was changed to Illinois Northern Hospital for the Insane and in 1910 to Elgin State Hospital, by which name it is now known.

The Anna State Hospital, formerly known as the Illinois Southern Hospital for the Insane, established the same year as the Elgin State Hospital (1869) and opened for the reception of patients December 15, 1873.

Kankakee State Hospital, established in 1877 as the Illinois Eastern Hospital for the Insane and located at Kankakee. The name of the hospital was changed in 1910 to Kankakee State Hospital. The first patients were received on December 4, 1879.

The Chester State Hospital, instituted in 1889 under the name of the Asylum for Insane Criminals, was opened for the reception of patients in November, 1891.

Peoria State Hospital, established in 1895, under the name of The Illinois Asylum for the Incurable Insane; this name was subsequently changed to The Illinois General Hospital for the Insane, and again to Peoria State Hospital, by which it is now known. It was opened for the reception of patients on February 10, 1902.

The same Legislature that established the Peoria State Hospital (1895) also established the Illinois Western Hospital for the Insane. This institution is now known as the Watertown State Hospital, and was opened on May 16, 1898.

On July 1, 1912, the State of Illinois assumed charge of the Cook County Insane Asylum and changed the name of the institution to the Chicago State Hospital. This institution was the development of a part of the county poor farm, established at the town of Jefferson, about 12 miles northwest of Chicago, in 1851, which had cared for the insane of Cook County from its opening in 1854 up to its taking over by the state.

The Alton State Hospital is the ninth institution for the care of the insane in Illinois. It is still in process of construction, although since December 28, 1914, small numbers of patients have been housed in farm buildings already in existence at the time the site of the hospital was purchased.

There are two other institutions for the care of the mentally diseased of Illinois.

The Lincoln State School and Colony, located at Lincoln, was established in 1865 for the "instruction and training of idiots and feeble-minded children in the State of Illinois;" originally located at Jacksonville, it was removed to its present location on October 4, 1883.

The Illinois Colony for Epileptics, now in process of construction at Dixon, Ill., was established by the General Assembly in 1913.

In 1907 the state established the Illinois State Psychopathic Institute, and located it on the grounds of the Kankakee State Hospital. Its object is to improve the general care and treatment of the insane in the State of Illinois, and to conduct research into the etiology of mental disorders.

The Chicago Detention Hospital is a Cook County institution and merely holds patients until they can be transferred to the state hospitals at Elgin, Kankakee or Chicago. No other Illinois city maintains a detention hospital.

Each of the nine state hospitals in Illinois is in a sense a receiving or detention hospital as, under the lunacy law, any person may be detained or held 10 days in any institution pending investigation as to his mental condition, and this without other legal process.

On January 1, 1910, the act creating the present Illinois State Board of Administration went into effect, and the board assumed the management of 18 state charitable institutions and the State Psychopathic Institute.[1] Since that date there have been added two new institutions, making 21 now under the control of this board. They are: Elgin State Hospital, Kankakee State Hospital, Jacksonville State Hospital, Anna State Hospital, Watertown State Hospital, Peoria State Hospital, Chicago State Hospital, Chester State Hospital, Lincoln State School and Colony, The Illinois School for the Deaf, Jacksonville; The Illinois School for the Blind, Jacksonville; The Illinois Industrial Home for the Blind, Chicago; The Illinois Soldiers' and Sailors' Home, Quincy; The Soldiers' Widows' Home of Illinois, Wilmington; The Illinois Soldiers' Orphans' Home, Normal; The Illinois Charitable Eye and Ear Infirmary, Chicago; The State Training School for Girls, Geneva; The St. Charles School for Boys, St. Charles; Alton State Hospital, Dixon State Colony for Epileptics, and the State Psychopathic Institute, Kankakee, Ill.

The combined population of all of these institutions for both inmates and employees is 24,349. Of this number, 20,947 are

[1] The portion of this article dealing with the Illinois State Board of Administration was prepared by Frank D. Whipp, fiscal supervisor, as of March 1, 1915.

inmates and 3402 are employees. The inmates are classified as: insane, 15,383; feeble-minded, 1635; deaf, 388; blind, 312; soldiers' institutions, 2104; eye and ear infirmary, 222; girls' and boys' training schools, 903. The ratio of the inmates to employees in the state institutions on a total basis is 6.16; for the insane group it is 6.05, and for all other classes 6.46.

Since the Board of Administration has been in charge of these institutions, covering a period of over five years, it has disbursed appropriations for operating expenses and permanent improvements amounting to over $21,250,000. Two years ago the General Assembly appropriated the sum of $11,346,551 for these institutions. These appropriations were for ordinary operating expenses and permanent improvements for the two years ending June 30, 1915.

In addition to the 21 institutions, the board also maintains five separate sub-departments, namely: Visitation and instruction of adult blind, visitation of dependent, neglected and delinquent children, support of inmates, supervising engineer, and deportation agent.

For over 40 years the state charitable institutions of Illinois, were managed by separate boards of trustees, consisting of three members in a majority of the institutions, and five members for the remainder. These trustees served without pay and usually held monthly or quarterly meetings for the transaction of their business. The combined membership of these boards was about 60, and in addition to the trustees each institution had a local treasurer, and all funds were deposited in local banks. When the act creating the Board of Administration went into effect the offices held by these 60 trustees and 18 local treasurers were abolished.

The origin of the Board of Administration dates back 15 or 20 years. The first step toward centralization of authority and management of state charitable institutions in Illinois was taken about this time in a recommendation made by the Illinois State Commissioners of Public Charities, the matter being under consideration and discussion from time to time by members of the General Assembly and the state officials. The proposed legislation first took concrete form in 1908, when the Illinois State Commissioners of Public Charities reported to the Governor of Illinois, recommending the change. The bill introduced into the General Assembly was prepared by a committee appointed by the president of the State Board of Charities, made up as follows: Frank H. Armstrong, Chicago; Jesse A. Baldwin, Chicago; A. C. Bartlett, Chicago; Judge W. N. Butler, Cairo; John W. Bunn, Springfield; William Butterworth, Moline; James B. Forgan, Chicago; H. A. Haugan, Chicago; Prof. Charles R. Henderson, University of Chicago; C. E. Hull, Salem; F. T. Joyner, East St. Louis; R. A. Keyes, Chicago; Sherman C. Kingsley, Chicago; Judge Julian W. Mack, Chicago; William B. Moulton, Chicago; Dr. Harold N. Moyer, Chicago; Dr. Frank P. Norbury, Jacksonville; Dr. Hugh T. Patrick, Chicago; Byron L. Smith, Chicago; Charles A. Starne, Springfield; Bishop John L. Spalding, Peoria; B. E. Sunny, Chicago; Frank D. Whipp, department and institution auditor, Springfield. The framers of the bill collected expert opinions from various sources, studied systems of administration in America and abroad, and, as a result, submitted the bill, which was finally passed in a modified form by the General Assembly.

The members of the Board of Administration controlling these 21 institutions are five in number, serving six-year overlapping terms, each receiving a salary of $6000 per annum and necessary traveling expenses. One member must be qualified by experience to advise the board regarding the care and treatment of the insane, feeble-minded and the epileptic. One member is designated by the Governor to act as president, and the three remaining members must be citizens of Illinois, whose professions are not specified. Of the five members, not more than three can belong to the same political party. The law provides that members shall devote their whole time to the work of the state and not engage in any other gainful occupation or pursuit. The board is given absolute authority to administer the business affairs of these institutions, and has the power to appoint and discharge, subject to the rules of the State Civil Service Commission, all employees of the state charitable institutions. In addition to the Board of Administration, the law provides for the appointment of a Charities Commission, which is in no way responsible for the business affairs of the institutions. It is composed of five non-salaried members, serving five-year overlapping terms, and not more than three can belong to the same political party.

On July 31, 1909, the Governor of the State of Illinois appointed the members of the Board of Administration. They were: Lawrence Y. Sherman, Springfield, president; Thomas O'Connor, Peoria; Judge Benjamin R. Burroughs, Edwardsville; Dr. James L. Greene, Kankakee; and Frank D. Whipp, Springfield. Judge Sherman, president of the board, has held some of the most important offices in the gift of the people of this state; he has served continuously as a member of the State Legislature, has been Speaker of the House of Representatives, Lieutenant Governor of the State, and is now United States Senator from the State of Illinois. Dr. Greene was formerly connected with the state insane hospital service in the State of Nebraska, and at the time of his appointment was superintendent of the Illinois Eastern Hospital for the Insane, at Kankakee. He retired from the board in 1911 to become superintendent of the Arkansas State Hospital for the Insane at Little Rock, Ark. He has recently resigned from that position and is now practicing his profession at Hot Springs, Ark. Judge Burroughs is a lawyer, and for over 20 years was circuit judge in his district. For six years he was justice of the Appellate Court of the Third District of Illinois. He also retired as a member of the board in 1913 to engage in the practice of his profession at Edwardsville, Ill. Mr. O'Connor has been a member of the board since its creation. He was formerly in the plumbing business in the City of Peoria, and two years prior to his appointment was Mayor of the City of Peoria. Mr. Whipp, who has also been a member since the board was created, has devoted 25 years of his life to the charities service of the state. He was formerly connected with the State Board of Charities as assistant secretary in auditing accounts of the state institutions. When he was appointed a member of the board he held the position of department and institution auditor for the Governor of Illinois.

Since the original board was appointed Judge Sherman has been succeeded by Fred J. Kern, of Belleville, who is editor and proprietor of the Belleville *News-Democrat,* and for five successive years was Mayor of the City of Belleville. Mr. Kern has represented his district in Congress. Judge Burroughs has been succeeded by James Hyland, for several years engaged in business in the City of Chicago. Dr. Greene, who retired as a member of the board, was succeeded as alienist by Dr. Frank P.

Norbury, who was then superintendent of the Kankakee State Hospital. He has also retired to engage in private practice, and is now operating the Maplewood Sanitarium at Jacksonville, a private sanitarium for the care and treatment of mental and nervous diseases. On December 1, 1913, Dr. George A. Zeller, superintendent of the Peoria State Hospital, succeeded Dr. Norbury as alienist of the board. Dr. Zeller has had considerable experience in the medical service of the United States Army in the Philippines, and for 16 years, since the inception of the Peoria State Hospital, he was its superintendent.

The personnel of the Board of Administration at present is: Fred J. Kern, Belleville, president; Thomas O'Connor, Peoria; James Hyland, Chicago; Dr. George A. Zeller, Peoria; and Frank D. Whipp, Springfield.

Voluntary Patients.—Any voluntary patient may be admitted on his own written application, accompanied by a certificate from the county court of the county in which he resides. All voluntary patients have the right to leave on giving three days' notice to the superintendent.

Insane persons not residents may not be detained in any private institution unless committed in accordance with the laws of the state in which they are residents or with the laws of Illinois.

No private patient may be admitted to a state hospital until a bond with sureties has been filed with the superintendent and approved by the county judge to provide suitably for him and to remove him when required.

Legal Procedure in Commitment.—No person not legally adjudged insane may be restrained of his liberty except during temporary detention for a reasonable time, not exceeding 10 days, pending a judicial investigation of his mental condition.

Any reputable citizen of the county in which a person supposed to be insane resides or is found may file with the clerk of the county court a sworn statement that the person named is insane and requires restraint or commitment to some hospital. When the person has not been examined by a physician the judge may appoint a qualified physician of the county to make such examination. The hearing may take place with or without the presence of the person affected, but not until he has been notified.

Inquests in lunacy must be by jury or a commission of two licensed physicians. If no jury be demanded, the judge must appoint a commission of two qualified physicians in regular and active practice, residents of the county and of known competency and integrity, to make a personal examination of the patient and file a sworn report of the result of their inquiries with conclusions and recommendations. The commissioners have power to administer oaths and take sworn testimony. Inquests by jury must consist of six persons and one of them at least must be a qualified physician. Inquests in lunacy may be in open court or in chambers or at the home of the person alleged to be insane. The judge may require all persons other than the patient, his friends, witnesses, licensed attorneys and officers of the court to withdraw from the room during the inquest.

The jury or commission must furnish answers to the interrogatories that may be prescribed by the commission of public charities and certify to their correctness. The interrogatories must be submitted to the medical member or members of the jury or commission by the court. The court may set them aside and order another inquest.

Upon the return of the findings of the jury or commission the court must enter the proper order for his discharge with or without conditions, or remand him to the custody of friends, or commit him to some hospital or asylum.

Appeal from Commitment.—Every person is entitled to the benefit of the writ of *habeas corpus* and the question of insanity must be decided at the hearing. If the person is adjudged sane the court must rescind the judgment of insanity.

Costs of Commitment of county patients are paid by the county treasury; in cases of private patients, by the guardian or conservator out of the estate. When the person is found not to be insane the court may require the costs to be paid by the person filing the application for commitment.

JACKSONVILLE STATE HOSPITAL.[1]

JACKSONVILLE, ILL.

The first movement for the public care of the insane in the State of Illinois was inspired and inaugurated by Dorothea Dix, who visited the state in 1846, traveling through the northern, central and southern districts, informing herself as to the conditions then and there prevailing. Miss Dix was then near the completion of the great mission of service and self-sacrifice in the cause of humanity to which her life had been devoted for many years.

After her first visit to Illinois in the summer of 1846, Miss Dix returned in December of that year. She came from New England to the state capital at Springfield, by a circuitous route; first journeying to Pittsburgh by rail and going thence by boat on the Ohio and Mississippi rivers to St. Louis, then to Springfield by stage.[2] The fatigue and exposure of this protracted journey rendered her an invalid much of the winter.

When the Legislature assembled in January, 1847, Miss Dix presented an eloquent and effective memorial at a special hearing given for the purpose before the House and Senate. William Thomas, of Jacksonville, prepared and introduced the bill to incorporate an institution for the insane. Miss Dix established herself for the time being at Springfield. She was not well enough to go out to meet and talk with members of the Legislature, so she made daily lists of names of the members and invited them to come to her hotel, that she might converse with them regarding the bill.[3] She thus met all, or nearly all, of the members of the Legislature. She set forth what she termed "a just claim," rather than an appeal to "charity." She protrayed eloquently the condition of

[1] By Richard Dewey, M. D.

[2] Encyclopedia Britannica, 11th ed., Vol. VIII, p. 346: As an illustration of Miss Dix's resourcefulness, a friend of hers (Mrs. Margaret Mewill, of Portland, Me.), related to the author that when Miss Dix was starting for the West, in order to be prepared for contingencies, she carried with her a box containing carpenter's tools, nails, rope, leather, etc., things likely to be needed in case of accident to vehicle or harness in that unsettled country.

[3] Twenty-third biennial report of Dr. H. F. Carriel, p. 17.

these helpless fellow beings, denied the light of reason and hidden from the light of day in jails and almshouses. She also described even more dismal abodes which she had seen and learned of in her tour of Illinois; noisome pens and cages unfit for human habitation.

Miss Dix's public presentation of her memorial in Illinois and the directing of attention to these afflicted people, who, to the careless world, were "out of sight" and "out of mind," met with the same interest and success she had achieved in other communities. Her labors resulted in the passage through the Legislature of the act of incorporation creating the "Illinois State Hospital for the Insane,"[1] which became a law by the signature of the Governor in March, 1847.

The act creating the new hospital provided that it should be located within four miles of Jacksonville, in Morgan County, Ill. It is worthy of note that even in that early day the name "hospital," rather than "asylum," was employed. The act of incorporation provided that in the admission of patients preference should be given to "recent cases," and also that the "indigent insane in this state shall always have precedence." A tax levy, expected to yield $20,000 per year for each of three years, was provided for in the law, which further required that 250 patients should be provided for in the buildings to be erected. The per capita allowance on this basis was $240 per patient, a sum hardly sufficient even in that day to build in a substantial manner and provide the necessary furniture, fixtures, heating apparatus, etc., but the state was at this time burdened with debt, the result of financial mismanagement.

On March 20, 1847, seven of the nine men named in the act of incorporation as trustees, to-wit, Nathaniel English, James Dunlap, Bezaleel Gillett, Samuel D. Lockwood, Owen M. Long, Joseph Morton, and William Thomas, met and organized. Samuel D. Lockwood was elected president, William Thomas was made secretary, and John J. Harden, one of the incorporators, having died, the Governor appointed Wm. W. Happy his successor. John Henry, of the original nine, who was not present at the first meeting, subsequently qualified and thus made the board complete.

[1] The legal name was changed to "Illinois Central Hospital for the Insane" in 1875, and to "Jacksonville State Hospital" in 1910.

James Jackson was subsequently elected treasurer and John Henry was appointed steward. One hundred and sixty acres of land were purchased for the sum of $3631.42. This land was situated south of the City of Jacksonville, one and one-half miles from the court house of Morgan County. A beginning upon the foundation of the central structure was made in the fall of 1847, the plan of the state hospital at Indianapolis being adopted largely as a model. In August, 1848, Dr. J. M. Higgins, of Griggsville, Ill., was appointed medical superintendent. His duties which did not begin until April 16, 1849, consisted mainly of the supervision of building operations.

In 1848 and 1849 various hindrances operated to prevent the completion of the building; in five years' time nearly 50 independent contracts were made in expending $80,000. It was not until November, 1851, that patients could be received. The second biennial report of the trustees for 1849 and 1850 feelingly alludes to the difficulties encountered, as follows (page 68): "How, then, shall we, a people of yesterday, expect to rear an asylum for our insane fellows upon the ground from which we have but just now frightened the panther and the prairie wolf, without delays and disappointments?" Allusion is made in this report to the fact that investigation of the cost of existing institutions in the United States shows that $800 to $1000 per capita is the rule, while here $240 was a limit fixed by law. Even this amount had not been realized from the tax levy provided in the act of incorporation.

Reception of patients began November 3, 1851, and from that day to December 1, 1852, 138 were received. Two wards only were complete, all males being congregated in one and all females in the other, without regard to mental state. The report for 1851 and 1852 presents a list of six instead of nine trustees, owing to a change in the law. The inability to classify the patients and the fact that work was still progressing on the building, which as yet had no heating apparatus except cast iron stoves, occasioned many difficulties. The trustees, however, present in the report covering this period a table showing that the hospital under their direction as compared with 10 institutions in other states had a larger percentage of cures, except one, the smallest death-rate and lowest per capita expense; and their pride is perhaps pardonable in feeling that these results are most creditable to "our infant institution." At this time there were already 240 applications for admission on file which could not be granted for want of room. There were 82 patients under care December 1, 1852, and eight attendants. An unfortunate patient lost her life from her clothes catching fire by contact with the stove. This accident hastened the introduction of steam heat. There is a description of the new apparatus, and the superintendent remarked, " one is reminded of the delightful atmosphere of summer " by the " fresh, warm air, agreeable to the feeling and eminently conducive to health " produced by the heating system. During this period the hospital barn was set on fire by a patient who had been considered harmless. These difficulties, in some measure inseparable from the period of inception, led to criticism, reasonable and unreasonable.

A " table of causation " of insanity in the 138 patients received is presented and one is reminded, by seeing " spiritual rappings " given as the cause in two cases, that the cult of " table turning " and mediumistic wonder-working as developed by the " Fox Sisters " was then in its ascendancy. Beginning in 1853, a time of unrest for the administration was experienced. The Board of Trustees had not been wholly unanimous in the first election of a superintendent and further differences having arisen, in June, 1853, they declared the office of superintendent vacant and ordered that the assistant physician assume the superintendent's duties. This action was taken with one dissenting vote; no reasons were assigned for it. It is known that the differences arose from the same source that has made many an institution trouble, namely, the question of local patronage. Half the board were in favor of making all purchases locally, while the other half wanted to throw purchases open to competition from other localities. Dr. Higgins declined to resign and the matter of retirement remained in dispute until March, 1854, when the trustees, having been sustained on an appeal to the Supreme Court, removed the superintendent.

Dr. H. K. Jones remained in charge and a committee of the Board of Trustees then visited Eastern institutions, and after inquiry and investigation in New York and New England, heard favorable reports of Dr. Andrew McFarland, late superintendent of the New Hampshire Asylum for the Insane. He was indorsed for the position by the superintendents of the well-known institutions of Utica, N. Y., and Hartford, Conn. After due consideration Dr. McFarland was appointed medical superintendent for the term of 10 years in May, 1854, and entered upon his duties June 16 of the same year. During this biennial period an entirely new Board of nine Trustees was appointed. In December, 1854, Dr. McFarland presented his first report as superintendent. From December, 1852, to December, 1854, the capacity of the hospital had risen from 82 to 166. During this biennial period the evil of a deficient water supply was experienced and showed itself with increasing severity year after year. The hospital was wholly dependent upon four wells and two cisterns. In 1854 two additional wells and two cisterns of 600 barrels capacity each had been dug, but the supply was still deficient to such an extent that the patients often lacked the baths necessary for cleanliness, to say nothing of the therapeutic use of water. The "never failing supply of water" called for in the act of incorporation was neglected in this, as in so many other instances.

The biennial report of 1856 takes up even in that early day the familiar story of overcrowding and tells of the occupation by patients of quarters in the main building intended for employees. It was also necessary to refuse admission to many chronic cases. The number of patients had now risen from 166 two years previously to 214 on October 14, 1856. Eight per cent of the 203 patients admitted in the two years were reported as "puerperal" patients, amounting really to a percentage for the female sex alone of 16 per cent. In December, 1858, the population had risen to 229 cases, and great economy was necessary to keep within the appropriations. The order for return of 45 patients to the counties had also been made, so as to provide room for acute cases. The percentage of recovery upon number discharged was 32. A table was given showing average per capita cost of maintenance of eight other institutions, which was $235 per annum—the corresponding figure for the Illinois Hospital was $144.

In 1860 30 cases of typhoid fever were reported, with three deaths. In this connection it is to be noticed that the water famine from which the institution suffered was such that closets and sewers were insufficiently flushed. In consequence of this serious difficulty as to water supply, Hydraulic Engineer E. S. Chesbrough, of Chicago, who planned and executed the tunnel under Lake Michigan to furnish a water supply for the City of Chicago, was called in consultation and later elaborated a plan for relief. In the biennial report the deaths from tuberculosis amounted to 20 per cent of total deaths. Another familiar subject is that of overcrowding. The superintendent stated that two more institutions equalling the then present capacity of the Illinois Hospital would not be sufficient to provide for the insane at that time needing accommodations.

The number of patients remaining December 1, 1862, was 302. The new arrangements for water supply, consisting of a reservoir with a capacity of 2,500,000 gallons, had been completed. This reservoir was designed to be kept filled by a pumping engine from Mauvaisterre Creek, about a third of a mile east of the hospital.

Dr. Andrew McFarland was re-elected medical superintendent for a second period of ten years June 16, 1864.

In the table of causes of insanity 23 cases are given in which the Civil War is supposed to have acted as a factor. Of these 14 were soldiers brought from camps, hospitals, etc., and the other nine were cases of civilians. Over-anxiety, grief or war excitement had been apparently the immediate cause of the mental overthrow. The number of patients treated in the biennial period ending in 1864 was 710, and there remained in the care of the hospital December 1, 1864, 301 patients.

The mortality had increased in consequence of a patient with smallpox having been admitted; 12 cases resulted, with two deaths. In the summer of 1864 an epidemic of dysentery, resulting in 14 fatalities, occurred. There were 27 "puerperal" cases among 408 patients admitted. There were again also two cases in which "spiritualism" was the assigned cause and 16 attributed to "war excitement."

In 1857 an appropriation was made for an extension of the west wing, which was completed in 1858. The extension of the east wing was commenced but was not finally completed and occupied till 1867.[1] The buildings had now cost fully $400,000, and afforded accommodation for 450 patients. This was a per capita allowance

[1] In 1867 Miss Mary J. Lincoln from La Harpe, Hancock County, was admitted suffering from "dementia." Her father was said to be a cousin of Abraham Lincoln. She had been insane 13 years; was a native of Kentucky. Her features resembled those of Lincoln. She died of phthisis pulmonalis, August 30, 1888.

of about $1000, although the original per capita allowance was only $240. The table of mortality showed a percentage of 29, upon the total deaths, due to tuberculosis. Extreme need of means for repairs was felt at this time. The sewers, the heating and ventilating apparatus and the plumbing were all exceedingly defective.

The "jury law," so-called, for commitment of the insane, had been recently enacted and an eloquent discussion of its hardships and injustice was given by Dr. McFarland. The appointment of Dr. H. Artemus Gilman, as assistant physician, occurred this year. The death of Alexander McDonald had ended his long and honorable service as treasurer; he was succeeded in that office by Edward P. Kirby, of Jacksonville. The act for protection of "personal liberty," referred to above, approved by Governor Oglesby, March, 1867, contained a clause which required that all inmates then in the hospital should be examined and their sanity or insanity passed upon by a court of record. This remarkable legislation resulted in the necessity of bringing from the hospital and presenting before the court of Morgan County some 300 individuals previously committed to the insane hospital from all parts of the state. This proceeding proved useless, if not farcical. The action here referred to was largely a result of the activity of Mrs. E. P. W. Packard, a former inmate, who was then conducting a statewide agitation against the State Hospital for the Insane and against Dr. McFarland personally. The authors of the new law had doubtless anticipated that other cases like that of Mrs. Packard (*i. e.*, of alleged wrongful commitment) would be brought to light, but this anticipation was not realized. Nor was Mrs. Packard's commitment itself technically illegal, for the reason that a clause in the law of February 15, 1851, then in force (clause No. 10) expressly provided authority for a married woman to be committed by her husband. This was a mischievous and unconstitutional provision, and was largely the cause of the whole trouble. A legislative investigating committee had championed the cause of Mrs. Packard and with "star chamber" methods had conducted what was really a personal attack upon Dr. McFarland. The trustees requested that Dr. McFarland be allowed to appear and to meet his accusers face to face. This request was refused. This refusal and the hasty publication in the press of the committee's report, containing much that was false, clearly showed their personal hostility. The trustees then conducted a careful investigation and published their report, expressing their full confidence in Dr. McFarland's integrity and ability. The trustees making this report were E. G. Miner, president, Fernando Jones, Joseph E. Eccles, Francis A. Hoffman, Richard C. Dunn and Isaac L. Morrison.

Dr. McFarland had previously expressed his intention to resign, and at the meeting of the board on June 8, 1870, presented his formal resignation. At this same meeting Dr. H. F. Carriel, previously assistant superintendent at the State Hospital at Trenton, N. J., was appointed medical superintendent.

Dr. Andrew McFarland at the time of his resignation had been 16 years in charge of the State Hospital, and the service rendered by him was and is worthy of recognition, as able, assiduous, and successful in a high degree, especially when the difficulties with which his position was surrounded are considered. In a pioneer stage of the evolution of the work of caring for that difficult class of fellow-beings—the insane—where problems of organization and of finance were constantly presenting themselves and there were few precedents for guidance, it was inevitable that errors should occur. Dr. McFarland's integrity was not brought in question nor was any serious accusation against him proven, but the clamor resulting from the fact of Mrs. Packard's detention in the hospital against her will and the fact that she now appeared not only sane, but unusually bright and capable, and alleged that she had *never* been insane, and was fervently believed by the masses of the people, produced a situation where retirement from his position was regarded by him as the lesser of two evils. Dr. McFarland was an able, eloquent writer and enjoyed the confidence of those immediately associated with him. It was his misfortune that statewide agitation led to much injustice being done him personally.[1]

The report for the two years ending December 1, 1870, shows some changes in the government of the hospital. The size of the Board of Trustees had been legally reduced in 1857 from nine to six and in 1869 from six to three and a new board had been

[1] See the "Jury Law for Commitment of the Insane in Illinois" (1867-1893), American Journal of Insanity, Vol. LXIX, No. 3, January, 1913.

appointed. Dr. H. F. Carriel was installed as superintendent in July, 1869. He had been chosen by the board after extensive correspondence and visits to other state institutions and after conferring with men of high standing in public philanthropy.

Dr. Carriel's record for the next several years is largely one of a struggle for adequate repairs and improvements in an equipment confessedly antiquated and imperfect. The sewerage, the water supply and the heating of the buildings were all in an unsatisfactory condition. Some of the walls of the main building were cracked and needed to be taken down and built over. A system of downward ventilation for the water-closets, the substitution of tile for wooden floors in these, and the construction of ventilating flues for wards and rooms were planned and gradually carried through.

No rain had fallen during five months ending in December, 1871; the reservoir upon which the institution was dependent for water had proved leaky and soon was entirely empty. A new floor and sides of brick and cement were at once constructed for the reservoir. During the summer a fatal epidemic of dysentery had occurred, affecting 60 patients, nine of whom died.

On November 30, 1872, it was possible for the first time to report the hospital out of debt. At this time, by new fiscal regulations, it was arranged to pay the appropriation for current expenses in advance instead of at the end of each quarter. A resolution commending Dr. Carriel for his success in the various repairs and betterments was passed by the Board of Trustees. The new hospital at Elgin was ready for occupancy and 40 patients were transferred to that institution.

The perpetual problem of water supply again presented itself, and a new reservoir was built, of 5,000,000 gallons capacity.

Efforts were made in the direction of employment and amusement. A paint shop and a broom shop were provided, giving occupation to many of the patients.

In 1874 the hospital was crowded 20 per cent beyond its proper capacity. Isaac Scarritt, the capable, highly respected president of the Board of Trustees, died in 1873.

A carpenter shop was put in operation; many improvements were made in the equipment. Food cars were introduced, the dining rooms reconstructed. It had long been necessary to carry water to 600 patients and employees daily for drinking purposes, but in 1874 there was a sufficient supply from the creek; not, however, of as pure quality as was desirable, this water being surface water. At this time a filter-bed was projected with capacity of 70,000 gallons per diem, and was soon in operation.

Transfers of 94 patients to the Northern Hospital at Elgin and 46 to the Southern Hospital at Anna were made. The supervision of the recently created State Board of Commissioners of Public Charities was found helpful and stimulating to the management, new powers having been given this board by the act of 1875. Much interest was manifested by the public in the institution, over 11,000 people being conducted through it in the biennial period. On one occasion a man appeared at the office with 300 Sabbath school children, whom he desired to have shown about, and when informed this was impracticable, insisted that tax payers were entitled to this privilege. A baseball club had been formed and furnished much interest to patients and employees. In the biennial period ending in 1878 there was a controversy with the City of Jacksonville in consequence of the sewers of the institution becoming a nuisance and legal proceedings were threatened. This matter was adjusted by the Legislature of 1880.

Two new wings for 75 patients each were completed in 1880, the number of patients being 534. The percentage of recovery on the patients discharged whose insanity was of three months' duration or less was 59 per cent. The percentage on the whole number was 28 per cent.

In the report of 1880 it is shown that much had been done for the occupation and diversion of patients. Shops had been supplied for various trades, also farm buildings which provided for more farm industry and gave employment to increased numbers of patients. A green-house of moderate dimensions was added for the patients' pleasure and diversion. The report of the State Board of Charities stated that in the past 10 years about $100,000 had been judiciously expended for various repairs and improvements, and highly praised Dr. Carriel's wise and economical administration and successful reconstruction of the institution and its service.

In the fall of 1882 Dr. H. A. Gilman resigned the position of assistant physician, which he had held creditably for 16 years, having received the appointment of medical superintendent to the State Hospital for the Insane at Mt. Pleasant, Iowa. The superintendent argued in the report of 1882 for additional provision for the insane either by providing new institutions or making additions to the old ones. The number of insane at that time in the State of Illinois was not less than 5000 and less than half of these were provided for.

In the legislative session preceding the report of 1884 an appropriation of $135,000 to enlarge the capacity of the hospital was made, requiring provision to be completed for that sum for 300 patients, the per capita allowance being $450. This building was then under construction. In the report of 1886 the new "annex" is reported completed, and Dr. Frederick C. Winslow, formerly assistant physician, who had been in private practice, had returned as assistant-in-charge. The new accommodations had been rapidly taken up and the number of patients had reached 926. A 7,000,000-gallon reservoir had been completed, giving the institution 12,000,000 gallons storage capacity for water.

In the biennial period of 1888 Dr. J. D. Waller resigned after six years' creditable service, and Dr. Frank P. Norbury was appointed in his stead.

The General Assembly, meeting in 1891, increased the capacity of the Elgin, Anna and Jacksonville institutions by 300 patients each, appropriating $120,000 to each institution for that purpose. The net cost per week for maintenance of 898 patients in 1890 was $2.97 1-6.

In the construction of the new annex an amusement hall, 60 feet by 90 feet, was provided.

The second annex building was finished in 1892; one was devoted entirely to male patients, with Dr. Norbury in charge, and one to female patients under Dr. Winslow. In this period 15 cases of insanity were admitted in which "la grippe" was given as the exciting cause. The water supply was again a source of anxiety, general bathing being suspended during a few weeks of severe drought. Incandescent electric lighting was installed during this period, 1200 lamps for the buildings and 20 arc lamps for the grounds.

The inauguration of John P. Altgeld as Governor in January, 1893, and the coming of the Democratic party into power for the first time in over 30 years, led to a complete change in the Boards of Trustees and the other officers of the state institutions. Dr.

H. F. Carriel having filed his resignation, to take effect July 1, Dr. J. F. McKinzie, of Leroy, McLean County, was appointed in his stead. Dr. Carriel had served the institution with distinguished success for 23 years and was universally recognized to have given the Central Hospital an enviable reputation at home and abroad. The only reason for accepting his resignation was the political exigency created by the "outs" and "ins" of party politics. An appropriation of $43,200 which had been made by the Legislature for an infirmary building was vetoed by the Governor, as he was of the opinion that provision should be made for a new institution.

The report of 1896 shows a surplus of $56,000 and a reduction of $15,000 per annum is made in the amount requested for running expenses. Aside from economy that may have been practiced, the general depression in prices of goods and in wages succeeding the panic of 1893 had made it possible to conduct the institution at a considerable reduction in expense.

February 1, 1895, Dr. McKenzie resigned as medical superintendent and Dr. Walter Watson, of Mt. Vernon, was elected his successor. A room previously used as a chapel was converted into an assembly hall for the social meeting of attendants and employees when off duty. Enlarged freedom at night for patients was secured by leaving the doors of seven of the least disturbed wards unlocked at night and employing additional night help. At this time the operation of the new commitment law, which went into effect July 1, 1893, was shown by the fact that 206 out of 846 commitments in the two years were by medical commission instead of juries. Twenty cases of typhoid fever occurred in this period; 17 were employees and three were patients. One patient died.

John R. Tanner becoming chief executive of Illinois in January, 1897, appointed a new Board of Trustees, accepting the resignation of the former board. The new board took charge March 25, 1897. Dr. Frederick C. Winslow was elected medical superintendent, succeeding Dr. Walter Watson, of Mt. Vernon, in that position.

The trustees state in their report for 1898 that they found indebtedness and overdrafts upon the treasury amounting to $19,000. They reported that in 15 months they had removed the indebtedness and at the close of the period had a cash balance of $10,000. The hospital again needed remodeling of its plumbing; fire escapes were seriously needed, the floors and stairways being of wood in the new buildings and in the old also to some extent. An infirmary was badly needed for patients physically ill. The report of 1900 by Dr. Winslow gives account of many improvements; a new heating, ventilating, lighting and power plant had been installed.

In 1902 Dr. Winslow, having taken charge of the institution at Peoria July 1, was succeeded as superintendent by Dr. Joseph Robbins, of Quincy, who, after serving from July 1, 1901, to July 1, 1902, was succeeded by Dr. Henry B. Carriel, who for four years had been assistant physician. Dr. Carriel was the son of Dr. Henry F. Carriel, who was in charge from 1870 to 1893.

In this report the trustees speak of the desirability of improving the diet and also of increasing the compensation of nurses so as to secure better service. Erysipelas, an old enemy, was present again in 1901. In the report of 1904 the increase of the number of patients to 1342 is recorded. Two hundred and sixty-nine deaths from all causes are reported. The death rate on the number of patients remaining June 30, 1904, was 20 per cent. It was 10 per cent on the total number treated. Fire protection was provided through efficient apparatus, a new water tower giving adequate pressure, and through replacing wooden stairs with fireproof material. The percentage of recoveries had fallen greatly; 75 per cent of the patients admitted were incurable.

The corrosive action of the water continued to destroy the pipes and boilers and $24,000 was asked for new boilers. The disproportion between service plant and numbers accumulated by continual additions for patients, was seriously felt in inadequate heating, bathing and laundry facilities, in the kitchen and bakery and in an insufficient amount of land for agriculture, etc.

In 1908 the trustees reported they had not more than 50 acres for tillage.

Evidences of a progressive spirit are shown in the abolition of mechanical restraint; in the training school courses, introduced with lectures as prescribed by the State Commission of Public Charities; also by a school for demented patients, which had been in operation four years, being conducted by a former patient with most gratifying success. A pathologist was added to the medical staff, Dr. George H. Stacy having been selected for the place, and Joseph Tormey, D. D. S., filled the newly created position of dentist.

In 1910, the newly appointed Board of Administration having taken charge of all the state hospitals for the insane, the report of the superintendent of this hospital, as of all the state charitable institutions, is incorporated with that of the new board. A. L. Bowen, secretary, reported the hospital greatly overcrowded, with a population of 1471 patients.

A new one-story tubercular hospital had been completed and occupied by 24 patients. This building was found to answer its purpose admirably and was very attractive in appearance. Of the two hospital buildings provided for by appropriation, the one for female patients was ready; that for men was changed in plan by building three stories instead of two, and was not yet ready for occupation. A building to cost $50,000 for quarters for nurses and attendants had been contracted for.

Much valuable assistance in the care and treatment of patients needing surgical advice or operations had been rendered by Dr. Carl E. Black, of Jacksonville. In general a spirit and atmosphere of progress, of scientific activity and of more complete and elastic adaptation of means to ends seemed to pervade the institution.

June 28, 1911, the graduating exercises of the training school occurred. A class of four was graduated. It is noted that a training school class of six had been graduated in 1910, and that five of these graduates still remained in service in June, 1911. Mr. Bowen, the secretary of the Board of Administration, on his visit of December 10 and 11, 1912, reported as follows:

> A plan to convert one whole floor of the main building from tip to tip to reception service is being worked out and gives promise of success. The east side will be occupied by men and the west side by women. There will be four wards on each side, each ward being designed for a special class of acute patients. The wards furthest from center will be the hospital wards, in the new extensions recently completed and thrown open.
>
> There will be a ward for the quiet, a ward for the semi-restless and disturbed, a ward for the disturbed and excited and the hospital ward, all on the same level and adjoining each other. Hydrotherapy is located in each hospital, so that it will be convenient and easy of access for all sections of the reception service.

The women attendants were reported comfortably housed in the side of the nurses' home intended for them, and the other half for the men was ready for occupation. This was the first institution in Illinois to provide complete housing for all ward help.

Mr. Bowen, on his visit April 11-12, 1913, reports among other things: "No seclusion or restraint in use. The male home for employees is now occupied. The old ladies have been given the first floor of the infirmary building, which will be known as 'Woman's Building.'"

The hydrotherapeutic apparatus had been installed on both sides at that time, but no one had been secured to operate it, such help, as well as help for attendants and nurses, being difficult to obtain. The number of patients was 1687.

PRESIDENTS BOARD OF TRUSTEES.

Samuel D. Lockwood.... 1847-1848
Rev. J. B. Turner....... 1849-1850
J. T. Holmes........... 1851-1852
Fleming Stevenson 1853-1856
William Ross 1857-1860
L. S. Church 1861-1864
W. H. Brown 1865-1866
E. G. Miner 1867-1868
Isaac Scarritt 1869-1872
Gen. John Tillson 1873-1874
Daniel R. Ballou........ 1875-1882
David E. Beatty........ 1883-1892
Joseph M. Page........ 1893-1896
Frederick L. Sharpe.... 1897-1900
Henry Miner 1901-1902
John R. Davis 1903-1906
Dr. G. W. Ross (acting pres.) 1907-1908

SECRETARIES AND TREASURERS.

William Thomas (secretary) 1847-1849
James Jackson (treasurer) 1847-1850
Alex. McDonald (sec. and treas.) 1854-1866
Edward P. Kirby 1868-1874
B. F. Beesley 1876-1890
Thomas B. Orear 1892-1893
Millard F. Dunlap...... 1894-1896
John R. Robertson 1898-1900
Annie C. Dickson 1902-1906
John R. Robinson....... 1908-1909

In August, 1909, there was a reorganization under the State Board of Administration, the State Treasurer acting as hospital treasurer.

Frank D. Whipp (fiscal supervisor) 1908-1909

BOARD OF TRUSTEES.

Name	Years
Joseph Morton	1847-1852
Owen M. Long	1847-1848
Nathaniel English	1847-1848
William W. Happy	1847-1850
Joseph Dunlap	1847-1848
James Gordon	1847-1850
Aquilla Becroft	1847-1852
James Lurton	1849-1850
John Croker	1849-1850
A. C. Dickson	1849-1852
William S. Hurst	1849-1852
J. B. Turner	1851-1852
W. B. Warren	1851-1852
William Butler	1853-1856
Simeon Francis	1853-1858
Chas. H. Lanphier	1853-1856
Benjamin Pyatt, Jr.	1853-1856
William L. Craven	1853-1856
Richard Henry	1853-1856
Pleasant L. Ward	1853-1856
Darius Dexter	1853-1854
James Ward	1855-1856
Samuel Clubb	1857-1862
E. G. Miner	1857-1866
John T. Cassell	1857-1866
H. E. Dummer	1857-1864
W. H. Brown	1861-1866
J. T. Eccles	1863-1864
Francis A. Hoffman	1865-1868
R. C. Dunn	1865-1866
Fernando Jones	1867-1868
Isaac L. Morrison	1867-1868
Gen. John Tillson	1869-1870
Jonathan B. Turner	1869-1872
Dr. W. W. Sedgwick	1873-1874
H. G. Whitlock	1873-1876
Wm. H. Ellis	1875-1876
John Gordon	1878-1880
David E. Beatty	1878-1882
Edward P. Kirby	1882-1892
R. W. Willett	1884-1890
Wm. R. Newton	1891-1892
Owen P. Thompson	1893-1896
Reddick M. Ridgeley	1893-1894
John McCreery	1894-1896
Morris Emerson	1898-
J. A. Glenn	1898-1900
Kenneth M. Whitham	1900-
F. W. Menke	1892-1904
W. L. Fay	1902-
Henry Miner	1904-
Dr. G. W. Ross	1906-
Charles H. Williamson	1908-

Board of Trustees legislated out of existence by law of 1909, creating Board of Administration.

MEDICAL SUPERINTENDENTS.

Name	Years
Dr. James M. Higgins	1848-1853
Dr. H. K. Jones, acting	1853-1854
Dr. Andrew McFarland	1854-1870
Dr. Henry F. Carriel	1870-1893
Dr. J. F. McKenzie	1893-1895
Dr. Walter Watson	1895-1897
Dr. Frederick Winslow	1898-1901
Dr. Joseph Robbins	1901-1902
Dr. Henry B. Carriel	1902-1915
Dr. Edward L. Hill (in office)	1915-

ASSISTANT PHYSICIANS.

Dr. H. K. Jones (acting supt. to 1854) 1851-1852
Dr. Charles F. Cornett.. 1854-1859
Dr. Asa P. Kenny 1860-1864
Dr. Charles Dutton 1864-1868
Dr. Samuel S. Emery... 1866-1868
Dr. H. Artemus Gilman. 1866-1880
Dr. Elias C. Neal 1871-1875
Dr. Frederick C. Winslow 1876-1892
Dr. Louis A. Frost 1882-1894
Dr. John D. Waller 1882-1886
Dr. James F. Graham .. 1884-1886
Dr. Wm. K. McLaughlin 1886-1890
Dr. Frank P. Norbury.. 1888-1892
Dr. O. H. P. McNair .. 1890-1892
Dr. Frederick O. Jackson 1892-1894
Dr. Samuel H. Sheppard 1892-1894
Dr. William L. Grimes.. 1894-1896
Dr. Charles C. Sater.... 1894-1896
Dr. Charles E. Chapin.. 1894-1896
Dr. Lillian Nuckols..... 1896-1896
Dr. Henry B. Carriel... 1898-1900
Dr. Elmer L. Crouch....1903-1909
Dr. Alonza F. Burnham. 1898-1900
Dr. Edward Peters 1898-1904
Dr. Louis H. Clampit.... 1902-1905
Dr. William C. Cole (died during service) 1902-1904
Dr. H. A. Potts 1904-1906
Dr. E. F. Leonard 1905-1913
Dr. F. A. Stubblefield .. 1906-1915
Dr. Ralph T. Hinton 1908-1912
Dr. Joseph Tormey (dentist) 1908-1910
Dr. F. J. Sullivan 1907-1907
Dr. George H. Stacey (pathologist) 1908-1910
Dr. F. E. Munch 1909-1912
Dr. W. L. Treadway ... 1909-1913
Dr. Thomas E. Charles (interne) 1909-1910
Dr. F. W. Nickle 1911-1912
Dr. Elizabeth D. Carroll 1912-1913
Dr. R. P. Pratt.......... 1912-1913
Dr. Charles A. Oaks.... 1913-1913
Dr. C. G. Thomas...... 1913-1913
Dr. E. A. Foley (in office) 1911-
Dr. C. R. Lowe (in office) 1913-
Dr. E. J. Strickler (in office) 1913-
Dr. Minerva Blair Pontius 1912-1915
Dr. T. G. McLin (in office) 1913-
Dr. Wm. Babcock (dentist) 1914-1914
Dr. Anny M. Peterson (in office) 1915-
Dr. L. G. Wright (in office) 1915-

CHAPLAINS.

Rev. J. M. Sturtevant.... 1853-1860
Rev. W. S. Russell...... 1862-
Rev. J. G. Roberts 1864-1868
Rev. E. A. Tanner 1870-1880

After 1880, duties assumed in rotation by pastors of Jacksonville.

ELGIN STATE HOSPITAL.[1]

Elgin, Ill.

The "Northern Illinois Hospital and Asylum for the Insane"[2] (so called in the first appropriation bill) was created by an act of incorporation passed by the Legislature at the session of 1869. The sum of $125,000 was appropriated by this act, which also called for the appointment of a Board of Commissioners to select a location.

This commission was duly appointed by the Governor, consisting of: Samuel D. Lockwood, of Kane County; John H. Bryant, of Bureau County; D. S. Hammond, of Cook County; Merritt L. Joslyn, of McHenry County; Augustus Adams, of De Kalb County; Benjamin F. Shaw, of Lee County; William Adams, of Will County; S. M. Church, of Winnebago County; and A. J. Matteson, of Whiteside County. The commission selected a site on the Fox River about one mile south of the City of Elgin, in Kane County. There was a proposal by the City of Elgin to donate 80 acres or more if deemed necessary, of the "Chisholm Farm," which was the tract of land decided upon, and an agreement was also made to furnish free freight for all material to be used in construction. A spring was included in the offerings of the city, situated about three-quarters of a mile from the proposed site, which was supposed to be capable of furnishing the water supply. The Locating Commission having fixed upon the site, Governor John M. Palmer appointed C. N. Holden, of Chicago, Dr. Oliver Everett, of Dixon, and Judge Pleasants, of Rock Island, as a Board of Trustees. Judge Pleasants failed to qualify and Henry Sherman, of Elgin, was later appointed in his place.

On December 23, 1869, the first regular meeting of the board was held. C. N. Holden, of Chicago, was elected president; Orlando Davidson, of Elgin, treasurer; and R. W. Padelford, of Elgin, secretary. The trustees' first decision was that the entire "Chisholm Farm" of 155 acres would be a necessity for the purposes of the hospital. Even this, it was believed, would be hardly

[1] By Richard Dewey, M. D.

[2] Legal name changed to "Illinois Northern Hospital for the Insane" in 1875, and "Elgin State Hospital" in 1910.

sufficient, as the board were of the opinion that "both the cottage and the congregate systems of construction should be finally adopted."[1] The law under which they were acting expressly provided that either of the two systems might be utilized and on this account they felt the more liberal-sized tract of land would be needed. The trustees expressed the opinion that a large class among the insane "should receive the more domestic and home-like treatment secured by the cottage system." For these reasons 323 acres were procured at $100 per acre, and paid for by the City of Elgin.

Plans and estimates for buildings were now sought. Conferences were held at which the members of the Board of Charities, Dr. Andrew McFarland, formerly superintendent for many years at the State Hospital at Jacksonville, Dr. R. J. Patterson, formerly superintendent of the State Hospital at Mt. Pleasant, Iowa, and of the State Hospital at Indianapolis, then of "Bellevue Place," a private hospital at Batavia, Ill., and many others assisted. The plans of Colonel S. V. Shipman, of Madison, Wis., were finally selected for a main building on the "congregate" plan. Colonel Shipman had previously furnished the plans for state hospitals for the insane at Madison and Oshkosh, Wis. These plans were of traditional "Kirkbride" type, and closely followed that of the Government Hospital at Washington; with central building and symmetrical wings *en echelon.*

It was proposed at this time to build the north wing only, leaving the central building and the south wing to be added later. The amount appropriated ($125,000) was only sufficient to construct one wing and the necessary service buildings. The location that had been chosen upon this tract of land, gently sloping toward the river, was sightly and attractive, commanding a pleasant and extensive landscape.

In the summer of 1870 the work of construction upon the proposed north wing was begun, and the building was enclosed late in that year. It remained still necessary that the central building and the service buildings should be provided and that the heating

[1] This provision in the law grew out of much general discussion of the so-called "cottage" system for the insane and advocacy of this idea before the Legislature. The State Board of Charities had taken an active part in favor of this "cottage" or "detached-ward" idea.

apparatus be procured and installed. The following spring and summer the interior finishing was proceeded with and contracts were made for the construction of the service buildings, in the rear, also for the heating apparatus.

In September, 1871, Dr. Edward A. Kilbourne was elected medical superintendent. Dr. Kilbourne was at the time practicing medicine in Aurora, Ill. He was a man of ability and wide experience. He had interrupted his medical studies to serve in the army during the Civil War as a captain in a regiment of volunteers from his native state, Vermont, and after obtaining his medical degree in New York City in 1868, at the College of Physicians and Surgeons, he had seen some months' service in the city asylum of New York on Blackwell's Island. He then served a year in the Brooklyn City Hospital as resident physician and surgeon, and later went abroad, acting as ship's surgeon, and visited clinics and hospitals in London and Paris.

The completion and occupation of the new hospital were seriously interfered with by the Chicago fire October 9, 1871. Various contractors lost in the fire both material and means to finish their work and the task of furnishing, which Dr. Kilbourne had just begun, was brought to a standstill for a time. The heating apparatus could not be obtained and put in place until about four months later than the time called for by the contract.

In December, 1871, Dr. Richard Dewey was appointed assistant physician and entered upon his duties January 1, 1872. In February, 1872, a formal opening and inspection occurred. The Governor, John M. Palmer, the State Board of Charities, and large delegations from the House and Senate, with numerous distinguished visitors, participated.

Another serious delay in the reception of patients was caused by the failure of the spring upon which the hospital was dependent for its water supply. In the spring of 1872 the flow was only sufficient to feed the boilers, and it became necessary in April, 1872, to employ two teams in hauling water. Fortunately, however, a comparatively easy solution of the difficulty was found in the Fox River, flowing 800 yards away.

A reservoir was dug near the river and both river and spring water flowed in. A water main was laid to the building. A pumping station was provided, and an inexhaustible supply of water was thus made available, although the Fox River as a water supply could not perhaps be considered above reproach.

On April 3, 1872, the first patients were received, and as rapidly as possible the most urgent cases were provided for. They came from the State Hospital at Jacksonville, from the county almshouses and from homes. The waiting list was a long one, and the great majority were chronic cases.

The building was three stories in height and the two lower stories were given to male patients, while the third was arranged for women. What was to be eventually the first ward was taken for offices and living rooms for the officers and employees. There were 183 patients on November 30, 1872. This number occupied every bed available. Indeed the capacity was already overtaxed.

The report of November, 1874, records the completion of the hospital buildings July 1, 1874, some months *in advance* of the date agreed upon in the contract.

In their report for 1874 the trustees, in discussing the "detached-ward" or "cottage" construction provided for in the act establishing the Northern Hospital, expressed themselves as having become satisfied, on further experience, that this style of construction is "inadvisable," stating, among other arguments, that detached buildings will "cost more per patient."

The superintendent presented the details of construction and occupation of the new central building and south wing which rendered the hospital complete as originally planned. The south wing, although completed, remained unoccupied by patients, as the previous Legislature failed to provide for the maintenance of the additional number.

Col. S. V. Shipman's final report as architect was presented and the trustees bore testimony to his honesty, ability and efficiency both as architect and building superintendent.

The report for 1876 records the increasing completeness and efficiency of the work. The period was marked by a redistricting of the state into southern, central and northern districts and by extensive transfers and exchanges of patients. Dr. Henry J. Brooks, of Dixon, Ill., was added to the medical staff as assistant physician.

The natural beauty of the ornamental grounds, embracing some 75 acres, was enhanced under the direction of Mr. John Blair, landscape architect, by extensive grading, planting and seeding of the lawn, by setting out trees and shrubs, and by the addition of an ornamental basin and fountain of rustic-rock work in front of the main building. Rustic arbors and settees were also added in large numbers. Fruit trees were set out and large additions made to the kitchen garden. The need of provision for a pathological laboratory was again urged upon the Legislature.

A fatal accident to a patient, occurring in December, 1876, led to a public investigation by the State Board of Charities to establish the facts with regard to conduct of attendants and correctness of the medical treatment. On this point, the statement of the board, after most thorough and extended investigation, was as follows: "The testimony was unanimous that it (the medical treatment) was abundantly justified by precedent and by high medical authority." And the result of the inquiry as a whole was stated in the closing sentences of the report: "As to general humanity and success of the institution, nothing was developed that would bring it in question."

The trustees in their report for 1878 presented a statement regarding a bequest by Jonathan Burr, of Chicago, left in trust to be given to an asylum for the insane, "when such asylum shall have been established" in the northern part of Illinois "possessing a character of permanence and stability." This bequest conveyed property amounting at that time to $35,000, the net income of which was to be used "in and towards keeping and maintaining such asylum in a condition to relieve those who are so unfortunate as to need its treatment and care." After prolonged litigation this fund had been secured to the hospital. The trustees' interpretation of the intent of the bequest was that it should be "used to furnish such surroundings in the shape of amusements and comforts as would tend to make them (patients) enjoy the asylum as a home." C. N. Holden, former president of the Board of Trustees, rendered valuable service in securing this bequest. Dr. Kilbourne recommended the employment of this fund in maintaining a greenhouse and this recommendation was later carried out, giving to the institution this permanent and beautiful attraction in front of the north wing.[1] The dimensions of the building were 113 by 38 feet, the point of the Gothic arched roof being 34 feet in height. By wise and ingenious economy a large room, intended for a work-

[1] The greenhouse was finally completed in 1886.

shop, was secured in making the authorized changes in laundry and boilerhouse. Much literary activity was developed among the patients by the efforts at this time of two lady patients, who personally made and secured from others contributions of interest and merit, combining them in a periodical which they called *The Attempt.* On one occasion, when Governor and Mrs. Beveridge were visiting the hospital, readings were given from this periodical. The Governor suggested the periodical be renamed *The Success.* His suggestion was acted upon.

The work of changing the public road in front of the hospital was done in 1879 and 1880 by removing it away from the buildings and toward the river, some 300 feet; at the north and south entrance to the grounds lodges were erected. Dr. Richard Dewey, assistant physician since 1872, having been appointed superintendent of the new Eastern Hospital at Kankakee, resigned and took up his new duties in August, 1879. The average number of patients was 520.

A beginning of pathological work and a report on the technique of hardening brain tissue and making microphotographs, together with a report of cases and cuts of microscopic slides, prepared by Dr. O. C. Oliver, recently added to the medical staff,[1] was appended to the report for that year.

The wearing out of heating apparatus hastened by the scale deposited in boilers and pipes from hard water, and the efforts made to better the water supply, are worthy of mention. We learn from the 1882 report that another serious complication was the extravagant consumption of fuel. A three-inch artesian well was sunk over 2000 feet in depth. The installation of the telephone, then a new invention, is recorded in this period. An effort to reduce the amount of mechanical restraint had resulted in lessening it to a "minimum." Reports of daily use of restraint then made corresponded to those introduced two years earlier at Kankakee. (See report of Kankakee Hospital for 1880.)

In the period of 1884 incandescent electric light was substituted for gas in interior lighting with an increase of safety and a saving of $500 per annum. Twenty cases of typhoid with three deaths are recorded. The system of forced ventilation by two

[1] Dr. Oliver died of typhoid fever in December, 1880.

12-foot fans for the north and south wings had been completed and the heating apparatus renewed throughout by installing new boilers and substituting "low" for "high" pressure steam heating. Dr. Archibald Church was appointed an assistant early in 1884.

The artificial lake, 400 to 150 feet in extent, in front of the south wing, forming at the same time a storage reservoir for water, was reported as completed in 1886. It was irregular in shape, spanned by a rustic bridge and dotted with several islets. In December, 1887, Dr. Church terminated his services at Elgin, with a view of study in Europe.

Important provision against fire was made in 1888 by the erection of a hose-house and tower, by putting in fireproof partitions running to the roof and fireproof doors between the sections of the main building.

The discharge and return to Du Page County in 1889 of two female patients, whose condition was such that they were unfit for care in the county almshouse, and the scandal and newspaper sensationalism resulting therefrom, led to an investigation by the Board of Charities early in 1890.

The view of the State Board of Charities, after careful consideration of all circumstances, was that, in consideration of the fact that the county authorities were altogether unprovided with means of caring for such cases, it was an error to have ordered the discharge of these patients. They were returned to the State Hospital.

The unfortunate scandal of this case and the misunderstanding it gave rise to were productive of one good effect, namely, that of showing to the public the evils resulting from county care and the desirability of such provision for state care as to avoid such conditions.

The additional building to accommodate 300 patients, a duplicate of a building erected at Jacksonville for the same purpose, was contracted for, to be completed on January 1, 1891.

Dr. Edwin A. Kilbourne after a severe illness died at the hospital on February 27, 1890. He had given 19 years' faithful and able service to the institution.[1]

[1] See biographical sketch *American Journal Insanity*, Vol. 46, p. 571.

Dr. Henry J. Brooks, of Dixon, Ill., who in 1875 and 1876 was assistant physician at this hospital, was appointed superintendent to succeed Dr. Kilbourne.

After 23 years of faithful service R. W. Padelford resigned as secretary to the board in February, 1892. The new "annex" was occupied April 8, 1892, adding 300 to the capacity of the hospital. The two new associate dining-rooms were also put in service on April 10, one for the women on the north side and one for the men on the south, both connected conveniently with the main kitchen. The capacity of each was for about 300 patients, and all except the highly disturbed were able to enjoy the new arrangement. The patients go and come to the dining room in the open air, that is, without covered passageways.

During this period the new stand-pipe was completed. It occupied an eminence west of the main building, 95 feet above the river. It was 75 feet in height and 16 feet in diameter, and with its capacity of over 100,000 gallons, provided storage and fire pressure.

The meat supply was provided for by installing a slaughter-house, in which in one year 184,918 pounds of beef, veal, lamb and pork were furnished at a net cost per pound of a fraction over 5 cents. Three hundred and twenty head of live stock were purchased and 218 furnished by the hospital farm. The second year's operations made even a more favorable showing.

The report of 1894, addressed to Governor John P. Altgeld, whose election in 1892 resulted during the year 1893 in an entirely new Board of Trustees taking charge of all the state institutions, announces extensive changes. The superintendent, Dr. Henry J. Brooks, was succeeded June 12, 1893, by Dr. Arthur Loewy as "acting" superintendent and on October 4, 1893, Dr. Loewy was appointed superintendent. Dr. Wm. G. Stone, first assistant physician, resigned May 1, 1893, after 13 years' honorable service. The second and third assistant physicians were also replaced by new men. These removals were understood to be solely for political reasons. A new building for the combined purpose of amusement hall and gymnasium had been completed and the old hall converted into additional sleeping quarters for employees. Dr. Loewy introduced a new custom in regard to the night care of patients, namely, that of leaving the doors of their rooms open at night; first in the annex and later in the main building. To do this he added eight to the number of night attendants. He reported beneficial results from the change.

The following paragraph is from the superintendent's report for July 1, 1896:

At this time I desire to refer to table No. 25[1] in which is shown the percentage of recoveries and deaths since the opening. . . . . In 1872 the percentage of recoveries was 3.17 per cent. *For the year ending June 30, 1896, we have brought the percentage up to 53 per cent, which is 23 per cent above the average of institutions in the United States.*

Perhaps no further comment than the italics (which are ours) is needed. It is not intended for a moment to imply that Dr. Loewy's statement as to percentage of recoveries is not entirely honest. It is only one more instance of the fallibility of statistics and of the "rosy" coloring enthusiasm will give to prosaic arithmetical calculations.

A striking increase in paretic dementia was shown in the ratio of cases admitted. In the two years ending June 30, 1896, this was 6.8 per cent as compared with 1.28 per cent for the two years ending June 30, 1890. The death rate on the average attendance for this period was 13.75. In the biennial period ending July 1, 1898, the return of the Republican party to administrative control caused another upheavel, which was reflected in the administration of the hospital. Dr. John B. Hamilton, of Chicago, editor of the *Journal of the American Medical Association,* was appointed medical superintendent. Dr. Hamilton continued his editorial duties and spent much of his time in Chicago. The then newly appointed Board of Trustees when first taking up their duties in 1893 complained that no inventory of the state property was furnished them by their predecessors and that the financial condition of the institution was unsatisfactory. Now precisely the same complaint was made of themselves by their newly appointed successors. (P. 5. Trustees' report dated July 1, 1898; p. 7, report dated July 1, 1894.)

Dr. Hamilton died December 24, 1898. His administration was able, honest and efficient in many ways.

Dr. Frank S. Whitman, of Belvidere, was appointed January 12, 1899, as successor to Dr. Hamilton. Dr. Whitman was a graduate

[1] The tables are not numbered; evidently the table referred to is on p. 38.

of the Hahnemann Medical College of Chicago, and had been in practice in Belvidere, Ill. During his administration the infirmary for women with a capacity of 100 beds was completed. Richard Yates being elected Governor, in 1900, appointed a new Board of Trustees early in 1901. Dr. Whitman continued his services as superintendent, being reappointed by this new board. In this period the room formerly used as chapel in the central building was converted into dormitories for the employees, the amusement hall being enlarged and beautified and devoted to both chapel services and recreations. Dr. Frank H. Jenks, an assistant physician, after four years' valuable medical service resigned to enter private practice in Aurora.

Records of laboratory work and of a large number of autopsies are given in this report. For the 1902 and 1904 periods the percentage of recoveries was 30 per cent and 26 per cent respectively (a contrast to the *53 per cent of recoveries* shown in the report of 1896). C. W. Marsh, first appointed a trustee in 1874, 30 years previously, and president in 1876 and for many years not connected with the board, was reappointed by Governor Yates and again made president of the board.

In July, 1906, Dr. Whitman having tendered his resignation, after eight years' service, Dr. V. H. Podstata succeeded to the place. The trustees reported that the civil service law, passed by the previous Legislature, was fairly satisfactory, but that the wages they could afford to pay were insufficient to attract the grade of attendants and nurses desirable. Dr. Podstata inaugurated a training school for nurses and showed at once a keen appreciation of the medical side of the work. He advocated advanced methods of curative treatment and the creation of a psychopathic hospital in the strict sense, especially emphasizing hydrotherapeutics, a separate provision for the tubercular and for the chronic class of patients, also uniform and persevering efforts at re-education. Finally he emphasized the need of a laboratory in which valuable pathological and bacteriological work could be done. The familiar story of defective heating, plumbing, ventilation and water supply was again rehearsed; also the congested condition in offices and living quarters, resulting from such quarters, originally planned for the service of 500 inmates, being compelled to serve for over 1200.

In writing of the probable and possible increase of numbers of patients, the superintendent recommends that if numbers are to be increased, "cottages" rather than a large building be added.

In the report of 1908 the superintendent reported that the hospital was provided with three sources of water supply: the springs, which yield pure and wholesome water for drinking, but inadequate in amount for other purposes, the water from the Fox River, and the city water of Elgin. These were made available for fire protection and for use in boilers, flushing sewers, etc., and all could be drawn upon at once in case of fire, by an automatic fire pump, with a capacity of 1000 gallons per minute and pressure sufficient to throw a stream over all the buildings. The ventilating and heating had been remodeled and the 12-foot fans, "unused for 15 years past," had been put in commission. A farm ward and a "modern cottage" for women, built of concrete, pressed brick and interlocking tile with best modern plumbing and no guards or bars on the windows, had been built and occupied.

Dr. Podstata reported a new feature in the medical staff—the employment of internes. The medical staff consisted of four senior physicians, four internes and one laboratory assistant. The internes under the seniors examined patients and acquired more efficiency than was developed by the assistants when they had an unvarying routine and the total care of 250 or 260 patients each. The assignment to each of the nine physicians was 160 patients. The daily staff meetings proved a great aid toward professional advancement and the development of power in observation and study. The problem of mechanical restraint had been carefully studied. The superintendent limited such restraint in every possible way, but found a certain amount necessary; how much he does not say nor is a record of it presented. An effort was made to give continuous baths, but the supply of hot water was so irregular and uncertain as to seriously impair their utility.

Dr. Podstata resigned March 15, 1910. He had rendered valuable service since July 1, 1906, having shown great professional ability and zeal. His ideals were high and he labored zealously to attain them. Dr. Sidney D. Wilgus, having taken office as superintendent May 1, 1910, made a brief report to the newly constituted Board of Administration on July 1, 1910. He found the institution overcrowded. Patients were sleeping in the hallways, while the new industrial building, intended for shops, was occupied by 40 beds for patients instead of by industrial machinery and tools. A deplorable condition of insufficiency of attendants and nurses was noted. Dilapidation of the plumbing existed in many buildings. The need of separating the tubercular was emphasized. Twenty-five per cent of the deaths were from tuberculosis. There were 40 positive and 60 suspected cases on the female side, and 25 positive and 80 suspected cases on the male side. Thirty-three per cent of the deaths were from paresis.

The report of the newly created State Charities Commission for 1910, in its survey of the Elgin State Hospital, spoke of the newer buildings being admirable in construction, mentioned improvements in lighting, etc., and criticised the hospital building, which had been utilized for men, stating it was badly equipped and was not built for its then present purpose. The new receiving ward was approved. The new storage building, though good in itself, was badly located, being far from the railroad switch; and it had a basement eight inches below the sewer level, which could not be drained. The continuous bath fixtures provided for men and women "in small rooms" had not been used for over a year because "hot water is not to be had in proper quantities and there is no apparatus for properly mixing hot and cold water. Hot water generally is lacking, one of the women's cottages being entirely without it." The commissioners state: "The kitchen and laundry cannot be too severely condemned."

In January, 1911, smallpox became epidemic in the hospital; eight cases occurred, some of them fatal. In November, 1911, diphtheria obtained a foothold and up to the spring of 1912, 15 cases occurred—apparently without fatality. From September to the latter part of December, 1911, seven cases of typhoid fever occurred, apparently originating with a "bacillus carrier" who worked in the women's dining room. A report upon pellagra states that in 1911 26 cases with 15 deaths occurred, and in 1912 16 cases with one death.

Dr. Hinton's report of October 1, 1912, for the preceding two years showed much efficient activity in the medical service. An improved classification of the psychoses, corresponding to advanced ideas, had been adopted and re-examination and reclassification of previously admitted cases inaugurated, so that a card index or catalogue of all cases complete and modern could be prepared. Daily staff meetings and discussions were held and conferences two evenings in each month. Diagnosis and treatment received careful discussion, and clinical and therapeutic work was placed upon a higher plane.

Daily ward reports and night reports had been introduced. Clinical observation and data were thorough and accurate. A large amount of valuable laboratory work had been done, chemical, bacteriological and pathological. The organization of the "State Hospitals Medical Association" had been found a factor of great advantage in arousing the scientific spirit and creating an honorable emulation.

Another significant index of advancement was the training school for nurses, inaugurated by Dr. Podstata. In July, 1911, five nurses were graduated and in 1912 three completed their course. These were the first to have completed their course of training at the Elgin State Hospital and all remained in the service of the hospital.

The "psychopathic building for women," with its hydrotherapeutic equipment, facilities for rest treatment, attractive exterior and interior, was spoken of with enthusiasm. The detached location was an advantage. Dr. Hinton remarks, "In short, we are able to segregate these patients; a condition which is so necessary for their successful treatment."

At an inspection by A. L. Bowen, executive secretary of the State Charities Commission, on February 25-27, 1913, the following improvements were noted:

> There are now no patients anywhere sleeping on floors. The new "psychopathic building for women" is now in use. It is liberally provided with bath-rooms. The windows are not screened but were blocked at seven inches at first, but a patient slipped through a window and fell, fracturing her spine. The space was then reduced to five inches.[1]
>
> This building gives such satisfaction that the superintendent, Dr. Hinton, asks to duplicate it for males and put a kitchen for both between the two. The kitchen in this building, fitted at first with electric cooking apparatus, proved a failure and gas was substituted.

[1] The space allowed for raising the windows at Kankakee cottages was fixed at five inches in 1879 and this was the rule up to 1893. (See third biennial report of Kankakee Hospital October 1, 1882, p. 18.) In the "open" cottages the windows were left the same as in any house.

The new laundry, bakery, laboratory, and cottage for tubercular patients are completed. The new laundry has a "conning tower" from which the whole interior is visible. The building is well lighted and ventilated and well equipped. The new bakery is complete. All walls in oven room are of white glazed brick; floors of terrazzo; machinery and store rooms well designed. The cottage for tubercular patients accommodates 20 of each sex; faces south. It is patterned after the attractive building at Jacksonville. Interior finish is white. These four buildings have been completed for the appropriation of $65,000 and enough remains to supply the necessary apparatus in the laboratory. From the $27,000 appropriation $7000 was used to complete the acute female cottage, and the remaining $20,000 has provided a one-story yellow-bricked and slate-roofed structure, accommodating 80 men. In these buildings 170 patients can be housed very comfortably. All buildings are now connected by tunnels.

A new fire service has been completed which gives direct pressure to the pipe lines inside the buildings as well as to the fire-hydrants. Provision has been made for laying 175,000 feet of new floors and a good part of the work is already done; the wooden stairways are to be replaced by concrete.

The pumping station at the river has been supplied with electric motive power, thus obviating the necessity of hauling coal a mile and effecting a decided saving. There is still great danger of fire originating in the old boiler house, from which it would inevitably travel over the kitchen and be very likely to spread to the whole service buildings and central building.

At an inspection made by A. L. Bowen, executive secretary of the State Charities Commission, on July 21 and 22, 1913, it was found that the new general bath-house was about completed and ready for use. It is termed "excellent" in construction and equipment. It will be used on certain days for men and certain other days for women. It is liberally provided with tubs and showers. There was found practically no restraint, either day or night, and three or four patients only in seclusion. The windows of nearly every building are now provided with fly screens.

The new building for untidy, demented males is occupied and accomplishing its object well. The laboratory and morgue are now very completely fitted out. The labor of patients is being employed in making cement blocks for a two-story building to be erected on the foundation of the vegetable cellar. The first story will be a carpenter shop and the second story will furnish sleeping rooms for 27 persons—all is being done from the repair fund.

TRUSTEES.

C. N. Holden, president. 1869-1874
C. W. Marsh 1874-1904
Oliver Everett, M. D.... 1869-1872
Henry Sherman 1869-1874
Edwin H. Sheldon 1876-1878
F. C. Bosworth 1878-1884
George P. Lord 1876-1878
Frederick Stahl 1878-1882
S. P. Sedgwick, M. D.[1].. 1884-1890
D. F. Barclay[1] 1886-1888
L. L. Hiatt 1892-1894
John Neuman 1893-1897
Dennis J. Hogan[1] 1893-1897
J. D. Donovan.......... 1893-1897
Charles Neiman 1894-1896
Frank B. Brookman..... 1896-1898
A. S. Wright[1].......... 1897-1900
W. S. Cowan 1898-1900
J. C. Murphy 1898-1900
J. B. Lane[1] 1902-1904
W. S. Bullock 1902-1904
E. S. Eno 1904-1909
Robert Rew[1] 1906-1910
P. M. Woodsworth 1906-1908

TREASURERS.

Orleander Davidson 1869-1874
S. S. Mann 1876-
J. A. Carpenter 1878-
W. H. Wing 1880-1884
George P. Lord 1886-1892
Philip Freiler 1893-1897
David F. Barclay 1898-1900
D. E. Wood 1902-1909

SECRETARIES.

R. W. Padelford 1869-1890
Edward Wellinghoff ... 1892- / 1902-1904
Annas Hathaway 1894-1896
Charles A. Miller 1898-1900
H. O. Hilton........... 1906-1908
H. J. Slagle 1908-

SUPERINTENDENTS.

Dr. E. A. Kilbourne[1] ... 1871-1890
Dr. H. J. Brooks 1890-1893
Dr. Arthur Loewy 1893-1897
Dr. John B. Hamilton[1].. 1897-1898
Dr. F. S. Whitman 1899-1906
Dr. V. H. Podstata 1906-1909
Dr. Sidney D. Wilgus... 1910-1911
Dr. R. T. Hinton....... 1911-1914
Dr. H. J. Gahagan (in office) 1914-

ASSISTANT SUPERINTENDENTS.

Dr. F. H. Jenks 1909-1911
Dr. C. B. Dirks 1911-1913
Dr. M. C. Hawley (in office) 1914-

---

[1] Died in office.

ASSISTANT PHYSICIANS.

Dr. Richard Dewey 1871-1879
Dr. Henry J. Brooks 1876-1878
Dr. John J. Crane 1878-1882
Dr. O. C. Oliver 1880-1880
Dr. Wm. G. Stone...... 1880-1893
Dr. Allen Fitch 1882-1883
Dr. James Mills 1883-1885
Dr. Archibald Church .. 1884-1886
Dr. William Cuthbertson 1888-1889
Dr. Albin Young 1889-1893
Dr. William T. Patterson 1890-1892
Dr. Walter S. Haven... 1892-1893
Dr. Walter R. Robinson 1892-
Dr. A. L. Loewy 1893-1893
Dr. C. H. Franz 1893-1897
Dr. Henry J. Gahagan.. 1893-1897
Dr. John E. Hogan..... 1893-1895
Dr. Ella V. Tinnerman.. 1895-1896
Dr. Frank H. Jenks.... { 1896-1901, 1905-1911 }
Dr. E. A. Foley 1896-1905
Dr. Lucius F. Foote 1898-1900
Dr. Charles Kahn ...... { 1898-1899, 1903-1905 }
Dr. J. M. Kearney .... { 1898-1901, 1903-1907 }
Dr. C. A. Buswell 1900-1902
Dr. Charles E. Sisson .. 1900-1904
Dr. George W. Lucas... 1901-1910
Dr. M. F. Clark 1901-1906
Dr. P. F. Gillette........ 1901-1903
Dr. H. G. Hart 1905-1907
Dr. F. A. Walls 1906-1906
Dr. Clara Dunne 1906-1907
Dr. F. J. Sullivan...... 1907-1907
Dr. Wilma Jacobs....... 1907-1907
Dr. R. B. Hoag......... 1907-1908
Dr. Addison Bybee 1906-1909
Dr. C. O. Bolger........ 1907-1908
Dr. Thos R. Foster 1908-1910
Dr. Joy Rickets......... 1908-1909
Dr. G. W. Morrow...... 1908-1909
Dr. E. J. Greer.......... 1908-1908
Dr. H. C. Miller 1908-1908
Dr. Paul Hess 1908-1909
Dr. Roy Cox 1909-1909
Dr. P. F. Becker 1909-1910
Dr. Robert McLallen.... 1909-1909
Dr. H. J. Smith........ 1909-1911
Dr. Olive Hughes....... 1909-1914
Dr. C. B. Dirks......... 1911-1913
Dr. C. C. Atherton...... 1911-1913
Dr. A. G. Wittman...... 1910-1914
Dr. C. R. Bell.......... 1910-1912
Dr. E. V. Dale.......... 1910-1910
Dr. R. R. McCarthy..... 1911-1913
Dr. H. S. McCarthy..... 1911-1913
Dr. E. Erickson........ 1909-1910
Dr. I. F. Fremmell..... 1909-1912
Dr. S. L. Gabby........ 1910-1912
Dr. Fay Spangler ...... { 1911-1911, 1913-1914 }
Dr. Charles Stevens.... 1910-1911
Dr. W. R. Tutt.......... 1912-1913
Dr. Victor A. Bles (in office) 1912-
Dr. D. C. Kallock....... 1913-1913
Dr. E. Y. Levitin........ 1914-1914
Dr. Louise M. Abbott (in office) 1914-
Dr. E. W. Fell......... 1913-1914
Dr. R. M. Ritchey (in office) 1914-
Dr. G. C. Stimpson (in office) 1914-
Dr. J. K. Pollock (in office) 1914-

ANNA STATE HOSPITAL.[1]

ANNA, ILL.

The Anna State Hospital was formerly the Illinois Southern Hospital for the Insane. It was created by act of the General Assembly of 1869, and formally opened for receiving patients on December 15, 1873, by proclamation of Governor John L. Beveridge.

The grounds of the hospital consist of 569 acres, of which about 30 acres are in lawn, 290 acres under cultivation, and the remainder in pasture and woodland.

In 1881 fire completely destroyed the north wing of the main building; again in 1895 fire visited the institution, destroying the center or administration building and the south wing. The portions destroyed were promptly replaced.

The buildings include the administration building, four stories, with two wings; the annex, three stories, with two wings; a male cottage, two stories, with two wings; a cottage for infirm female patients; an infirmary of 100 beds, two stories; a hospital for the care of the physically ill and for giving hydrotherapy, 100 beds, two stories; and in course of construction a cottage for the care of tuberculosis patients and a new modern dairy barn.

In addition there are a laundry, machine shops, stables, cold storage and ice and power plants, also a modern bakery, general kitchen and store room.

On July 1, 1911, there became available, as provided by the Forty-seventh General Assembly, an appropriation of $135,000 for the purpose of furnishing a water supply for the institution. As a result the hospital has fully equipped water works, with pumping station and filtering plant, an impounding reservoir and dam of a capacity of 30,000,000 gallons, from which the water is forced to a naturally elevated reservoir capable of holding 2,000,000 gallons.

The ordinary operating expenses are approximately $300,000 per annum. The average number of patients enrolled at present (1914): males, 948; females, 796; total, 1744. Number of admis-

[1] Prepared by Ralph A. Goodner, M. D., superintendent.

sions since the receiving service was opened, 11,096; number of employees at present, 280.

The superintendent, an assistant superintendent, two physicians, three assistant physicians, one dentist and a chief nurse compose the medical staff.

A training school for nurses was established in 1907 and is still maintained. Standard and modern scientific methods in the care and treatment of the insane have been introduced and followed. Much original and research work is now being done. A well-equipped laboratory is in charge of a competent pathologist. Seclusion and mechanical restraint have been abolished.

There are 15 open wards, mostly female. About one-fifth of the population is upon parole. More than one-half of the male patients are under the care and supervision of female attendants. An eight-hour system of service for attendants, nurses and employees has been established.

Entertainments of various kinds are frequently given, in addition to a picture show each Tuesday, matinee and night, and a dance each Friday night. Religious services are held every Sunday in the chapel by the local clergy of Anna in rotation, and Catholic services are held each Wednesday.

The following were the first Board of Commissioners, appointed by Gov. John M. Palmer: Lieutenant Governor John Dougherty;[1] D. R. Kingsbury, Dr. G. L. Owens,[1] Colonel H. W. Hall and Colonel Benjamin M. Wiley.[1]

TRUSTEES SERVING FROM 1873 UNTIL THE DISCONTINUANCE OF THE TRUSTEE SYSTEM IN 1910.

Amos Clark.[1]
W. R. Brown.[1]
C. Kirkpatrick.[1]
J. C. Boyle.[1]
W. N. Mitchell.[1]
John E. Dietrich.[1]
E. H. Finch.[1]
Wm. T. Bruner.[1]
James A. Viall.[1]
James Bottom.[1]
John C. Baker.[1]
Wm. H. Boicourt.[1]
Walter H. Wood.
Marshall Culp.
John Spire.[1]
Albert Smith.[1]
Alva Blanchard.[1]
Scott Matthews.
Thomas W. Gannon.
James C. Mitchell.
Samuel Hastings.[1]
Colonel L. Krughoff.[1]
L. E. Sunderland.[1]
Judge John Lynch.
H. H. Kohn.
P. H. Eisemayer.

[1] Deceased.

SUPERINTENDENTS FROM 1873 TO THE PRESENT TIME.

Dr. R. S. Dewey........	1873-1873	Dr. W. A. Stoker........	1897-1900
Dr. A. F. Barnes[1].......	1873-1878	Dr. R. F. Bennett.......	1900-1903
Dr. Horace Wardner[1]..	1878-1890	Dr. Wm. L. Athon......	1903-1913
Dr. E. B. Elrod[1]........	1890-1893	Dr. Ralph A. Goodner..	1913-
Dr. Wm. C. Lence[1].....	1893-1897		

MEMBERS OF THE STAFF FROM 1873 TO THE PRESENT TIME, IN ORDER OF THEIR APPOINTMENT.

Dr. Converse.
F. W. Mercer.[1]
L. Stocking.
W. W. Hester.[1]
A. B. Beattie.
N. J. Benson.
M. D. Baker.
Ralph A. Goodner.
R. M. McCall.
S. C. Hall.[1]
Jessie L. Carrithers.
Samuel C. Dodds.
D. R. Sanders.[1]
P. H. McRaven.
J. E. Groves.[1]
C. B. Caldwell.
Eugene Cohn.
G. W. Morrow.
E. Louise Abbott.
E. A. Foley.
R. M. Ritchey.
Thomas R. Foster.
Bernard Lemchen.
P. S. Waters.
Angelina G. Hamilton.
W. W. Mercer.
A. L. Jacoby.
A. B. Beattie.
Thos. H. Mulvey.

SUPERINTENDENT.

Ralph A. Goodner.

ASSISTANT SUPERINTENDENT.

Whedon W. Mercer.

MEDICAL STAFF.

George W. Morrow, physician.
Angelina G. Hamilton, physician.
A. B. Beattie, assistant physician.
P. S. Water, assistant physician.
A. L. Jacoby, assistant physician and pathologist.
D. L. Woodworth, D. D. S., dentist.
Elizabeth Donovan, chief nurse.

---

[1] Deceased.

KANKAKEE STATE HOSPITAL.[1]

KANKAKEE, ILL.

FIRST SYSTEMATIC DEPARTURE IN THE UNITED STATES FROM CONGREGATE CONSTRUCTION.

It is necessary to recall briefly the status and tendency of opinion and action with reference to the insane in the 60's and 70's of the last century in order to appreciate the circumstances which led to the adoption at Kankakee (in 1879) of a system of completely detached wards, and which originated a movement that had somewhat far-reaching results in influencing construction for the insane in several states of the Union.[2]

We can refer here only to the more or less immediate results of legislative action and trace the development of building plans as determined by enactment in Illinois, which in their turn were related to legislation in other states—particularly New York.[3]

The act of 1877 creating the state hospital, later located at Kankakee, provided that the State Board of Public Charities should have the power of approval or disapproval of any building plans that might be adopted. This provision of the law really committed the matter into the hands of one man. That man was

[1] By Richard Dewey, M. D.

[2] The following circumstances may be noted as illustrating the direct effect: The Governors of Ohio and Indiana, each accompanied by a state commission and an architect or engineer, inspected the detached wards at Kankakee in 1883. Later the institutions at Toledo (capacity 1000), at Logansport (capacity 380), and at Richmond (capacity 400), all on the detached ward plan, were constructed. North Dakota employed Major Willett, architect at Kankakee, and in 1885 had 160 patients in three detached wards.

[3] Anyone interested in the views on building plans held at that period can find documents and discussions in the files of the *American Journal of Insanity*, and in the "Propositions and Resolutions" collected and published in 1876 by the Association of Superintendents; also the reports of the Board of Public Charities of New York, Massachusetts, Pennsylvania and Illinois (the only State Boards of Charities in existence up to 1869). The report for 1884 of the Illinois Board of Public Charities, Chapter III, page 65, has a very full *resumé* of the subject from the pen of Secretary Fred. H. Wines.

WILLETT & PASHLEY
ARCHITECTS

KANKAKEE STATE HOSPITAL.

the secretary of the board, Rev. Fred. H. Wines. The State Board of Public Charities had been created and organized and Mr. Wines was chosen as its secretary in 1869. In the same year the act for the new hospital, later located at Elgin, was before the Legislature. A clause was inserted in this act through the efforts of Mr. Wines which would have enabled the trustees of the new institution to adopt the so-called "cottage system" had they so elected, but no action in this direction had been taken up to 1877. Therefore, in 1877, when the new Eastern Hospital was created, Mr. Wines procured the insertion of a clause in the appropriation bill which made the approval of the Board of Charities to any building plans which might be adopted at Kankakee *obligatory*. Mr. Wines had become a convinced advocate of the "segregate" as against the "congregate" style of construction for the insane and the provision of the law above referred to made him the arbiter of the plans for that institution, and he acted the part in an original and forceful way. Mr. Wines, formerly a Presbyterian clergyman at the state capital, and during the Civil War a chaplain in a Missouri regiment on the Union side, had become secretary of the State Board of Commissioners of Public Charities at the request of Governor John M. Palmer. He was a brilliant writer and speaker, a man of broad sympathies and humanitarian motives. He was also possessed of a grasp of economic principles and administrative details unusual for a clergyman. He had familiarized himself with the question of further provision for the insane in Illinois and in other states, and his study of the problems involved had made him an advocate of greater freedom and elasticity in constructive and administrative matters.

The situation at this time with regard to the insane was such as to arouse anxiety in the public mind. While the nation had been absorbed in the Civil War, a great accumulation of this class as public charges had taken place throughout the land, and when this fact seemed to come to light all at once, the people rather suddenly became aware of a heavy public burden and menace. Various states confronted with this question had attempted to meet it by erecting new institutions or adding to old ones. Millions had been poured out in this way, with the result that institutions were no sooner provided than they were filled to overflowing and still hundreds remained unprovided for in the almshouses and jails. All these institutions had been built upon the congregate plan of construction and had cost from $1000 to $1500 for each patient accommodated, indeed in some instances $3000 and even $4000 had been expended per capita for every individual that could be received. It began to be seen that this state of things could not continue and many expedients for relief were proposed. The question of separation of the acute from the chronic insane came up and a controversy resulted between those, on one hand, who insisted that chronic cases should be separately and more cheaply provided for, and those, on the other, who averred that it was a vicious principle to separate the insane into curable and incurable classes.

The plan of separation, however, prevailed for a time, as in a notable instance in the State of New York, where the Asylum for the Chronic Insane at Ovid (named later in honor of Dr. Willard) came into existence in the same year, 1865. In 1866 Dr. George Cook, of Canandaigua, presented at the Washington meeting of the Superintendents' Association a paper on "Provision for the Insane Poor of the State of New York," advocating separate provision for the chronic insane, a policy which was strenuously opposed by the general sentiment of the Association, as shown by the debate which followed. The only policy on which the Association would agree was that of providing for all the insane buildings of a congregate type built in conformity with the "Propositions" of 1851 and 1852.[1]

The instructive facts about the buildings at Ovid were that the cost of them was only about $500 for each patient accommodated, less than one-half the amount previously customary; and that they were in reality "detached wards," though each of a capacity of several hundred patients and built upon the linear or congregate plan.[2]

Returning now to the inception of the institution at Kankakee, we find that all these problems of cost of buildings and of separation of the acute and chronic classes had been carefully studied by the Board of Public Charities of Illinois and by Secretary Wines.

[1] Propositions and Resolutions of the Association of Medical Superintendents of American Institutions for the Insane, published by the Association, 1876.

[2] Later additions were two and one-story buildings, an entire departure from the congregate plan.

The opinion arrived at, as expressed in their report,[1] was "that the classification demanded (for the insane as a whole) was not in separate wards of one building, nor in separate institutions (for acute and chronic), but in separate or detached buildings for the care of both recent and chronic cases in a single institution under a single head."

The genesis of the departure from congregate buildings can now be further shown. A great task was before the State of Illinois, as before all the states, namely, that of providing quarters decent and reasonable in cost for thousands of insane. Expense of construction must be reduced. All must be taken care of. The so-called acute and chronic cases must not be separated, since there was no knowledge obtainable for determining, concerning a large minority, which were and which were not curable, and since the association of the two classes under proper conditions of classification not only need not be harmful, but might be beneficial. The "congregate" style of building had prevailed in this country and the men in authoritative positions and expert in these matters united in the opinion that further extension in providing for the insane must be upon the same lines. When in 1869 the appropriation was made for a new institution in Illinois and the plans were under consideration, the newly-created Board of Charities issued a call for a conference, at which the views of three superintendents were presented, Dr. Andrew McFarland, then superintendent of the State Hospital at Jacksonville; Dr. R. J. Patterson, of Illinois, and Dr. Woodburn, of Indiana. An extensive correspondence had also been held with the leaders of thought in this direction throughout the country. There seemed to have been a crystallization of two opposed opinions; one party held that buildings approximating more to the "house" than to the "institution" type should be adopted; the other that the "central buildings with wings" should be adhered to under all circumstances. Dr. McFarland expressed himself at the meeting above referred to as follows:

> The present system of architectural construction adapts the entire institution to the demands of its smallest and worst class, while for the great majority all these appliances are utterly unnecessary. We need more of the element of home life. I would not abolish the old form of institution. The two systems may exist side by side. I would have the central hospital

[1] Report of the Board of Public Charities of Illinois, 1884, p. 81.

in the foreground. At a little distance I would have a group, not of cottages. They should be houses of two stories in height. Under this system the facility of extension would be great. Classification would be more complete.[1]

Mr. Wines, in stating the case for detached construction in the report of the board for 1882, employed the following language (p. 112):

To Dr. McFarland, therefore, more than to any other man, belongs the credit of planting the germ which has developed into the hospital at Kankakee. His words passed unnoticed at the time, but they made a deep impression upon the State Board, and especially upon its secretary, Mr. Wines, in whose brain they ultimately took practical shape.

A resolution was adopted at the meeting referred to, to the effect that a combination in insane asylums, as far as practicable, of the "cottage system" with that at present in vogue was desirable.[2]

There was no immediate result from this meeting, or from the discussion and declaration of principles, but they bore fruit later in 1877 and 1878, when the Kankakee Hospital was under construction. The trustees of the new institution hesitated to take the responsibility of a radical innovation in construction, but consented to accept a plan which was so devised as to admit of development upon either congregate or segregate plan and to leave it to the next General Assembly to decide whether detached buildings should or should not be constructed. In the year 1878 Secretary Wines, being delegated by the state to attend the Prison Congress at Stockholm, was able to study European institutions for the insane, which further convinced him of the practicability of the "detached ward," and on his return he submitted to the Legislature a report which resulted in the first appropriation for detached buildings at Kankakee. In the session of 1879 the sum of $30,000 was appropriated to accommodate 100 patients. The

[1] Report of the Board of Public Charities of Illinois, 1882, p. 111.

[2] In the preceding year, at the meeting of the Western Association for the Promotion of Social Science in Chicago, Dr. McFarland had read a paper entitled "What Shall be Done with the Insane of the West?" in which he said: "A single type has given impress to all our institutions. The radical fault of this system is that the individuality of the subject is stifled and lost. Insane asylums must be, as it were, decentralized." Report of Board of Charities of Illinois, 1884, p. 83.

legislative approval, for which the trustees had waited, was thus given for the first time to the "detached ward" idea.

It now became necessary to prepare plans for "detached wards" and to study the development of an institution on these lines. The attitude of mind in which the undertaking was approached may be understood from the following quotation:[1]

> The foundation of this experiment was laid in fear and trembling. The so-called "cottage system" of organization of hospitals for the insane had been for many years a topic of discussion among theorists, but the general sentiment of that branch of the medical profession engaged in the actual care of the insane was adverse to it.

The Board of State Charities, in justifying its efforts and in the assumption of responsibility for building plans, made the following claim with some show of reason:

> We are familiar with the conditions of the insane in the county almshouses. If the superintendents of hospitals can claim for themselves peculiar knowledge of insanity from the medical point of view, we too may claim a peculiar knowledge of the insane from the administrative and governmental point of view, gained by observation outside as well as inside the state institutions. In planning the institution at Kankakee we had especially in mind the chronic incurable cases, who are inoffensive and harmless; who do not require locked doors or barred windows, and who can sleep in large associated dormitories.[2]

Having thus described the genesis of the "segregation" movement in Illinois, we will take up the order of events as they occurred from the passage of the bill creating the institution at Kankakee.

The Eastern Hospital for the Insane at Kankakee was created by an act of the Legislature enacted May 25, 1877, appropriating $200,000 "for land and for the construction of buildings." This act provided for the appointment of a Board of Commissioners by the Governor to select a location. Under this act Governor Shelby M. Cullom appointed John H. Addams,[3] William A. McConnell, John Thomas, A. P. Bartlett, William M. Garrard, Myron C. Didley and Dr. Joseph Robbins.[4]

[1] Report of the Board of Public Charities, 1882, p. 111.

[2] Report of Illinois Board of Public Charities, 1882, p. 115.

[3] Called by Abraham Lincoln, who was his friend, "The Addams with the two D's." Father of Jane Addams.

[4] Afterwards medical superintendent of Central Hospital, Jacksonville, in 1901-02.

The commissioners visited nine cities where locations were offered, and, after careful consideration of the merits of each, on August 2, 1877, selected the site known as the "Cowgill Farm," situated on the left bank of the Kankakee River about one mile south of the City of Kankakee. The farm comprised 251 acres of land; the cost to the state was $14,000.

After the location was determined the Governor appointed the following Board of Trustees to have charge of the institution: John H. Clough, William Reddick and W. F. Murphy. It is worthy of note here that this board was appointed under unusual conditions as to party control in the State Senate of Illinois. Confirmation by the Senate of all Boards of Trustees after appointment by the Governor was required by law, and to secure such confirmation at this session of the Legislature it was necessary to appoint "non-partisan" boards, as the minority party held a controlling balance of power in the Senate. There were therefore two Republicans and one Democrat on the Board of Trustees of the Kankakee Hospital. In the light of subsequent events this representation of both political parties may be regarded as fortunate, since, partly in consequence of the minority representation and partly by reason of the disposition of all three members of the board to ignore partisan politics and to hold the superintendent alone responsible, a policy in accordance with civil service principles was maintained. Such principles were faithfully enforced from 1879 up to 1893, in which year a reversal of political party control occurred.[1]

John H. Clough was chosen president when the Board of Trustees organized at Springfield, August 8, 1877. Haswell C. Clarke, of Kankakee, was elected treasurer. Frank E. Leonard, of Kankakee, acted as secretary *pro tem.* Major James R. Willett,

[1] The writer having been the first superintendent, well recalls one of his official acts—the securing of a carpenter. After thorough inquiry, the man found by all odds best qualified was selected, but when later the appointment became known to the local "boss" of the political "machine" a period of consternation ensued, and the superintendent discovered that he had appointed a *Democrat* instead of a *Republican,* carpenter. In local political circles this was felt to be a serious blunder. There was no interference with the appointment, however, and that same good craftsman remained in full exercise of his functions until 14 years later, when a new Governor (Altgeld) decapitated all the Boards of Trustees, in order to secure at each institution a superintendent who would do his bidding.

of Chicago, was elected architect and superintendent of construction, September 13, 1877, and was directed forthwith to prepare plans and estimates for buildings.

Colonel Clarke, who had been made treasurer in August, 1877, was also given the additional duties of secretary to the Board of Trustees at a meeting held December 19. At a meeting held January 29, 1878, at Springfield, Major Willett, architect, presented his plans for the buildings which it had been determined to erect, namely, a central or administrative building and one section of the south wing to accommodate 75 patients; also a kitchen, laundry, boiler house, etc. The plans, as prepared by the architect in frequent consultation with Mr. Wines, were approved by the trustees and then submitted to the Governor and the Board of Public Charities, by whom they were also approved. The general arrangements of buildings and the laying out of the grounds were very largely determined by Mr. Wines. It had been settled that the first provision for patients should be a central building of the typical "congregate" character, with a capacity when complete of 300 beds. It was the decision of the trustees that they would leave the matter of construction of "detached wards" for the coming session of the Legislature to determine, as they did not wish to make a radical departure from approved and customary plans for such institutions.[1]

It is convenient here to anticipate events by mentioning some features of the buildings as then planned and afterwards constructed. The material of all buildings was to be limestone in rock-faced range work. This work was very suitable for the "blue limestone" quarried at Kankakee. The caps and sills were to be of "Bedford" cut stone.

The main building was massive and stately, yet pleasing in outline, built in sections, three stories high with one-story connecting corridors; the roofs were of blue slate, the chimneys of "cherry-red" brick. The central building and wings were absolutely fireproof, all partitions being of stone or brick and all floors and roofs were laid over brick arches. The central building had a well-proportioned tower over 100 feet in height, bearing a white marble clock face 10 feet in diameter. One admirable feature of the buildings was the natural ventilation, devised by Major Willett in

[1] Legislative approval with an appropriation for "cottages" was given in 1879.

order to do away with forced ventilation, always expensive and at that date often unsatisfactory. Every room, small or large, had one or more complete continuous flues, each running to the top through its own chimney. Some one gave the institution when completed the name of "Chimney Village" as describing the unusual number of massive chimneys visible everywhere above the roofs.

On March 19, 1878, the contract for the erection of the buildings described above was awarded to the Commissioners of the Illinois State Penitentiary. A main sewer, 18 inches in diameter, over a mile in length, was also contracted for and built to empty into the river below the dam at Kankakee City. A pump-house and gas-house were erected at the river, together with a stone tower 70 feet high for furnishing water pressure. The water supply was from the river, then a pure water, though somewhat muddy at times.

During the year 1879 the building operations went forward favorably. It was found that the shop building and the tower of the central building could also be completed within the appropriation. There had been some doubt of this when the main contract was let.

In June, 1879, two acres of additional land were purchased, which gave a right of way for a side-track to the grounds from the Illinois Central Railroad.

Dr. Richard Dewey, previously for some years first assistant physician at the Northern Hospital, was appointed medical superintendent on June 13, 1879. One of his first duties was the preparation, jointly with Mr. Wines, of sketches for plans of the first group of "detached wards." An appropriation of $30,000 had just been made, calling for buildings of this class with a capacity for 100 patients.

Before speaking in detail of these detached wards, a brief statement should be made as to the general lines which the development of the institution was intended to follow. The distinctive feature was the construction and grouping of buildings as dwellings for the insane which should approximate ordinary houses as nearly as the limitations of insanity would allow. It was felt that a departure was desirable from the too-great uniformity heretofore prevailing, which did not seem to take sufficiently into account the wide variations among different classes of the insane.

The several buildings were to be adapted to all forms of insanity except the extreme degrees of mania. For these the central or congregate structure was at the time still considered necessary. The general plan consisted of a square site about 1200 feet on each of its sides. Avenues were laid out, forming each of the four sides of the square, intended to be like the streets of a town. The east side of the square fronted upon the Kankakee River and was occupied by the main hospital building; the avenues upon the other three sides were intended to be lined with detached two-story dwellings. This square, as ultimately built up, gave to the institution the appearance of a town or village. The detached buildings for female patients were upon the north half; those for men upon the south half. At the center of the west line, where the railroad spur entered the grounds, the business of the institution was concentrated; here were the business offices, stores, supply department, cold storage building, heating plant, etc. The medical headquarters were at the central building upon the opposite side of the square containing the medical offices, the reception-wards, and the equipment for medical care of acute insanity. The service buildings, kitchen, laundry, boiler and engine house, shops, etc., were all located upon the central line dividing the square into two halves, devoted respectively to men and women patients. A general dining-room, accommodating about 400 male patients, was also planned and later constructed at the center of the west line. Each of these buildings was to stand strictly detached; there were no fences, no enclosures and no connecting corridors. Some of the groups of patients intended to be accommodated were the feeble or infirmary cases, which would have their own dining room, but it was believed that the physically able-bodied patients could for the most part come and go more as people do who live in houses in the outside world. A hospital building for each sex formed part of the plan, as well as buildings especially arranged for those employed in farm labor and gardening in proximity to their own work. A building for the employees was planned at the outset and later built at the center of the west avenue. The wing for the women employees was separated from that for the men by the great general dining-room. In connection with the wing for women employees was an extension for sewing room and workshop for women's handicrafts. A like provision for employment of men was secured by the shop building 100 feet long and two stories in height, which was built in connection with the engine house and carpenter shops. Bath houses for each sex were a part of the scheme and were duly provided; at the bath house for men was a barber shop. A completely equipped fire department, with four hose carts, hook and ladder truck and companies of employees to man them, was suitably provided for in a central location in 1885.[1]

Where the "general plan" above described differs from ideas previously prevailing, it will be found that one or other of the following motives determined the changes made:

1. Diminution in expense of construction and administration.

2. Securing of a greater amount of beneficial employment among the inmates, primarily for their own good.

3. Introduction of a more domestic or natural and homelike mode of life and lessening rigor of confinement and restraint.

We return now to the preparation of plans for the first detached wards for 100 patients, which engaged the attention of Mr. Wines and the superintendent at the outset. These were the buildings numbered "one," "three" and "five," south. Some details of the plans of these buildings may deserve a word of description. The central of the three was a double house accommodating 23 inmates in each half. The two other buildings, one on each side, had a capacity of upwards of 30. The rear portion of the central building contained a dining-room for all. The general plan of these, as of all detached buildings, consisted of day rooms and service rooms on the first floor and associated dormitories on the second floor. Of the three buildings, the one at the east, No. 1, was designed for paroled convalescent or "trusty" patients and was intended to be an "open" ward. It contained six single rooms. These buildings were almost wholly for patients of the able-bodied class, harmless and largely industrious and reliable. The central of the three, however, was to receive some patients not physically robust, who could thus go to their meals without going out-of-doors. Also in this building a few "fugacious"

[1] It required the fire in January, 1885 (described elsewhere), to bring from the Legislature the appropriation for this improvement; to their previous refusal (or cutting down of an appropriation for fire protection from $2500 to $1000) the fire above mentioned with loss of life had been attributed, not without some show of reason.

patients were domiciled, whose day room and dormitory had guarded windows. In this connection mention may be made of the "relief" building and of one section of No. 1 north, later constructed, as these were the only ones of all the detached wards, as finally completed, which had any guards or bars at the windows. All other detached buildings, accommodating in the end over 2000 patients, had ordinary double-hung wooden sashes without guards or bars. The panes of glass were large enough (16 by 20 inches) to give egress to anyone who wished to break out. Windows were arranged to open at top and bottom five inches, except in the "open" wards, where they were the same as in any house. Practically no difficulty was experienced from beginning to end from window-breaking. The purposes of the "relief" building and of the one section of No. 1 above referred to was the separation of epileptic and so-called criminal insane (especially insane convicts) from contact with the general body of the patients.[1] One section of No. 1 north was in reality a ward for maniacal female patients for a time before the main building for female patients was completed. This section of No. 1 north at the time mentioned had window guards. The first six buildings were supplied with heat from the central boiler house, carried in an underground tunnel. The other 12 buildings were heated by hot air furnaces. The water and gas and sewerage of all the detached buildings were provided for by mains running in the avenue in front, just as in a town or city. The food supply was provided from the main kitchen. Food cars were used in which food could be kept hot. There was a small kitchen connected with each detached ward dining-room in which tea and coffee were made.

The main hospital building having reached the point of readiness for occupation, the superintendent took up the work of furnishing, and in November, 1879, officers and employees first occupied their several quarters. On December 4 the first patients were admitted; on January 13, 1880, a formal opening and inspection occurred, attended by Governor Cullom and many guests from Illinois and other states.

[1] It was for the general welfare rather than their own that the epileptic and criminal cases were separated; and their association together, though objectionable, was expedient as a makeshift, since they could not then be provided for in a separate institution.

GENERAL GROUND PLAN,
KANKAKEE STATE HOSPITAL,
KANKAKEE, ILL.

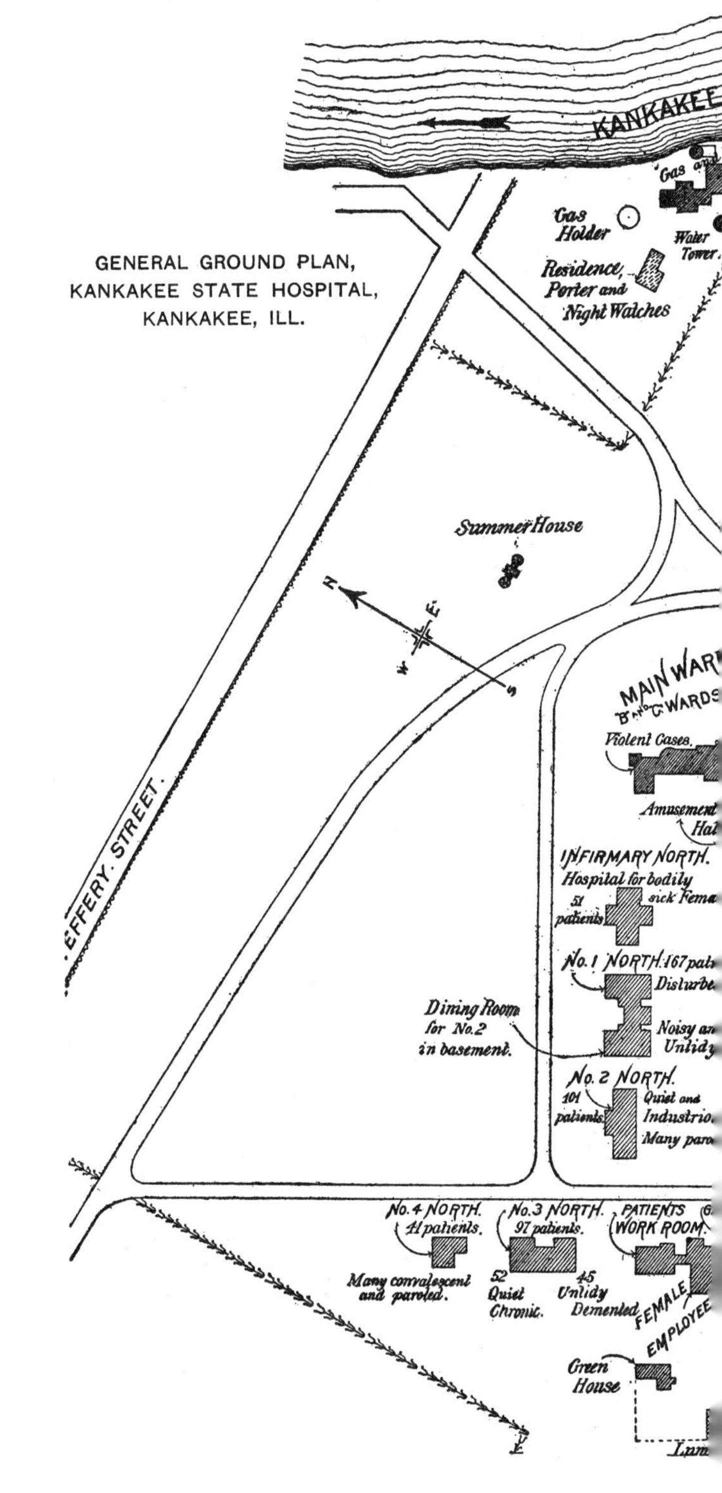

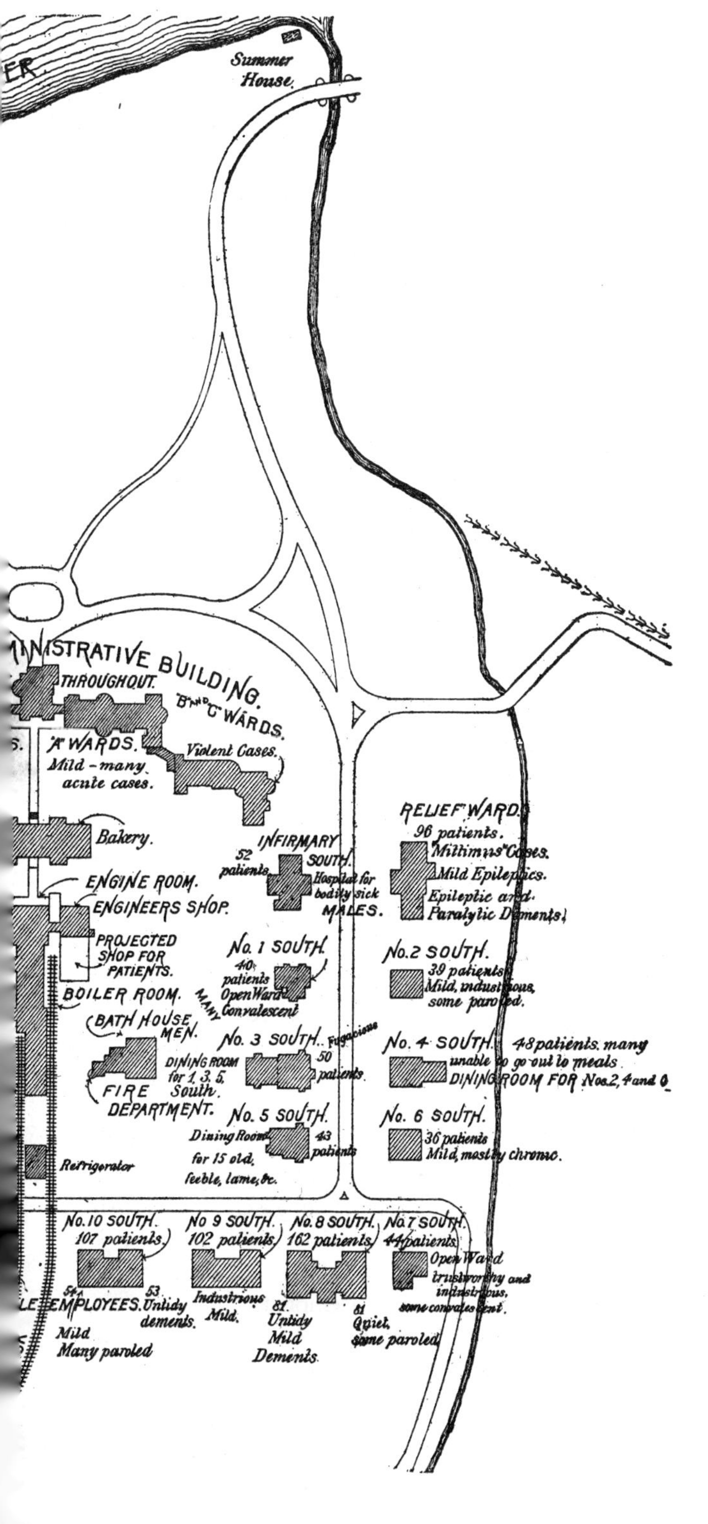

Summer House
ADMINISTRATIVE BUILDING.
THROUGHOUT.
"B" AND "C" WARDS.
Violent Cases.
"A" WARDS.
Mild - many acute cases.
Bakery.
ENGINE ROOM.
ENGINEERS SHOP.
PROJECTED SHOP FOR PATIENTS.
BOILER ROOM.
BATH HOUSE MEN.
FIRE DEPARTMENT.
DINING ROOM for 1, 3, 5, South.
Refrigerator
INFIRMARY SOUTH.
52 patients
Hospital for bodily sick
MALES.
RELIEF WARD.
96 patients.
"Miltimus" Cases.
Mild Epileptics.
Epileptic and Paralytic Dements.
No. 1 SOUTH.
40 patients
Open Ward
Convalescent
MANY
No. 2 SOUTH.
39 patients
Mild, industrious, some paroled.
No. 3 SOUTH.
Fugacious
50 patients.
No. 4 SOUTH.
48 patients, many unable to go out to meals
DINING ROOM FOR Nos. 2, 4 and 6
No. 5 SOUTH.
Dining Room for 15 old, feeble, lame, &c.
43 patients
No. 6 SOUTH.
36 patients
Mild, mostly chronic.
No. 10 SOUTH.
107 patients.
No 9 SOUTH.
102 patients.
No. 8 SOUTH.
162 patients.
No. 7 SOUTH.
44 patients.
Open Ward
trustworthy and industrious, some convalescent.
54
53
Unlidy dements.
EMPLOYEES.
Mild
Many paroled
Industrious
Mild.
81
Untidy
Mild
Dements.
81
Quiet,
some paroled

Dr. Harold N. Moyer was appointed assistant physician in November, 1879. Early in 1882 John H. Clough, who had acted as president of the Board of Trustees from the beginning, tendered his resignation. Mr. Clough's service had been of great value to the institution from his sound business views and his great probity and independence of character. In June, 1882, Ezra B. McCagg, of Chicago, was appointed as successor to Mr. Clough and elected to the presidency of the board. Dr. Henry M. Bannister was appointed first assistant at the April (1881) meeting. In July, 1882, Dr. Moyer was given leave of absence without pay to travel and study in Europe. In January, 1882, a contract was made for three additional detached wards (Nos. 2, 4, 6, south), accommodating 100 patients, to be located opposite the three already in use on the south avenue. In March, 1882, a contract for the first section of the north wing of the main building was executed.

In that day the question of using restraint and seclusion in the case of violent patients was a somewhat vexed one. The plan adopted from the start at Kankakee to keep mechanical restraint and seclusion at a minimum was as follows: All apparatus was kept in the dispensary. If need for its use seemed to arise, this was reported to the physician, who then visited the patient and personally investigated all the circumstances. This often of itself resulted in obviating restraint; but if the physician decided to order its use, it was prescribed definitely in writing as to form and length of time and the hour fixed at which the apparatus must be returned. The same rule was applied to seclusion. A record was kept in a book maintained for that purpose at the office; it was also entered by the attendant upon the daily ward report. Each record was independently checked with the others, so that a reliable record was kept. Further comment on these records will be found in following pages.

In June, 1883, the action of the Legislature laid upon the trustees the considerable task of erecting buildings for "not less than 1000 additional patients," for which purpose an appropriation was voted of $400,000. While this was a vindication of the system of detached wards after four years of trial by the state, the vindication seemed almost too emphatic to those who, without having been consulted, were suddenly charged with the carrying out of this "large order." A total capacity of 800 or 1000 was as great as had ever been contemplated or provided for in the service buildings and other arrangements. Now the addition of 1000 would bring the capacity to over 1600. The preparation of plans on a more extensive scale than had ever been anticipated was now necessitated. These buildings were required by law to correspond to the detached wards already in use, to be "not more" than two stories high, to be built of "brick and stone." The furniture, plumbing, heating, water, gas and sewer were all to be included within the amount of $400 per capita; also all provision for the additional employees.

It became evident, after a very little study, that the new buildings, in order to come within the appropriation, must be of large capacity[1] and of absolute simplicity in construction; any great amount of variety and all elaboration with regard to tastefulness of design or ornamentation would have to be renounced; dining-rooms would mostly have to be arranged in the basement, except one large general dining-room. It would also be necessary to arrange to construct a building for employees' quarters, which would need to accommodate about 150 persons.

On August 30, 1883, a contract was made for the construction and completion of 12 new detached wards, and these buildings were built, furnished, and occupied from time to time as they reached a state of readiness. In June, 1886, the number of patients had reached 1500 and the buildings for 1000 additional patients were completed and in use.

A woman assistant physician, Dr. Delia Howe, was appointed in 1885, this being one of the earliest additions of a woman to the medical staff of a hospital for the insane. A large amount of benefit to the female patients resulted from Dr. Howe's service.

Electric lights were introduced in the fall of 1885, thus doing away with gas for lighting purposes.

In 1885 an emblem and colors, a white cross upon a blue shield, were adopted as the "coat of arms" of the hospital and used in the decorations for festive occasions. In May, 1886, uniforms for attendants were adopted, navy blue with emblematic brass buttons for men and blue seersucker for women.

[1] Two of the buildings as finally constructed were each for 160 patients (four divisions of 40 each) and four were of 100 capacity (in two divisions of 50 each).

On January 18, 1885, the destruction by fire of the south infirmary, with a loss of 17 lives, produced a painful shock. The building had just been occupied, being one of the 12 new buildings for 1000 aditional patients. There had been no opportunity to organize fire service and the efforts at rescue were impromptu in character.

William A. Reid, attendant in charge of the infirmary, bravely secured the removal to safety of every bedridden patient, and John Coyne, an ex-patient then in the employ of the hospital, assisted four men down a ladder to safety by going up into the burning building. (These two men were later awarded gold medals bearing the emblem and color of the hospital and appropriately inscribed.) The fire seemed to originate from the hot air furnace and was probably the direct result of using this cheap method of heating a non-fireproof building, which was necessitated by the requirement of the state to construct and complete buildings at the rate of $400 per capita. The succeeding Legislature appropriated $18,000 for building and apparatus for a fire department, fire escapes and fireproof floors over furnaces, besides the necessary fund for rebuilding the infirmary ($12,000).

The ultimate result was a most complete equipment for fire protection; and for a day and night fire-alarm service. A hose house 33 x 36 feet, with tower for drying hose, was constructed; hose carts and hook and ladder truck were procured and a hook and ladder company and four hose companies were formed among the employees; 57 fire hydrants and 33 iron fire escape verandas were installed, and fireproof brick arches were laid over all furnace rooms. Great assistance was rendered in organizing this institutional fire department by Dr. Lawrence H. Prince, of the medical staff, whose natural talent for such work had been supplemented by service in the famous "Fire Insurance Patrol" under Captain Bullwinkle, of Chicago.[1] Dr. Prince acted as fire marshal until October, 1887.

The infirmary fire caused some discussion on the question of results from fire in a hospital on the "detached ward" plan as

[1] On May 1, 1887, when an extensive fire occurred in Kankakee City, the four hose companies of the hospital fire department were taken to the fire by the hospital teams and rendered service which was recognized by a resolution of thanks by the City Councils, also by checks sent by appreciative citizens.

compared with the results of fire in an institution on the "congregate" plan, and some opponents of the "cottage" idea were inclined to look upon this fire as an outgrowth of the "system"; but a little reflection served to show that fire is no respecter of "systems," congregate or segregate, and that buildings that are not fireproof are legitimate prey to fire.

On November 5, 1886, the attendants' training school was organized. The only schools of this character then in existence were at the McLean Asylum, of Massachusetts, the Buffalo State Asylum, New York, the Hudson River Asylum, at Poughkeepsie, N. Y., and the Indiana State Asylum, at Indianapolis. It was intended at Kankakee to include in the course of instruction all the attendants of both sexes and to give such teaching and training as could be applied to the entire body. Training school courses in that day were given only, or chiefly, in the general hospitals to women. Such training, being mainly for cases of bodily sickness, surgical operations, confinements, etc., included some instruction only partially applicable to the work of a hospital for the insane, while there were many things of the first importance for attendants upon the insane which were not taught the nurse in a general hospital training school.

A class of 36 was graduated from the training school in June, 1888.[1] Up to March 31, 1893, 130 attendants had been graduated —66 women and 64 men. Sixty were still in the employ of the hospital, eleven men and six women employed in other capacities having been promoted for merit.

The circumstances of the development of the hospital were such that when the buildings for the additional 1000 patients were completed the total population numbered 1000 men and 600 women. This inequality of the sexes was inconvenient and inequitable to the district assigned the hospital, which required room for an equal number of each sex for its proper relief. Moreover, the north half of the hospital square, which was for women, had been only partially built up, the north avenue having buildings fronting only on one side. An appropriation of $150,000 was therefore asked of the Legislature to enable detached wards for 300 more women patients to be put up. This appropriation was granted by the Legislature of 1889 and the capacity of the hospital

[1] The writer retired from the superintendency of Kankakee in April, 1893, and the training school then came to an end for a time.

was thus raised to 2000 patients, which number was attained early in 1893.

In 1890 a large diversification of employment had been brought about by assiduous attention. The manufacture of all brooms, baskets, mattresses, harness, slippers and repairing of boots and shoes, were done on the premises; also caning of chairs. All socks and stockings required for both sexes were knit by the women patients; all underclothing for men and under and outer clothing for women were made in the sewing room; also "jeans" suits for men. The wards were abundantly supplied with rugs, doormats, and strips of rag carpet. A scroll-saw, turning lathe, blacksmith forge and anvil were in constant use, and a tinshop was kept in constant operation; a hand printing press was employed to do all minor jobs of printing.

A patient who was a skilled engraver made very satisfactory plates for cards and stationery for the institution. In addition to the above, the farm of 840 acres was kept in a good state of cultivation; the garden and ornamental grounds supplied employment for a large force. In connection with all of this work only one extra man was employed for oversight, as the regular attendants and nurses or domestic employees accompanied these patients to their work and worked with them. There were many "trusty" patients who required little or no supervision.

Mr. G. P. A. Healy, the celebrated American protrait painter, gave to Mr. McCagg, president of the Board of Trustees, in Paris in 1891 about 80 of his paintings. It was understood that Mr. McCagg would bestow these for the most part upon the hospital at Kankakee, retaining any he might choose for himself, but Mr. McCagg gave them all without reserve to the hospital.[1]

[1] The paintings were distributed through the wards and their beauty and attractiveness furnished a new interest and enjoyment to the patients. A catalogue of these paintings was prepared and they were placed upon exhibition in the new shop building for a few days just previous to the occupation of the shop for its proper purpose. The public were invited to view them for a small fee and a convenient little sum was realized for the patients' amusement fund.

Among the paintings which were of especial interest we note No. 4, the portrait of the Count of Paris; No. 5, portrait of Monsieur Barbedienne, the bronze founder; No. 7, a portrait of Mary Anderson, the famous tragedienne; No. 12, a portrait of President Arthur; No. 25, a study of Cardinal Gibbons. There were many copies from the old masters, Rem-

In January, 1893, John P. Altgeld was inaugurated as Governor. The Democratic party was now in power for the first time in Illinois since the Civil War. The result was a change in all the governing boards of the state institutions. Edmund Sill, F. D. Radeke and J. W. Orr formed the new Board of Trustees, who accepted the resignation of Dr. Richard Dewey as superintendent in April, 1893. Dr. S. V. Clevenger, of Chicago, was appointed his successor. Dr. Clevenger remained in charge only about three months, as the condition of his health led to his early resignation and to the appointment of Dr. Clarke Gapen, July 12, 1893.

One important act of Dr. Clevenger, however, was the appointment of Dr. Adolf Meyer as pathologist. Dr. Meyer had recently come to Chicago from Zurich, Switzerland, and had become known to Dr. Ludwig Hektoen, formerly assistant physician at Kankakee and later professor of pathology at Rush Medical College, Chicago. Dr. Hektoen wrote to Dr. Dewey of Dr. Meyer's rare qualifications and the letter had been turned over to Dr. Clevenger. Dr. Meyer's service at Kankakee was the beginning of a career of distinguished honor and success, culminating in 1913 in the directorship of the Henry Phipps Psychiatric Institute, Baltimore, Md. Dr. Meyer served from May, 1893, continuing under the superintendency of Dr. Gapen; and with the co-operation of the latter a laboratory was finally equipped, in which valuable work was done in original research and in instruction of the medical staff. At first Dr. Meyer worked under great difficulties, the only available space for laboratory work being small and badly lighted, but in the course of the year 1893, while the World's Fair was in progress in Chicago, there was obtained by purchase from the German University exhibit an equipment with which at least a beginning could be made in establishing more adequate laboratory service. Later two rooms were set apart in the tower of the main building which were fairly well adapted for the work. A course of instruction was inaugurated for the medical staff, and the patho-anatomical findings in 192 cases were reported in 1895.[1] Staff meetings were systematically held and valuable progress was made. Dr. Meyer also greatly improved the case-taking system,

brandt, Velasquez and others; also copies of a Turner landscape; of a portrait of a lady by Gilbert Stuart; of Sir Joshua Reynolds' "Heads of Angels"; also a portrait of King Charles of Roumania.

[1] Pathological Report, Illinois Eastern Hospital, 1896.

preparing blanks of an admirable and comprehensive character for the anamnesis.

The report of 1896 speaks of a general state of bad repair, walls, roofs, woodwork and plaster having become seriously deteriorated. A general process of renovation was carried out. The time was favorable for this, a time of great business depression, unemployment and low prices. It was possible in consequence of these conditions to employ $95,000 from the ordinary fund for repairs and improvements so that a degree of benefit to the hospital was realized from the general unfortunate financial conditions. The low figure of $138 per capita per annum was reached during this biennial period.

The plan was adopted of keeping newly arrived patients in bed for a considerable time. Women nurses were employed in some of the male wards with advantage. Separate provision for tubercular cases was provided; No. 3, south, was made a hospital ward. Dentistry where needed was provided for the patients through the appointment of a dental specialist. The bath house was remodeled and showers and individual stalls constructed.

In this period, tuberculosis having been found among the dairy herd, pasteurization of the milk supply was adopted and a system of irrigation for the kitchen garden was installed.

In 1897 a new Board of Trustees was appointed by Governor Tanner, whose accession placed the state again in Republican control. The resignation of Dr. Clarke Gapen was accepted wholly or largely from partisan considerations. His service had been generally regarded as able and assiduous. Dr. William G. Stearns was promoted from the position of pathologist to the superintendency. The example set by the previous administration was followed and a "clean sweep" occurred with the resulting confusion, including charges and counter-charges of mal-administration. The board now in charge alleged that the bookkeeping was found defective and instead of a surplus in the treasury of $8000 or more, as reported, there was indebtedness of over $22,000. There was litigation with the city on a charge that the hospital sewerage contaminated the river. All the boilers were condemned and a plan for a central heating plant was adopted. The issue of a publication called *The Psychiater* was begun. It was to contain advanced studies and to be issued four times a year. Mention is made that under the new commitment law 31 "voluntary" commitments had occurred in the biennial period.

Dr. Stearns was superseded in 1899 by Dr. J. C. Corbus, of Mendota, formerly for some years member of the State Board of Charities. Dr. Stearns had shown ability in his short incumbency, but was hampered by unfavorable political conditions.

The report of 1900 records the creation of a new postoffice named "Hospital" for the institution mail. The policy was adopted at this time of purchasing no supplies and employing no person outside the State of Illinois. A new amusement hall with a seating capacity of 1000 was completed and put in use. The old amusement hall was taken for a dormitory for the night attendants and nurses. Tuberculosis was found to prevail in 73 milch cows of the hospital herd.

The report of 1902 showed 2200 inmates, an increase of 200 for the biennial period. The monthly pay-roll had been reduced by the sum of $2000. A new sewer 30 inches in diameter and a mile in length, replacing the old one, had been completed.

The report of 1904 represents the training school as flourishing, the number of applicants being in excess of the number that could be received in the classes. The water being reported as unsuitable for drinking purposes, special arrangements were made to supply the patients with water obtained from melting ice manufactured in the hospital ice-plant.

In 1906 Dr. J. C. Corbus, being now 75 years of age, expressed his willingness to retire, and his resignation being accepted, the trustees on July 21 appointed in Dr. Corbus' stead, Dr. James L. Greene, who had previously been in charge of the State Hospital at Lincoln, Neb.

When Dr. Greene became superintendent he found many conditions producing perplexity and solicitude. There were 40 cases of typhoid among the patients and employees. The physical property was in a dilapidated condition. The proper heating of many of the buildings was impossible from deterioration of apparatus. Furniture and fixtures were worn out or entirely lacking. The domestic department was so destitute that it was impossible to prepare suitable meals; 1800 of the patients' beds had no springs, these having rusted and having been replaced by wooden slats. Hair mattresses had been replaced by straw ticks; only 900 pillows could be found for over 2000 patients. An extensive process of renovation was immediately necessary and was carried through as rapidly as means at hand would permit.

Under the lead of Dr. Frank Billings, of Chicago, the State Board of Public Charities sought advancement all along the line. Bernard E. Sunny, Alba M. Jones and Henry H. Troup formed the new Board of Trustees. The new boards were charged with the duty of placing the institutions upon a higher level. The Board of State Commissioners of Public Charities met in Springfield in 1906 and drew up a program, some of whose items were as follows:

1. To establish a state psychopathic institute.
2. To favor the installation of hydrotherapeutic apparatus.
3. To encourage industrial re-education.
4. To establish uniformity, that is, to "standardize" the service in the state hospitals.
5. To adopt uniform medical records.
6. To establish training schools in all hospitals for the insane and to draft a uniform curriculum.

In addition to these proposals the commissioners advocated "complete state care" (*i. e.,* the removal of all unfortunates from county almshouses and jails); also abolition of mechanical restraint and soporifics. Finally, they announced the principle of using "the cottage plan" in new institutions, thus endorsing segregate instead of congregate construction.

The State Psychopathic Institute was founded by the General Assembly in 1907, upon the urgent representations of the Governor and the Board of State Charities, and $25,000 was appropriated for its equipment. It was understood it would be located at the Kankakee State Hospital; its operations began in September, 1907, although the building provided was not completed until July, 1908. Work was at first limited to teaching the medical officers of the state service and the inauguration of systematic examinations and records of cases.[1]

The scope of the more strictly Psychopathic Hospital department was enlarged by a new building, completed in 1908. This building was of pleasing exterior and attractive interior. Its capacity was 123 beds. Seventy thousand dollars were appro-

[1] For fuller description of the Psychopathic Hospital see page 259.

priated for it in 1907; $20,500 additional in 1909. The building was arranged with facilities for the care of acute cases, elevators, examining and operating rooms, sterilizers, solaria, etc. Provision for hydrotherapeutic apparatus was made in the basement.

Hydrotherapeutic apparatus was introduced in the main building for male patients in 1908, duplicating that which had been in use for female patients since 1906.

In July, 1909, Dr. James L. Greene was appointed by the Governor to the newly-created position of " alienist " upon the " State Board of Administration " and Dr. J. F. WenGlesky was made acting superintendent. He served in this capacity until October 18, when Dr. Frank P. Norbury, of Jacksonville, was appointed superintendent, and assumed the duties of the position.

The new State Charities Act had become effective July 1, 1909. This law provided for " state care." It was the intention of the law that all the insane remaining in county care should be transferred to the state institutions. When this was done in the Kankakee district serious overcrowding resulted. Dining and day rooms were converted into dormitories and a large number still unprovided for could only be given beds upon the floors. In the matter of " state care " an exception was made of Cook County, since of the 2700 inmates at Kankakee there were already 1700 who were residents of Cook County. It was evident that " state care " was impossible for the 2000 still remaining under the custody of the county asylum at Dunning. The law was so framed, however, that the Cook County Asylum might be converted into a state hospital in the event of the county transferring the property of the asylum to the state, and this was afterwards done.

The inauguration of training schools in all state hospitals in 1911 was a very considerable step in advance.[1]

A large amount of earnest work was expended upon this enterprise under the initiative of Dr. Frank Billings, of the State Board of Charities. Dr. Frank P. Norbury, the alienist member of the Board of Administration, supervised in an able manner the laying out of the course of instruction and the schedule for lectures, demonstrations, practical drill, etc.

[1] At Kankakee this was only a revival of what the first superintendent established a quarter of a century earlier. See report of Kankakee Hospital for 1888, pp. 18, *et seq.*

In the *Institution Quarterly* of September, 1912, is found a paper by Dr. Frank P. Norbury, alienist of the State Board, on "Standard of Seclusion and Restraint" (mechanical), which states:

> The Board of Administration, in response to these newer ideas in hospital management, has sought to supervise restraint by having it ordered "on prescription" and reported in regular form as a part of the activities of hospital management. The object is to define restraint, seclusion, etc., and to place responsibility in its regulation in each hospital. The forms herewith shown, together with the special order issued by the Board of Administration, represent, it is believed, an adequate regulation and a permanent record "worth while" as a step in advance in hospital management.[1]

The establishing of this system for regulation of mechanical restraint was also a revival so far as Kankakee was concerned.[2] It was adopted in all the state institutions in 1911 and has, we understand, resulted largely in the discontinuance of restraint.

On September 1, 1911, Dr. Wilgus, the superintendent, stated there was not one patient under restraint at Kankakee.

During the same period (1910-1912) regulations were adopted for standardizing the medical service, three grades being adopted: first, "assistant superintendent"; second, "physicians"; third, "assistant physicians." Examinations were held for admission as assistants and for promotion to the higher grades under civil service rules. The effect of civil service rules and of instruction in the Psychopathic Institute was such as to raise the level of attainment; friendly rivalry and emulation were thus created between the hospitals. A medical society was also formed, which tended to promote professional attainment and alertness in the professional work. During the above named period the Board of Administration also adopted methods for systematic purchase of all supplies.

The laboratory of the Psychopathic Institute was fully equipped,

[1] There follow definitions of "restraint" and "seclusion" which were to be employed in preparing records in each institution. We note that "prolonged or continuous baths" are included under forms of "restraint."

[2] This "step in advance," although quite forgotten (or never known) by the newer generation, had in 1880 to 1886 been precisely formulated, administered and reported under the writer's direction. See reports of Kankakee for 1880, p. 19, *et seq.*; also for 1882, p. 22, *et seq.*; also 1884 and 1886.

but the work of research lagged, owing to shortage of the staff. To adapt the staff fully to the requirements of the work it was found desirable to provide for internes.

At the visit of the executive secretary, 1911, there was found in No. 1 north an appalling state of overcrowding, disorder and unsanitary conditions. There was scarcely room between the beds for the patients to stand. Straw ticks were in general use as mattresses. The doors were kept locked at night. The main building was found at this time in excellent order in all parts. As other examples of overcrowding, the case of A-3 south is given. In 1906 it contained 29 patients; in 1911, 41. Cottage No. 3 south, which had 74 patients in 1906, had 107 in 1911.

January 11, 1913: The visit is recorded of a class of 50 students in sociology from the University of Illinois, with the professor under whom they are studying, for the purpose of gaining conception of the outward aspect of insanity and of the methods of the state in caring for its insane.

The census of the patients at that time amounted to 2950. There were 12 physicians, nine of whom were on regular day duty, one on night duty and two engaged in research; there were on an average 330 patients in the care of each of the nine.

April 4, 1913, the hospital bakery was partially burned. In the efforts to bring the fire hose into use and employ the high pressure pump the pressure suddenly ceased entirely and it was afterwards found there was an extensive split in a length of water main. The split had evidently existed when the pipe was laid, as it had been partially plugged with wood and rags.

The water is a source of anxiety, not as to quantity but quality. All water has been taken lately from two deep artesian wells, one of which furnishes soft and pure water; the water of the other tends to corrode pipes and boilers. The river water is now used for most purposes except drinking, and the better of the two wells is taken for drinking purposes. The use of river water for drinking had formerly been found to result in frequent cases of typhoid.

In April, 1913, the population reached 3085; over 200 were sleeping on the floor.

In this year the general dining-room heretofore used for 500 patients from the west row of cottages was completely renovated and is now used for the employees' dining-room, while the basement underneath, formerly used as the employees' dining-room, is now remodeled and enlarged and used for the patients. The *Quarterly* states it is a badly lighted room and will require artificial light even in the daytime. No. 5 north has had an addition made to it for 60 female nurses.

In December, 1913, an order was issued closing the hospital to promiscuous visiting. It had been found that such visiting very easily degenerated into an abuse and had reached such a stage that the grounds had been used like a public park for picnics on Saturdays and Sundays and disorderly crowds had wandered about. This was objectionable, particularly with reference to the north cottages for disturbed and untidy female patients. Even railroad companies advertised excursions to Kankakee, giving the hospital for insane as one of the "attractions."

In this connection an improvement is announced in the rules about visits of patients' friends. It is ordered that friends shall be taken promptly to the patient in the department where he is without bringing him to some other ward or waiting to "dress him up."

The measures taken by the secretary under the instruction of the State Board of Administration in thoroughly investigating and following up every clue to alleged misdeeds of employees, especially where there is a charge of abuse or cruelty to a patient, and the entire freedom in seeking to throw all possible light on any alleged misdeed; to welcome inquiry and conceal nothing—all these things indicate a healthy tone and atmosphere in the administration of the state institutions, which is illustrated by several cases detailed in the December, 1913, *Institution Quarterly*.

In January, 1914, the *Quarterly* makes record of an interesting transformation in the male hospital ward, which had been a "storm center of trouble" for more than a year. It had been the recommendation of the executive secretary of the Board of Administration that women nurses should be placed in charge, and this step has now been taken. Seventeen women are now employed in the care of male patients. The results of this change will be watched with interest.

The following notes are taken from the June-September *Quarterly:*

June, 1914: At this time there are 1000 paroled patients. There are 12 "open" cottages, whose doors are never locked and whose windows are not barred or screened. No patients are now sleeping on the floor. Some day-rooms have been taken for dormitories and two patients have been put in certain single rooms. This is not allowed except as a necessity, growing out of the overcrowded condition. Women attendants on male wards have been increased in number. Ten additional male wards have been put in the charge of women nurses. Eight hundred of the most demented and untidy are taken to the hall for a picture show once each week. Every screen door has been taken off. In two months no patient's door has been locked at night. There has been no seclusion and only one case of restraint. The changes for the better have been cordially and unanimously supported by doctors and employees. The water supply has now been made ample and unobjectionable. The new laundry is nearing completion.

As the hospital at Kankakee was avowedly a departure from methods previously prevailing in architectural construction and was administered with the purpose of putting to the test certain progressive ideas, a few words may be given in conclusion as to the results attained.

Was the more domestic style of construction, the so-called "cottage" or detached ward, successful, and did it win general approval?

This question is answered by results, immediate and remote, so well known as to require but the briefest statement. This more simple, segregated and less expensive style of architecture employed in the detached buildings at Kankakee as a substitute for the many-storied, congregate "central building, with wings" (previously considered necessary), was given immediate recognition and is accepted to-day as a matter of course. The change in constructive ideas had begun in a rudimentary way before Kankakee existed and would doubtless have developed in any event, but Kankakee served as an impetus, a point of departure and an object lesson. Ohio, Indiana, Dakota, New York at Ogdensburg and Central Islip, departed from the congregate "center building with wings" after the experimental stage had been passed and all frankly availed themselves of the experience here recorded.[1] Later Massachusetts, the General Government Hospital at Washington, D. C., Canada at Mimico near Toronto, and many other states and municipalities built extensively on the detached plan.

[1] For details see biennial reports of the Kankakee Hospital for 1886-1888; 1890-1892.

Illinois continued to extend in the same line as shown at Peoria in the resolution of its Board of Public Charities adopted in 1909, "to use the cottage plan for new institutions,"[1] and the *Quarterly* of June, 1914, in reporting the visits of the State Board of Administration to institutions in New York, Washington, D. C., Maryland, Ohio and Indiana, remarks: "The new institutions and the additions to the old are all on the cottage plan. The 'cottage'-plan hospital at Kankakee, the first of its kind in the world, had served during these years to demonstrate the foresight of its designers."[2]

Perhaps it may be said that individuality rather than any stereotyped form of building grew largely from the experience at Kankakee, and the truth coming to recognition there, was freedom in construction. It was established as a fact that the insane can be well cared for in any good building and that the spirit pervading the buildings is even more important than their outward form. Bound up with the freer construction are elements of freedom in other points. No one would object to less rigorous and more indulgent management for the patients provided this were compatible with safety and economy. This was the point to be tested. Order, efficiency, industry and economy must accompany the giving of greater indulgences and privileges to the patients.

The first report of the medical superintendent in 1880 contained the following statement of the purposes kept in view at Kankakee:

This hospital, while seeking the good results usually accomplished by such institutions, is especially committed to a course of careful experimentation and effort in the direction of determining—

First. How moderate the expense of erecting suitable buildings for the insane can be made.

Second. Whether occupation which will be beneficial in every sense cannot be secured for a majority of the inmates.

Third. To what extent the rigor of confinement and restraint can be removed and a natural and somewhat domestic mode of life be introduced among our patients.

And first referring to the cost of buildings: It had been, as is well known, the general experience prior to 1880 that the cost of the congregate style of building throughout the country had ranged from $1000 per capita up. In many instances double and even treble this amount had been expended for every patient

[1] Report for 1909.

[2] *Institution Quarterly,* June, 1914, p. 60.

accommodated. One notable exception had attracted attention; this was the cost of the additions made by Dr. Chapin to the Willard Asylum at Ovid, N. Y. Some of these additions had been built for $500 per capita, not including, however, the cost of the general service buildings, land, furniture, etc. These buildings were still, however, on the congregate plan.

At Kankakee in 1883-1884 detached buildings for 1000 patients were completed for $400 per capita, including furniture. The total per capita cost at Kankakee, when a capacity of 1600 had been reached, was $754.50. This figure included the congregate fireproof main building for 300 patients, which alone had cost upward of $1000 per capita. It also included cost of land, service buildings, etc., for the institution as a whole, furniture and every expense in fact except actual running expenses. These latter items are, as is well known, often not included in reckoning per capita expense; hence a notable reduction in expense of construction is seen. It is also true that still further extension at Kankakee continued to lower the proportional expense. Thus a reduction in building expense bordering upon 50 per cent is shown, which is a realization of one of the aims at Kankakee above mentioned.

Coming now to the question of occupation for insane, it is to be said that the development of Kankakee showed an expansion in industries of many sorts, and a percentage of employment not hitherto attained or reported, so far as known. Something of the variety of industries is shown in the preceding pages and in the record here presented as Appendix A (see p. 253) of the articles made in the year ending June 30, 1891. This would not be an unusual record at the present day, but at that time was a distinct advance. The record of general percentage of employment was accurately kept from the beginning and steadily rose from 42½ in the first biennial period to 57 per cent in 1888; 68 per cent in 1890 and 73 per cent in the last period of the writer's superintendency (1892). This record was kept with accuracy, no person being counted twice (see Appendix B) and only the actual number of persons employed was reckoned; whether given to only one or to several kinds of work.[1]

[1] See tables of employment biennial reports 1880-1892. As also Appendices A and B.

In this connection it is also to be noted that in the period under discussion the running expense of the institution per capita generally averaged lower than that of any other of the Illinois state hospitals, as shown by the annual comparative statements of the Boards of Charities.

Now taking up the question of increased privileges to patients and removal to some extent of the "rigor of confinement and restraint" and the introduction of a "natural and somewhat domestic mode of life," we may refer first to the record of "open" wards and of patients on parole, which exceeded in that day the records of other institutions. Indeed the limits of parole and of privileges were not determined by the limit of numbers of patients to whom such privileges could be extended with safety, but by other considerations of the welfare of patients themselves. It did not take long to discover that scores of patients who could have the parole with entire safety were in nowise benefited thereby, but were prone to give themselves up to loitering and insolence; therefore in the case of the able-bodied a reasonable amount of work was made a condition. The parole was limited to certain times and places for the patient's own good.

The diffusion of a homelike atmosphere and the promotion of amusement and employment were an important part of the effort to give greater contentment and satisfaction to these persons, and of course what was accomplished in non-restraint comes under this head.

In this direction the effect also of living in a "house" rather than a "ward," of going and coming to meals, to work and to entertainments more as people in the outside world, must be seen or experienced to be appreciated.

In this connection we may refer to the status in the present year (1914), described on page 246, showing that 1000 patients were on parole; that there were 12 "open" cottages never locked in the day and without bars or screens at windows; 10 male wards were in charge of women nurses; 800 of the most demented patients were taken to a weekly picture show. In two months there had been no seclusion and only one case of mechanical restraint.

The reader is now, I hope, in a position to form his own opinion concerning the institution at Kankakee and in closing my account, as the individual through whom its plans and progress were carried out, in its formative years, I desire to pay a tribute of honor to the memory of Frederick Howard Wines. His ability and force of character were the originating and sustaining power in the inception of "segregated" construction at Kankakee, as opposed to the "congregate" style previously prevailing. His ideas, ably and eloquently presented, were the source of much that was new and valuable in the evolution of greater freedom, adaptability, intelligence and efficiency in constructing and organizing institutions for the insane in the United States.

TRUSTEES.

Name	Years
John H. Clough (president)	1877-1881
William Reddick	1877-1885
William F. Murphy	1887-1891
Ezra B. McCagg (president)	1881-1893
John L. Donovan	1881-1893
Lemuel Milk	1885-1889
Walter W. Todd	1889-1893
Edmund Sill (president)	1893-1897
J. W. Orr	1893-1897
F. D. Radcke	1893-1897
Len. Small (president)	1897-1906
George T. Buckingham	1897-1902
J. J. Magee	1897-1900
Almette Powell	1900-1906
A. M. Jones	1906-1909
P. Whalen	1904-1906
C. E. Robinson	1905-
Bernard E. Sunny (president)	1906-1909
Harry H. Troup	1908-1909

Board of Trustees superseded by State Board of Administration, July, 1909.

MEDICAL SUPERINTENDENTS.

Name	Years
Dr. Richard Dewey	1879-1893
Dr. S. V. Clevenger (April 1-July 12)	1893-1893
Dr. Clarke Gapen	1893-1897
Dr. Wm. G. Stearns	1897-1899
Dr. J. C. Corbus	1899-1906
Dr. J. L. Greene	1906-1909
Dr. Frank P. Norbury	1909-1911
Dr. Sidney D. Wilgus	1911-1913
Dr. P. M. Kelly (in office)	1913-

ASSISTANT SUPERINTENDENTS.

Name	Years
Dr. Julius F. WenGlesky	1907-1910
Dr. Francis J. Sullivan (acting)	1907-1911
Dr. T. R. Foster	1910-1911
Dr. Charles F. Read	1911-1914
Dr. Eugene Cohn (in office)	1914-

DIRECTOR OF STATE PATHOLOGICAL LABORATORY.

Name	Years
Dr. Adolf Meyer	1893-1895
Dr. Wm. G. Stearns	1895-1897
Dr. V. Podstata	1897-1903

DIRECTOR OF STATE PSYCHOPATHIC INSTITUTE.

Dr. H. Douglas Singer.. 1907-

ASSISTANT PHYSICIANS.

Dr. Harold N. Moyer...	1879-1882	Dr. Chas. Ricksher......	1912-1913
Dr. Henry M. Bannister.	1881-1892	Dr. H. T. Child.........	1912-1913
Dr. Elmore S. Pettyjohn	1882-1885	Dr. Chas. R. Lowe......	1912-1913
Dr. Cassius D. Westcott.	1884-1886	Dr. Otis Like...........	1913-1913
Dr. Lawrence H. Prince	1885-1887	Dr. W. G. Murray (in office)	1912-
Dr. Abraham L. Warner	1886-1894	Dr. E. C. Pratt (in office)	1912-
Dr. Delia Howe........	1885-1888	Dr. D. Fish (in office)..	1912-
Dr. M. M. Crocker......	1887-1889	Dr. J. T. Rooks (in office)	1912-
Dr. Edward Howard....	1887-1889	Dr. H. J. Freemmel.....	1913-1914
Dr. Ludwig Hektoen....	1887-1887	Dr. A. H. Deppe........	1913-1914
Dr. Anne C. Barnet.....	1888-1893	Dr. Elizabeth Carroll (in office)	1913-
Dr. Louis R. Head......	1888-1888	Dr. T. J. Riach (in office)	1913-
Dr. B. L. Riese.........	1888-1890	Dr. G. F. Haig (in office)	1914-
Dr. J. P. Houston.......	1889-1889	Dr. F. J. Sullivan (in office)	1914-
Dr. L. L. Shelton.......	1889-1891	Dr. J. T. Rooks (in office)	1914-
Dr. J. Chambers Dodds..	1889-1889	Dr. Elizabeth D. Carroll (in office)	1914-
Dr. Samuel Dodds......	1890-1891	Dr. Drury L. Fish (in office)	1914-
Dr. Charles H. Bradley..	1891-1893	Dr. Jos. Cooperstein (in office)	1914-
Dr. George Boody.......	1891-1893	Dr. H. T. Childs (in office)	1914-
Dr. H. D. Valin.........	1892-1892	Dr. O. G. Kibler (in office)	1914-
Dr. T. R. Foster........	1892-1892; 1897-	Dr. E. C. Davis (in office)	1914-
Dr. Isabel M. Davenport	1893-1893		
Dr. Wm. G. Stearns....	1894-1897		
Dr. O. A. Kell..........	1901-1910		
Dr. C. G. Rydin.........	1905-1910		
Dr. E. A. Foley.........	1907-1910		
Dr. R. H. Rea..........	1909-1910		
Dr. Wm. T. Lorenz......	1910-1910		
Dr. W. W. Mercer......	1910-1911		
Dr. C. F. Sanborn.......	1910-1911		
Dr. T. G. Charles........	1910-1912		
Dr. W. H. Holmes......	1911-1912		

SECRETARY AND TREASURER.

Col. Haswell C. Clarke..	1877-1893	Alexis Granger	1896-1897
Daniel C. Taylor.......	1893-1896	C. R. Miller............	1897-1906

TREASURER.

Clarence E. Holt 1908-

APPENDIX A.

The following list is presented, showing articles manufactured by the patients in the shops and wards during the year ending June 30, 1891:

Article	Number
Dresses, cotton and woolen	1006
Underwear, men's and women's	5274
Sheets and pillowcases	3308
Table cloths, napkins and towels	3802
Window curtains and lambrequins	925
Woolen rugs and husk mats	439
Coats, vests and blouses	161
Pants and overalls	197
Aprons, caps and mittens	1535
Shirts	1511
Mattress-ticks and blankets	77
Socks and stockings, pairs	2802
Sunbonnets and bibs	300
Hats, trimmed	230
Pictures, framed	419
Brooms	6352
Baskets, farm, laundry and market	56
Chairs repaired, all kinds	292
Settees, camp stools and bedrests (repaired or made)	44
Carpet, yards (rag)	528
Harness, made, sets	6
Harness, repaired and extra parts made	296
Tinware made (pieces)	3933
Tinware repaired (pieces)	971
Upholstering, hair mattresses, new and made-over	175
Pillows, made over and renovated	2000
Shoemaking, pairs repaired	1293
Slippers, made	126

Printing, programmes for entertainments and chapel service, cards, bills, forms, etc.

Copper-plate engraving, wood-turning, scroll saw work, wood carving, locksmithing, light blacksmithing, and a large variety of ladies' fancy work.

An exhibit of arts, crafts and fancy work was made at the State Fair at Peoria in 1891 and the above list distributed to visitors. The list was printed on the hospital press.

APPENDIX B.

Table Showing Number of Patients Employed in all Departments, November 8, 1884.

This table is absolutely correct as to number employed and kinds of employment, but counts the same person in some cases *twice over,* when such person happens to be employed in two or more departments.

The ratio of employment if computed from this table would be 88 per cent for men and 76 per cent for women, whereas the actual percentage, counting *persons* employed, was 60 per cent for men and 49 per cent for women.

Males.	
On farm	10
In garden	3
On grounds	34
Assisting supernumerary	4
Assisting engineer	6
Assisting mason	4
In laundry	8
Taking care of stock	2
Stable work	1
Teaming	6
Assisting blacksmith	1
Filling straw beds	10
In boiler rooms	2
Assisting porter	14
Assisting druggist	1
Assisting matron	4
In kitchen	8
In bakery	3
In dining rooms	58
Ward work	83
Digging ditches for tile drain	50
Shoveling coal	13
Assisting store keeper	1
Shoe making	1
Assisting carpenter	3
Assisting butcher	1
Assisting plumber	1
Furnace work	2
	334
Percentage of patients shown to be employed by above list	80
Percentage of patients actually employed	60

Females.	
Ward work	87
Kitchen work	24
Laundry work	6
In ironing room	10
In sewing room	28
Ward mending	22
Fancy work	8
Mending room	7
Carrying clothes and general choring	20
Knitting	5
	217
Percentage of patients shown to be employed by above list	76
Percentage of patients actually employed	49

The above table, compiled in 1884, shows a much lower percentage of employment than was later regularly maintained.

From 1884 to 1893 (when the writer ceased to be superintendent) it was found possible to steadily increase the average number employed.

NOTE.—The method of counting both persons and kinds of work in making percentage of employment is fallacious, as shown in this appendix, as the apparent ratio of employment here shown is over 25 per cent in excess of the real ratio.

APPENDIX C.

POLITICAL INFLUENCE IN THE STATE HOSPITAL, 1893.

A few words may not be out of place with regard to the presence or absence of partisan political motives in the administration of Kankakee Hospital during the 14 years covered by the writer's superintendency. Mention has been made of the appointment at the beginning of a carpenter who, to the consternation of the local political boss, was found to be a Democrat. And it should be stated that, although the local party managers were disturbed by this lack of attention to the party labels, the Board of Trustees had no share in this political sentiment. They were, as has been stated, a non-partisan board—two Republicans and one Democrat —but all agreed wholly in disregarding partisan political questions so far as the business and administration of the hospital was concerned.[1]

[1] The only occasion during the 14 years on which political questions received attention or discussion in the trustees' meetings was in 1889 or 1890, during the term of Joseph W. Fifer as Governor. On one occasion the private secretary of the Governor spent two or three days at the hospital and on the day of his departure stated to the superintendent he wished to ask a favor for a brother of the Governor. This brother of the Governor was in need of employment and it was desired that a position which would pay about $60 per month should be found for him. After the departure of the secretary the superintendent, thinking it best to have the advice of the trustees on a question of this kind, arranged a meeting and made known to the trustees the views of the Governor's secretary. The superintendent requested instructions in the matter, but the trustees asked first for the superintendent's views. They inquired whether a position such as that described was available and were

Toward the end of the 14 years above named, when some question was raised about the politics of people employed in the hospital, a tabular statement was prepared of the male employees—about 150 in number—and they were found to be nearly equally divided between the Republican and Democratic parties. No employee, when applying for work, was ever questioned as to his politics nor later as to his manner of voting. The trustees, superintendent, and possibly two others of those in charge, made small contributions to the campaign fund from their own pockets, as was a very prevalent custom in that day, but no assessments were ever levied upon the whole list of employees, as happened at a later date.

If I speak of the successive Governors, it is absolutely with reference to the effect of their methods upon the efficiency of the state hospitals, whose history I am seeking to write in an impartial spirit. John P. Altgeld, though he swept away (in 1893) all Boards of Trustees and through them practically all the Republican incumbents of office, high and low, was seriously desirous of honest and efficient administration, but his methods could not fail of mischievous results. The men to whom he gave power at Kankakee were not as disinterested or public spirited as himself or as men in public office ought to be. Some of them were actuated by personal motives rather than desire for public welfare. When the Republican party again regained power, in 1896, another "clean sweep" followed with its inevitable evil consequences, and the successive Republican Governors, John R. Tanner (1897-1901) and Richard Yates (1901-1905), were known to be given to partisanship. Many of the men entrusted with power in the state hospitals under their rule had little conception of public office as a public trust—in fact, methods prevailed under their administra-

---

informed that it was not. The superintendent was then asked what he proposed to do about the matter, and his reply was that if the decision were left to him he should inform the secretary that a position of the kind desired did not exist in the institution and he regretted his inability to comply with the wish expressed. The trustees thereupon instructed the superintendent to advise the Governor through his private secretary as above stated in as diplomatic manner as possible. Nothing further was heard from the Governor's office in regard to it, and indeed it seemed probable, in the light of subsequent events, that the private secretary had taken upon himself more than the Governor knew of or desired.

tion that were productive of abuses. Partisan work was expected of the persons given employment. In political campaigns, the hospital band and glee club were sent to furnish music at party rallies. Assessments were directly collected in some cases; in others withheld from wages of employees for the promotion of partisan or personal aims. Places were given to unfit individuals. Business transactions were determined rather by favor than by merit. Of the recurring scandals, it is unnecessary to speak. They were sufficiently well known and susceptible of abundant proof. The superintendent from 1899-1906, a man over three score and ten, was superintendent only in name. The trustees, instead of fulfilling their trust, directed the operations of the "machine" they created. They assumed functions that did not rightly belong to a board of trustees. Their omissions and commissions brought disgrace and scandal. Their misdeeds served as an object lesson to their successors, and after Governor Deneen assumed office (1905) an improvement occurred. Governor Deneen sought to establish a higher standard, and during his first term a civil service law was enacted. The Board of Public Charities appointed by him endeavored to secure improvement, both in a practical and a scientific sense.

At this point mention may justly be made of services of especial value to the hospital which came to an end in 1893. Both John H. Clough, the first president of the board, and Ezra B. McCagg, his successor, brought exceptional knowledge, experience, fidelity and ability to the discharge of their duties. William Reddick was also a man of admirable qualities of heart and mind. From humble beginnings he rose to the attainment of much honor and of wealth which his humanitarian impulses led him to distribute generously. A beautiful and stately public library was given by him to his home city and 100 acres of land were added by him to the county farm.

The secretary and treasurer from the beginning in 1877 till 1893, Col. Haswell C. Clarke, was a man whose services the hospital was especially fortunate in securing. He was a veteran of the Civil War, having enlisted while still under age, and without the knowledge of his parents, being then a student at Harvard College. He was attached to the staff of Gen. Ben Butler and gave gallant service during the occupation of New Orleans as well as in Virginia, where he was for a long period frequently exposed to the enemy's fire while daily riding to convey dispatches between the field headquarters. Col. Clarke's high sense of honor, geniality, fair-mindedness and absolute fidelity in his duties as treasurer and secretary were notable.

The architect, James R. Willett, who also served uninterruptedly for 16 years, was another exceptionally forceful and capable man in the performance of his duties. He was a thorough engineer as well as architect, and always made soundness and stability his first consideration, seemingly leaving appearances to take care of themselves. Yet his work somehow produced an effect of admirable taste and good judgment.

James Lillie, the builder and contractor who carried out the entire series of building operations from 1877 to 1893, involving an outlay of $1,250,000, was thoroughly competent in his calling and a man of sterling character. In the face of very active competition he knew how to estimate closely enough to distance other bidders, and yet honorably make a reasonable profit.

Another man who contributed very materially to the practical success at Kankakee was John C. Burt, supervisor of the male wards, afterwards "business assistant to the superintendent." He had been associated with Dr. Dewey at Elgin as pharmacist. His grasp of the essentials of the problems of establishing diversification of industries, enforcing humane supervision, judiciously enlarging privileges of the patients, all in the exercise of economy and safety, was thorough. In the later years, as "business assistant" from 1886 to 1893, Mr. Burt most ably assisted the superintendent in the executive management of the business, as distinguished from the medical affairs of this institution.

Mr. S. N. Calkin during more than 11 years carried on the farming operations with marked ability. It was not a simple task to successfully cultivate over 800 acres of land and maintain a milking herd of over 100 cattle; also a kitchen garden of nearly or quite 100 acres. There were 10,000 or 15,000 bushels of grain to harvest every year; there was a great ice harvest in the winter, and more than all the rest were the slaughtering and packing for a population of over 2000. Nearly 1000 head of cattle were slaughtered for beef each year, a rendering plant was also attached and from the tallow of the slaughter house the hospital was supplied with laundry soap.

Several faithful craftsmen who served through the 14 years deserve honorable mention: James Bradbury, the engineer; Gerhard Paulissen, the foreman of carpenter work; William E. Toler, the shop foreman, and Anna, his wife, a housekeeper of no ordinary ability, served nearly the whole period, and the latter is still serving in the same capacity (1914).

ILLINOIS STATE PSYCHOPATHIC INSTITUTE.[1]

KANKAKEE, ILL.

This institution was founded in 1907, with the object of improving the general care and treatment of the insane in the State of Illinois and of conducting research into the etiology of mental disorders. It is located upon the grounds of the Kankakee State Hospital. During the first three years of its existence attention was devoted almost entirely to the functions of teaching and reorganizing the medical service, because of limited appropriations for its upkeep. During this period systematic instruction in psychiatry was given to all medical officers in the service; a uniform system of examination and records of patients was formulated and later adopted in all the state hospitals; and the present graded system of medical officers was outlined and recommended to the Board of Administration. Staff meetings for the consideration of all patients admitted to the hospitals were inaugurated, medical societies were established in each hospital and an inter-hospital medical association was founded, to which all medical officers belonged. The laboratory work was limited to the routine blood, urine, spinal fluid, bacteriologic and pathologic work of the Kankakee State Hospital.

Since July 1, 1910, larger appropriations have been available and it has been possible to employ assistants. The teaching has been maintained partly by courses of instruction given at the institute and partly by visits to the different hospitals.

The research work has been divided into four departments: (1) Clinical; (2) clinical pathology; (3) biologic chemistry; (4) histology. Each of these departments has now an assistant in charge and technicians are gradually being added. The clinical

[1] By H. Douglas Singer, M. D., director.

department has control of two wards, each with a capacity of about 35 beds, by the courtesy of the Kankakee State Hospital. The clinical pathologist has until the last three or four months been required to perform the routine laboratory examinations for the Kankakee State Hospital, but this duty has now been largely eliminated. Wassermann reactions are performed upon specimens sent from all of the state institutions, penal as well as charitable. The histologic department receives material mainly from the Kankakee State Hospital, but all the state hospitals have been requested to furnish material from disorders selected for special study whenever possible.

Prior to 1913 the position of physician to the institute was filled by the detail of a physician from one of the state hospitals for varying periods. The following have served in this capacity: Dr. C. F. Read, 1910-1911; Dr. A. H. Dollear, 1911-1912; Dr. M. C. Hawley, 1912; Dr. Treadway, 1912; Dr. Morrow and Dr. S. N. Clark. On July 1, 1913, Dr. Clark was appointed on the staff of the institute.

The position of clinical pathologist has been held successively by Dr. A. Bybee, 1910-1911; Dr. W. H. Holmes, 1911-1912; Dr. S. L. Gabby, 1912, and Dr. K. M. Manougian. Mr. A. F. Wussow was the first biologic chemist, 1911-1912, and was succeeded by Dr. E. L. Ross, 1912, and later by Dr. W. B. Quantz. The pathological department was organized in 1912, when Dr. L. J. Pollock was appointed; he was succeeded by Dr. E. B. Jewell, 1912, and later by Dr. C. Ricksher.

The present (1914) officers are:

H. Douglas Singer, M. D., M. R., C. P., director.
S. N. Clark, M. D., physician.
Chas. Ricksher, M. D., clinical pathologist.
W. B. Quartz, biologic chemist.
K. N. Manougian, M. D., pathologist.

CHESTER STATE HOSPITAL.[1]

MENARD, ILL.

The Chester State Hospital, formerly the Asylum for Insane Criminals, was created by an act of the Legislature approved June 1, 1889, and was opened for the reception of patients in November, 1891. The act provided for the transfer to this institution of all the insane convicts in the penitentiaries at Joliet and Chester. Committals are also made under the mittimus of any of the several courts of the state. The homicidal and dangerous patients confined in the other state hospitals for the insane may be transferred to this institution by order of the Board of Administration.

The institution is situated on a high bluff commanding a fine view of the Mississippi River and surrounding country. The main building is "T" shaped, and consists of the administration offices, the superintendent's and employees' quarters, four wards for the patients, the employees' and patients dining room, and a general kitchen. There are the usual outlying buildings, such as laundry, stables, dairy, barn, etc.

The site comprises 17 acres owned by the state; 43 acres adjoining are rented for farm and garden purposes, where most of the vegetables and fruit used by the patients are grown.

The institution is accessible by the St. Louis, Iron Mountain and Southern, the Illinois Southern, the Cotton Belt, and the W. C. & W. railroads.

The medical organization consists of a superintendent and an assistant. The patients are given a thorough, uniform mental and physical examination in accordance with the general outline furnished by the clinical director of the State Psychopathic Institute, who makes regular visits to this hospital to review all doubtfully classified cases, and to conduct lecture courses. There is a clinical and pathological laboratory sufficient for the needs of the hospital. Inasmuch as the inmates are all males, the attendant force is composed of men. There is one supervising nurse who has received special nursing training in the care of the insane.

Inasmuch as this hospital is for the care of the criminal insane, discipline requires greater restriction of the freedom of the patients than is the case in the average hospital for the insane.

[1] By George Knapp Farris, M. D., superintendent.

During the summer months about 16 per cent are employed out of doors, and during the winter months about 10 per cent. Every effort is made to encourage employment, especially in the occupation department, which is conducted under a skilled mechanic. Wherever possible, inmates are encouraged to assist in the several departments of the institution. From 50 to 60 per cent of the patients are employed.

Few of the patients committed to this institution are paroled. They are either discharged when recovered, in accordance with the provisions made in the commitment papers, or upon recovery returned to the prison from which they have been received.

The present (1914) number of patients is 228. The capacity of the institution is 150.

The appropriation for the ordinary expenses of the institution for the years 1915 and 1916 is $50,000 per annum; for repairs and improvements $3000 per annum; for library purposes $200 per annum.

TRUSTEES.

J. B. Messick	1889-1893 1897-1899 1900-1901	James E. Jobe	1897-1901
		H. F. Bader	1899-1900
		J. H. Duncan	1901-1906
John J. Brown	1889-1893	James E. McClure	1901-1903 1904-1910
James A. Rose	1889-1893		
E. C. Kramer	1893-1897	Thos. J. Clark	1901-1909
W. V. Choisser	1893-1897	J. B. Blackman	1903-1904
J. J. Schueder	1893-1895	Rufus Neely	1906-1910
C. S. Hearn	1895-1897	L. L. Emerson	1909-1910
Thos. W. Scott	1897-1901		

SUPERINTENDENTS.[1]

Dr. Patterson.
Dr. E. S. Benson.
Dr. Auten.
Dr. R. T. Higgins.
Dr. Walter E. Songer.
Dr. C. H. Anderson.
Dr. G. K. Farris.
Dr. Jerome L. Harrell, in office.

ASSISTANT PHYSICIANS.[1]

Dr. A. F. Telford.
Dr. Duncan.
Dr. Blackman.
Dr. Smith.
Dr. Meade.
Dr. R. M. Ritchey.
Dr. R. F. Windsor.
Dr. W. L. Hercik.
Dr. I. F. Frisch.
Dr. Otis Like.
Dr. I. F. Freemmel, in office.

[1] In order of their appointment.

PEORIA STATE HOSPITAL.[1]

PEORIA, ILL.

(FORMERLY THE ILLINOIS GENERAL HOSPITAL FOR THE INSANE; ORIGINALLY THE ILLINOIS ASYLUM FOR THE INCURABLE INSANE.)

As the various titles imply this institution is an evolution growing out of the needs of the incurably insane, who were cared for in almshouses or consigned to the custodial wards of the other institutions for the care of the insane.

The movement that gave being to the Illinois Asylum for the Incurable Insane dates back many years.

The State of Illinois maintains eight state hospitals for the exclusive care of the insane, which had an average daily population of more than 14,000 during the year 1912. It is probable that, as each institution became filled to its capacity and a new one was projected, someone advanced the idea that an institution for the incurables would relieve the situation. It is likely that such action would have been greatly hastened had it not been for a provision of the Illinois Lunacy Law which said to the officer conveying a patient to a state institution:

> . . . . that if there is no room in such hospital for the admission of the person committed thereto, and that such county shall have its full quota of patients in said hospital, the superintendent thereof shall return to said county one quiet, harmless, chronic patient, but should said county not have its full quota of patients in said hospital, the superintendent shall return one quiet, harmless, chronic patient to any county which may be in excess of its quota; and should no county be in excess of its quota, the superintendent shall select the most quiet, harmless, chronic patient in said hospital and return him to the county from which he was committed, in order to make room for the patient recently adjudged insane.

This law gave such easy egress for the excess over the quota of the various counties that the immediate necessity of a separate state institution for the care of the incurables was for a long time obscured.

The institution at Kankakee was founded solely to care for the incurably insane, but before it was fairly occupied it became a dis-

[1] By Geo. A. Zeller, M. D.

trict asylum for the Eastern Illinois territory, and for the growing number of commitments in the Chicago courts. In the meantime, the advocates of county care for incurables found themselves compelled to build annexes to the almshouses or, in the absence of such facilities, to board their insane in the neighboring counties, where the authorities had made provision for this class of inmates. During all these years there was a determined coterie of philanthropists constantly urging upon the Legislature the necessity of erecting an asylum for the incurable insane. Conspicuous among these was Dr. Frederick Howard Wines, whose many years of service as secretary of the State Board of Charities of Illinois permitted him to present the claims of these unfortunates as no other person could.[1]

During the administration of Governor Oglesby some headway toward the founding of this institution was made, but the time was not yet opportune.

The birth of the women's club movement in the decade 1880-1890 brought new pressure to bear on the subject. In Peoria, in particular, the question was energetically pushed by Mrs. Clara P. Bourland, Mrs. Anna Petherbridge and Mrs. S. O. Loughridge. The writer recalls that at the request of these ladies he introduced a resolution in the Republican County Convention of 1892, urging upon the legislative nominees the necessity of providing state care for the insane inmates of the almshouses. A similar resolution was adopted in the conventions of the other parties that year. It was not, however, until the middle of the administration of Governor John P. Altgeld that the movement gained sufficient headway to become a law. Many members of the Legislature were, or had been, members of county Boards of Supervisors and, as such, were aware of the deplorable conditions under which the insane were kept in the almshouses. When the bill was presented in the session of 1895 it speedily became a law.

That Governor Altgeld had a tender regard for the interests of the insane is shown by the fact that the session of 1895 established this institution and the Illinois Western Hospital for the Insane as well. Few states have organized two state hospitals during a single legislative session. It was a time of intense financial dis-

[1] Mr. Wines was not an advocate of separating the insane into curable and incurable classes, but of treating all for benefit or recovery in one institution.

tress and it may be that the inability of the average citizen to extend private aid made the public officials all the more heedful of the needs of the unfortunates.

As this movement had its greatest strength in Peoria, there seemed a settled conviction that the institution should be located there. When Governor Altgeld stipulated that the city obtaining the institution should donate the site, the public spirit of the city speedily rose to the occasion and a half section of land, situated in the village of Bartonville, was tendered to the state free of charge. Mr. Joseph B. Barton headed the subscription with a part of his homestead and was generously supported by the citizens in general. The commission named by Governor Altgeld, consisting of John Finely, of Peoria, Henry Alexander, of Joliet, and John McAndrews, of Chicago, after inspecting a number of sites selected the Barton site and immediately closed a contract for an octagonal building, with radiating wings capable of indefinite extension. The laying of the corner-stone in August, of 1895, was an imposing ceremony, the Governor with full staff being present.

The election of 1896 brought John R. Tanner into the gubernatorial chair. He at once saw that the partially completed building was wholly inadequate for the purpose it was to serve. Coupled with this was a faulty construction and the discovery that the building stood over an abandoned coal mine. After consulting expert advice, it was decided to raze the entire structure. It required courage to do this, but this was a quality conspicuous in John R. Tanner. He called Dr. Wines back to the secretaryship and gave him a free hand in planning an up-to-date institution upon the cottage plan.

Clothed with this authority, Dr. Wines caused the erection of a nurses' home, domestic building, power house and supply building.

Much criticism was aroused by the failure to erect buildings for patients, but Governor Tanner was proceeding along a fixed policy and laid his foundation wisely. The construction of these buildings and the subsequent cottages occupied the whole of his administration. Although he did not live to see them completed or occupied, the institution stands as a monument to his broad-minded conception of public necessities. In July, 1898, he appointed Dr. George A. Zeller superintendent in order that he might co-operate and advise with the commissioners during the constructive period. Dr. Zeller, who received no pay from the state, went to the Philippines as a surgeon of the United States Volunteers late in 1899.

In 1900 Richard Yates, the first native-born Governor, came into office and pushed to completion what had been so long building. He urged liberal appropriations and on February 10, 1902, had the satisfaction of seeing its doors thrown open for the reception of 700 patients. In the second half of his administration he signed a bill appropriating $300,000 for an additional row of cottages and when he retired from office in 1905 the institution contained a population of 1400 inmates.

In December, 1901, Governor Yates reappointed Dr. Zeller superintendent, and recalled him from the Philippines. The exigencies in the islands were such, however, that it was not until nearly a year later that the doctor was able to report for duty and personally take charge of the recently opened institution which, in the interim, had been managed by Dr. Carriel, of the Jacksonville State Hospital, and Dr. W. E. Taylor, of the Watertown State Hospital.

The advent of Governor Charles S. Deneen in 1905 marked a new epoch in the care of the insane. Hospitalization and scientific research now became dominant factors, and he authorized the erection of two fireproof hospitals of a capacity of 125 patients each.

The name "incurable" no longer appealed to the modern conception of the function of a state hospital, and the Legislature of 1907 changed the name to that of The Illinois General Hospital for the Insane. This name it retained only two years, when, in the general adoption of the new nomenclature, it became, in the legislative session of 1909, The Peoria State Hospital, which title will probably adhere to it permanently.

Governor Deneen also caused the erection of a psychopathic hospital, a dormitory for male employees, added three farms, and caused the erection of extensive buildings for the detached farm colony and the establishment of extensive dairy and farming economies.

The entire plant as it stands in 1912 represents an outlay of more than $2,000,000 and houses 2300 patients and 350 employees.

The administration building has yet to be erected. One of the cottages, up to the present time, has served that purpose admirably, but will eventually give way to a specially adapted building, which will occupy a site on the brow of the bluff, overlooking the Illinois River valley.

The plant consists of 20 cottages in three distinct groups, a hospital group for the physically ill, two extensive open air colonies for the all-year treatment of consumptives, a hospital for advanced consumptives, a psychopathic hospital, a general dining room, capable of seating 760, detached farm colonies and workshops, the whole numbering 42 distinct and detached buildings.

The entire land area consists of 570 acres, of which 183 acres constitute the institutional site, the remainder consisting of three detached farms. The acquisition of these farms marks the beginning of the detached colony plan. Although located more than a mile from the parent plant, one of the farms has a modern dormitory for the accommodation of 70 male patients who are thus provided with ideal rural surroundings and are engaged in the usual agricultural pursuits, including the care of 100 cows and several thousand chickens. A similar colony building for women will soon be erected and a third for the garden colony will follow.

The policy of this institution has been to keep every able-bodied patient at work and the character of the earlier inmates, many of whom were exceedingly violent or advanced in dementia, made it obligatory to secure the maximum of effort from a class of patients seldom seen at work in an institution for the insane.

In the earlier operation of the institution, when it was said that the cottage plan was ideal but too costly to be feasible, the per capita cost of maintenance was easily brought down to $130 per annum, a figure as low as that of any other institution in the state. The higher standard of care demanded by an enlightened public opinion, the large infirm population, the extensive tent colonies for consumptives and the extension of individual treatment to each patient as well as an advance in the price of the commodities of life, brought the per capita cost of maintenance up to $175 per patient, at which figure it remains at the present time (1912).

The purchasing system is that adopted by the Board of Administration and is uniform in all of the 18 institutions governed by that body. Quarterly estimates are prepared by the chief clerk after consultation with the heads of departments. These are forwarded to the office of the board in the capitol and bids are opened publicly and contracts awarded to the lowest bidder, after extensive advertising.

The reception and examination of patients is conducted according to the outlined program of the director of the State Psychopathic Institute.

A staff meeting is held every morning at 8 o'clock, attended by all members, and a case is invariably presented. The complete history is read and the patient is re-examined, after which the case is freely discussed with or without the presence of the patient, as indicated by his mental condition.

A second staff meeting is held in the staff office at 1 o'clock every afternoon. At this meeting the superintendent presides and reads the report of the officer of the day and of each member of the staff. Every occurrence of the previous day is carefully considered and discussed by the members and recommendations for the betterment of the service are freely invited. This meeting lasts from 30 minutes to two hours, but seldom adjourns without all feeling that something has been learned, or that an improvement in some feature of institutional life will result.

The staff is reassigned quarterly, thus giving each member a tour of duty in the receiving service and at the same time keeping him in touch with every other department of the institution.

The medical and scientific work has kept pace with the times. In the earlier years of his incumbency the superintendent addressed many official and philanthropic bodies on the necessity of complete state care, segregation, classification and the extension of the field of public charity. Later he appeared before many medical societies with papers on the various institutional phenomena. In particular, he advocated non-restraint and non-imprisonment, and on November 1, 1905, the last vestige of restraint was cast aside and the last bar and grating were removed from the doors and windows. The knowledge that 2000 patients were cared for in this manner attracted interested visitors from all parts of the country, and the influence of the institution in modifying the trying conditions under which the insane were kept was widespread.

In 1904 the writer began the accumulation of a museum of discarded restraint apparatus, which included shackles, wristlets, camisoles, blind sleeve dresses and, in fact, everything from the straitjacket to the so-called Utica Crib. This museum was visited by thousands and the pictures of it, published in successive biennial reports, are said to have had a marked influence in the curtailment of mechanical restraint in every state in the Union. The printed report of the official board of one state calls attention to a reduction of mechanical restraint to the extent of more than 80 per cent after a visit to a "certain Northern institution." We well recall the warm commendations of the gentlemen comprising this commission and their surprise at seeing in the exhibit of antiques the identical apparatus in daily use in the institutions they were seeking to modernize and which they did modernize in a manner that makes them rank with the most progressive in the land.

The members of the staff also prepared and published many scientific papers. The creation of the Illinois Association of Hospital Physicians with monthly meetings in each institution and triennial meetings at some designated point, insures constant interest in scientific and professional matters.

Recognizing that in the treatment of the deranged mind the patient was entitled to every agency that might in the slightest degree exert a beneficial influence, extensive solaria were attached to each hospital. These sun parlors are flooded with blue, violet, amber or opal light and patients are assigned to them according to the psychosis. While no great claim is made for phototherapy, the experiment is considered well worth while, being both harmless and inexpensive.

Leucodescent lamps with globes of various colors are also available and the color treatment is thus applicable throughout the night as well as during the day.

The agitation for the segregation of consumptives and their treatment in the open air led the superintendent to enclose a large porch with canvas, in 1905. This constituted the so-called porch colony. In the year following tents were annexed to each hospital and 25 consumptives of each sex were thus segregated and treated. Later these tents were assembled in a connected pavilion and an independent hospital was conducted. Soon after it was determined to construct a separate tent colony for each sex and in 1910 a hospital for advanced consumptives was also built. At present 140 consumptives are thus segregated. The result of this segregation has been marvelous. Whereas there were 60 deaths per annum for a number of years, the number has dropped to 15 and the tent colonies are now filled with run-down patients who are there as convalescents rather than as consumptives. No difficulty has been experienced in securing nurses for consumptives. Their pay and hours are the same as in the other wards and the timidity that prevailed at the outset has entirely disappeared.

There are 60 epileptics of each sex and two distinct colonies are maintained for them. Dietary treatment has been attempted; the non-salt treatment, the excessive salt treatment, the limitation of nitrogenous foods, the absolute withdrawal of bromides and later the graded drop-dose system, together with a careful study of elimination, have all been applied with the usual disappointing results. The epileptic colonies, both on the male and female side, are wholly presided over by women attendants. They take a keen interest in the patients and have taught them to help themselves and each other. They maintain many diversions and among other employments have the care of several hundred chickens. The epileptic men have a billiard table and have enjoyed its unrestricted use for years without the occurrence of an untoward incident.

Illinois maintains a separate hospital for the criminal insane and those of known criminal instincts are committed there direct by the courts, although many have been brought to this institution; among them two lifetermers and a number of others who had served terms in prison. This institution does not concede that there is such a thing as a dangerous insane person. There is no cell or place of confinement. Seclusion is never practised and all patients in each cottage are kept in the general sitting room, under the eyes of the attendants during the day and sleep in dormitories or two in a room at night.

The dietary is prescribed by the Board of Administration and is sufficiently varied to insure proper nutrition. The food is prepared in a general kitchen capable of providing for ten times the number of patients and is conveyed in bulk to the various dining-rooms in specially built carts drawn by patients. The large central mess hall seats 750 at each meal. Each hospital, infirmary, tent colony, receiving cottage and farm colony has an individual diet kitchen.

The training school was organized in 1906 with a three-years' graded course. Thirty-eight nurses have graduated and passed the civil service examination as well. All the members of the first, second and third classes, 1909-10-11, have attained high rank as supervising nurses here and elsewhere and two of them recently passed the examination as chief nurse and are now serving as such in two of the leading institutions of the state. Since the new registration law of Illinois does not recognize a state hospital diploma unless it has been supplemented by a year in a general hospital, the course has been reduced to two years and the classes of the future will be very large.

The economic features of this institution are founded upon the centralization of its various departments. One kitchen, one power house, one store, one mechanical department, and stipulated and variable staff assignments as well as the employment of patients wherever a sane person can be replaced, have made it possible to maintain a universal eight-hour tour of duty throughout with a force no greater than is maintained in the other institutions under the 13 and 15 hour schedule.

The substitution of female for male attendants is so general that only one cottage is in the hands of men. Attendants are taught to use their minds rather than their muscles. They are expected to spend their entire eight hours in developing and interesting their patients. As rapidly as patients show an aptness for a higher class of work, they are transferred to a more useful field. The "wall flower" is not encouraged. Patients have individual places at the dining room table but in the cottages are free to select their own seats or move about at will.

The report of the Peoria State Hospital covering the two years prior to 1908 opens with the following paragraph:

> We take pride in presenting the observations of a complete biennial period, during which 2000 of the most violent, destructive and dangerous insane in the world have been cared for without once having to resort to mechanical restraint; without using a single grain of narcotic on any ward, except in the hospital for the sick; without a screen or bar on any door or window, and without once turning a key upon a single patient night or day and with women caring for more than 800 insane men.

The innovations in successful operation during the period were as follows: Abolition of narcotics, non-restraint, non-imprisonment, the eight-hour tour of duty, women attendants for the insane men, segregation of consumptives, colonization of epileptics, phototherapy and industrial re-education.

In spite of the many successful advances in institutional methods emanating from the Peoria State Hospital and which gave it more than local prominence, it is probable that its greatest contribution to medical knowledge was in connection with pellagra. When the disease was first recognized here in 1909 the superintendent at once realized its significance and through his former connection with the army medical service was able to enlist the co-operation of the Surgeon General of the Public Health Service, who detailed Captains Siler and Nichols, two of the ablest men in the Medical Corps, to spend a month in the institution. The disease had been recognized elsewhere, especially in the South, but many officials did not grasp the full meaning of the invasion and it remained for this institution to arouse the public mind, as well as to interest the profession. The presence of 200 cases, 100 of whom died, afforded ample material for research and study.

The corn theory of causation being the only one with any standing, it was determined to inaugurate an extensive feeding experiment. Consequently 50 patients were placed on an absolute corn diet and 50 on a diet where corn and corn products were greatly in excess. The experiment was continued an entire year and was surrounded by every safeguard. A physician was assigned to oversee the experiment and to make observations. The results were negative except to demonstrate that the amount of corn eaten was not a factor in the causation of pellagra.

The publicity given to the subject of pellagra drew to the institution many of the leading medical men of the nation and prompted Governor Deneen to appoint the Illinois Pellagra Commission. The report of this commission, covering two years' work and embracing a most searching inquiry into every feature of the disease, has just been published and is regarded as the most valuable contribution ever made to the subject.

The changes in the personnel of the medical staff of a large institution are so numerous that a tabulation of the scientific contributions of each is difficult. Promotions have not infrequently followed, and a writer who is given credit for work done in one institution might in the meantime have gone to another, which might feel itself entitled to the credit. In this connection, it is proper to state that many able contributions have been made by the members of this staff and many valuable comparative statistics tabulated and published.

Dr. Zeller resigned the superintendency of the Peoria State Hospital on December 1, 1913, in order to accept the position of state alienist and member of the Board of Administration. He was succeeded by Dr. Ralph T. Hinton.

The committee has been unable to obtain a list of the assistant physicians attached to this hospital prior to 1914.

The number of patients 1914 were: Men, 1080; women, 1120; total, 2200. The number of employees: Men, 126; women, 228; total, 354.

MEDICAL OFFICERS.

Ralph T Hinton, M. D. .... Managing officer.
H. J. Smith, M. D. .... Assistant superintendent.
H. L. Krafft, M. D. .... Physician.
Clara E. Hayes, M. D. .... Physician.
Fred A. Causey, M. D. .... Assistant physician.
A. G. Witman, M. D. .... Assistant physician.
W. S. Osborn, M. D. .... Assistant physician.
Henry E. Randolph, M. D. .... Interne.

WATERTOWN STATE HOSPITAL.

East Moline, Ill.

The Watertown State Hospital for the Insane was established by an act of the Legislature approved May 22, 1895, by which act the usual board of three trustees was created and $100,000 appropriated for the construction of the hospital.

After considering various propositions, the trustees finally selected a site five miles above Moline, near the village of Watertown, in Rock Island County, on an elevation about a quarter of a mile from the Mississippi River.

The corner stone was laid September 5, 1896, Governor Altgeld delivering the dedicatory address. Owing to the unfavorable weather, the insolvency of the contractors, and an inadequate appropriation, the work proceeded slowly and when, on March

18, 1897, new trustees were appointed, they found the buildings incomplete. With additional appropriations granted by the Legislature, they were enabled to resume operations and on May 16, 1898, the front wards were ready for occupancy and 336 patients were received from the Jacksonville Hospital. Since that time each Legislature has made an appropriation for construction until the institution has a capacity of 1200 patients.

The hospital grounds consist of approximately 400 acres. One hundred acres on the hills, immediately surrounding the institution, provide a healthy location and afford a magnificent outlook over the Mississippi Valley. The farm and garden are in the bottom to the south and east of the institution, the farm buildings being about a half mile from the hospital proper. Access to the hospital is furnished by a switch running to the top of the hill from the C. B. & Q. Ry., which follows the south line of the farm.

The buildings are of fireproof construction, the wards being built entirely of stone, and detached buildings such as the power house, store, dormitories, etc., being of pressed brick.

In their primitive condition the grounds surrounding the buildings were very irregular and the soil was of such a character that each rain caused considerable damage. These natural difficulties have been in a large measure overcome and the institution is now provided with concrete walks and macadam roads and considerable has been done toward beautifying the grounds.

Although within easy distance of the Mississippi River, the institution has its own wells, from which it draws an abundant supply of pure water. A sewage disposal plant has been constructed, into which enters the sewage from the entire establishment. In this sewage box all solid matter is destroyed by a natural process and nothing passes out except a stream of clear, odorless water which finds its way to the river.

The institution is well equipped and could carry on its existence in a large measure independent of the outside world, having its own electric light and steam plant in addition to water supply and sewage system, carpenter shop, machine shop, shoe shop, store building, printing office, laundry and refrigerating plant.

Electricity is furnished by three direct-connected dynamos, which furnish light and power for the various departments. The buildings are heated with steam, both by the direct and indirect system. Four large boilers with a capacity of 1000 horse power are equipped with chain grate mechanical stokers, the Johnson heat regulator and the Paul vacuum system, all of which have been very economical to the state.

The institution has an infirmary with a capacity of 75 patients. Two cottages for tubercular cases have been established, together with tent colonies; a chapel and theatre with a capacity of 1000, a large recreation and amusement hall equipped with billiard tables, bowling alleys, apparatus for gymnastic exercises, with a seating capacity of 1500 where band concerts, dances and other forms of amusement are held. The institution has a parole ward with accommodations for 100 patients. The farm is well equipped in every way.

The site, valued at $40,000, was paid for by the citizens of Rock Island County, one-half in subscriptions and one-half by the sale of county bonds. The fact that the institution has never had a case of malarial or typhoid fever more than compensates for its being somewhat inaccessible.

The total appropriation made by the Legislature for construction and other purposes, exclusive of maintenance, up to 1905 was $600,604, this including not alone the main ward building, but the annex, the recreation hall, store, dormitories for male and female employees, infirmary, society hall, detached buildings for parole patients and all the barns and other buildings on the farm.

September 30, 1905, there were 1170 patients in the institution. The quarterly statement ending September 30, 1905, shows a surplus of $27,480.55 in the ordinary expense fund and a net per capita cost of $26.21, gross $29.62.

The first superintendent was Dr. W. E. Taylor, of Monmouth, who was elected in January, 1897.

Since 1905 various improvements have been made from time to time. These include in 1904-1906: An artesian well, 1391 feet deep; an amusement hall 200 feet long and 100 feet wide, with a seating capacity of 1500, equipped with three bowling alleys, billiard and pool tables, a stage for theatrical performances, and main floor where the weekly dances are held; the old amusement hall remodeled and converted into a chapel; two cottages for tubercular patients, with a capacity of 20 patients each, and each cottage with a wide porch around it where patients can sleep during both summer and winter; a band stand in front of the administration building, having a floor space of 900 square feet; tile floors with marble wainscoting in place of wooden walls; a number of rooms remodeled, tile floors and marble walls being used in place of plaster and wood, and the wooden floor on ward No. 8 replaced with tile and marble base, at a cost of $1600. A camp in the grove was established during the summer, where 100 untidy and violent patients are kept. Approximately one mile of cement sidewalk was laid and considerable hard road built; a large and more efficient septic tank with a capacity of 125,000 gallons, which was necessary on account of the increased population; approximately two miles of deep drain tile in the low land of the farm, making it very productive.

During 1906-1908 the "C" building was constructed at a cost of $100,000. This building has 43,992 square feet of floor space and is used exclusively for a receiving ward for the treatment of recent and acute cases. It is fireproof, and every room where patients are kept receives light. The building is thoroughly equipped with a complete hydrotherapeutic outfit and electrical and all appliances for the use of light energy. In this building is a morgue, post-mortem room, private chapel, sewing room, gymnasium, smoking and lounging rooms, school rooms and industrial department. The laboratories and operating room are well-equipped.

An industrial building was erected, with a floor space of 8300 feet; in this building are the dressmaking department and tailor shop, in which all clothing worn by patients is made; a broom factory, mattress factory, printing shop, shoe shop (in which many of the heavier shoes are made and a repair department), a weaving department where rugs, carpets, hammocks, etc., are manufactured. There are also a basketry and an entensive tin shop, and extensive blacksmith and machine shops.

On the camp ground there have been erected 13 frame cottages, a large dining-room and an amphitheatre with a seating capacity of 2000.

Beginning in 1906 a fair has been held each year, which continues for a period of three days, where the products of the farm and articles manufactured by the industrial departments, as well as by the culinary department, are exhibited. The patients are stimulated to take great interest in this enterprise, for two reasons: First, they take great pride in doing something, and second, they are rewarded by receiving premiums for superior work. Each year they have exhibited about 7000 articles and approximately $7000 in premiums are awarded.

Many improvements have been made in the way of beautifying the grounds by grading, building hard roads, planting shade trees and shrubbery. Ten thousand eight hundred square feet of sidewalk was laid, one-half mile of sewers and one concrete tunnel 6 x 7 feet and 546 feet long, and one tunnel 324 feet long, 3 x 4 feet. The tunnels are utilized for water mains, steam pipes, electric wires, etc., the object being to preserve heat, protect wires and render them accessible in case of breakage.

During this period 90½ acres of very productive land were added to the farm and a contract made for the purchase of 150 acres additional.

In 1908-1910 the improvements consisted of one 265 H. P. boiler installed; 500 feet terrazzo laid in dining-room used by wards 6 and 8, at a cost of $1000; tile floor laid in main hall of administration building, $1000, and a clinical laboratory at a cost of $500.

During the period 1912-1914 the improvements comprised a cement floor under ward 8, a new trunk room, a shower bath for male wards in the administration building, and a shower bath under ward 4 for the use of the working men in the power house and on the farm. A tile floor was laid in the living-room of ward 3, a toilet room placed in the carpenter shop, and two in the basement of the administration building. A male tubercular ward was created by utilizing the parole ward, which is isolated from the group of buildings; a dining-room was made in the basement, and the food is prepared in the C kitchen. This cottage is known as Hospital No. 2.

Ward No. 2 was made into a parole ward, the dining-room discontinued and the space used for a dormitory, thus accommodating about 25 more patients; the doors of this ward are not locked and patients go and come at will. Their meals are served in the basement of the administration building.

Two small cottages from the camp ground were attached to B-4 cottage, increasing the sleeping capacity 12 patients; the dormitory formerly in use was converted into a large dining-room, thus eliminating one of the objectionable features existing there. This cottage is occupied by old men.

A new dining-room for attendants was made in the basement of the C building; attendants take two meals a day in this dining-room—the other meal being taken on the ward. A larger dining-room was also made for the doctors in the C building.

A meeting of the heads of departments was called for Tuesdays, thus enabling the superintendent to keep in touch with the workings of all departments; at these meetings anything pertaining to repairs or the good of the institution is discussed.

Upon the recommendation of the Board of Administration and the approval of the Governor, the eight-hour system for attendants and mechanics has been installed and is now working very satisfactorily.

With the appropriations made for the period 1912-1914 there are under construction the following buildings: An assembly hall, at a cost of $25,000; also a building known as the men's infirmary, which will adequately care for about 100 patients; a nurses' home for female employees, at a cost of $50,000; this building is located on the hill immediately at the rear of the annex; the location is very desirable, inasmuch as it is a considerable distance from the main group of buildings; a building for the care of male tubercular patients, the cost being $18,000.

The water supply system from the Mississippi River and a reservoir have been completed at a cost of $8500; a sanitary cow-barn, for which $10,000 was appropriated, has been constructed, and a tool and implement house, for $1500.

A concrete tunnel 7 x 6½ x 275 feet has been constructed from the administration building to the annex, this being done by hospital labor. This tunnel is sufficiently large to accommodate pipes and wires, and there is also room for the food wagon to pass, carrying food from the administration building to the annex. Electric wires have been placed in metal conduits, thus increasing the power one-third over what it was while the rubber conduits were in use.

Number of patients: Men, 820; women, 690; total, 1510. Number of employees: Men, 110; women, 125; total, 235.

ORIGINAL BOARD OF TRUSTEES.

Frank W. Gould, president.
Allan M. Clement.
J. I. McCawley.
C. F. Lynde, treasurer.

J. I. McCawley was succeeded by D. E. Munger, and Mr. Munger by William Trembor. Upon the death of F. W. Gould, J. W. Simonson was appointed president of the board.

SUPERINTENDENTS.

Dr. W. E. Taylor.
Dr. W. A. Crooks.
Dr. J. A. Campbell.

ASSISTANT SUPERINTENDENTS.

Dr. W. A. Crooks.
Dr. A. H. Dollear.
Dr. H. J. Smith.
Dr. C. F. Read.
Dr. M. C. Hawley.
Dr. C. C. Atherton.

PHYSICIANS AND ASSISTANT PHYSICIANS.

Dr. Francis M. Soule.
Dr. C. A. Goodwin.
Dr. G. W. Dishong.
Dr. W. L. Hercik.
Dr. Ester H. Stone.
Dr. E. A. Soule.
Dr. F. B. Clarke.
Dr. M. C. Hawley.
Dr. R. F. Winsor.
Dr. W. H. Gambrill.
Dr. T. F. Neil.
Dr. W. W. Mercer.
Dr. W. A. Cook.
Dr. W. S. James.
Dr. W. A. Ford.
Dr. W. K. Dyer.
Dr. Lewis J. Pollock.
Dr. H. S. Seiwell.
Dr. Olive F. Hughes.
Dr. P. S. Winner.
Dr. F. A. Causey.
Dr. Leaf Knight.
Dr. Alice Smith.

CHICAGO STATE HOSPITAL.[1]

Dunning, Ill.

In 1851 the county poor farm was established at the town of Jefferson, Ill., about 12 miles northwest of Chicago. The farm consisted of 160 acres of fairly improved land, and was formerly owned by Peter Ludby, who located it in 1839. Additional land was purchased in 1860 and in 1884. At the present time (1915) the land consists of 234 acres.

By November, 1854, the county poorhouse was nearly finished. The building was of brick, three stories high and basement, and cost about $25,000.

In 1858 Dr. D. B. Fonda was physician for the poorhouse and insane departments. At that time the building of the insane asylum, 200 feet south of the almshouse hospital, was contemplated.

In the first biennial report of the Board of State Commissioners of Public Charities of the State of Illinois, dated December, 1870, occurs the following:

> Although the keeper of the Cook County almshouse seems to be a humane, conscientious man, who conducts the institution to the very best of his ability under the circumstances and surroundings, it is nevertheless for so wealthy a county a miserably planned and badly managed institution.
>
> The capacity is probably not over 450, while the number of inmates is sometimes as great as 700.
>
> Of the manner in which the insane have hitherto been cared for nothing need be said. A new insane asylum in connection with the almshouse has been built.
>
> The farm of 160 acres is worked in the interest of the county, the superintendent receiving a salary for his services. The inmates do nearly all the farm work, also the housework and make most of the clothing. There is a school upon the premises, which is attended by the greater part of the children between the ages of eight and 14.

The old insane department was of brick, with small barred windows, iron doors, and heavy wooden doors outside, with apertures and hinged shutters for passing food. The cells were about seven by eight feet; they were not heated, except by a stove in the corridor, which did not raise the temperature in some of them above the freezing point; the cold, however, did not freeze out the

[1] By Geo. Leininger, M. D., superintendent.

vermin with which the beds, walls and floors were alive. The number of cells in this department was 21, 10 on the lower floor and 11 on the upper floor; many of them contained two beds.

The other buildings were all frame; they were more like barns or barracks—immense areas of bare floors, crowded with cheap iron strap bedsteads.

The heating was insufficient; there was no ventilation; the arrangements for bathing were so imperfect, there being no hot water, that during the winter months the inmates were not bathed; even in summer the number of tubs was too small and they were inconveniently located.

There were no halls in these buildings, the entire space being divided into rooms; the stairways were either on the outside or in the center of the room.

In the report for 1878 it is stated that the Cook County poorhouse "is a rookery and should be torn down."

The plans for additional buildings for the infirmary were drawn by John G. Cochrane, the architect, and the designs submitted by him were adopted by the county on the 22d of September, 1881.

The contract for the erection of the buildings was awarded in June, 1882, to Messrs. McGraw & Downey, who completed their part of the work in time for the institution to receive inmates by June in the following year.

They consisted of nine separate and distinct buildings, connected by corridors arranged in a semi-circular form, with a frontage generally to the south. In front of the circle were the administration and the four dormitory buildings; immediately in the rear was the central building, and on either side of this the hospitals and dining rooms; in the rear of these were the kitchens and laundry houses, all connected by corridors. The construction was of brick and three stories in height.

In 1884 the infirmary had accommodations for 1000 patients. The patients were transferred to the county infirmary at Oak Forest, Ill., in December, 1910, and the buildings of the infirmary were used to house the insane.

In January, 1912, fire destroyed the central portion of the building, which contained six wards, operating room, two congregate dining-rooms, kitchen, chapel and the corridors leading from the east to the west wings. However, the fire did not destroy the two west wings, which were not in use, nor the three east wings, which were occupied by the insane patients. The two west wings were wrecked during the early part of 1913 in order to provide sites for cottage wards 13 and 14.

The east wings continued in use as wards for insane patients until January 9, 1914, when a fire started in the ruins at the western end of the buildings; shortly after this fire the buildings were abandoned and the contract was let to have them wrecked. The buildings were leveled during the year 1914.

The boiler room and pump house connected with the infirmary remains in use at the present time (1915).

The ice-house, which was built at the same time as the infirmary buildings in 1883, is in use at the present time (1915) as a paint shop.

The Cook County Insane Asylum.

The constantly increasing number of insane cases in the wards of the poorhouse soon made manifest the necessity of providing separate and suitable quarters for this class of county charges. Accordingly in 1870 the insane asylum was built. This institution was erected on the county farm, a little over a block northeast of the infirmary, on ground dotted with forest trees and gradually sloping to an artificial lake. L. B. Dixon, of Chicago, was the architect.

The asylum building had a frontage to the east of 272 feet and was divided by a center building, in which the offices were situated; the two wings were divided into wards. Each ward was 116 feet long from north to south. The central building had a frontage of 50 feet. At each extreme end of wings was a projection 20 feet to the rear for bathroom, water closets and stairs to the yards. The building was of brick, with cut stone trimmings, and was three stories high above the basement. Each wing had a center corridor 13 feet wide, with three windows on each end. The patients' rooms were on each side of the corridors. Especial pains were taken to secure a thoroughly efficient system of warming and ventilation. The heating was by high pressure steam, and ventilation was forced by two double-bladed iron fans, eight feet in diameter. The water closets were at the end of each ward. The bathrooms were adjoining at the end of each wing. There was a soiled clothes drop from each bathroom to a room in the basement. There were two bathtubs and three water closets on each floor. Each wing had a dining-room on each floor with attendants' room adjoining. A dumb waiter extended to the basement from each dining-room. There was a linen room for each story of each wing near the attendants' room. At the end of each wing there was a separate stairway with separate exits into yards for inmates.

In the rear of the insane asylum at a distance of 100 feet was the laundry building, 60 by 60 feet in size, built of brick with shingle roof two stories above the ground, with a cellar. This building was divided by a hall through its center with laundry, drying room and ironing rooms on one side, and kitchen and bakery on the opposite side. The second story was subdivided into apartments for servants employed in rooms below. This laundry building was connected with the main building by a brick corridor 10 feet wide.

All food for patients in the asylum was brought into the basement of the asylum in an iron car from the rear building, and was carried to the various dining-rooms by a dumb waiter.

The boiler, engine and fan rooms were next to the laundry building and were of brick. The fuel shed was next to the boiler house and the flour shed in the rear of the laundry building. The smokestack for the boiler was 85 feet high and 9 feet square at the base.

Pure water was supplied these buildings by an artesian well 756 feet deep. The cost of these buildings completed was $135,-000. They furnished accommodations for 200 patients, giving a room to each.

In 1871, on account of the overcrowded condition of the hospital, cells were fitted up in the basement.

In 1872 a new library was fitted up for the patients at a cost of $500. One of the large rooms in the rear building was fitted up as a sewing room, and this room was also used for a dance once or twice a week for the patients.

In 1873 a fourth story addition was added to the main building for the insane which was occupied during the early part of January, 1874, as an amusement hall for the patients and quarters for about 50 patients.

In 1874 a piano was purchased for the hall and a bowling alley was fitted up in the basement for the use of the patients. A reserve reservoir was built, to be used in the event of fire, the two reservoirs in the basement being used to collect rain water from the roofs for use in the boilers. A gas house was built, which introduced the lighting of the building by gas; and a small infirmary was arranged for on each ward to care for the sick and helpless patients.

During 1877 a new steam drying room was constructed next to the laundry and a new artesian well, 2107 feet deep, was bored.

In the report for this year the medical superintendent complained that he was not backed up by the warden, and that he was insulted when he tried to obtain the proper amount of nourishment and its proper preparation for the patients; also that patients were not sufficiently clothed.

In a report made in 1878 by the State Board of Commissioners of Public Charities the following occurs:

> The insane department is a large and well built establishment constructed substantially on the principles and methods approved by the American Association of Medical Superintendents of Hospitals for the Insane. The number of wards is 16; there are four floors and four wards on each floor. There are 437 inmates, with 100 sleeping on the floor.

There was a small amusement hall which would hold 100 persons. A few books served as a library, but no periodicals were taken. The upper floors were occupied by women, the lower floors by men. The drug room was in the basement and averaged about 100 prescriptions daily. There was an icehouse on the grounds holding 300 or 400 tons. At a little distance from the main building were the barns and piggery.

Dr. John Spray was medical director from January 1, 1878, to September 1, 1882, and he was superintendent (in sole charge) from September 1, 1882, to September 1, 1884.

Of the inmates under treatment during March, 1884, there were 285 males and 325 females. Out of this number only 72 were native-born Americans.

Until 1882 the nearest railway station at which one could take the cars to or from the county farm was at the village of Jefferson, two miles away, on the Wisconsin division of the Chicago & Northwestern Railroad. However, the commissioners of Cook

County, seeing the necessity of having railroad communication direct from the city, built some three miles of line running across the poor farm in a southerly direction, and intersecting the St. Paul road at Galewood. This was done and the first train from the city to the county farm was started on the 11th of September, 1882.

The county also erected at its terminus of the line a handsome depot building at a cost of $2100, and the station was named Dunning, in honor of one of the oldest and wealthiest settlers in the vicinity.

The infirmary and insane asylum up to 1882 were under one management, a committee of five county commissioners, which had entire control. This committee appointed a medical superintendent over the asylum, and a warden, matron, engineer and storekeeper, but none of these officers had any power except as directed by the committee, nor had either institution any head. Quoting from a report of the State Board of Charities dated 1878: "The warden is not head, and the superintendent is not head; the real head is the committee, which has five heads."

In 1882 the county board adopted new rules, which provided that the warden and superintendent should be elected by the Board of County Commissioners. These officers were placed more directly in charge of their respective departments and given enlarged powers of management and control.

This asylum was the first in the West to appoint female physicians. It was the first in the state to appoint graduate and trained female nurses in charge of the particular nursing and administration of all drugs. The female physicians were Dr. Delia Howe, appointed May 1, 1884, and Dr. Harriet Alexander, appointed February 1, 1885.

Dr. James D. Kiernan was appointed medical superintendent September 1, 1884, and was replaced by Dr. Spray September 1, 1885.

The present (1915) detached ward buildings were completed in 1885, at a cost of $135,000. They are two stories in height, built of brick. A large basement houses at the present time (1915) the general bathroom for patients, with a swimming pool of about 20 by 25 feet; also the carpenter shop, machine shop and mattress shop.

In 1885 there were many complaints made against the appointing of employees through the political friendship of the appointing power, which resulted in the presence of many inexperienced and incapable attendants.

Dr. Kiernan, who had been medical superintendent from September 1, 1884, to September 1, 1885, read a paper before the Chicago Medical Society complaining of abuses and mistreatment of patients; and as a result a committee from the State Board of Charities investigated the institution. Several county commissioners, ex-county commissioners and about 14 contractors were indicted by the grand jury. The heads of the institutions were removed and the institutions were thoroughly investigated, and it was demonstrated that extravagant management and graft existed.

In 1887 the present amusement hall was completed, having been designed as a cottage ward for patients. This building is two stories in height; the upper floor is used for an amusement hall at the present time, a large stage having been built at the north end of the building.

In 1890 Dr. John A. Benson was medical superintendent. During this year the present cottage wards 1, 2, 3 and 4 were completed. The buildings are built of brick and are two stories and basement high. A biological laboratory and autopsy house was also erected. The lower floor of the amusement hall was fitted up as an industrial department for re-educational purposes for patients, and a teacher employed to teach industrial arts. During this year there was only one artesian well in use, which had a flow of 36,000 gallons a day, collected in two cisterns and pumped throughout the buildings. A pond behind the main building supplied the laundry, but the pond was almost dry and the artesian water supply was low, resulting in not enough water for the proper cleansing and bathing of inmates.

In 1891 Dr. Brown was superintendent, followed by James Pine as warden in 1892. In 1892 the present cold storage building was completed. This building is of brick construction and is one story high; it is situated about 100 feet east of the south end of the present store building.

In 1893 Mr. Sawyer was warden. During this year the present (1915) store building was completed. This building is of brick construction and is about 40 feet by 150 feet, two stories and basement high. The south end of the building was fitted up and has been used as a drug store ever since. The present druggist, Mr. Henry Lindlade, was appointed assistant druggist February 24, 1894, and was the first civil service appointee as druggist July 1, 1895.

In 1894 Mr. O. W. Nash was appointed warden; he resigned June 1, 1895, being succeeded by George F. Morgan. Mr. Morgan remained until January 1, 1897.

On January 2, 1895, the laundry building burned. The present building was completed in 1896. It is one story high and of brick construction.

During the year 1895 civil service was instituted, and the control and treatment of patients in the insane asylum was for the first time under the sole management of an able corps of physicians appointed by reason of their fitness. A medical supervising staff was appointed September 23, 1895, consisting of Dr. Richard Dewey, Dr. Sanger Brown, Dr. Archibald Church, Dr. D. W. Lewis and Dr. William Cuthbertson. This staff made the rules and regulations for the hospital resident staff.

The hospital grounds were connected with the city water mains by an 8-inch pipe, and fire plugs, with connections, were installed about the grounds.

In 1897 Mr. Albert N. Lange was appointed general superintendent. It was during this year that the present (1915) cottage wards 5 and 6 were completed. These buildings are constructed of brick, with a large day room in the center, a dormitory on each side and the dining room in the rear. The buildings face west and are on the avenue with other cottages.

During 1898 the consumptive hospital was completed. This building is situated near the southeast corner of the grounds. It is of brick construction, three stories and attic high. It has three wings like the letter T and faces south. The longest wing runs north and south. However, the west wing is longer than the east wing. In 1903 this building was remodeled and used for the physically sick insane and continues as such at the present time (1915).

Mr. A. N. Lange resigned as general superintendent November 17, 1902. On November 30, 1902, Dr. John R. Neely was appointed general superintendent.

The working force of the institution was under the supervision of the general superintendent, the assistant general superintendent being in charge of the infirmary.

Dr. John R. Neely resigned as general superintendent June 1, 1903. In 1903 the present (1915) cottage wards 7, 8 and 9 were completed. These buildings were known as Group No. 1 and are located at the end of the avenue leading north from the main building for the insane. The group completes and closes the avenue. For this reason the Renaissance architectural treatment was employed to mark the middle building. A large portico is surmounted by a classic pediment supported by Ionic columns, and the apex of the roof of the middle building is marked with a colonial lantern. A covered colonade or veranda connects the three buildings and provides a passageway for the inmates of the two side cottages to and from the dining-room located in the middle building. These cottages are faced on all sides with dark red shale common brick and have cut-stone trimmings. The roofs are covered with red tile. The ornamental colonade and the veranda are of cement and painted white. The two cottages on the sides are duplicates. They are each 100 feet long by 48 feet wide. On the first floor of each is a large day room, 42 feet by 48 feet in size, which is lighted on four sides and opens up on the rear. The middle building is 102 feet long by 31 feet wide. On the first floor are two dining-rooms, with a common kitchen and serving room.

Dr. V. H. Podstata was appointed general superintendent June 1, 1903, in order to modernize the institution.

A training school for nurses was established. The pathological department was re-established, with Dr. M. H. McHugh in charge. The fire department was reorganized and drilled by Captains Figg and Hand, of the Chicago Fire Department. The county board authorized the appointment of internes. The cottage in the vicinity of the infirmary which was formerly used for maternity cases and cases of infectious diseases was remodeled into a nurses' home; this building was wrecked during 1914.

Mr. George P. Smith was appointed business manager September 18, 1903, as a civil service appointee.

The consumptive hospital was built during this year. It is situated 1500 feet west of the infirmary buildings on the Dunning Farm. It is of wooden construction and consists of five buildings, connected by spacious corridors, facing south. The middle building is two stories high and was used as the administration building for offices and living quarters.

In the year 1907 a two-story building was completed at the west end of these buildings and was used as a hospital ward for the more advanced cases of tuberculosis. These buildings became the property of the State of Illinois July 1, 1912, but the county was allowed the use of them until March, 1914.

In 1904 the hospital staff consisted of, in the insane department, three senior physicians and three internes; in the infirmary, one senior physician and three internes; in the consumptive hospital, one senior physician and two internes.

During this year the present (1915) pathological building and morgue were occupied. This building is situated about 100 yards south of the main building for the insane. It is of brick construction, two stories high, and contains a large amphitheatre, where clinics are held. The present farm cottage building was also completed during 1904. This building is situated near the center of the farm, about 1400 feet west of the main building for the insane. The building fronts east and back of it are grouped the barns, chicken houses, etc. The building is 80 feet long, 54 feet wide and two stories in height; there are two one-story extensions in the rear, 27 feet by 22 feet. The construction is of brick and artistic in appearance. It was designed to accommodate 45 patients. At the present time (1915) there are 75 patients housed in the building.

The biological laboratory, which was erected in 1890, was torn down during 1904, when the new building was occupied.

During 1904 the present cottage wards 10 and 11 were completed. These buildings were known as Group No. 2, and are situated 125 feet north of the detached ward buildings, facing east. They consist of two two-story cottages and one one-story cottage, connecting the group surrounding a court. The two larger cottages are 84 feet long by 74 feet deep. The middle cottage is 58 feet long by 38 feet deep. The open court is 58 feet long, enclosed by an ornamental fence.

In 1905 the first graduation exercises of the training school for nurses were held.

Dr. V. H. Podstata, general superintendent, resigned July 16, 1906, to become superintendent of the Elgin State Hospital. Dr

O. C. Willhite was appointed general superintendent July 16, 1906. In 1906 hydrotherapeutic and electrical appliances were installed in the west basement of the hospital ward.

In 1907 a psychopathologist was appointed, and semi-weekly meetings of the staff were held for presentation of cases and discussions. The old picket fence separating the infirmary and insane asylum was torn down; 1500 small trees were purchased and placed in a nursery for transplanting. A large open ditch, which ran through the grounds, was laid with five 15-inch tile and covered over.

Four 250 horse-power water-tube boilers, equipped with traveling chain grates, were installed in 1907. Two 500 horse-power boilers were also installed, with traveling chain grates. A new smokestack, 180 feet high, was built during the year.

A system was developed for re-educational purposes for the insane. Two attendants were sent to the school of civics and philanthropy with pay. One of these attendants, Miss Myra Henderson, continues at the present time (1915) in the employ of the hospital.

A consulting staff of 12 physicians from Chicago was attached to the institution. Dentist T. W. Schnell visited the hospital one day each week in order to look after the dental needs of the patients.

In 1912 cottage ward No. 1 was established as an art cottage for female patients, in charge of Miss Ingborg Olson, and continues as such at the present time (1915). A gynecological service was also established.

In January, 1912, fire destroyed the central portion of the infirmary buildings, which contained six wards, operating room, two congregate dining-rooms, kitchen, chapel and the corridors leading from the east to the west wings. The fire did not destroy the two west wings which were not in use, nor the three east wings which housed insane patients.

In the year 1909 the General Assembly passed a law entitled "An Act to Revise the Laws Relating to Charities, etc." Section 20 of this act provided for the removal of the insane and feeble-minded from the county almshouses to state institutions. All of the provisions of Section 20 were complied with except that part relating to the insane and feeble-minded in almshouses in counties of over 150,000 population.

An appropriation was made by the General Assembly in 1911 to provide for the insane and feeble-minded in the Cook County Hospital for the Insane at Dunning, Ill.

On July 1, 1912, the County of Cook transferred to the State of Illinois all lands, buildings and equipment known as the Cook County Institution at Dunning, Ill., the name to be changed to Chicago State Hospital.

The details of the transfer to the state were made by a committee composed of three members of the Cook County Board of Commissioners, in joint session with the Board of Administration of the State of Illinois. The committee of the Board of Cook County Commissioners was composed of Peter Bartzen, ex-officio member, Bartley Berg, chairman, Joseph Mendel and Lawrence J. Coffee. The state was represented by the Board of Administration. The appraisement of buildings, lands and furniture was made under the direction of the Cook County Board of Commissioners, and the valuation is given as follows: Buildings, $983,518.06; lands, $500,640; furniture, $34,970.

The buildings consisted of the administration building, the detached ward buildings (2), hospital, infirmary buildings, cottage wards 1, 2, 3, 4, 5, 6, 7, 8, 9, 10, 11, farm wards, tuberculosis cottages (6), nurses' cottage, amusement hall, store building, laundry, pathological laboratory and morgue building, power house, fire hall, horse barn, cold storage, paint shop, tool house, oil house, smoke house, hay barn, hog shed, slaughter house, chicken house and greenhouses Nos. 1 and 2.

The land consisted of 234 acres and was appraised at $2100 an acre. Of the 234 acres contained in the tract which comprises the site of this hospital, 100 acres are under cultivation. The soil is black loam, about 14 inches deep, and is peculiarly adapted to the growth of fruits and vegetables.

The State of Illinois assumed charge of the Cook County Insane Asylum July 1, 1912, and the name was changed to the Chicago State Hospital.

The Chicago State Hospital.

When this hospital was taken over by the state Dr. F. B. Clarke, formerly medical director under the county management, was appointed acting superintendent and served as such until the time of his resignation December 15, 1912, when Dr. R. H. Rea became acting superintendent, serving until April 7, 1913. Dr. George Leininger was appointed superintendent April 7, 1913, and continues as such at the present time. Dr. H. J. Smith was transferred from the Watertown State Hospital, where he was serving as assistant superintendent, to a like position in this hospital April 17, 1913. On March 15, 1914, Dr. Smith was transferred to the Peoria State Hospital as assistant superintendent. Dr. C. F. Read, formerly assistant superintendent at the Kankakee State Hospital, was transferred to this hospital March 16, 1914, as assistant superintendent. Dr. R. H. Rea remains in the hospital as physician, having served continuously since April 21, 1910.

The medical staff was increased and additional stenographers were added in order to keep complete records of the history, etiology, diagnosis, prognosis and treatment of each patient.

In December, 1913, a small one-story cottage of brick construction was opened as an unlocked cottage, and accommodates 40 female patients. This new building is cottage ward No. 12. Cottage wards 13 and 14 were completed and occupied in February, 1914. Cottage ward 14 is a parole ward and accommodates 125 male patients. Cottage ward 13 is a closed cottage for male patients. Both buildings are two stories and basement in height, of brick construction and very pleasing to the eye. In cottage ward No. 14 a billiard table has been installed and is quite popular with the patients.

The following new buildings are under construction at the present time (1915): An administration building, three stories in height, 187 feet long and 75 feet deep, of brick construction. It occupies the site of the infirmary buildings which were torn down in 1914. The building will contain the offices and living quarters of the hospital staff. Two receiving wards, both identical, of brick construction and two stories in height, one for the female and the other for male patients. The buildings are 238 feet long by 65 feet deep, and are situated opposite each other on the main driveway to the present administration building. Two infirmary cottages, to be known as Cottage Wards 15 and 16. These buildings are of brick construction, two stories in height, and situated just west of the poorhouse boiler room, fronting south on the driveway leading to the old tubercular hospital.

An untidy cottage, one story in height, of brick construction, situated just west of the nurses' home, near the main track of the Chicago, Milwaukee and St. Paul Railroad.

A nurses' home, three stories high, of brick construction, and situated directly west of the present paint shop, facing west. It is 187 feet long and 75 feet deep and will accommodate about 150 employees.

In the spring of 1914 the buildings which housed the consumptives under county management were thoroughly overhauled, cleansed, disinfected and calsomined, and are now occupied by insane patients. The wards in these buildings are known as the detached wards, 5, 5A, 6, 7, 8 and 9. The furnace heating plants have been removed and steam heating is now used.

A small root cellar or vegetable house was constructed for $2000. The building is 60 feet by 40 feet and situated just west of the main building for the insane.

On July 1, 1912, the nursing service consisted of four supervising nurses, 78 male and 72 female attendants. At the present time (1915) the nursing service consists of one chief nurse, two male supervising nurses, two female supervising nurses, one acting supervising nurse (female), 145 female attendants, 135 male attendants. In February, 1914, the eight-hour system was installed for the nursing service in part of the hospital, and as it proved a success it was rapidly extended, so that by the middle of May, 1914, all the employees were working on eight-hour shifts.

The present training school for nurses under state management was organized September 1, 1912, at which time 20 pupil-nurses were enrolled, nine of whom remained for the full course and graduated in June, 1914.

Under the supervision of an industrial art teacher, the female patients are instructed in plain sewing, hemstitching, drawn work, embroidery, crocheting, knitting, etc., reed and raffia work, fancy weaving, etc. The male patients are instructed along re-educational lines under the supervision of a manual training instructor. The work consists in making brushes, window shades, carpenter work and fret-saw work. Many patients are employed on the farm and in the garden.

The patients have a weekly dance which they look forward to and enjoy very much. Moving picture shows have been given. Entertainments have been given by various fraternal organizations. Baseball and other games during the summer between patients are held almost daily. Elaborate entertainments are given on holidays, *e. g.*, Fourth of July, etc.

Insane patients present in the hospital December 1, 1871, 216; in the hospital March 19, 1915, 3019.

Officers of the Cook County Insane Asylum, the Cook County Infirmary and the Cook County Consumptive Hospital, from 1868 to the Taking Over of the Institutions by the State, July 1, 1912.[1]

PHYSICIANS FOR THE POORHOUSE AND INSANE DEPARTMENT.

Dr. C. B. Fonda........	1868-1872	Dr. J. W. Tope........	1872-1874

MEDICAL SUPERINTENDENTS.

Dr. Geo. P. Cunningham	1876-1878	Dr. John C. Spray......	1885-1890
Dr. John C. Spray (in sole charge 1882-1884)	1878-1882	Dr. John A. Benson.....	1890-1891
Dr. James D. Kiernan..	1884-1885	Dr. Brown	1891-

WARDENS.

George S. Kimberly.....	1872-1874	James Pine	1891-
John D. Walsh (acting)	1876-	M. Sawyer	1893-
H. M. Peters...........	1877-	O. W. Nash...........	1894-1895
H. A. Varnell...........	1885-		

GENERAL SUPERINTENDENTS.

George F. Morgan (assistant 1903)	1895-1897	Dr. Chas. Eberlein (acting)	1910-1911
Albert N. Lange........	1897-1902	Dr. J. P. Percival.......	1911-1911
Dr. John R. Neely......	1902-1903	Henry J. Lynch (acting)	1911-1911
Dr. V. H. Podstata......	1903-1906	Dr. S. R. Pietrowicz....	1911-1912
Dr. O. C. Willhite......	1906-	Dr. F. B. Clarke........	1912-1912

[1] In a number of instances the date of assuming office only has been obtained.

ASSISTANT SUPERINTENDENTS.

Dr. Alexander Theummler 1884-1885
Chauncey F. Chapman.. 1890-

ASSISTANT PHYSICIANS.

Dr. J. C. Kelly.......... 1872-1874
Dr. A. W. Hagenback.. 1876-
Dr. James Lawless...... 1876-
Dr. S. V. Clevenger..... 1883-1885
Dr. Delia E. Howe...... 1884-1885
Dr. Harriet Alexander.. 1884-1885
Dr. Charles Keller...... 1884-1884
Dr. Thomas Cauley..... 1885-
Dr. Rosa Engelmann.... 1890-
Dr. C. B. Hauvey....... 1890-
Dr. G. W. Johnson...... 1893-
Dr. Clara Ferguson..... 1895-
Dr. M. H. McHugh..... 1903-
Dr. Elizabeth Kerney....
Dr. Charles Eberlein.... 1908-1912
Dr. Minnie Finch....... 1908-1909
Dr. Goodrich Snow..... 1908-1909
Dr. Clara Dunn......... 1908-1912
Dr. Charles Inghert..... 1908-1909
Dr. Louis J. Pollock.... 1908-1910
Dr. Henry W. Miller... 1908-
Dr. John T. Turner..... 1909-1910
Dr. Earl B. Jewell...... 1909-
Dr. Henry B. Bernhardt. 1909-1910
Dr. W. C. Speidel...... 1910-1911
Dr. Robert H. Rea......1910-
Dr. C. F. Sanborn...... 1911-1912
Dr. J. A. Smith........ 1911-
Dr. J. Cooperstein...... 1911-
Dr. Faith Spangler...... 1911-
Dr. D. I. Paradine...... 1911-
Dr. K. M. Manougian... 1912-1914
Dr. William W. Wood.. 1912-
Dr. P. S. Winner........ 1912-
Dr. I. J. Frisch.......... 1912-
Dr. T. J. Riach......... 1912-

INFIRMARY: CHIEF MALE PHYSICIANS.

Dr. J. J. Crowe......... 1895-
Dr. Ralph C. Hamill.... 1908-1910
Dr. Louis J. Pollock..... 1910-

ASSISTANT PHYSICIANS.

Dr. P. Crowley......... 1895-
Dr. J. O. Spray......... 1895-
Dr. John W. Turner..... 1910-

INTERNES.

Dr. Charles Solomon.... 1908-1909
Dr. Mannie A. Bernstein 1908-1909
Dr. John W. Turner.... 1908-1909
Dr. H. C. Mix......... 1909-1910
Dr. David E. Nelson.... 1909-1910

CONSUMPTIVE HOSPITAL: SENIOR PHYSICIAN.

Dr. Ernest S. Moire.... 1908-1912

ASSISTANT PHYSICIANS.

Dr. James A. Farren.... 1908-1909
Dr. Thomas McEachron 1909-1910
Dr. Edward M. Mikkelson 1910-1912
Dr. George J. Kruk.... 1912-1912

Officers of the Chicago State Hospital from the Date of the Taking Over by the State of the Cook County Asylum, Infirmary and Consumptive Hospital, July 1, 1912.

SUPERINTENDENTS.

Dr. F. B. Clarke (acting) 1912-1912
Dr. R. H. Rea (acting). 1912-1913
Dr. George Leininger (in office) 1913-

ASSISTANT SUPERINTENDENTS.

Dr. I. F. Fremmel...... 1912-1913
Dr. H. J. Smith........ 1913-1914
Dr. C. F. Read (in office) 1914-

PHYSICIANS.

Dr. R. H. Rea (in office) 1912-
Dr. Barnett Lemchen (in office) 1912-
Dr. C. C. Ellis (in office) 1912-
Dr. K. M. Manougian.. 1912-1914
Dr. F. J. Sullivan....... 1912-1912
Dr. I. F. Fremmel...... 1912-1914
Dr. J. C. Cooperstein... 1912-1913

ASSISTANT PHYSICIANS.

Dr. I. J. Frisch......... 1912-1913
Dr. John Peters........ 1912-1913
Dr. Faith E. Spangler... 1912-1913
Dr. P. S. Winner....... 1912-1914
Dr. W. W. Wood....... 1912-1912
Dr. T. V. Riach......... 1912-1913
Dr. R. R. McCarthy (in office) 1913-
Dr. Harriet S. McCarthy (in office) 1913-
Dr. G. M. Lisor (in office) 1912-
Dr. Otis Like (in office). 1914-
Dr. R. B. Kershaw (in office) 1914-
Dr. L. G. Wright (in office) 1914-
Dr. Alice M. Smith (in office) 1914-

INTERNES.

Dr. H. S. Seiwell....... 1913-1914
Dr. F. N. Cliff.......... 1913-1914
Dr. A. J. Fertick........ 1913-1914
Dr. J. C. Kaczkowski (in office) 1914-

ALTON STATE HOSPITAL.[1]

ALTON, ILL.

The Alton State Hospital is the ninth institution for the care of the insane in Illinois. Its ultimate capacity will be 1500 inmates. Five buildings, costing in the aggregate more than $200,000, are now in process of construction, and others will be provided for during the 1914-1915 session of the Legislature.

[1] By George A. Zeller, M. D., alienist, Board of Administration.

The site embraces 1000 acres and contains eight sets of farm buildings. As the tenant leases expired it was determined to anticipate the completion of the big new modern plant, and occupy the vacated buildings as a colony for chronic patients transferred from other state institutions. Accordingly on December 28, 1914, 20 patients arrived at the Alton State Hospital, having been transferred from the Anna State Hospital by the Board of Administration, which was represented on the occasion by Hon. Thomas O'Connor. These 20 patients formed the nucleus of the Alton State Hospital. Two weeks after their arrival 15 additional patients arrived, having been likewise transferred from the Anna State Hospital. They are housed in a farm building of almost baronial proportions, and their surroundings are ideal. As one observes their daily life and notes the harmony of their surroundings and the ease with which they have adapted themselves to their new environment, one is led to the conclusion that it will be a happy day for the insane when no ward or cottage will contain more than 35 inmates.

Dr. Henry S. Seiwell, assistant physician at the Watertown State Hospital, was transferred to the Alton State Hospital under the title of medical director, and will so continue until the appointment of a superintendent is deemed justifiable.

When the patients were transferred their attendants were likewise transferred, so that Dr. Seiwell had from the outset both a trained corps of attendants and a well-disciplined group of patients.

Other buildings will be occupied as soon as equipped, and it is hoped to have 100 patients present by early summer. It is the policy of the Board of Administration to pay considerable attention to geographical distribution, hence the patients selected for transfer are all former residents of the vicinity of Alton.

The water supply of the institution is that of the City of Alton, and mains have already been laid. The tracks of the Alton Street Railway are now being extended to the site and a railroad switch track leads directly to the new buildings. The public highway dividing the tract is a popular automobile route, and passing machines will do much toward relieving the monotony of institutional life.

LINCOLN STATE SCHOOL AND COLONY.[1]

LINCOLN, ILL.

The Lincoln State School and Colony, located at Lincoln, was first established at Jacksonville by an act of the General Assembly, approved February 15, 1865, entitled "An Act to Organize an Experimental School for the Instruction and Training of Idiots and Feeble-minded Children in the State of Illinois." The directors of the Institution for the Education of the Deaf and Dumb at Jacksonville were authorized to take such measures as might be suitable for the purpose of accomplishing the benevolent object of the Legislature. The first meeting of the directors was held March 1, 1865, at Jacksonville, at which time Dr. Philip G. Gillett was appointed, ex-officio, superintendent. The selection of the mansion and grounds of ex-Governor Joseph Duncan was decided upon and they were leased for the temporary home of the new institution. At the regular session of the General Assembly in 1871 an act was passed incorporating the Asylum for Feeble-minded Children as one of the permanent charitable institutions of the state. In April, 1875, appropriations were made for land and the construction of buildings for the asylum. After a careful survey of the state, Lincoln was selected as the permanent location.

On December 13, 1865, Dr. Charles T. Wilbur was elected superintendent of the experimental institution at Jacksonville. Dr. Wilbur served in this capacity through the change of location to Lincoln and up to October 4, 1883.

Dr. T. H. Leonard, the present incumbent, assumed his duties in August, 1913.

On January 1, 1910, the Board of Administration took over the control of the Institution for the Feeble-minded and shortly afterwards the name was changed to Lincoln State School and Colony. Simultaneously the Board of Trustees was automatically abolished.

The main building and grounds were occupied in 1878, and the enlarged accommodations greatly facilitated the work of the asylum. The original design and object of this institution

[1] By Dr. Thomas H. Leonard, superintendent.

were not to care for cases of custodial character; but the growing necessity of providing and caring for custodial cases became so apparent that the Thirty-sixth General Assembly made appropriations for the construction of a custodial building, which was completed in 1890. This building was soon found inadequate and further appropriations were made in 1899 for the erection of two cottages, the boys' cottage, completed in 1901, and the girls' cottage in 1902. The various buildings comprising the main institution at the present time are the administration, or main building, the school building and gymnasium, a building housing the older working boys, the boys' cottage, the girls' cottage, the North Hospital, the South Hospital, Forest Home, a wooden building occupied by women employees, the barn, two houses for employees, the boiler and engine rooms, the laundry, two industrial buildings, and the bake-shop. These buildings are situated on a tract of 94 acres in the southwest corner of the City of Lincoln. The main building faces south State Street, and a line of the street railway passes the front gate.

Three miles by road to the southwest is the Lincoln State School and Colony Farm, which is composed of a tract of 432 acres. On this farm is the farm cottage, with the outlying dairy barns and buildings to accommodate the various activities.

The object of the institution is to provide care for feeble-minded children, and in addition to prepare them for self-support as far as possible. The great majority of children can never by their efforts, even after education, do more than partially compensate the state for their keep.

The school accommodates 500 children, some of whom can only attend part of each school day. The general scope of the school is to educate the children manually and industrially, but to some who show more than usual ability in such lines instruction in literary branches is given. The girls are taught lace-making, plain and fancy sewing, reed and raffia work, basketry, art, music and literary branches. It is the intention of the school to so instruct the younger children that as they grow older and show fitness they may be promoted to the industrial shops, where the girls find useful occupation in the sewing room, the laundry mending room and the various fields of domestic science. The boys receive instruction in reed and raffia, basketry, sloyd and carpentry, manual work and the literary branches while in school. They are thus trained so that they may enter the tailor shop, the shoe shop, the brush shop, the mattress shop, the garden and the various skilled industries of the institution for which they are available. All children on their entrance into school, if of suitable age, begin school work in the kindergarten.

The farm is a garden as well as a farm. It has hot-houses and suitable plots for raising food crops for the institution. The field crops are grown not so much for sale as to feed the large dairy herd, the hogs, the sheep and the horses that are required by the institution. The farm cottage is occupied by 75 boys, who show particular adaptability to this kind of work.

Children eligible for admission must be feeble-minded and so deficient mentally as to be incapable of being educated at the ordinary public school. They should not be epileptic, insane, paralyzed, extremely helpless or afflicted with contagious disease. When admission is desired for a child, application is made to the superintendent. He returns an application blank which is self-explanatory. Cook County cases are handled through the Cook County agent's office. When the application of a given child is accepted, those interested are notified by letter and directed to file a personal bond to pay the expenses or to secure a county certificate, according as the financial circumstances dictate.

During the decennial period from 1905 to 1915 many changes were made at the Lincoln State School and Colony. The year 1906 saw the completion of substantial additions to the boys' cottage and the girls' cottage. In 1908 the completion of the gymnasium, a building capable of use as an auditorium and seating 1000 people, was a marked addition to the school and entertainment feature. In 1909 a new and modern bakery was finished and occupied. In 1910 a second industrial building, which was much needed, was finished, and a substantial addition was made to the greenhouse in South Park. The new South Hospital was completed in 1912 and occupied in the spring of 1913. It is a fine, well built, fireproof building.

In 1914 the new dairy barn of hollow tile construction was completed, and the building of the new hospital for tuberculosis cases was started. Also in 1914 the cottage additions were begun, and their completion, with that of the hospital for tuberculous children, served to relieve the congestion.

In the early part of 1906 electrical power was supplied for the shop machinery, the sewing machines in the tailor shop, shoe shop, sewing room, mending rooms and brush factory, and other special machinery. In 1907 an extensive reorganization of the mechanical equipment of the institution was started. This was inaugurated by the completion of a cement tunnel from the main building to the central building, to carry all heat and water pipes, cables for telephone and electric wires. With this work finished, the whole heating system of conduits throughout the institution was replaced and enlarged. The following year a telephone system was installed, as was also a Gamewell fire alarm system. Lawn swings, miles of cement walks and a neat iron fence around the institution were added. In 1912 was begun a renewal of the boiler system, with an enlargement amounting to a rebuilding of the boiler and engine rooms. Four modern water-tube boilers with automatic stokers replaced nine of the old style fire-tube boilers. At the same time new coal-sheds and the work of housing in these boilers went along, new concrete bases being made for the various engines and other heavy machinery. The plumbing, steam-fitting and sewerage work about the institution kept pace with the other improvements.

Following the inauguration of the civil service law in 1906, a complete reorganization of the medical department of this institution took place in 1907. The medical staff was increased to four members, an assistant superintendent, two assistant physicians and an interne, besides the superintendent. The system of record keeping was made modern with files for correspondence, card indexes for cases and the record of complete medical examinations. Systematic business staff meetings were held daily, and this change has been progressive up to the present time. Vigorous effort has been made to give a comprehensive and scientific study of the feeble-minded, with such laboratory and diagnostic aids as modern medicine has produced.

The nursing service was also reorganized, beginning in 1907, when a chief nurse was placed in charge, neat uniforms for the nurses and attendants being adopted, and a training school for nurses inaugurated. This training school has been kept up-to-date and has been recognized as a means of bettering the conditions of care and sanitation, as well as for the introduction of modern methods. A number of the graduates of the training school have remained in the service to teach the newer pupils.

In 1909 a department of psychology was added to the other departments of the institution. Dr. E. B. Huey, late of Johns Hopkins University, was in charge. Following Dr. Huey's resignation in 1911, Dr. C. H. Town had charge of this department and so remained until she was succeeded by Dr. and Mrs. George Ordahl in 1914. Dr. and Mrs. Ordahl both hold the degree of Ph. D., and under their direction this department is broadening out so that it now includes not only a routine psychological examination of each child so that he may be properly graded mentally, but also the pedagogical feature of directing a child's school activities after he has once been properly classified mentally.

A dental department was established in 1911, the dentist staying one day each week. It was found in 1913 that the dental conditions of the children demanded more attention than they had been receiving, and since that time a resident dentist has been employed.

In 1908 the substantial wooden structure known as the Old Hospital was emptied of children, who were sent to the North Hospital; the building was then thoroughly fumigated, painted, overhauled, and converted into pleasant quarters for female employees. It was re-christened "Forest Home." In 1908 a central dining-room was made in the central building to accommodate all employees. This change was coincident with the completion of a modern sanitary kitchen. The library, with a number of modern volumes comprehending many varieties of reading, has at all times been accessible and much used. The crowning achievement was reached in the latter part of 1914, when the eight-hour system of employment was adopted.

As late as early 1907 the form of restraint known as "Utica Crib" was in use at this institution. Straps, ropes, wristlets, belts, camisoles and various other forms of mechanical restraint were also freely used. It remained for the year 1914 to see the last of such methods. A steady trend of public sentiment in the school system has been for kindness to take the place of punishment as a disciplinary measure. The former "jail-rooms" are no more; punishments of a physical nature, whippings, etc., have been abolished. The amount of seclusion necessary in children of a wild and excitable type has been reduced to an absolute minimum.

The amusements of the children are given constant study. New games have been adopted, weekly picture shows inaugurated, new gymnasium apparatus bought, roller-skating, dancing and entertainments introduced on the gymnasium floor. When the weather is seasonable in summer and the days are warm and the duties of the children irksome, they have an hour or two every evening on the front lawn of the institution, where they may enjoy rest and diversion under the trees.

Seventeen teachers in the school are employed to teach these children, not only what may be learned industrially and mentally but also to instruct them in social amenities and the correct use of utensils in the dining-room. One hundred and sixteen attendants help in this work, and an extension service of the school, with teachers in charge, has been placed recently on the various wards within reach of crippled, maimed and deformed children, and those who are otherwise physically or mentally incapable of attending the regular school.

BOARD OF TRUSTEES.

Name	Term	Name	Term
William Thomas[1]	1865-1870	Wm. B. Fish, M. D.[2]	1884-1894
Isaac G. Wilson	1865-1870	Benson Wood	1886-1892
L. E. Worcester	1865-1870	C. R. Gittings[1]	1890-1894 1898-1902
R. Boal, M. D.[1]	1865-1872	A. B. Nicholson[1]	1890-1894
John R. Woods	1865-1870	T. N. Green	1894-1898
James N. Brown	1865-1868	C. M. Dunlap	1894-1898
Philip G. Gillett[2]	1865-1872	C. A. Purdunn[1]	1894-1898
John A. Chestnut	1868-1872	S. C. Smiley	1898-1902
Wm. P. Barr	1870-1872	Z. K. Wood[2]	1898-1900
Graham Lee[1]	1872-1878 1878-1890	G. D. Corwine	1900-1902
David Prince, M. D.	1872-1876	John F. Regan[1]	1902-1904
C. T. Wilbur[2]	1872-1884	Edward Stubblefield	1902-1904
Rev. Wm. J. Rutledge	1874-1876	Jacob F. Swank	1902-1904
C. R. Cummings[1]	1876-1880	Judge James W. Gibson[1]	1904-1908
A. B. Nicholson	1876-1878	Carl F. Bartling	1904-1910
E. Callahan	1878-1886	John Wagner	1904-1908
J. C. Warnock	1878-1882	Joseph Desilva, M. D.[1]	1908-1910
E. D. Blinn[1]	1882-1890	W. H. C. Smith, M. D.	1908-1910

[1] President. [2] Secretary.

TREASURERS.

A. E. Ayres	1865-1872	Stephen A. Foley	1894-1896
William S. Hook	1872-1878	George Wendell	1896-1898
W. R. Randolph	1878-1884	H. C. Quisenberry	1898-1902
John D. Gillett	1884-1890	John T. Foster	1902-1904
John A. Hoblit	1890-1894	John S. Haller	1904-1910

SUPERINTENDENTS.

Dr. Charles T. Wilbur	1865-1883	Dr. S. H. McLean	1901-1903
Dr. W. B. Fish	1883-1892	Dr. C. B. Taylor	1903-1907
Dr. A. M. Miller	1893-1895	Dr. H. G. Hardt	1907-1913
Dr. J. W. Smith	1895-1897	Dr. Thos. H. Leonard (in office)	1913-
Dr. W. L. Athon	1897-1901		

ASSISTANT SUPERINTENDENTS.

Dr. W. H. C. Smith	1889-1907	Dr. C. B. Caldwell (in office)	1907-
Dr. John R. Barnet	1897-1902		
C. B. Taylor	1902-1903		

ASSISTANT PHYSICIANS.

Dr. R. L. Frisby	1901-1905	Dr. Olga Bridgman	1912-1913
Dr. Wm. Young	1902-1907	Dr. J. J. Mendelsohn (in office)	1912-
Dr. Robert B. Hoag	1905-1907	Dr. K. H. Elting (in office)	1913-
Dr. C. J. T. Rochow	1907-1909	Dr. H. J. Freemmel (in office)	1914-
Dr. Harriet Hook	1907-1908	Dr. Geo. Ordahl (in office)	1914-
Dr. A. G. Hamilton	1908-1912	Dr. Wilson K. Dyer (in office)	1915-
Dr. J. T. Black	1909-1910		
Dr. Roy H. Cox[1]	1910-1910		
Dr. C. C. Atherton	1910-1911		
Dr. W. W. Mercer	1911-1913		
Dr. S. A. Smith	1911-1912		
Dr. Ruth Alexander[2]	1912-1912		

PSYCHOLOGISTS.

Dr. Geo. Ordahl	1914-1915	Mr. Harrison L. Harley (in office)	1915-

---

[1] Two weeks only.

[2] Four months only.

THE ILLINOIS COLONY FOR EPILEPTICS.[1]

DIXON, ILL.

In 1894 the State Board of Commissioners of Public Charities presented a report to the Governor of Illinois, recommending that the General Assembly take steps to create an epileptic colony. The board at that time stated that there were 8000 epileptics in the State of Illinois and of this number 434 were in hospitals for the insane.

In the report to the Governor, made by the same board in 1896, the creation of the colony was again urged and statistics were shown relating to the number of epileptics in the state.

In 1898 the board repeated its recommendation for the creation of this institution, and stated that: "we trust the present General Assembly may give this crying need recognition by the creation of an institution for this unfortunate class."

During the year 1896 the Forty-first General Assembly passed an act authorizing the establishing of the Illinois State Colony for Epileptics, making an appropriation of $2500 for the expenses incident to the location of the colony. The Board of Commissioners of Public Charities was empowered to make the selection, but no appropriation was made to pay for the site. The Board of Commissioners of Public Charities located the colony at "Notch Cliff," Jersey County, Ill., on the bluffs overlooking the Mississippi River, near the town of Elsah. Recommendations were repeatedly made by the Board of Commissioners of Public Charities for an appropriation necessary to establish this institution, but without avail.

In 1902 a bill was introduced in the Forty-third General Assembly providing for an appropriation of $100,000 for the purchase of the site. The bill passed the House, but the Senate failed to concur.

In 1907 the Forty-fifth General Assembly had up for consideration a bill appropriating $265,000 for such a colony, and the Forty-sixth General Assembly in 1909 was presented with a bill appropriating $100,000 for this purpose, but these bills also failed to pass.

[1] By Frank Whipp, fiscal supervisor and member of Board of Administration.

The agitation for the creation of the colony was revived at a meeting of the Illinois State Conference of Charities and Corrections held in October, 1912, which recommended the establishment of a colony to care for 2000 inmates. After this long campaign by the charity boards and organizations, the colony was finally established by an act of the Forty-eighth General Assembly in 1913, at which time an appropriation was made of $500,000 for the purchase of site, drawing of plans and preliminary construction of new buildings. The Board of Administration of State Charitable Institutions was empowered to select a new site for this colony. The board invited applications from localities in the State of Illinois desiring the location of the colony, and 21 sites were offered, located in 11 different counties.

All of the sites were inspected by the Board of Administration, and in February, 1914, the State Colony for Epileptics was located on a site three miles north of Dixon, Lee County, Ill. This site contains approximately 1100 acres of land, and is bordered on one side by the beautiful Rock River and is so situated that the colony will have good drainage, an abundance of water and adequate railroad facilities. Aside from the geographical advantages of this location, the colony is in one of the most healthful communities of the state. Contracts have been made which insure the building of a switch track from the Illinois Central Railroad and the extension of the electric line from the City of Dixon to the entrance of the colony grounds. The location is considered an ideal one, it being convenient to the large population of the state, and in a territory which has not been heretofore favored with a state institution.

The Board of Administration has paid the sum of $234,912.24 for the site and the expenses in connection therewith, leaving a balance of $265,087.76 in the appropriation available for new buildings and other improvements. Contracts have been let for the erection of nine buildings to cost $243,289, and the construction of these buildings will be commenced as soon as the weather permits.

An act creating the colony provides that accommodations shall be provided for the care and comfort of 1500 inmates. The preamble of this act states that there are at least 10,000 persons of all ages and conditions suffering from epilepsy who reside in Illinois.

The name of the institution will probably be changed to that of The Dixon State Farm.

THE ANDREW McFARLAND OAK LAWN RETREAT.

Jacksonville, Ill.

This is a sanitarium for treatment of mental and nervous diseases and was founded by Dr. Andrew McFarland in 1871. Dr. McFarland was born in New Hampshire and educated at Jefferson Medical College. He was appointed superintendent of the New Hampshire Asylum for the Insane in 1845. In 1854 he was appointed superintendent of the Illinois Central Hospital for the Insane, which position he held until 1870, when he resigned and established this sanitarium. After his death the institution was left in charge of his granddaughter, Dr. Anne McFarland-Sharpe. Dr. Wm. K. McLaughlin is now the medical superintendent of the institution. The institution has seven acres of grounds; the main building is a copy of Melrose Abbey. It is divided into wards, each containing five rooms, with separate dining-room, bath and closet. There are also five private rooms for patients in the administration building. The capacity is limited to 40 patients. There is a detached building for the care of epileptics.

OFFICERS.

Dr. Wm. K. McLaughlin................Superintendent.
Dr. Anne McFarland-Sharpe............Resident physician.
J. Thompson Sharpe....................Business manager.

KENILWORTH SANITARIUM.

Kenilworth, Ill.

This institution is located in a park of 10 acres. The building is a three-and-a-half-story structure, the exterior being finished in Portland cement. The rooms are so arranged that six independent suites may be furnished if desired, with special parlor, bathroom and bedroom. The heating is by steam and lighting is by electricity, there being also an electric passenger elevator. There are four pavilions, which open toward the south and which have concrete floors and concrete walks leading to them, which can be utilized for exercise in bad weather. There are eight muffled rooms, so constructed that any noise made by the occupant is not heard outside the room.

Hydrotherapy, massage, calisthenics and medical remedies are employed. The most approved diagnostic methods, including the

Wassermann test, are utilized. The proportion of nurses is 25 nurses to 21 patients. In the way of out-door sports there are golf, croquet and tennis.

A woman physician, who is also a graduate nurse, acts as superintendent of nurses in addition to her other duties.

The cost of the plant as it stands at present was $152,000. Cases of chronic alcoholism and drug addiction are received as well as nervous and mental cases. The institution is organized as a stock company, but is entirely controlled by Dr. Sanger Brown, physician-in-charge. Chicago office, Mallers Building, 59 E. Madison Avenue.

MEDICAL STAFF.

Dr. Sanger Brown, president.
Dr. H. W. Powers, medical superintendent from 1905 to 1912.
Dr. Sherman Brown, medical superintendent from 1912 to present date.

ASSISTANT PHYSICIANS.

Dr. Lillian Mitchell, from Februray, 1905, to March, 1906.
Dr. Wilma Jacobs, a few months in 1906.
Dr. Esther Ryerson, December, 1907, to March, 1908.
Dr. Thyra Josselyn, June, 1908, to August, 1908.
Dr. Anna Mulholland, March, 1909, to July, 1909.
Dr. Ella Blackburn, November, 1909, to May, 1912.
Dr. Katheryn Driscoll, May, 1912, to present time.

PRIVATE HOME FOR THE FEEBLE-MINDED.

WHEATON, ILL.

This institution was established by Mrs. E. B. Howe about 1908. It is licensed by the State of Illinois and cares for the feeble-minded and mildly insane. The capacity is limited to seven or eight patients. The institution is small, the grounds being limited to one and a half acres. The investment is estimated at $6000.

DR. BROUGHTON'S SANITARIUM.

ROCKFORD, ILL.

This institution is confined to the treatment of drug and alcoholic patients and does not care for mental cases. The present physician is Dr. G. J. Werrick.

THE CARE OF THE INSANE IN INDIANA.[1]

The benevolent and correctional institutions, including the hospitals for the insane, of Indiana, are now and have always been administered by individual boards. These boards consisted of three members until 1907, when the number was increased to four members. They have usually been appointed by the Governor, but in two or three instances during the period of high partisanship before 1892, when the Legislature and Governor happened to belong to opposing political parties, the Legislature relieved the Governor of the responsibility of this appointing power and itself exercised it by electing the members of these boards. The method was, of course, never successful; was always opposed by public opinion, and, being a matter of party expediency, was not permanent and the power was always restored to its proper place with the Governor just as soon as the Legislature and executive departments were in harmony. Since 1893 this action has not been repeated, notwithstanding the fact that the two branches of state government have not always been in political accord.

In 1883 the Legislature, in depriving the Governor of the appointing power, enacted the most extreme law in the history of the state, by creating for the three state institutions located at Indianapolis—the hospital for the insane, the asylum for the blind and the institution for the education of the deaf and dumb—a board of two members for each, and one president in common for the three boards; and all were elected by the Legislature. The action was purely partisan, with nothing else to commend it, and, as was expected and intended, all belonged to the same political party. The administration was a failure and developed so much scandal that the law was soon repealed.

In 1889 Indiana took its longest forward stride in the management of its benevolent institutions by creating a board of state charities and clothing it with advisory powers only. This board consisted of six members, three each from the two leading political parties, who were appointed by the Governor. This law still stands, and, while the functions of this board have been increased and broadened into a great work covering all the state, county and

[1] Prepared by Samuel E. Smith, M. D.

township charities, its authority over the state institutions remains advisory only and not executive. The members serve without salaries and the Governors have exercised unusual care and judgment in the many appointments. Without exception they have been, both as men and women, representative of the state's highest citizenship, and have devoted their time and labor without personal remuneration to the development of the state benevolent work. Likewise has this board been most fortunate in the selection of its secretary. During a period of 23 years only three men have served in this position, and they were Alexander Johnson, Ernest P. Bicknell and Amos W. Butler, the present incumbent. All three have won national fame in this field of work.

When this board was created in 1889 the trustees of the state hospitals and other institutions consisted of three members elected by the Legislature, but this appointing power was again lodged with the Governor in 1893, where it has properly remained to this day.

Prior to 1889 the boards of trustees, with the authority of law, not only appointed the superintendent, but also all officers and employees, not omitting the scullery maids. The superintendent was permitted, as an act of courtesy, to nominate in some instances, but the power of appointment and discharge as well was legally and usually exercised by the boards.

In 1889 a law was enacted providing for the organization of the three additional hospitals—the Northern Hospital at Logansport, the Eastern Hospital at Richmond, and the Southern Hospital at Evansville—and for the first time the medical superintendent was empowered to select and appoint his officers and employees subject only to the confirmation of the Board of Trustees. By an unfortunate oversight the author of the measure failed to give also to the medical superintendent the rightful power of discharge of his subordinates. This duty was not mentioned in the law, and afterwards, in a few instances, it was claimed and exercised disadvantageously by certain boards. However, the act of 1889 was distinctly an advance, and it was believed by the author of the bill and a few others actively interested in the cause that the thus broadened powers, although incomplete, of the medical superintendent would become, as they did in a short time, the entering wedge to still better things. While the management was still partisan, because the members of the boards were elected by the Legislature (by the party in power), the popular demand for non-partisan control was in the air and growing stronger year by year. The Board of State Charities was beginning to exercise influence for good, and the members of the professions and a few of the newspapers were fostering and encouraging the new doctrine.

The first hospital organized under a bi-partisan control, which in this instance was non-partisan in spirit, was the Northern Hospital at Logansport, and this was accomplished under peculiar circumstances. The Board of Commissioners of the three additional hospitals was composed of four members, two representing each of the two leading political parties, and Governor Porter was in 1887 *ex-officio* president of the board. This board was authorized by its organic act to organize, open for the admission of patients and manage, pending action by the next succeeding Legislature, any or all of the new hospitals when completed. Efforts were directed towards the completion of the Northern Hospital to meet a specially urgent demand for the accommodation of the insane in need of hospital treatment, and in the autumn of 1887 it effected its organization by the appointment of Dr. Joseph G. Rogers, medical engineer of that board, to the position of medical superintendent, and on the latter's nomination appointed also the members of the staff as assistant physicians. This board continued in control only about 18 months after the new hospital was opened on July 1, 1888, when the Legislature convened and the usual partisan board was elected under the act of 1889 and took charge. This new board fortunately was composed of good men, who soon felt the spirit of the new methods and supported the non-partisan management, which has continued to this day.

The Eastern Hospital was the next to inaugurate, without support by law, the non-partisan management. It was opened in August, 1890, with a partisan organization which did not succeed, and six months thereafter the Legislature abolished the board and elected a new one. Dr. Samuel E. Smith, then assistant physician in the Northern Hospital, was promoted to the position of medical superintendent of the Eastern Hospital and assumed his duties May 15, 1891. As rapidly as possible he established the new order of non-partisan management, which has stood the test without change for nearly 21 years.

The effort to maintain these two hospitals under non-partisan management was not done with a blare of trumpets. The system was not popular enough for that, but those actively interested had sufficient faith in its virtues to believe that, while the methods might not strike a popular chord in those partisan days, they were confident the results would justify them and, if continued a few years without attracting too much attention to the means, the results would receive popular commendation; and this view proved correct.

Then the Central Hospital in 1893 came under the management of Dr. George F. Edenharter as superintendent, who was progressive and sympathetic with the new order, which he established as rapidly as possible under most unfavorable conditions on account of his proximity to the state capital, the storm center of political activity.

The popularity of non-partisan management grew apace, although it seemed slow enough until 1896, when the minority party embodied the principle in a plank in its platform, and while this plank was not a prominent issue, this party was successful in the election and came into control of state affairs in January, 1897.

The principle supported by popular favor and submitted at an opportune time was crystallized into law by the Legislature of 1897. The bill was drawn by Charles E. Shiveley, of Richmond, then a member of the Indiana Senate, who stood sponsor for it and, after a good fight, won.

This law provided for individual boards of three members each, appointed by the Governor, no more than two of whom should be affiliated with the same political party, and in addition two sections vital to the cause of non-partisan management, which read as follows:

SEC. 6. Said persons so appointed upon said Boards of Trustees shall serve without any compensation, save and except their necessary traveling expenses and other expenses while engaged in performing their duties under this act, which expenses shall be paid, as other expenses of said institutions, quarterly.

SEC. 7. Said Board of Trustees shall, in the employment of superintendents and confirmation of assistants and other employees, take into consideration only the qualifications and fitness of the persons selected to fill such places, and no person shall be selected or employed to fill any of such positions on account of his political belief or affiliations, and no superintendent, assistant or employee shall be dismissed from service on account of his political belief, faith or affiliations, and in the employment or dismissal of such superintendent, assistant or employee, the qualifications, character, merit and fitness shall be the only matters to be considered by such Board of Trustees in the selection or retention of such employees.

When the bill for the act was printed after first reading Dr. Samuel E. Smith observed an important omission, which he feared to attempt to correct by the usual amendment, and at his suggestion the author agreed to endeavor to make the correction by unanimous consent of the Senate without discussion, by interlining in line 2 of Section 7 the words "*confirmation of.*" His effort was successful and the right of the medical superintendent to appoint his staff and employees was legalized.

This law was quite satisfactory and worked admirably, and, while the representation on the board was bi-partisan, it was in effect non-partisan. It was a long stride in the affairs of the public institutions of Indiana and fixed firmly the principle of efficiency as the basis of employment and tenure. It resulted in better treatment and care of the state's dependents and unfortunates, as well as more economy in administration.

The fact that the minority was represented by only one member on each board brought forth an occasional criticism and for this reason the law was strengthened, broadened and much improved under the direction of Governor J. Frank Hanly by the Legislature of 1907. The sections important for present purposes are as follows:

SEC. 1. *Be it enacted by the General Assembly of the State of Indiana,* That the Board of Trustees of the Central Hospital for Insane, the Northern Hospital for Insane, the Eastern Hospital for Insane, the Southern Hospital for Insane, the Southeastern Hospital for Insane, the Indiana Village for Epileptics, the Indiana Soldiers' and Sailors' Orphans' Home, the Indiana Institution for the Education of the Deaf and Dumb, the Indiana Institution for the Education of the Blind, the Indiana School for Feeble-minded Youth, the Indiana Boys' School, the Board of Control of the Indiana State Prison, the Indiana Industrial School for Girls and the Indiana Women's Prison, shall hereafter consist of four trustees each. One additional trustee shall be appointed by the Governor to each of said boards as the same are now constituted, within 30 days from the taking effect of this act, and each of such additional trustees so appointed shall serve for a term of four years. The Board of Managers of the Indiana Reformatory shall continue to consist of four members, as now constituted, and after the first expiration of term of office which shall occur in the Board of Trustees of the Indiana State Soldiers' Home, said board shall consist thereafter of four members only. Upon the expiration of the term of any member of any of said boards, or upon a vacancy occurring in any of said boards, the Governor shall appoint a successor to such member, except as herein otherwise provided. All appointments shall be for a term of four years respectively, excepting in case of vacancy by death, removal or resignation they shall be for the unexpired term. In making all appointments referred to in this section the Governor, in addition to the qualifications hereinafter mentioned, shall take into consideration the political affiliations and belief of such appointees, so that not more than two of the members of said boards respectively shall be members of the same political party or have the same political affiliation or belief. The names of said Board of Control of the Indiana State Prison, the Board of Managers of the Indiana Reformatory, the Indiana Industrial School for Girls and the Indiana Women's Prison shall each be known hereafter as the Board of Trustees of said institutions respectively: *Provided,* That this act shall not be construed as abolishing any of the present governing boards of said institutions, but the present members of all of said boards shall serve out their respective terms thereon, under the appointments already made.

SEC. 5. Such trustees shall receive as compensation three hundred dollars ($300) a year each and their reasonable expenses, not to exceed one hundred and twenty-five dollars ($125) a year each, which shall be paid quarterly as other expenses of the institutions are paid. No person shall be eligible to be appointed a member of any of the Boards of Trustees referred to in this act who is a contractor with the institution of whose board he or she is a member, or who is interested, either directly or indirectly, in any contract with or in furnishing any of the supplies for such institution, and if any person appointed under the provisions of this act shall become so interested during his or her term of office, such interest shall vacate his or her office, and his or her successor shall immediately be appointed as hereinbefore provided, to fill his or her unexpired term.

SEC. 6. Such boards shall have the legal custody and supervision of their respective institutions. Three members of a board shall constitute a quorum for the organization of the board and for the transaction of all business. The trustees shall give so much of their time and attention to the affairs of their respective institutions as shall insure the wise, efficient and faithful management thereof. Each board shall appoint a superintendent or head of the particular institution when there is a vacancy, to be known by the same name as that now applied to such officer in each of the respective institutions mentioned in this act, and such board shall have the power to remove him or her for any cause impairing faithful, efficient or intelligent administration of the office, after opportunity is given him or her to be heard upon written charges. The superintendents of the Indiana Girls' School and of the Indiana Women's Prison shall be women; the superintendent of any hospital for the insane and of the Indiana Village for Epileptics shall be a reputable physician. No person shall be appointed superintendent of a hospital for the insane unless he has had professional experience in an institution for the insane, and no person shall be appointed superintendent of the Indiana Village for Epileptics unless he has had professional experience in a similar institution or in an institution for the insane. All other officers and employees of each institution named herein shall be selected and appointed by the superintendent or head of the institution and shall be removable at his or her pleasure, and all of such officers and employees shall be appointed regardless of political or religious affiliation on the basis of fitness, after examination as to their qualifications for the duties to be performed, under such rules and regulations as may be prescribed by the board of the institution. The annual compensation of the superintendent or head of the institution, and the number of officers and employees, their duties and compensations, shall be fixed by the Board of Trustees at its discretion, and said trustees are hereby forbidden to solicit or request or in any way interfere with the appointment or discharge of any officer or employee. It is hereby made a misdemeanor for any person to solicit or receive from any officer or employee of said institutions any money for campaign assessments, or for any officer or employee of said institution to pay any such assessment, to any person or organization or political party. Upon conviction such person so soliciting, receiving or paying such assessment shall be fined in any sum not less than fifty dollars ($50) nor more than five hundred dollars ($500), to which may be added imprisonment in the county jail or workhouse for not less than sixty (60) days nor more than one year; and any person so offending who is an officer or employee of an institution named in this act shall be immediately removed from such position and shall not be eligible for reappointment for a period of five years.

Sec. 7. In the purchase of supplies that enter into the maintenance of any of the institutions covered by this act, it shall be the duty to invite competitive bids through sealed proposals to the president of the board of each institution, and the lowest and best responsible bidder shall be awarded the contract, and the same provision shall apply to the construction and equipment of all buildings for any such institution. Public notice of such bids shall be given by publication in the two leading newspapers in the county where such institution is located, and otherwise if considered beneficial. If such board deems it advisable and in the interest of economy to buy certain articles in quantity to last for a longer period, it shall have the right to do so. Such fact, however, shall be particularly stated in the notices. Blank bids shall be furnished for all applicants, but bids shall not be rejected because not contained on such form. Any or all bids may be rejected.

This law is still in force and, it is believed, has fixed certain principles of management in Indiana for many years to come. While it is in advance of any previous legislation in this commonwealth, as well as most others, it contains one retrogressive feature, which is embodied in Section 5, providing small salaries for the trustees. There is some division of opinion on this point. It appears, however, that the state can with propriety call upon a few of its successful citizens who are interested in public benevolence, who would feel honored by the trust, to administer these great charities without personal compensation.

The government of the state hospitals and other public institutions in Indiana is therefore by individual non-partisan boards of four members appointed by the Governor, and supervised by a Board of State Charities of six members and a secretary, with advisory functions and powers only. To this system Indiana is wedded and believes the progress of the past 20 years justified its faith. As opposed to the system of the Central Board of Control, its conviction is strong. It believes that it has effectually set aside the strong argument of economy of management universally claimed by the Central Board of Control by Indiana's showing in the report of the studies of Henry E. Wright, of the Russell Sage Foundation, in 1910, and at the same time has preserved to the state's service and its unfortunates the benefits of individualism in management, both in power and responsibility. The independent Board of State Charities, with its unpaid service, is in a sense a citizens' committee, and, while enjoying the full confidence of the people, it is the buffer between the state institutions and public opinion, and always stands ready, as both people and officers know, to correct or protect as the quality of management may require.

Source of Support.—The state hospitals are supported entirely by legislative appropriations from the state treasury made biennially. Recommendations are made by the Board of Trustees and medical superintendent to the Governor, who refers them for investigation to a legislative committee of three members, one from the Senate and two from the House, appointed by the Governor 60 days before the Legislature convenes. The two leading political parties must be represented on this board and usually the members are experienced in this or similar work. This committee visits, inspects and inquires into the needs of the hospitals and other institutions and requires special financial reports and estimates for its information. The recommendations of this committee, which devotes nearly all of its time both 60 days before and throughout the legislative session, is usually final and guides legislative action.

There are three regular funds provided—maintenance, clothing and repairs—and specific funds cover major repairs, new construction and other permanent improvements.

The maintenance funds vary slightly with the local conditions of the several hospitals and are fixed sums for a given number of patients, to which a per capita allowance of $180 per annum is allowed for any daily average number in excess of the given number. This allows some elasticity in the amount of funds for a changing population, such as would follow by any increase in capacity from new construction and the like.

The repair and clothing funds are fixed.

The clothing furnished patients in a hospital is charged to the counties in which the patients have a legal settlement; is reported to the Treasurer of the state, who reimburses the state treasury for the amount from collection from the counties.

The estate, if any, of a patient, or his family if able, is expected to provide necessary clothing for the patient while under treatment in the hospital, and about 50 per cent do so, although the law is not mandatory. When not otherwise supplied, it must be furnished by the hospital in the manner heretofore described.

Otherwise there is no charge for the care and treatment of any insane citizen in a state hospital and all are received and treated on exactly the same plane. This method is in consonance with a principle of the state constitution of 1851, set forth in a section which reads as follows:

> It shall be the duty of the General Assembly to provide by law for the support of institutions for the education of the deaf and dumb, and of the blind; and, also, for the treatment of the insane.

In 1889 a law was enacted requiring the medical superintendent to collect from the estates of patients an amount equal to the cost of their maintenance. It was speedily repealed at the next session of the Legislature as the result of an effort to make such a collection by legal process in an instance where such a collection would have worked a serious hardship. No other attempt of this kind has been made.

One court has, also, held that under the constitution the state is under obligations to provide clothing for all insane persons while under treatment in a state hospital.

Under the Indiana constitution and laws it is therefore apparent that no private patients can be admitted to the state hospitals.

The state is committed to the policy of state care, both by its constitution and all subsequent legislation relating to the subject. It has never, however, made sufficient provision in its hospitals for all of its insane, although it has approached it twice. At the present time there are 5500 insane persons in the state, and of this number approximately 5200 are enrolled in the state hospitals. The 300 are in county infirmaries and at large. One county, under a law authorizing such when necessary, has a small hospital for its chronic insane and a few others have made special provision for small numbers in connection with county infirmaries.

Pending commitment to the state hospital an insane person, when not provided for in the family, is held in the city hospital, county jail or county infirmary, depending upon the tendencies shown by the patient. Special effort, which no doubt will soon prove successful, is being made to prevent the temporary detention of any case in a city or county jail.

Indeed, the day is near at hand when the state hospitals will be able to furnish accommodations for the state's insane.

Commitment.—Prior to 1881 insanity inquests for the purpose of commitment to the state hospital were conducted by two justices of the peace. A statement of the attending physician or one medical examiner was required, and also a sworn statement by at least one witness that the person alleged to be insane was insane and also dangerous to the community.

In 1881 the law was revised requiring a preliminary statement before a justice of the peace from one reputable citizen of the county, alleging the condition of insanity and at the same time giving some history of the person, together with any witness.

This justice appointed another justice and a medical examiner other than the medical attendant and all were required to visit and examine into the condition of the person alleged to be insane at his home or wherever located. The justice then fixed a day for the inquest and directed the clerk of the circuit court to issue subpœnas to the medical attendant, medical examiner, the person alleging the insanity and any other witnesses named in the preliminary statement, or not, to attend the inquest and give testimony under oath. It was not necessary for the person alleged to be insane to be present, and he was not barred from attendance. The finding of the justices was then certified to the clerk of the circuit court, together with a complete record of the evidence. If the justices found the person insane and he could be conveyed to a state hospital for the insane without danger to life, application for his admission was made by the clerk to the medical superintendent of the hospital and with the application was transmitted a complete record of the insanity proceedings.

On receipt of the application for admission and the transcript of the record the medical superintendent determined upon the information furnished whether the case was "recent and presumably curable, or chronic and less curable, or idiotic and incurable." If "recent and curable" he at once issued an acceptance to the proper clerk. If "chronic, whether curable or incurable," an acceptance was issued by the medical superintendent conditioned upon room in the hospital and the quota of room apportioned to the county based upon its population.

Another and older statute is more specific in the order of preference when, for want of room, all cannot be admitted:

1. Recent cases, *i. e.*, when the disease is of less than one year's duration.
2. Chronic cases (*i. e.*, when the disease is of more than one year's duration) presenting the most favorable prospect of recovery.
3. Those of whom application has been longest on file.
4. Each county should be entitled to its just proportion according to its population, but preference may be given to the recent cases of one county over the chronic cases of another county.

In no event, it should be noted, could a warrant be issued for conveying a patient to a state hospital until an acceptance had been issued by the medical superintendent. If, however, a sheriff should convey a patient to the hospital without the medical superintendent having issued an acceptance, no fee whatever for service could be allowed.

This statute of 1881 remained in force until 1901, when it was amended, authorizing one justice of the peace to conduct the inquest and sit in judgment in the court house of the proper county and authorizing him to subpœna as witnesses the attending physician, *two* medical examiners, the persons alleging the insanity and any and all other witnesses to appear on a fixed day and give testimony under oath. All are required to examine the person within five days preceding the inquest, and the sworn certificate of the two medical examiners must be made jointly. If found insane by the justice, certification is made to the clerk of the circuit court, as under the act of 1881, heretofore described. In all other respects the statute of 1881 is still in effect.

In executing the warrant for conveying an insane woman to and from a hospital the sheriff must be accompanied by a woman. If a friend or relative requests of the clerk the privilege of conveying the insane person to the hospital it is mandatory that the clerk issue to the relative or friend the necessary warrant and pay out of the treasury the necessary traveling expenses therefor if demanded.

Discharge.—The discharge of a patient from a state hospital is based wholly on the judgment and discretion of the medical superintendent. Two laws are in force, one applying to the Central Hospital, the oldest institution, and a later one to the other four hospitals.

The superintendent of the Central Hospital may discharge any patient upon restoration to health; and incurable and harmless patients shall be discharged whenever it is necessary to make room for recent cases.

The law governing the discharge of patients from the Eastern, Northern, Southern and Southeastern hospitals reads as follows:

SEC. 15. The medical superintendent may discharge a patient from the hospital whenever in his opinion the mental and physical condition of such patient shall justify it, and may furlough patients to their homes whenever in his opinion they may be benefited thereby, but he shall retain in hospital such inmates thereof as may in his judgment be unfit to be at large or may require special medical care: *Provided,* That in no case shall the exercise of the right of the writ of *habeas corpus* as regulated by law in such cases be denied.

The medical superintendent is authorized to discharge a patient:

1. To the clerk of the circuit court, who must issue a warrant to the sheriff for the patient's removal from the hospital and deliver him to his family or friends.
2. To the patient's friends if ready, able and willing to remove him.
3. To the patient himself when restored to "perfect health of mind and body and in every way able to provide for himself."

Recommitment.—In the event of a recurrence of insanity or a delay of over six months in the admission of an insane person to a state hospital, application for readmission or a renewal of the application for admission may be effected by recommital proceedings, which consist of a sworn statement by the attending physician to the clerk of the circuit court, who makes application for admission to the medical superintendent as in an original inquest. A second inquest is never necessary.

Dangerous Insane.—An old statute of 1855 is still in force but rarely invoked, which permits a person alleged to be insane and dangerous to the community to be tried by jury in the circuit court, and, if found dangerous, the clerk is authorized to provide safe care at the expense of the county.

Insane Criminals.—In 1889 a law was enacted authorizing the establishment, in connection with the Indiana Reformatory, of the Indiana Hospital for the Criminal Insane, but, on account of a technical omission, its provisions were never carried out.

In 1909 another law was enacted with substantially the same provisions as that of 1889, authorizing the establishment of the Indiana Hospital for Insane Criminals as a department of the Indiana State Prison at Michigan City. The law is effective and the necessary construction is now completed.

It provides for the commitment of criminals in the reformatory or state prison to that hospital on insanity proceedings ordered by the Governor on information from the general superintendent of the reformatory or warden of the prison, before a justice of the peace in substantially the same manner as insanity inquests for commitment to a state hospital for the insane.

Provision is also made for the commitment to that hospital of persons found guilty of a felony, when also found insane by the trial court. The form of commitment is the same as above described.

Unsoundness of Mind and Guardianship.—Proceedings by insanity inquests for commitment to a hospital for the insane do not in Indiana invalidate any rights of citizenship, except the restriction of liberty for treatment and safety.

A guardianship to conserve an insane person's property rights and interests is based upon a finding of "unsoundness of mind" by jury trial before a judge of a circuit court.

Private Patients and Private Hospitals.—Indiana has no laws governing the commitment of patients to private hospitals. Admission to private or non-state hospitals is either voluntary or on order of a court.

No private or voluntary patients can be admitted to a state hospital. All admissions to the state hospitals must be by commitment, and not otherwise.

CENTRAL INDIANA HOSPITAL FOR INSANE.[1]

INDIANAPOLIS, IND.

In a paper read by Dr. Joseph G. Rogers to the Seventh Conference of Charities we find that "the first step towards institutional care of the insane in Indiana was a memorial to the Legislature of 1832. A favorable report was made, but nothing further was done until 1844, when Governor Bigger pressed the matter in his message and Dr. W. S. Cornett, of the Senate, moved an amendment to the revenue bill, "that one cent on the hundred dollars be levied as a fund with which to erect a lunatic asylum," which was adopted. This levy produced $12,000 during the year and was continued.

During the session of the Legislature of 1844-45 an "Act to Provide for the Procuring a Suitable Site for the Erection of a State Lunatic Asylum" was passed and approved January 13, 1845.

Section 1 of said act reads as follows:

Be it enacted by the General Assembly of the State of Indiana, That John Evans, Livingston Dunlap and James Blake be, and they are hereby, appointed a Board of Commissioners to select and purchase such a tract of land, not exceeding two hundred acres in quantity, as may be most suitable in regard to health and convenience for the location of a state lunatic asylum.

Under Sections 3 and 4 of the same act the commissioners were instructed "to obtain all the information possible, by correspondence and otherwise, concerning the best plans and specifications and methods of managing an asylum for lunatics," and submit the results of their investigations to the Legislature of 1846.

The first meeting of the commissioners was held in the City of Indianapolis, at the office of Dr. Dunlap, on February 1, 1845. At this meeting Dr. Evans was appointed an agent of the board to gather such information as he may think necessary to lay before the board on the subject of the location, plans and buildings and modes of managing hospitals for the insane.

On May 30, 1845, the commissioners again met at the office of Dr. Dunlap, and Dr. Evans submitted his report of his trip to

[1] By George F. Edenharter, M. D., superintendent.

"numerous institutions," etc. This report contains the following paragraph:

> Again it is important that an institution which depends upon the benevolence and liberality of the Legislature for its erection and must continue to do so year after year for its support, should be so situated that these legislators may see the blessed fruits of their philanthropy; and, again, it should be so situated that they can exercise a guardian care over it—to guard against, detect and correct abuses, if any arise. Nor is this all; it is most necessary that they should be able to inspect and thoroughly understand its wants that, knowing, they may supply them. He also reports that the wants of our state will probably demand at present an insitution for from 100 to 150 patients.

At this meeting "it was agreed that a general survey of the county adjacent to the City of Indianapolis be made by the Board of Commissioners for the purpose of selecting the most advantageous site in its vicinity." On August 28, 1845, the commissioners had another meeting and "it was decided that the farm belonging to N. Bolton, lying two miles west of Indianapolis, on the macadamized National Road, possessed more advantages for a site for a hospital for the insane than any other that could be obtained; and it was unanimously agreed that the same be purchased at the rate of $53.12½ per acre."

The property (160 acres) passed to the State of Indiana on August 29, 1845.

On December 22, 1845, the Board of Commissioners drew up a full report for the Legislature of their plans and recommendations. On January 21, 1846, they met for the purpose of considering the new law passed by the Legislature entitled "An Act to Provide for the Erection of Suitable Buildings for the Use of the Indiana Hospital for the Insane," which act was approved January 19, 1846.

Section 1 provides "that the Commissioners of the Indiana Lunatic Asylum are hereby authorized to cause to be erected upon the grounds heretofore purchased for that purpose, suitable buildings for the use and accommodation of said institution, which shall hereafter be called and known by the name of the Indiana Hospital for the Insane, and also to make such improvements upon and about said grounds as they may think expedient and proper."

Section 9 provides that "the sum of $15,000 is hereby appropriated out of the fund set apart for the lunatic hospital for the purpose of defraying the expenses incurred under the provisions of this act."

At a meeting of the Board of Commissioners held January 24, 1846, "after free discussion of the propriety of different plans of prosecuting the work, it was decided that it should be done by letting contracts for furnishing materials and for the different kinds of work."

On February 11, 1846, the board awarded the contract for brick, paying an average of $3.31½ per 1000.

On May 5, 1846, the superintendent was authorized "to let by contract the excavation for the foundation of the hospital."

On June 4, 1846, the board authorized the signing of a contract with Z. R. Clark for the brickwork of the hospital. Contracts for lumber and other materials were awarded soon after.

Under date of October 31, 1848, the superintendent, in his report to the board, says that "the two wards of the south wing, now nearly in readiness for the reception of patients, have been plainly but neatly finished and will be furnished in a similar manner. Notice will in a few days be given to those applicants who by law have precedence to fill the apartments prepared to the extent of their capacity."

According to the hospital record the first five patients were admitted on November 21, 1848.

To quote again from the paper of Dr. Rogers: "In 1855 the hospital had a capacity of 225 inmates, in 1857 of 300. In April of this year, the Legislature having failed to provide means for maintenance, all the inmates (303) were sent back to their counties; some went into the poorhouses, some into jails, and the remainder to their homes. Of the latter many were kept in isolated cabins hastily erected for the purpose. Twenty were subsequently returned to the hospital and cared for at the expense of their counties. In October the state officers agreed to make legal provision of funds, and the hospital was reopened. In 1863-4 a similar condition obtained, but no inmates were discharged and the general fund provided means without legislative enactment."

On Tuesday, May 15, 1866, the Board of Commissioners advertised for proposals to erect the north wing at the department for men.

The official records of the hospital from November, 1870, to March, 1879, cannot be found. In the absence of this record it is impossible to furnish preliminary details concerning the construction of the department for women. Therefore, suffice it to say that "An Act Increasing the Capacity of the Indiana Hospital for the Insane by Additional Buildings, Creating Different Departments and Declaring an Emergency" was passed by the Legislature in 1875. The plans of the department for women were presumably in accordance with the views of the then superintendent, Dr. Orpheus Everts, if not actually drawn under his supervision. On June 2, 1884, the Board of Commissioners ordered the following spread upon the record:

> WHEREAS, The building contemplated and authorized by the act of March 11, 1875, having been finished and being now ready for occupancy, it is ordered by this board that said buildings be now placed in charge and control of the trustees for the Indiana Hospital for the Insane, and this board, pursuant to the terms of said act, is now dissolved and ceases to be.

Since this time the state has added a number of new buildings, viz.: The store building, 1885; boiler house and plant, 1886; power house and electric plant, 1892; carpenter shop, 1894; fire department, 1894; laundry, 1894-5; engineers' mechanical department, 1894; pathological department, 1895; kitchen women's building, 1897; bakery, 1897; congregate dining room (W.), 1899; congregate dining room (N.), 1899; congregate dining room (S.), 1899; greenhouse, 1899; hospital for "sick insane," 1901; cold storage plant, 1901; upholstering department, 1911; amusement hall and chapel, 1912, and other minor buildings.

The patients in the institution are cared for in the two main buildings, viz.: the department for men and the department for women. The men's department is built on what is known as the straight block system, and the women's department is constructed on the Kirkbride plan.

All of the mechanical departments are in separate buildings, and the buildings are heated from a central plant in accordance with legislative enactment.

The original building for the Hospital for the Insane, with its additions, is at present used for the department for men.

The entire group of buildings is four stories high. The outside and principal inside walls are of brick. The general construction of all these buildings is the common wooden joist construction; the same may be said of the kitchen and accessory departments in the rear of the main building. This building contains over 600 rooms and the area of floor space is 206,341 square feet.

The department for women consists of one center building containing the general offices, the quarters for the superintendent and other officers, and of side wings, three on the north and three on the south side of the center or administration building. All of these buildings are four stories high, over a full basement used for the distribution of steam heat. To the west of the center building and in direct communication therewith is the general kitchen, the rooms for the employees and the chapel.

The entire building is constructed on a stone foundation; all exterior and interior walls are of brick; all stairways are fireproof. Its length is 1046 feet; its circumference is 4240 feet. Its cost was about $800,000. As before stated, its construction was authorized in 1875.

In the superintendent's (Dr. Edenharter) report for the fiscal year ending October 31, 1894, the following announcement was made:

> It affords us much pleasure to announce that plans have been matured and perfected whereby we will be enabled to completely reconstruct and reorganize our pathological department. It will be placed on such footing as to meet the requirements of the most exacting pathological investigation. Its accessories will be of such character as will satisfy any demand for necessary laboratory work.

It should not be inferred from the name that the work therein is purely of a pathological character, because, in addition thereto, all methods of clinical investigation—psychical, physiological, chemical, bacteriological, etc.—are employed.

This department had its inception in a desire to establish the work of this hospital upon a scientific basis—to provide the medical staff with facilities for the accurate determination of the character of the diseases met with in institutional life.

It was also the ambition to create a scientific department—a medical center—for the use of the physicians and medical students of the state, wherein the diseases of the mind and nervous system could be clinically studied and, if possible, to determine their cause and formulate methods for their prevention and cure.

Students who interest themselves in this specialty are urged to visit this department, where every effort is made to assist them in obtaining a knowledge of the laboratory and clinical methods in vogue. When requested, the pathologist properly directs their efforts in research in any desired direction. All facilities for clinical study are extended to the physicians and medical students of the state.

This pathological building was erected in 1895 and the equipment completed in 1896. It was dedicated on December 18, 1896, by the Marion County Medical Society; Professor Ludvig Hektoen, M. D., of Chicago, delivered the dedicatory address.

It is two stories high, constructed over stone foundation, and built of brick and stone. It contains 19 working rooms, with toilet rooms, etc. The first floor contains the following rooms: General reception, reception for relatives, viewing, mortuary, dissecting, furnace, supply, chemical laboratory, anatomical and pathological museum and lecture room. The latter has a seating capacity of 160 persons.

The second floor has the following rooms: Pathologists' study (private), records, photography and accessory, models, charts, diagrams, etc., library and conference, microscopical laboratory, bacteriological laboratory, pathologists' research (private).

In the superintendent's (Dr. Edenharter) report for the fiscal year ending October 31, 1895, the following language was used:

> A hospital entirely separate from the main buildings is necessary. We not only need the room now occupied as "sick wards," but from every view it is the duty of the state to care for the sick in a separate building; she owes it not only to those afflicted but to those who have no intercurrent disease.

The General Assembly of 1899 appropriated $110,000 for the erection of a hospital building—capacity, 100 patients.

This hospital consists of five distinct buildings, all of which are connected by corridors. The administration building forms the central feature and is directly connected with the department for men and the department for women; it contains the reception room for visitors, the various offices, supply rooms and lavatories on the first floor, and the sleeping rooms for the clinical assistants on the second floor.

The department for men and the department for women, to the right and left of the administration building, contain the surgical wards on the first floor and the medical wards on the second floor. Each ward consists of a day sitting room, adjacent to the large dormitory, and of 10 separate bed-rooms, also of a nurses' day

24

room, clothing room, linen and supply rooms, lavatory and bathrooms for patients, and lavatory and bathrooms for the attendants. All bathrooms and lavatories throughout are in separate buildings, independent of the wards.

The operating department is on the first floor, in direct communication with the men's and women's surgical ward. It consists of an operating room, rooms for general diagnosis, anæsthetizing, instruments, etc.

The rooms for sterilizing, for drugs, supplies, bandages, etc., are near at hand. The building is also provided with bathrooms and lavatories for the operator and for the nurses or attendants.

Directly connected with the department for men and the department for women, in the rear of the entire group of buildings, are the general dining rooms, storage rooms, sculleries, dishrooms, linen rooms and the kitchen. This connection is by means of corridors amply provided with cross ventilation. Under this arrangement the odors from this department cannot permeate the wards. On the second floor of this building are the sleeping rooms for the attendants. A basement of eight feet in the clear extends under the entire group of buildings. The construction in all of its details and the selection of the materials throughout were well considered. All outer and inner walls rest upon a concrete foundation. The outer foundation walls are of hard limestone; all inside partition walls are of brick.

The superstructure, from the top of the base course to the roof line, is of selected brick, trimmed with oolitic stone. All outer walls are of hollow construction, ventilated from basement to roof. All bathrooms and lavatories are lined with enameled brick. The entire building is wired for electric incandescent light, with iron-armored conduits. The plumbing and ventilating system throughout is based on modern sanitary methods. As no other method than that of impelling air by direct means with fans is equally independent of accidental natural conditions and equally efficient for the desired result, this method of heating was adopted. The ventilation is accomplished by means of flues for each room connected with the ventilating turrets in the attic. The building faces southwest, and every room, therefore, has the advantage of sunshine and air.

The airing roofs provided are of ample size to permit the taking of all patients out in the open air whenever deemed desirable.

The feature of this building arrangement is that none of the wards wherein patients are detained have any sewer connections; as before stated, all bathrooms and lavatories are absolutely separated from the wards, neither do the sewer lines pass under any of them. The equipment of this building cost $15,000.

The general store is located between the departments for men and women, and is used for general store purposes, the trustees' office, and the second floor for sleeping rooms. It is built of brick.

The power house and engineer's department are located at the rear of the general store. The electrical machinery is in the building and consists of three engines and six dynamos, with all necessary accessories. Also two G. E. turbines of 125 kw. each. Connected with, but yet separate, are the engineer's building and machine shop. Here the general stock for this department is kept, as well as the machines used in this work, viz., lathes, drill, forge, pipe-cutter, etc. Adjoining the power house is the boiler house, which contains the apparatus necessary for the operation and heating of the institution. This equipment has been remodeled in its entirety, and consists of eight (250 h. p.) Stirling boilers, eight Roney stokers (improved), four boiler feed pumps (Stilwell), one feed water heater (Webster), and other accessories. A coal crushing and carrying apparatus has also been installed. The engineer's repair shop is a separate building, located in the rear of the boiler house.

The laundry, erected in 1894-5, is a well constructed one-story brick and steel frame building, perfectly lighted and ventilated by side lights, skylights and openings. The equipment of this building consists of 12 brass washing machines, 3 sterilizing machines, 1 electrolyzer, 1 galvanized iron sterilizer, 4 centrifugal extractors, 1 1-100-inch mangle, 5 ironing machines, 1 starcher and kettle, 1 all-metal drying room, 1 dampening room, 2 soap kettles, 1 tumbler, 1 water heater, 24 ironing tables, provided with electric irons, and many other accessories which are necessary to make up a laundry equipment capable of handling the clothing of 2300 persons. The General Assembly of 1903 made an appropriation for an addition to this building for drying-room purposes; it is of the same construction as the main building.

The storage plant is a partly one and two-story brick building, with stone foundation and slate roof. It is divided into two parts, one for meats, which contains two rooms, and the other for produce and vegetables—this part has three rooms. In addition there are the machine room and meat-cutting room. It has a refrigerating capacity of 16 tons.

The bakery is a one-story brick structure, with slate roof and stone foundation; its four rooms are used in mixing, bake ovens, storage and miscellaneous purposes.

The two new dining rooms for the department for men, each with a seating capacity for 400 persons, are well constructed buildings, located at the north and south of the general kitchen and in close proximity to the main building. These buildings, in addition to the dining room, have sculleries, food departments, lavatories, etc. They are constructed on stone foundations, heavy brick walls with stone trimmings, encaustic tile floor, enameled and pressed brick wall linings, steel ceilings, skylights, and slate roofs. The dining room at the department for women has a seating capacity of 600 persons; it is similar in construction and arrangement to the dining room at the men's building.

The carpenter shop is a frame structure, in good condition. Here lumber, hardware and a great many other materials are stored; it has an equipment of machinery as follows: 1 planing machine, 1 friezing machine, 1 mortising machine, 1 sticking machine, 1 band saw filing machine, 1 swing cut-off saw, 1 band saw, 1 turning lathe, 1 joining saw and table, 1 rip saw, 1 teneting machine, 1 emery grinding machine, 1 mitering machine, 2 drilling machines, and other implements which make the outfit complete.

The greenhouse is constructed of steel frame and wood and consists of five separate departments.

The General Kitchens.—One of these is located at each department. The equipment in each is practically the same, viz., complete outfit of ranges, ovens, stock boilers, meat roasters, steamers, coffee, tea and hot water urns, warming ovens, refrigerators, and many other articles.

The fire department is a two-story frame structure, in good condition. It has on the first floor a large room, which contains the fire fighting apparatus, consisting of two hose wagons, each carrying 700 feet of hose, a hook and ladder truck with complete equipment, and a number of chemical fire extinguishers. A portion of this floor is used for club, bed and toilet rooms. The second floor is taken up entirely with bedrooms. All outside employees sleep in this building.

The upholstering department is a one-story brick building located west of the men's building. Here new mattresses are made and old ones sterilized, renovated and repaired, furniture upholstered and chairs caned.

The chapel and amusement hall, now under course of construction, embodies three distinct features: first, an auditorium of ample proportions in which to conduct chapel exercises and which is provided with all facilities for staging large entertainments; second, social quarters for the patients; third, social quarters for the employees.

1. The auditorium, a room 98 feet long and 70 feet wide, is designed to accommodate 1000 people. The roof is supported by iron trusses. A large stage, equipped for modern demands, is augmented by dressing and toilet rooms. A gallery extends along the rear of the auditorium and special provisions have been made to meet the demands of a moving picture apparatus. The auditorium is provided with ample emergency exits.

2. The basement of the structure is devoted entirely to the social quarters of the patients and includes recreation rooms, reading rooms and billiard rooms and bowling alleys. Access to these quarters is from the lawn grade and entirely separated from the doors to the auditorium proper.

3. The third distinct feature of the scheme is the social quarters for the employees. These quarters have been designed with a view of complete isolation, although an integral part of the structure. The sexes have individual quarters and include social rooms, the largest of which is 70 feet long and 22 feet wide.

The building is of the steel skeleton type of construction with a steel frame roof covered with slate. The foundation is concrete. It is of Gothic design; of red brick trimmed with stone. The total area of all quarters including the auditorium amounts to 12,500 square feet. The total cost of the structure, including heating, lighting, plumbing and seats, will be $50,000.

The name, square feet of floor space and the cubic feet of interior of all buildings and their estimated present value are given in the following tabulation:

Name of building	Floor area sq. ft.	Interior cu. ft.	Estimated value
Department for Men	206,341	2,269,751	285,000
Department for Women	337,234	3,865,344	850,000
New Hospital	84,834	983,148	110,000
Pathological Department	4,000	98,100	12,000
Chapel and Amusement Hall	12,500	513,000	50,000
General Store	8,352	49,920	5,000
Power House	3,308	75,384	25,000
Laundry	14,940	269,000	20,000
Cold Storage Plant	3,447	42,000	8,500
Bakery	2,016	24,000	3,500
Men's Dining Room (N.)	7,126	121,142	15,000
Men's Dining Room (S.)	7,126	121,142	15,000
Women's Dining Room	10,584	247,234	20,000
Carpenter Shop	8,204	90,256	5,000
Fire Department	5,540	55,400	3,500
Upholstering Department	3,000	30,000	3,500
Engineer's Department (store)	1,824	18,240	*
Boiler House	8,835	176,700	*
Repair Shop	960	9,600	500
Paint Shop	720	7,200	500
Oil House	192	1,920	200
Junk Shop	1,152	11,520	200
Officers' Barn	3,222	26,664	1,500
Farm Barn	2,100	32,400	1,000
Ice House	540	5,400	100
Pavilion for Men	1,824	18,240	1,000
Gate Lodge	399	2,400	300
Old Morgue	480	4,800	500
Pump House	330	3,500	330
Gas House	180	1,800	150
Greenhouse	5,000	60,000	8,000
Furnace	144	1,152	300
Total	746,454	9,236357	1,445,580

This table shows the total floor space of the institution to be 746,454 square feet—equal to 18 acres; and the interior or space to be heated 9,236,357 cubic feet.

IMPROVEMENTS (NOT OTHERWISE ENUMERATED).

Sewage System	$20,000.00
Water System	10,000.00
Gas System	2,000.00
Cement Walks	14,000.00
Tunnel	8,000.00
Total	$54,000.00

* Included in value of Power House.

GROUNDS.

One hundred and sixty acres of land, estimated value	$160,000.00

RE-TABULATION.

Value of Buildings	$1,445,580.00
Value of Improvements	54,000.00
Value of Grounds	160,000.00
Total	$1,659,580.00

INVENTORY BY DEPARTMENTS.

(September 30, 1911).

Housekeeping Department for Women	$7,505.00
Housekeeping Department for Men	4,692.35
Housekeeping Department Store House	1,651.00
Ward Property Department for Men	25,474.50
Ward Property Department for Women	26,799.58
Dining Department	2,466.80
General Kitchen Department for Men	3,909.29
General Kitchen Department for Women	6,667.86
General Store	8,107.31
Butcher Shop	1,767.59
Bakery	1,200.17
Clothing Department	9,113.89
Laundry	12,270.30
Engineer's Department	170,155.09
Electric Department and Telephones	51,847.93
Carpenter's Department	11,050.20
Painter's Department	878.00
Plasterer's Department	15.75
Fire Department	10,499.00
Police Department	50.00
Tin Shop	1,278.20
Upholsterer's Department	790.06
Barber Shop	284.75
Garden, Farm and Barn	2,024.60
Officers' Barn	2,473.00
Florist's Department	8,471.78
Library (General)	1,727.00
Chapel, Porter's Department	408.50
Drug Department	1,857.75
Surgical Instruments for General Use	186.55
Pathological Department and Scientific Library	9,437.25
Hospital for Sick Insane	10,531.06
Total invoice of above departments	$395,592.81

Re-tabulation.

Value of real estate, buildings and improvements	$1,659,580.00
Value of personal property	395,592.81
Total estimated value of all property	$2,055,172.81

Movement of Population from the Opening of the Institution October, 1848.

Year.	Admitted.		Discharged. Recovered.		Discharged. Improved.		Discharged. Unimproved.		Discharged. Not Insane.		Discharged. Idiotic.		Died.		Enrolled Close of Year.	
	M.	F.	M.	F.	M.	F.	M.	F.	M.	F.	M.	F.	M.	F.	M.	F.
Up to Oct. 31 1883..	6,814	5,361	2,960	2,555	541	783	1,112	890	....	....	....	....	786	622	618	496
1884..	481	585	190	139	51	37	41	44	....	....	....	....	81	31	643	750
1885..	453	321	234	147	26	71	78	12	7	7	....	....	70	57	677	777
1886..	416	371	163	148	48	49	117	14	6	4	....	....	62	41	697	892
1887..	391	386	208	137	65	106	108	54	6	4	....	....	51	33	649	864
1888..	353	325	141	170	67	45	82	35	4	3	....	5	55	60	655	871
1889..	337	237	151	91	37	70	70	28	8	3	....	....	42	43	684	873
1890..	380	284	77	63	110	108	130	80	....	....	....	....	35	35	712	871
1891..	302	259	33	89	61	40	116	153	1	....	....	....	55	55	748	793
1892..	200	199	47	80	82	45	55	28	....	....	....	....	50	50	714	789
1893..	198	202	107	67	83	47	23	4	....	....	....	....	51	54	693	819
1894..	246	206	74	81	76	39	25	31	....	....	....	....	70	70	694	804
1895..	269	210	59	71	73	39	45	11	....	3	....	1	81	51	705	838
1896..	251	232	80	70	68	51	19	16	....	2	....	....	78	56	711	875
1897..	290	232	79	102	82	38	58	5	1	2	....	....	71	57	710	903
1898..	304	264	74	95	55	55	73	10	....	1	....	....	73	65	739	941
1899..	342	282	103	68	38	33	105	12	....	....	....	....	79	82	756	1,028
1900..	385	265	97	96	78	77	37	9	1	....	....	....	84	59	764	1,052
1901..	313	269	99	81	73	74	34	13	1	....	....	....	98	80	772	1,073
1902..	388	228	113	77	89	53	19	15	....	....	....	....	89	52	800	1,104
1903..	349	240	102	85	87	72	17	15	....	....	....	....	84	85	859	1,087
1904..	387	250	119	52	98	71	39	24	1	....	....	....	125	72	864	1,118
1905..	322	231	74	49	80	55	10	3	....	....	....	....	110	84	912	1,158
1906..	262	179	99	113	72	50	25	13	1	....	....	....	100	62	877	1,099
Sept. 30 1907..	222	160	61	52	53	26	13	1	....	....	....	....	63	54	909	1,126
1908..	212	185	56	83	68	44	8	13	....	....	....	....	99	52	890	1,119
1909..	190	162	44	54	74	36	8	6	....	....	....	....	73	71	881	1,114
1910..	220	177	54	51	152	113	126	203	....	....	....	....	102	62	667	862
Total	14,267	12,142	5,698	4,966	2,442	2,327	2,593	1,742	37	29	....	6	3,817	2,195		

Regular Appropriation for Each Fiscal Year 1911-12 and 1912-13.

(Act approved March 4, 1911.)

Maintenance	$325,000.00
Repair	25,000.00
Clothing	15,000.00
Total	$365,000.00

Specific Appropriations for the Fiscal Years 1911-12 and 1912-13.

(Act approved March 4, 1911.)

Chapel and Amusement Hall	$50,000.00
Stairways	25,000.00
Fire Protection	5,000.00
Painting	5,000.00
Total	$85,000.00

SUPERINTENDENTS.

John Evans, M. D.	1847 (3d report).
Richard J. Patterson, M. D.	July, 1848, to June 1, 1853.
James S. Athon, M. D.	June 1, 1853, to Oct. 31, 1861.
James H. Woodburn, M. D.	Nov. 1, 1861, to 1865.
Wilson Lockhart, M. D.	1865 to 1869.
Orpheus Everts, M. D.	1869 to June 7, 1879.
Joseph G. Rogers, M. D.	June 7, 1879, to 1883.
William B. Fletcher, M. D.	1883 to Sept. 8, 1887.
Thomas S. Galbraith, M. D.	Sept. 8, 1887, to June 6, 1889.
Charles E. Wright, M. D.	June 6, 1889, to Feby. 22, 1893.
P. J. Watters, M. D. (acting)	March 4, 1893, to May 1, 1893.
George F. Edenharter, M. D.	May 1, 1893.

COMMISSIONERS.

January 13, 1845, John Evans, Livingston Dunlap and James Blake were constituted a Board of Commissioners to select a suitable site for the erection of a State Lunatic Asylum.

TRUSTEES.

John Evans	Jany. 13, 1845.
Livingston Dunlap	Jany. 13, 1845, to 1851.
James Blake	Jany. 13, 1845, to 1853.
John S. Bobbs	1847 to 1849.
Edwin J. Peck	1847 to 1860.
Stephen Major	1847 to 1852.
J. Evans	1848.
John Wilkins	1849.
James Ritchey	1850 to 1858.
William H. Goode	1850.
Henry Brady	1851 to 1860.
Samuel Grimes	1852 to 1858.

William H. Talbott .... 1853 to 1860.
H. F. West .... 1854 to 1856.
C. C. Campbell .... 1857 to 1858.
Andrew Wallace .... 1861 to 1867 (see report 1868).
P. H. Jameson .... 1861 to March 14, 1879.
J. W. Moody .... 1861 to 1866.
L. Humphreys .... 1867 to 1871 (see report 1870).
J. H. Woodburn .... 1869 to 1872 (see report 1868).
J. M. Caldwell .... 1871 to 1874 (see report 1870).
George F. Chittenden .... 1873 to March 14, 1879.
John F. Richardson .... 1875 to March 14, 1879.
John Fishback .... 1879 to 1883.
B. F. Spann .... 1879 to 1883.
R. H. Tarlton .... 1879 to 1884.
Thomas H. Harrison .... 1883 to April, 1889
P. M. Gapen .... 1883 to April, 1889.
B. H. Burrell .... 1885 to April, 1889.
J. L. Carson .... April, 1889, to 1897.
Z. H. Houser .... April, 1889, to 1895.
Thomas Markey .... April, 1889, to 1893.
John Osterman .... 1893 to 1902.
D. H. Davis .... 1895 to 1901.
Albert O. Lockridge .... 1897 to 1903.
R. L. Kennedy .... 1901 to 1904.
Eli Marvin .... 1902 to 1909.
Albert M. Adams .... 1903 to 1905.
Fremont Goodwin .... 1904 to 1905.
D. H. Davis .... 1905.
George B. Lockwood .... 1905 to 1907.
Adam Heimberger .... 1907.
Thomas Clifton .... 1907 to 1910.
Walter S. Chambers .... 1909.
Hugh Th. Miller .... 1910.

The following is the list of assistant physicians who have been in the service of this institution:

J. Nutt, M. D. .... Oct., 1848, to Oct., 1851.
Thomas B. Elliott, M. D. .... Oct., 1851, to 1856.
Thomas P. McCullough, M. D. .... 1853 to 1854.
George A. Torbett, M. D. .... 1854 to May, 1858.
N. C. Spann, M. D. .... 1856 (4 months).
Henry F. Barnes, M. D. .... Nov., 1857, to Oct., 1861.
John M. Dunlap, M. D. .... May, 1858, to 1863.
J. F. Cravens, M. D. .... Nov., 1861, to May, 1867.
Robert Charlton, M. D. .... 1864, unknown.
W. W. Hester, M. D. .... 1866 to Feb., 1879.

J. J. Wright, M. D. .... May, 1867, to 1869.
W. J. Elstun, M. D. .... Oct., 1879.
Charles L. Armington, M. D. .... Jany., 1871, to Oct., 1873.
John C. Walker, M. D. .... Feby., 1879, to 1883.
A. J. Thomas, M. D. .... Aug., 1879, to June, 1890.
W. H. Hubbard, M. D. .... Aug., 1879, to 1883.
J. N. Smith, M. D. .... Aug., 1879, to 1884.
John R. Brown, M. D. .... Sept., 1882, to 1887.
T. Davenport, M. D. .... 1884.
W. E. Brant, M. D. .... 1884.
Sarah Stockton, M. D. .... Dec., 1883, to 1889.
Wm. J. Browning, M. D. .... 1884; 1885 to 1887; and June, 1889, to 1890.
C. B. McClure, M. D. .... 1884 to 1886.
Christian H. Wiles, M. D. .... 1886 to June, 1889.
Edward F. Hodges, M. D., pathologist .... 1885 to 1887.
Frank M. Howard, M. D. .... 1887 to 1888.
E. C. Reyer, M. D. .... 1886 to 1888.
Wm. J. Burkhizer, M. D. .... Nov., 1888, to June, 1889.
P. J. Watters, M. D. .... Jany., 1889, to date.
A. M. Adams, M. D. .... April, 1889, to 1891.
John C. Curtis, M. D. .... June, 1889, to Nov., 1892.
F. M. Wiles, M. D. .... March, 1890, to June, 1913.
J. D. Simpson, M. D. .... 1890 to 1891.
F. A. Morrison, M. D., pathologist .... 1890 to 1896.
W. H. Rainey, M. D. .... Feby., 1891, to Feby., 1898.
Mary Smith, M. D. .... 1891 to May, 1898.
F. E. Ray, M. D., interne .... 1891.
F. E. Ray, M. D., asst. phys. .... 1892 to 1897.
Charles F. Applegate, M. D., interne ...... June, 1893, to Feby., 1895.
Edmund Ludlow, M. D. .... Sept., 1897, to Jany., 1901.
Robert Hessler, M. D., pathologist .... Sept., 1897, to Oct., 1898.
Fred L. Pettijohn, M. D., interne .... Jany., 1897.
Fred L. Pettijohn, M. D. .... Feby., 1898, to June, 1901.
Max A. Bahr, M. D., interne .... April, 1898; asst. phys., Jan., 1900; clinic psychiater, 1910 to date.
Sarah Stockton, M. D. .... Nov., 1898, to date.
Daniel Healey, M. D., pathologist .... July, 1899, to March, 1900.
John B. Briggs, M. D. .... July, 1900, to Sept., 1900.
Wm. Charles White, M. D., pathologist .. Dec., 1900, to Dec., 1901.
R. N. Todd, M. D., interne .... 1901; asst. phys., 1902-Oct., 1905.
A. R. Lemke, M. D., pathologist .... Jany., 1903, to Sept., 1903; asst. phys., 1904.
Elmer E. Mace, interne .... June., 1903, to Oct., 1903.
John A. McDonald, M. D. .... Oct., 1903, to June, 1907.
Charles F. Neu, M. D., pathologist .... Oct., 1903, to Oct., 1906.

Jos. J. Hoffman, M. D., interne .... June, 1905; asst. phys., 1906 to Sept., 1910.
Ernest D. Martin, M. D., asst. pathologist . Oct., 1906, to date.
Charles C. Manger, M. D., pathologist .... July, 1907, to July, 1908.
L. W. Tindolph, M. D., interne .... Aug., 1907, to Nov., 1907.
Paul M. St. Clair, M. D. .... Feby., 1908, to Feby., 1910.
Charles F. King, M. D. .... July, 1908, to April, 1909.
James A. Jackson, M. D., pathologist ..... Aug., 1908, to July, 1910.
C. Stanley Aitken, M. D. .... May, 1909, to Oct., 1910.
Ord Evermann, M. D. .... April, 1910, to date.
Sidney C. Niles, M. D. .... Oct., 1910, to Feby., 1911.
Edward J. Kempf, M. D. .... April, 1911, to Sept., 1912.
Patrick H. Weeks, M. D. .... Nov., 1912, to date.
James S. Rushton, M. D. .... May, 1913, to date.
J. E. Heatley, M. D. .... Nov., 1913, to March, 1914.

THE WORK OF THE BOARD OF COMMISSIONERS OF THE ADDITIONAL HOSPITALS FOR THE INSANE.[1]

The history of the following hospitals necessarily includes the history of the work of the Board of Commissioners of the Additional Hospitals for the Insane, who planned and built three hospitals, during the period 1883 to 1890.

From 1848 to 1888 one state hospital furnished the only accommodation for the treatment and care of Indiana's insane. This hospital, located at the capital, was known as the Indiana Hospital for the Insane, and was re-christened in 1889 the Central Indiana Hospital for the Insane. This one hospital proved inadequate, notwithstanding important additions made to meet the demands upon it. The insane were rapidly increasing in proportion at least to a growing general population. Indiana's rich agricultural land was filling up with a movement of immigration from other states. The number of insane kept step with this new population, and as a result of the insufficient accommodations in the one state hospital, the county poorhouses were filled to overflowing with this unfortunate class under conditions which add nothing to Indiana's fair name. Scant provision for even decent care was made by the political authorities. In the seventies partisan spirit ran high and the slogan which rang in everybody's ear was "to the victor belong the spoils." This principle touched every public office, not omitting the public treasury, down to the caretakers in county poorhouses and jails. This period of political high-handedness proved to be the state's period of preparation. Its very inhumanity brought humanity.

In 1880 it became apparent that one hospital, however largely it might develop, could not receive all the state's insane, and a demand for another hospital began to arise. It was quickened by directing public attention to the conditions of care, or rather neglect, of the insane by the counties, and in 1883 the movement crystalized into a legislative act authorizing the construction of another hospital and providing the necessary funds therefor. The manner in which this proposition was dealt with by the Legislature of that year was vexatious then and seemingly hopeless, but in a retrospect of 30 years it is amusing to think that out of it has come

[1] **By Samuel E. Smith, M. S., M. D., medical superintendent.**

good. The political situation was a "house divided against itself," but it did not fall. The Governor, the President of the Senate and certain state officers belonged to one party, the other state officers, the Speaker of the House and a majority of both branches of the Legislature belonged to another party. It was early apparent that both the Legislature and the Governor favored the new hospital, but the former could not see its way clear to give out of hand such a luscious plum to the latter. Moreover, a clamor arose from many sections of the state for the location of the coveted institution, resulting in a fatal combination of legislative votes against any promising site within any favored section, and so effective was this combination that the supporters of the measure were quickly convinced of the futility of the effort to secure another hospital. At this juncture a brilliant idea flashed from the fertile brain of some one, unknown, whose memory is deserving of credit for a good deed of humanity. The brilliant idea included two hospitals instead of one. This meant the union of two sections of the state against the field and gave much encouragement to the cause. When the legislative noses were counted, however, the combination against the favored sections was in the majority and therefore again fatal to it. The same fertile brain was again equal to the occasion and brought forth a suggestion of creating three hospitals instead of one or two. Thus the combination was broken, but not until a section in the southwestern corner of the state, of which the City of Evansville was the ruling center of activity and which held the key to the combination against the movement and was particularly and openly inimical to Indianapolis, dictated the generous conditions which were finally accepted, that "none of such hospitals shall be erected within 50 miles of the City of Indianapolis" and "that one of said hospitals shall be located at or near the City of Evansville."

The bill as then agreed upon passed both houses of the Legislature, but Governor Albert G. Porter declined either to sign or to veto it, and it became a law March 7, 1883, through lapse of time without the Governor's action. It provided for the location and erection of three additional hospitals for the insane and also provided for their management. Thus the effort to secure authorization and funds for one new hospital brought about the unprecedented result of the establishment of three additional hospitals, by taking advantage of the loyalty to local interests of the several members of the Legislature.

This organic act embodied some interesting features and a summary of it is given in Appendix A.

It is worthy of note that this Legislature of 1883, which took such a long stride forward in the care of the insane population by creating three new hospitals in one and the same act, to be erected by a bi-partisan board appointed by the Governor, stepped backward in another instance by enacting during the same session a perniciously partisan law for the government of the three state institutions located in and near the capital—the hospital for the insane, the asylum for the blind and the institution for the education of the deaf and dumb. This measure provided for a board of two trustees for each institution and one common president for the three boards, and all to be elected by the Legislature. Naturally, as was expected and intended, all the members came from the same political party and the inevitable happened. Out of the mismanagement of this organization, the most scandalous in the history of the state's public institutions, came the first step of the reformation which has progressed steadily from that day to this.

Pursuant to the provisions of the organic act Governor Albert G. Porter on March 21, 1883, appointed members of the Board of Commissioners of the Additional Hospitals and on April 11 it organized.

In July, 1883, the board engaged the services of Dr. Joseph G. Rogers as medical engineer. Dr. Rogers had served as superintendent of the Indiana Hospital for the Insane and was the best equipped man in the state for this special line of work. He devoted the remainder of his life to the care of the insane and did a noble work. He was president of the American Medico-Psychological Association in 1900.

In August, 1883, E. H. Ketcham, of Indianapolis, was appointed architect.

The board proceeded to select and purchase the necessary sites for the three hospitals. The law limited the purchase to 160 acres each, but permitted, unwisely, the acceptance of donations of land and money. The board was hampered somewhat in its selections by the spirited contests of the several sections of the state seeking two of the proposed hospitals, the third having been assigned at

Evansville by the organic act. Strange to say, the latter proved the most difficult because of the limitations of a relatively small area in which to find a tract of land combining the essentials of a hospital site. However, the question of sites was worked out rather promptly—possibly too hastily.

On August 3, 1883, the site for the Eastern Indiana Hospital was selected and purchased two miles west of the City of Richmond. This tract consisted of 160 acres and the purchase price was $20,000. An adjacent tract, consisting of 146.8 acres, was donated by the citizens of Richmond. The acreage of this site was therefore 306.8 acres. The land was rather level but broken across the eastern end by a ravine with a small stream, and was located alongside of the Pennsylvania Railway. It was named "Easthaven" by Dr. Samuel E. Smith.

On October 4, 1883, the site for the Northern Indiana Hospital was selected and purchased on the south bank of the Wabash River one and one-half miles west of the City of Logansport. This tract also consisted of 160 acres, costing $14,500, to which 121 acres were added as a donation by the citizens of Cass County, making a total of 281 acres. This tract was broken by a long rocky ridge running through its center, which affords a picturesque site for the hospital, and, although it fronts north, it overlooks the beautiful valley of the Wabash and the hills beyond. It was happily named "Longcliff" by Dr. Rogers, and by this name it is now generally known.

On January 3, 1884, the site for the Southern Indiana Hospital was finally selected and secured. The tract consisted of 160 acres and cost $17,400. Since the organic law determined the location of this hospital in the vicinity of Evansville, there was no inducement for a donation of additional land by the citizens of that community and none was tendered. The tract was not extended by purchase of additional land for a period of 24 years. It was a highly improved farm, fertile, well-drained and undulating in character. A ridge overlooking the surrounding country afforded a pleasing building site. It was named "Woodmere" by Dr. C. E. Laughlin, medical superintendent.

The planning of the three additional hospitals was placed in the hands of Dr. Rogers, the medical engineer. He was given a fair degree of latitude, and the essential features of these institutions should be credited to his skill and scientific judgment. He went into the study of hospital construction most thoroughly and investigated minutely the plans of the leading institutions for the care of the insane in this country, Canada, England, Scotland and France. His study included the various systems of heating, ventilation, plumbing, sewage disposal and illumination. In the end three several plans were adopted and worked out and each hospital embodied a different type of construction.

1. The cottage plan for the Eastern Indiana Hospital at Easthaven, near Richmond.

2. A modified block or pavilion plan for the Northern Indiana Hospital at Longcliff, near Logansport.

3. A radiate plan, with house-plan features, for the Southern Indiana Hospital at Woodmere, near Evansville.

The parent institution, the Central Indiana Hospital at Indianapolis, was built on the corridor or Kirkbride plan, and the three additional hospitals embodied severally the features of the cottage, block and radiate plans. Indiana, therefore, as early as 1884 had utilized in its four hospitals the four plans of hospital construction most in favor in the advanced thought of that day.

These new hospitals were built of the building materials of the land, common brick, terra cotta and oolitic lime-stone trimmings, slate roofs, oak finish and hard maple floors. Slow burning construction was applied throughout, and after nearly 30 years one must admire the exposed and heavy solid oak beams, the oak ceilings three inches thick without joists and the fine solid oak doors throughout the buildings. All were equipped with the best plumbing of that day, chiefly porcelain-lined iron fixtures. The heating was chiefly indirect radiation, with gravity ventilation. Each was equipped with Edison electric light plants, which, being new and untried, called for no little courage by public servants in their adoption. The cost was high and for several years the results were uncertain.

The total cost of the three hospitals when ready for occupancy was $1,328,800. One embarrassment to the board deserves special mention. The organic act stipulated a bond from the contractor in an amount not less than double the amount of the bid with freehold resident surety. This extraordinary requirement excluded many bidders and limited competition. Only a very few contractors could give such a bond and these few took some advantage of the absence of competition, and made the cost of some of the contracts higher than was otherwise necessary.

The Northern Hospital, at Logansport, was first completed with 366 available beds and was opened by Dr. Rogers, assisted by Dr. Samuel E. Smith, for the admission of patients on July 1, 1888. When the three hospitals were nearing completion the urgent need for more accommodations for urgent cases made it necessary for the board to concentrate its energies for the early completion of one of them, and it was then that the board tendered to Dr. Rogers the position of resident medical superintendent of the hospital of his choice. On account of conditions of climate he chose the Northern Hospital, at Logansport, and for this reason it was hurried forward and was first made ready for service. In point of construction this was not his choice, but his health, he then felt, called for the lower temperature of the northern part of the state. Dr. Rogers continued in charge of this hospital until his death, April 11, 1908.

A shortage of funds had delayed construction in all three hospitals for nearly two years, when in 1888 a fire destroyed the structures of the Indiana School for Feeble-minded Youth, at Knightstown. The Eastern Hospital, at Easthaven, near Richmond, was then rapidly put in condition for temporary quarters for this school, which occupied it for the two years pending a re-location and construction of its new buildings near Ft. Wayne. When vacated it was turned over to a new organization with a capacity of 390 beds, and opened for the admission of patients August 1, 1890, with Dr. E. F. Wells, medical superintendent, and a Board of Trustees consisting of George W. Koontz, John S. Martin and Milton C. Benham.

The Southern Hospital at Woodmere, near Evansville, was also seriously delayed for want of sufficient appropriation of funds and was closed two years, 1886 to 1888, but was finally opened for the admission of patients October 31, 1890.

SOUTHERN INDIANA HOSPITAL FOR THE INSANE.

EVANSVILLE, IND.

This institution was located and erected at Evansville, Ind., under provision of an act of the General Assembly in force March 1, 1883. The act provided for the appointment by the Governor of two commissioners from each of the two leading political parties, who, together with the Governor, should constitute a Board of Commissioners.

In accordance with this act Governor Albert G. Porter on March 21, 1883, appointed the following Commissioners: John C. Robinson, James R. Gray, William Grose and DeForrest Skinner. These commissioners appointed Dr. Joseph G. Rogers as medical engineer.

On the 3d day of January, 1884, this board bought of William Howard 160 acres of land situated on Newburgh Road, four miles east of the City of Evansville, in Vanderburgh County, Ind., and paid for it the sum of $17,400 as a site for the Southern Indiana Hospital for the Insane.

Plans and specifications for the buildings were adopted in February, 1884, and, pursuant to advertisement for bids thereon, the work of general construction was let to P. H. McCormack, of Columbus, Ind., for the sum of $286,585.20; subsequent changes in the work brought the amount paid to the contractor up to the sum of $300,896.47.

The Board of Commissioners conveyed the hospital to a Board of Trustees in April, 1890, but the institution was not completed and ready for the reception of patients until November 1, 1890.

The main buildings were erected near the center of the hospital domain, which consisted of 160 acres.

The original structure was built on the congregate-radiate plan and consisted of a central block, 66 x 112 feet, with two wings radiating at an angle of 30 degrees from each side; one wing extending north, affording quarters for employees, with an administration building on the south front. These buildings are three stories in height. An additional wing has been made to both the department for men and women. These additional structures are connected to the original buildings by colonnades, which are roofed and screened.

In the original plan each ward was provided with a dining room, but this plan was found in practice extravagant and unsatisfactory, and was remedied in 1908 by providing congregate dining rooms located between the north rear and middle wing in either department.

Detached buildings provided quarters for the power house, laundry, barn, stable and coachman's house.

The buildings erected since the opening of the institution are:

Carpenter shop	Constructed in	1890
Store room	" "	1891
Ward building for men	" "	1895
Well house	" "	1895
Railway station	" "	1895
Green house	" "	1895
Sewage station	" "	1898
Ward building for women	" "	1899
Assembly hall	" "	1899
Refrigerating plant and cold storage	" "	1901
Laundry	" "	1904
Bakery	" "	1905
Warehouse and fire department	" "	1905
Water tower and tank	" "	1905
Water softener	" "	1905
Heating system—remodeled	" "	1905
Septic plant	" "	1907
Power plant	" "	1907
Congregate dining rooms	" "	1908
Sanitary piggery	" "	1908
Dairy barn and two silos	" "	1911
Stock barn	" "	1911
Hospital for the sick	" "	1911
Hydrotherapeutic additions	" "	1912

The hospital district originally consisted of 16 counties in the southwest section of the state, from which recently one county has been deducted and the insane from these 15 counties constitute the hospital population.

The original capacity of the institution was 400; by changes and additions this has been increased to the present capacity of 810.

Persistent efforts for some years have at last been successful in providing the necessary hospital facilities and equipment which were omitted in the original plans, and there is now completed a splendidly equipped psychopathic hospital with 60 beds.

The appliances in every department are of the most modern type, including sterilizing apparatus, operating room accessories, complete hydrotherapeutic equipment, electric ranges, etc.

Since the opening of the institution, November 1, 1890, there have been admitted up to the close of the fiscal year ending September 30, 1911:

	Men	Women	Total
Admitted	1,773	1,505	3,278
Discharged—			
Recovered	426	455	881
Improved	297	208	505
Unimproved	88	55	143
Not insane	10	6	16
Total discharged	821	724	1,545
Total died	510	411	921
Total enrolled end of first year of institution			381
Total enrolled end of fiscal year 1911			807
Daily average attendance first year			235.444
Daily average atendance fiscal year 1911			746.538

CURRENT EXPENDITURES FOR FISCAL YEAR ENDING SEPTEMBER 30, 1911.

		Per Capita
Administration	$41,296.49	$55.284
Subsistence	45,322.04	60.672
Clothing, etc.	4,361.96	5.839
Office, domestic and outdoor departments	34,881.12	46.695
Ordinary repairs and minor improvements	5,993.54	8.023
Grand total of current expenditures	$131,855.15	$176.513
Less earnings paid into State Treasury	184.83	.247
Less amounts due from counties for clothing	4,851.41	6.495
	$126,818.91	$169.771

New buildings and furniture	$59,688.72
Permanent improvements	15,705.27
	$75,393.99

The following named physicians have served as medical superintendents since the opening of the institution:

Dr. A. J. Thomas ....Term of service, June 12, 1890, to July 15, 1897.
Dr. G. C. Mason ....Term of service, July 15, 1897, to March 13, 1900.
Dr. W. A. Stoker ....Term of service, October 9, 1900, to June 1, 1903.
Dr. C. E. Laughlin ....Term of service, June 1, 1903.

In the interim of six months between the incumbency of Dr. Mason and Dr. Stoker, Dr. John F. Glover, assistant physician, was appointed as acting superintendent.

PRESENT MANAGEMENT.

Board of Trustees.

Bird H. Davis ....President.
J. T. Akin ....Vice-president.
William S. Bogy ....Treasurer.
J. T. Stout ....Secretary.

At present (1912) the medical staff consists of:

Dr. C. E. Laughlin ......Medical Superintendent and Physician-in-Chief.
Dr. F. L. Lord ....Assistant Physician.
Dr. Arley I. Munson ....Assistant Physician.
One interne.

NORTHERN HOSPITAL FOR INSANE.[1]

LONGCLIFF, NEAR LOGANSPORT, IND.

Pursuant to the act of March 7, 1883, providing for the location and erection of three additional hospitals for the insane, Governor A. G. Porter on the 21st of March, 1883, appointed the following commissioners: John C. Robinson, Joseph R. Gray, William Grose and Deforrest Skinner. The board organized April 11, 1883, as follows: Governor Porter, president; Commissioner Grose, vice-president; Frank H. Blackledge, secretary; Dr. Joseph G. Rogers, medical engineer and superintendent of construction, and E. H. Ketcham, architect.

On October 4, 1883, the board bought of Andrew G. Shanklin 160 acres of land near Logansport and received as a donation to the state from the citizens of Cass County, 121 86/100 acres adjoining, constituting the site of the Northern Hospital for the Insane. In November, 1883, the board selected a preliminary sketch for this hospital, submitted by the architect and medical engineer, and ordered its elaboration with certain modifications. The plans were adopted May 26, 1884. After a public reception of bids on June 12, 1884, a contract was made with McCormack & Hege, of Columbus, Ind., for the construction of the buildings, for the sum of $362,802.29.

The work was commenced July 1, 1884, under the superintendency of Dr. Joseph G. Rogers. In 1885 bids were received for the steam boilers, heating apparatus, pumping engine, plumbing and sanitary fixtures, etc., according to specifications made by the medical engineer, and adopted by the board.

The boilers were awarded to the Babcock & Wilcox Co. for $9869.27; the heating apparatus to the Kelly & Jones Co., of Pittsburgh, Pa., for $14,087.40; the water distribution and sanitary fixtures to S. I. Pope & Co., of Chicago, for $12,524; as also the pumping engine for $767; the pipe tunnels to Price & Barnes, of Logansport, for $1.47 per lineal foot. On April 6, 1886, were awarded to the Yale & Towne Manufacturing Co. the locks and other door and window hardware for $4338.18; on May 4, 1886, the painting and varnishing to John T. Stevens, of Columbus.

[1] By Fred. W. Terflinger, M. D., Superintendent.

During 1887 contracts were made with the United States Electric Lighting Company for the lighting plant; with the Harrisburg Car Company and the Madison Machine Company for engines; with the A. M. Dolph Company for laundry equipment; with Duparquet & Huot for kitchen outfit; with J. B. Messenger for water works, and with various other parties for all necessary furniture and movable equipment.

The board was unable to expedite the work in hand on account of a failure on the part of the General Assembly of 1887 to make provision for sufficient revenue.

In November, 1887, the board appointed Dr. Joseph G. Rogers to be medical superintendent; George S. Forman, steward; Drs. F. B. Wynn and S. E. Smith, assistant physicians, and A. D. Ogborn, storekeeper; terms of service to commence when indicated by the board.

At a meeting held in the State House, January 3, 1888, a report submitted by Commissioners Robinson and Bundy (successor to Commissioner Grose, resigned) upon a report offered by the medical engineer and superintendent-elect on a system of organization for the Northern Indiana Hospital, recommending its adoption, was received and adopted.

The following is an abstract of the rules established:

1. For the management of the Northern Indiana Hospital for the Insane the Board of Commissioners for Additional Hospitals for Insane shall hold regular sessions at the hospital on the second Thursday after the first Monday of each month.

2. The medical superintendent shall be and act as the secretary of the Board of Management.

3. The medical superintendent shall sit with the board and have voice without vote.

4. The board shall elect a treasurer of the hospital, who shall give bond.

5. The medical superintendent shall cause to be kept a complete set of double entry books of account; also a hospital register, showing the name, date of admission, county, next friend, postal address, telegraph address, sex, age, etc., and diagnosis of each patient admitted; also a case book, recording the history of each patient while in the hospital. The board shall inspect the aforesaid books at each regular session.

6. The medical superintendent shall, at each regular session, make a report of the number of patients in the hospital at the beginning of the preceding month, the number received during said month, the number discharged and the condition and previous diagnosis, the number having died with causes of death and previous diagnosis, and the number remain-

ing at the end of the month; also a report of changes of officers and employees; also a report of the kind, quality and amounts of supplies received; also a report of revenue in money or kind from sales or donations.

7. The board shall provide from time to time such articles and materials as may be needed for the proper maintenance and care of the hospital and its inmates. The board shall also provide in the same manner furnished quarters, food, heat and lights for all persons employed in the care of the hospital, unless otherwise provided, including the family of the superintendent.

8. The board shall establish the pay of officers and employees of every grade not already indicated by law.

13. The medical superintendent shall be the chief medical officer as well as general director of the institution, and shall give personal attention to the medical care of the inmates as well as to the general management of the hospital, and shall be responsible to the board for such care and management. Therefore he is empowered to select and nominate to the board for formal appointment, according to the act of 1883, such officers as may be needed for the efficient performance of the work with the responsibility of which he is charged. The medical superintendent is further empowered by law to discharge any officer or employee without limitation other than a report to the board at the next session of his reasons therefor.

Rules for Admission.

1. The hospital for insane, near Logansport, shall be known as the Northern Indiana Hospital for the Insane.

2. The clerk of any circuit court in the state may, on and after the first day of June, 1888, make application to the medical superintendent of the Northern Indiana Hospital for the Insane for the admission to the said hospital of any insane citizen of the county pursuant to the proceedings and in the manner prescribed by law for the committal of insane persons to a hospital for insane.

4. Cases shall be preferred in the following order, environments being duly considered:

(a.) Cases of acute insanity, original or recurrent.

(b.) Cases of chronic insanity, dangerous to themselves or to the community.

(c.) Cases of chronic insanity, harmless, but requiring special medical and custodial care on account of mental disease.

(d.) Cases of chronic insanity, harmless and requiring special custodial care only.

The Northern Hospital, upon completion of the original buildings, consisted of the administration building, four ward buildings in the department for men and four in the department for women, a rear center building, boiler house and laundry.

The institution is situated on the south bank of the Wabash River, on a farm of 281 acres, the surface of which is broken by a long rocky ridge which passes through its center from east to west, affording a commanding site for the buildings with views in every direction over the broad and picturesque valley of the Wabash. Nearly half the land is densely wooded and the building site is adorned by a beautiful grove of maple trees. The opportunities for drainage are excellent.

Pursuant to a proclamation of the Governor, the hospital was opened for the reception of insane patients from all parts of the state, subject to the limitations prescribed by law and by a code of regulations established by the Board of Commissioners pursuant to law, on July 1, 1888. Dr. Joseph G. Rogers, who had been a member of the Board of Commissioners for Additional Hospitals for the Insane in the capacity of medical engineer, having been appointed superintendent, remained in the employ of the state in this capacity until his death, April 11, 1908. Under his supervision the able organization which took charge of the hospital at its opening was retained throughout the following years, and it grew and developed along safe and sound lines. As assistant physicians at the opening of the hospital, Dr. F. B. Wynn and Dr. Samuel E. Smith were appointed, and it is of interest to note that Dr. Wynn is now one of the leading practitioners in the state capital, Indianapolis, and Dr. S. E. Smith has for about 14 years occupied the position of superintendent in the Eastern Hospital for Insane at Richmond, Ind.

At the end of the first year of operation the available beds were all occupied, and we find the biennial report ending October 31, 1890, making request for additional accommodation. Up to the time of the opening of this hospital the only institution for insane in the state was located at Indianapolis, and for several years this hospital had been overcrowded and a large number of insane had accumulated in county almshouses and on poor farms, which accounts for the rapid influx of patients.

The Board of Commissioners on May 1, 1889, elected David Hough president; Dennis Uhl treasurer; and Lester F. Baker a trustee.

In the spring of 1889 Dr. S. E. Smith and a few months later Dr. F. B. Wynn, assistant physicians, resigned; the former to take the place of medical superintendent of the Eastern Hospital for Insane at Richmond; the latter to spend a year or two in Europe before entering general practice.

Dr. Smith's place was filled by the appointment of Dr. Alfred McNamee, who remained but a short time in the service, retiring in June of 1892 on account of ill health. His successor was Dr. Wm. H. Rogers, formerly an assistant physician of the Eastern Kentucky Asylum at Lexington, Ky. Dr. Wynn was succeeded by Dr. James W. Milligan, of Indianapolis.

On May 1, 1893, Lester F. Baker ceased to be a member of the board by expiration of term, and on the same date Governor Mathews appointed as trustees, each for a term of four years, John L. Forkner and Dennis Uhl.

Upon the urgent demand of the superintendent and the Board of Trustees the General Assembly of 1893 appropriated $20,000 for the purpose of increasing the capacity of the hospital. This was promptly used in building a new assembly hall, with sewing room and attendants' dormitory, converting the old assembly hall and sewing rooms into a central dining hall for patients and using the dining rooms thus vacated on seven wards as dormitories. At the same time a much-needed addition to the administration building was also made, including three rooms in the second story, built over the dispensary and dining room.

In June of 1892 Dr. Alfred McNamee left the service on account of recurrent ill health, but having regained his normal vigor he returned to his post again in February of the next year and filled it most efficiently until the spring of 1894, when once more he was obliged to seek health and strength from rest and change. Again, as on a former like occasion, Dr. William H. Rogers filled the vacancy efficiently and to the eminent satisfaction of the patients under his care for a term of six months, attendant upon Dr. McNamee's possible return; upon definite determination of this expectation he asked to be relieved. Thereupon Dr. Robert Hessler was tendered the appointment and assumed the duties of assistant physician in the department for men in August of 1894. Dr. James W. Milligan continued as assistant in the department for women.

On March 11, 1895, an act was passed abolishing the office of trustee of the various hospitals for the insane and other state charitable institutions, and provided that the Governor appoint separate boards for each institution, consisting of three members. In compliance with this act Jacob J. Todd, Dennis Uhl and Edward S. Scott were appointed to serve for a period of three years.

During the biennial period ending October 31, 1896, two annexes were constructed to the two terminal buildings of the hospital, providing additional accommodation for 84 patients.

In 1898 we find the former Board of Trustees succeeded by Charles W. Slick, Benjamin F. Keesling and Rufus Magee. Dr. Robert Hessler, after three years of service, on September 30, 1897, resigned to take the position of pathologist at the Central Hospital for Insane at Indianapolis. He was succeeded by Dr. Rolland F. Darnall.

The General Assembly of 1899 specifically appropriated $80,000 for the construction of two additional buildings containing two wards with a capacity for 200 inmates. The work was begun April 17, 1899, and completed in August, 1900; and we find the hospital at this time able to promptly care for all the insane of the northern district. This enlargement made additional members of the hospital staff necessary, and Dr. Lee H. Streaker and Dr. Catharine D. Johnson were appointed internes in the department for men and women, respectively. Dr. Rolland F. Darnall continued as assistant physician in the department for men, Dr. James W. Milligan having resigned and being succeeded by Dr. Samuel R. Cunningham. Dr. W. F. Willien, the original interne in the department for men, was followed in January, 1899, by Dr. Gilbert T. Smith, who served for one year and was succeeded by Dr. Lee H. Streaker. On January 1, 1902, Rufus Magee retired from the board on account of expiration of term. Henry A. Barnhart was appointed by Governor Durbin as his successor.

After a year's excellent service as interne, Dr. Catharine D. Johnson was promoted to the grade of junior assistant physician and placed in charge of three wards as a distinct division of the department for women. For personal reasons she resigned in April, 1902. Dr. Lee H. Streaker met with a like promotion after a like service, but at the end of his second year resigned to take the position of physician to the Indiana State Prison at Michigan City, where he rendered a signal service to the state by solving the problem, "What shall be done with the insane criminals?" by simply taking them out of a cell house and putting them in a ward of the prison hospital. In June Dr. S. R. Cunningham retired to enter general practice in Indianapolis. Dr. Bon O. Adams, late interne of the Indianapolis City Dispensary, occupied the position of junior assistant physician for three months, and Dr. Fred. Terflinger for two months. Dr. Edward C. Elder, of Indianapolis; Dr. Rebecca Parish, of Indianapolis; and Dr. John M. Pulliam, of Washington, were appointed to fill the vacancies created by these resignations.

Early in 1903 B. F. Keesling, trustee, retired on account of expiration of term and removed from the state. His place was filled by the appointment of Warren T. McCray.

Dr. R. F. Darnall, after six years of efficient service as assistant physician, resigned on July 20, 1903, to assume the duties of first assistant in the Woodcroft Hospital at Pueblo, Colo. Dr. Fred W. Terflinger, late interne at Indianapolis City Hospital, assumed the duties of asistant physician on August 1, 1903, in the department for women. Just previous to this appointment the medical service was divided into four sub-divisions, each in charge of a physician. This became necessary because of the growth of the institution, it having at this time a population of 929.

A mechanical workshop, storehouse, additional farm building and refrigerating apparatus were completed during this biennial period.

In June, 1905, Dr. Edward C. Elder, assistant physician, resigned to enter another field of practice. His place was filled by Dr. George E. Hoffman, of Rochester, Ind. In October, 1905, Dr. J. M. Pulliam resigned to enter general practice in Ft. Wayne. He was succeeded by Dr. M. C. Hawley, of Indianapolis. In October, 1906, Dr. Rebecca Parish retired to enter the missionary service. She was succeeded by Dr. Adele R. Emerson, of Boston, a graduate of the Woman's Medical College of Pennsylvania.

The General Assembly of 1905 appropriated $80,000 to build two additional houses, one for men and one for women, each having a capacity for 70 inmates. Excavations commenced March 12. The building for women comprises two wards, one in the lower and one in the upper story. The rooms and equipment are alike above and below and each affords accommodation for a variety of classes of patients. The building for men was designed with a view to its being used almost solely for patients whose pleasure it is to work in the open air on the farm, in the garden and elsewhere outside the general ward. It was intended that the routine of its daily life should be as nearly as possible like that of a large farm house, entirely independent and different, in many particulars from other parts of the hospital. It has an independent kitchen and dining room and meal hours. The appropriation for these buildings was called forth because of the again crowded condition of the hospital and the fact that many urgent applications could not be accepted because of lack of room. Temporary quarters for 30 men were provided in a tent located at the west end of the row of ward buildings. This tent was occupied for several years and was eventually replaced by a cheap wooden structure, which continues in service.

In 1907 the General Assembly passed an act increasing the number of members of boards of control for each institution from three to four, and pursuant to that act J. Frank Hanley, then Governor, appointed Wm. A. Morris as an additional member.

The most important progress of the year 1907 was the opening for use of the two additional buildings heretofore mentioned, which increased the capacity of the institution 150 beds. We now find the hospital has room for 1000 patients and, as a consequence, the management has been able to accept all cases in the northern district for insane properly admissible under the law. The cost of the two buildings was $80,000 appropriated by the General Assembly, and $6164.50 allowed by the Governor from his emergency fund. Dr. Adele Emerson resigned January 28, 1907, to return to Boston. Dr. Earl Palmer was engaged and assigned as junior assistant physician February 18, and on June 1 was promoted to be assistant physician and assigned to a division in the department for women.

On April 11, 1908, Dr. Joseph G. Rogers, medical engineer during construction and medical superintendent during the 20 years of the hospital's operation, died. He had been an invalid for more than two years, but his death was nevertheless a great shock and a deplorable loss to the institutional life of the state. On July 17 Dr. Fred W. Terflinger, who had been a member of the hospital staff for six years, was chosen to succeed Dr. Rogers as medical superintendent. The vacancy created on the staff by the appointment of Dr. Terflinger as superintendent was filled by the appointment of Dr. Mary L. Widdop as assistant physician in the department for women. On November 10, 1908, Henry A. Barnhart, of Rochester, who had been elected to Congress, resigned as trustee and was succeeded by Walter G. Zahrt, of Ft. Wayne, Ind., formerly steward of the institution.

On June 11, 1910, Dr. M. C. Hawley resigned from the staff to take up the general practice of medicine, and in February Dr. Lorne Yule was appointed junior assistant, and, after a satisfactory preliminary service, assumed the duties of assistant physician. On March 1, 1910, Dr. Frank L. Washburn was appointed pharmacist and pathologist.

The General Assembly of 1909 appropriated $15,000 for the erection of a mortuary, dispensary and pathological building. This was completed and occupied in the spring of 1911. It comprises a basement mortuary and storage rooms; on the first floor a library, dispensary, dental office and lecture room; and on the second floor two living rooms, a microscopical, chemical and electrical laboratory and a museum.

The capacity of the hospital, March 12, 1912, is 950 and the total enrollment 865. For the year and a half prior to September, 1910, the average population of the hospital had been in the neighborhood of 1000, but the completion and opening of the Madison institution and a redistricting of the state, whereby certain counties of the northern district were transferred to those of other hospitals, and a transfer of the patients from those counties to other hospitals, reduced the population to 800, enabling the management to accept all suspended cases.

There can be no voluntary admissions, nor can the hospital receive pay cases.

Dr. Clarence H. Burnette, Indiana College of Dentistry, was appointed resident dentist in October, 1912, and resigned his position June 1, 1913. From June 1, 1913, until April 1, 1914, this position was unoccupied, at which time Dr. P. L. Beale assumed the duties of the position.

N. B.—The names of all officers, with the dates of their service, are given in the body of this history.

EASTERN INDIANA HOSPITAL FOR THE INSANE.

EASTHAVEN, NEAR RICHMOND, IND.

Planned and constructed, 1883-1888.
Temporarily occupied by School for Feeble-Minded Youth, 1888-1890.
Opened for insane patients, August 1, 1890.

This hospital, when opened for the admission of patients August 1, 1890, was one of the very few cottage hospitals in the country, and was probably in advance of others in the grouping of its classification into small diversified cottages.[1] To be sure, it was small and far from complete as measured by the standard of to-day. It contained 390 beds for patients and its service building proved too small for even this number of inmates. It consisted of 17 structures arranged in and around the three sides of a quadrangle 1000 feet long and 700 feet wide. The third, or northern side, was closed by a grove of fine native trees, which later was made into a pleasant exercise park. Its southern side formed the front and in the center of this line of buildings was located the administration building, on either side of which was a detached cottage intended for infirmary purposes, one for men on the west

[1] An experience of more than 20 years as the medical superintendent of this hospital has convinced the writer that the cottage plan of construction for the treatment and care of the insane has most to commend it, and that it must grow in favor with future institutional construction. Small cottages in sufficient number to provide for nine classes, in sizes varying from 20 to 60 beds, and not more than two stories high, with ample porches on both floors, with day and night quarters entirely separated, without connecting covered corridors, except in the hospital group, with a central congregate dining room each for men and women, one general kitchen and with central heating and lighting systems with necessary conduit tunnels, will meet the highest requirements of such a hospital.

Not often is the opportunity vouchsafed to one after long years of experience in the development of one institution to be permitted to plan and supervise the construction of a new hospital along the lines of his own ideals, but the writer has been so honored and privileged lately by the confidence of his state and two of its chief executives, with the result, after three or four years of arduous labor, of a complete and fully equipped modern hospital known as the Southeastern Hospital for the Insane located at Madison. This will be described elsewhere.—SAMUEL EDWIN SMITH, M. S., M. D.

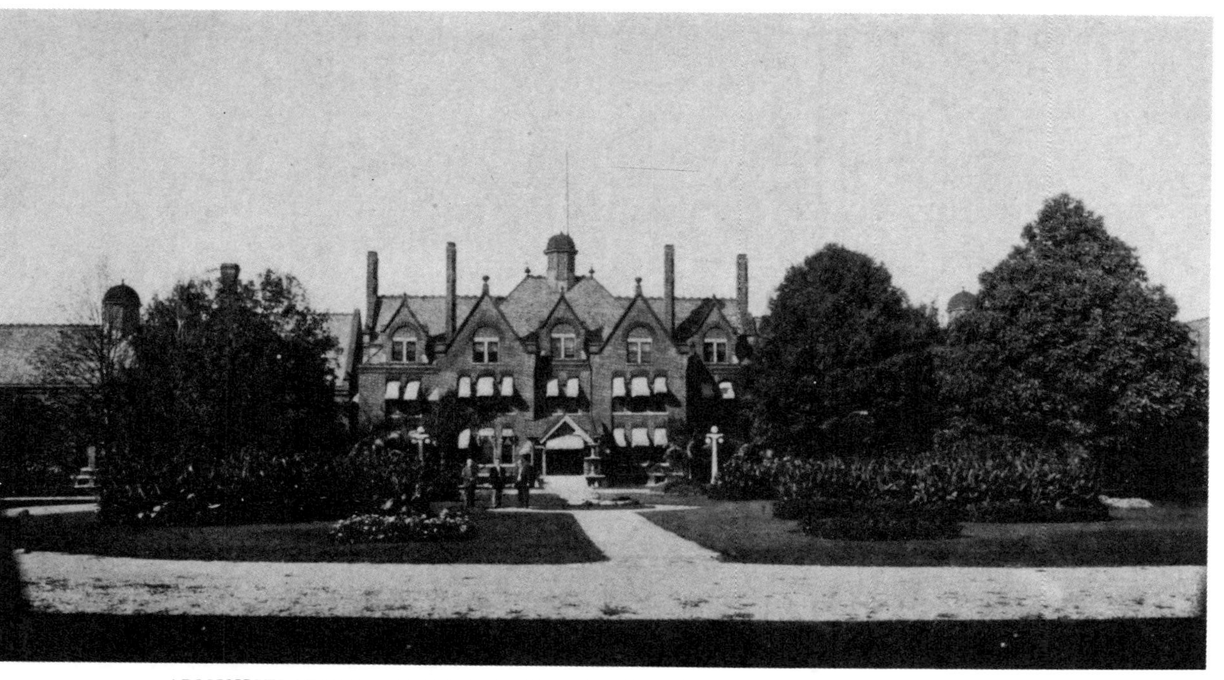

ADMINISTRATION BUILDING, EASTERN INDIANA HOSPITAL FOR THE INSANE.

and one for women on the east. In the rear of the administration building was the service building containing officers' and employees' quarters and dining rooms, general kitchen, bakery and cold store, and with an assembly hall on the second floor. In the rear were grouped the power house with its appurtenances and the laundry.

On the eastern side, located in a line and fronting the east, were five detached cottages for women patients, each with its own peculiar arrangement, external and internal.

On the western side was a line of detached cottages for men patients, similar in most particulars to those constituting the department for women.

No covered corridors between the cottages were built. Shallow brick tunnels radiated from the power house to the groups of cottages, in which were carried the steam, water and electric lines. The water mains, however, were placed in trenches in the ground.

The classification contemplated six groups in either department of six cottages for the infirm and mild acute, convalescent, melancholics and suicidal, quiet chronic and working, epileptics, and violent and maniacal classes. These were located in ten wards, two cottages having two horizontal wards each, one cottage three vertical wards, and three cottages one vertical ward each. The wards varied from 10 to 40 beds each. Ten per centum of the capacity was assigned to the violent and maniacal group and 85 percentum was dormitory construction. Each ward had a dining room and each cottage a kitchen. The aim was a family group.

The hospital was organized in 1890 and opened for the admission of patients August 1 of that year. The organization was dissolved by legislative action in March of the following year before all the cottages were occupied and a new board of trustees was selected. Samuel E. Smith, M. S., M. D., an assistant physician in the Northern Hospital since its opening, July, 1888, was made medical superintendent of the new hospital in April, 1891. He took charge May 15, 1891, and has remained in its continuous service to this day.

During the year 1891 all the beds were occupied and the test of actual service developed the weaknesses and inconveniences of plans and construction. These fortunately were not many, and most of them have been corrected by additional construction.

The most serious defect of plan was the individual kitchens with which each cottage was provided. Theoretically, a separate kitchen and dining room for each family group of patients is beautiful enough, but in practice the difficulties of supervision, the unnecessary waste from the numerous divisions of subsistence supplies, the lack of uniformity in the preparation of foods, the misapplication of the supplies by patients and attendants, the impossibility of maintaining a corps of competent cooks, the dangers from fire with the cooking utensils in proximity to all classes of patients, and constant presence of food and cooking odors throughout the cottages, rendered them impossible from an administrative point of view. Therefore in 1895 a large general kitchen and two large dining halls, one for men and one for women, were built and put into service, and the individual kitchens and most of the dining rooms were abandoned and, in most instances, utilized for small dormitories. The dining rooms in wards for the actively disturbed, sick and infirm have been maintained and served by wagons. The advantages of the general kitchen and congregate dining halls are many and are well known. In this hospital as high as 73 percentum of the patient population has been comfortably and safely taken to and from these dining halls for their meals.

This large kitchen and the dining halls were built with sanitary floors and are well lighted, heated and ventilated. On the second floor of the structure is an assembly hall with a seating capacity of 600, and employees' quarters, the men and women being segregated.

In 1898 a small detached kitchen and dining room were reconstructed for a few infirm patients on the first floor and the isolation of cases of tuberculosis on the second floor.

The single room capacity of about 15 percentum of the total capacity proved insufficient, and this deficiency was supplied by the construction of a single room cottage in each department, one in 1899 and one in 1902, at a total cost of $68,000. These increased the single room capacity to 29 percentum.

To meet another need not provided for in the original construction, two hospital cottages for sick were opened in 1900. These have a capacity of 30 beds each, with nurses' quarters and office and quarters for a medical interne. The bath-rooms are sanitary and commodious. The dormitories are well lighted and ventilated and the porches are ample and convenient. Operating rooms are conveniently located and fairly well equipped.

These two cottages cost $35,000 and proved of inestimable value in the care of the sick.

A woman physician was first added to the medical staff in that year and located in the women's hospital.

In 1907, at an outlay of $65,000, an infirmary cottage in each department with 40 beds was built. A special diet kitchen was erected at the same time and located between the infirmary and hospital cottage and connected with both by a covered corridor. These hospital groups have simplified and improved the nursing and care of the sick and infirm.

In the original construction only wooden floors were built in the bath-rooms, toilet rooms, sculleries and small dining rooms. These have all been removed and white vitreous tile and Venetian mosaic utilized.

The appurtenances have all been enlarged and improved from time to time to meet the needs of a growing population and later methods. The improvements include the power house, laundry, bakery, water system and tower and cold storage. The latter was built anew in 1899 and equipped with ice-making and refrigerating apparatus.

A sewerage purification plant was provided in 1903 at a cost of $15,000, which consists of a septic tank and four contact beds of gravel and sand enclosed with a concrete retaining wall. It automatically and satisfactorily oxidizes 85 percentum of the organic matter in 75,000 gallons of sewerage daily, and the effluent contains less organic matter than the brook into which it flows.

The grounds, a barren waste without tree, shrub or suggestion of a lawn in 1891, were carefully laid out and planted, and have developed in 20 years into a beautiful park, with exercise grounds in the rear and baseball grounds to the west.

The farm had some small additions made to it and has been well improved. A good dairy has been in operation many years. It now has a modern sanitary barn and a herd of 40 Holstein cattle. A brick stable and carriage house was built a few years ago, the farm houses all improved, and a sanitary piggery has been in service two years. The farm and gardens afford opportunity for the employment of many patients and supply, with the exception of potatoes, all the required vegetables.

The estate now consists of 323 acres, and hospital buildings, not including the farm appurtenances, number 30 brick structures. The total valuation of land, permanent improvements and personal property is $940,326.20.

The capacity is 830 beds, including certain small reservations in the hospital cottages for emergencies, and the daily average number present during the year 1912 was 794.

Since 1912 there has been added a new medical building for new laboratories, lecture-room and medical library, at a cost of $12,000; a new greenhouse at a cost of $5000; and a colony farm of 450 acres of fine land at a cost of $74,000.

COMMISSIONERS.

Governor Albert G. Porter.................Ex-officio president 1883-1885
Governor Isaac P. Gray....................Ex-officio president 1885-1889
Governor Alvin P. Hovey..................Ex-officio president 1889-1890

Joseph R. Gray......... 1883-1888
DeForrest Skinner 1883-1889
John C. Robinson...... 1883-1890
William Grose 1883-1886
Eugene H. Bundy...... 1886-1890
E. P. Richardson....... 1888-1890
Josiah Gwin 1889-1890

SECRETARIES.

Frank H. Blackledge.... 1883-1885
Pierre Gray 1885-1889
William B. Roberts..... 1889-1890

Dr. Joseph G. Rogers, medical engineer 1883-1890
Ed. H. Ketcham, architect 1883-1890

MEMBERS OF THE BOARD OF TRUSTEES.

George W. Koonts...... 1890-1891
John S. Martin........ 1890-1891
Milton C. Benham...... 1890-1891
Montgomery Marsh 1891-1895
James J. Smiley........ 1891-1895
Silas W. Halc.......... 1891-1902
William D. Page........ 1895-1901
E. Gurney Hill......... 1895-1900
Albert G. Ogborn....... 1900-1903
John W. Macy......... 1901-1902
Adam Heimberger 1902-1905
Warren Bigler 1902-1905
Thomas A. Jones...... 1903-1906
Carral K. McCollough.. 1905-1906
Joseph L. Cowing...... 1906-
John Detamore 1906-
John W. Hanan........ 1906-
Edward Barrett 1907-1910
Meredith Nicholson 1910-

MEDICAL SUPERINTENDENTS.

Edward F. Wells, M. D.. 1890-1891
Samuel E. Smith, M. S., M. D. 1891-

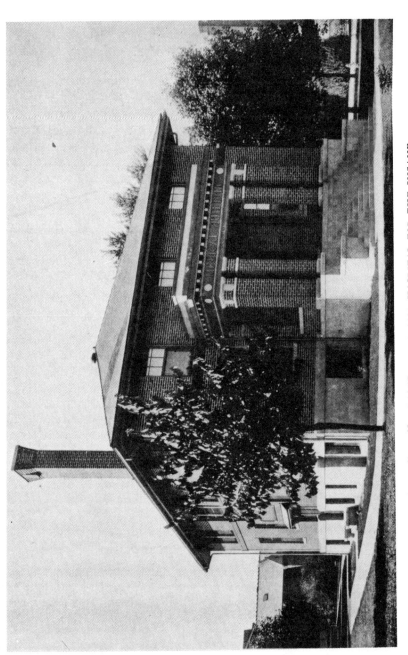

MEDICAL BUILDING, EASTERN INDIANA HOSPITAL FOR THE INSANE.

ASSISTANT MEDICAL OFFICERS.

Evan L. Patterson......	1890-1890	Carl W. McGaughey....	1904-1905
Oren E. Druley.........	1890-1891	J. Stillson Judah........	1905-1907
Samuel A. Gifford......	1890-1893	Larue D. Carter........	1907-1912
Lewis H. Gundry.......	1891-1893	Mary Wickens	1907-
Clinton T. Zaring......	1893-1898	William Spaulding	1907-1908
William S. Tomlin......	1893-1895	Fred W. Mayer........	1908-1908
Frank F. Hutchins......	1895-1901	Oscar A. Turner.......	1908-1912
Jediah H. Clark.........	1898-1900	Glenn E. Myers.........	1910-1911
Laura Mace	1898-1900	William V. Boyle.......	1911-1912
Mary H. Poole.........	1900-1902	Max A. Armstrong.....	1912-1913
Charles E. Cottingham..	1900-1903	Freeman R. Bannon....	1912-
Arthur J. McCracken...	1901-1904	Floyd F. Thompson....	1912-1913
M. Jennie Jenkins......	1902-1907	John A. Ritze...........	1913-1913
Paul S. Johnson........	1903-1910	Elbert W. Jackson......	1913-
Kenneth I. Jeffries......	1904-1907	Cecil G. Sutherlin.......	1913-

APPENDIX A.

AN ACT PROVIDING FOR THE LOCATION AND ERECTION OF ADDITIONAL HOSPITALS FOR THE INSANE AND PROVIDING FOR THE MANAGEMENT THEREOF.

Be it enacted by the General Assembly of the State of Indiana:

1. *Commissioners to Locate Hospitals for the Insane.*—That the Governor shall, immediately upon the taking effect of this act, appoint two commissioners from each of the two leading political parties, who, together with the Governor, who shall be *ex-officio* a member, are hereby constituted a board of commissioners to superintend the location, the letting the construction, and equipping of three hospitals for the insane; and none of such hospitals shall be erected within 50 miles of the City of Indianapolis. Such commissioners shall hold their office for two years, and until their successors are appointed, unless sooner released by order of the Governor: *Provided,* that one of said hospitals shall be located at or near the City of Evansville.

2. *Selection of Sites.*—It shall be the duty of such board of commissioners, after careful examination, to select, in parts of the state hereinbefore mentioned, suitable sites for the location of three several hospitals for the insane, which selection, when made, shall be the places at which such hospitals shall be erected.

3. *Purchase of Land, Conveyance, Advertising, Proposals, etc.*—When the places for the location of such hospitals shall have been fully agreed upon by such board, or a majority thereof, the said board of commissioners shall, without delay, contract for the purchase of a tract of land not exceeding 160 acres at each location, which they shall procure to be deeded

to the State of Indiana. . . . . Such board of commissioners shall, after selecting the locations for such hospitals, advertise for sealed proposals for the erection and completion of such hospitals upon such plans and specifications as may have been agreed on, embracing offices and buildings, as may be necessary to the complete establishment of such hospitals for the comfort and safekeeping of patients. . . . .

4. *Awards of Contracts—Bond Proviso.*—At the time specified in such advertisement for the opening and examination of bids the board shall meet at the places designated, and they, together with the Governor, shall open and examine the bids and award the contract or contracts to the lowest responsible bidder whose bond they deem sufficient, or they may award portions of the work to such bidders, if they shall deem it an advantage to the state to do so; and any and all bonds and sealed proposals contemplated by this act shall be accompanied by a bond, payable to the State of Indiana, signed by sufficient resident freehold surety, with a penalty in a sum not less than double the amount of the bid or proposal. . . . .

6. *Superintendent—Estimates—Warrants—Reserve.*—A competent and skillful person shall be selected by said board, with the approval of the Governor, for each of said hospitals, who shall remain on the hospital grounds and superintend the erection of said buildings and see that the work is well and faithfully done according to contract. . . . .

9. *Compensation of Commissioners.*—The Board of Commissioners and the person whose appointment is provided for in section six of this act, shall be allowed each $5 per day for all the time necessarily employed by them in the performance of the duties required by this act, and all necessary traveling expenses: *Provided,* That no commissioner shall receive more than $200 per annum for his services.

10. *Appropriations.*—In order to carry out the provisions of this act, there is hereby appropriated the sum of $300,000 for the year 1883, and $300,000 for the year 1884, out of any money in the treasury not otherwise appropriated.

12. *Appointment of Officers—Proviso—Compensation.*—The Board of Commissioners shall have authority to appoint a superintendent to take charge of the patients and hospital, to appoint a matron and such assistants and physicians, steward, and other officers as may be needed for the efficient and economical administration of the affairs of the hospitals. . . . .

15. *Capacity: 200 to 700 Patients.*—The capacity of such hospital mentioned in this act shall not be less than will accommodate 200 patients, and not greater than will accommodate 700 patients.

SOUTHEASTERN HOSPITAL FOR THE INSANE.[1]

MADISON, IND.

During the period from 1900 to 1905 there was a notable increase in the population of the State of Indiana, especially in the northern portions in proximity to Chicago. The proportion of insane having kept pace with this growth, the four hospitals became overcrowded and an excess of over 600 accumulated in the county infirmaries. To afford the necessary relief, a bill authorizing the establishment of a fifth state hospital was presented to the Legislature of 1905 and speedily became a law. This law became the organic act of the Southeastern Hospital for the Insane and was approved February 21, 1905.[2]

In accordance with the act, Governor J. Frank Hanly appointed George A. H. Shideler, John W. McCardle, Duane D. Jacobs and Ephraim Inman commissioners, who, on April 21, 1905, organized as follows: Governor J. Frank Hanly, *ex-officio,* president; D. D. Jacobs, vice-president; G. A. H. Shideler, secretary; Ephraim Inman, treasurer.

In April, 1907, John W. McCardle resigned to become a member of the State Board of Tax Commissioners, and Governor Hanly filled the vacancy thus created by the appointment of Walter H. Lewis, who assumed his duties May 29, 1907.

In August, 1905, Dr. Samuel E. Smith, at the request of Governor Hanly and the commissioners, inspected and reported on all the proposed sites. He was appointed expert medical adviser November 27, and on December 14, 1905, Herbert Foltz, of Indianapolis, was employed as architect.

In January, 1909, the term of office of Governor Hanly expired and he was succeeded by Governor Thomas R. Marshall, who became, *ex-officio,* president of the board. No other changes occurred.

Numerous sites were promptly submitted for the board's consideration, and all were visited and inspected by the board with as little delay as possible; all were eliminated as unfit, for various reasons, excepting seven located in several counties of the district.

[1] By Samuel E. Smith, M. S., M. D., medical adviser.

[2] See Appendix A for digest of act.

The seven sites each had something to commend them and the problem of final selection became difficult. At this juncture Dr. Samuel E. Smith was called by Governor Hanly and the commissioners and requested to inspect and report upon the several sites. He was reminded that the board was bi-partisan in personnel and non-partisan in purpose, and that it was in full sympathy with the motive of the organic act to select the site with reference to the best interests of the hospital and its patients only, and without bias by donation, gratuity, political or any other influence. This made the task an inviting one and Dr. Smith accepted the commission with the stipulation that he be permitted, in his own time and manner, to inspect the sites alone, accompanied only by some one local citizen who should be fully informed concerning property lines, local history, health conditions and the like.

Before making this survey Dr. Smith prepared a standard of measurement in which the essential natural requirements for a hospital site were given, according to his best judgment, a relative value on the basis of a scale of 100 units. By this standard the advantages of the several sites offered were critically and conscientiously measured and promptly noted on the completion of each inspection, and the comparison thus afforded enabled him to arrive at a conclusion founded upon scientific reasons and absolutely free from bias or prejudice and at the same time just and fair to all interests.

The standard and the grades of the several sites can be seen from table on following page.

On September 4, 1905, Dr. Smith submitted his report, which included the above standard and grades, and expressed the opinion that the totals of the tables proved the relative values of the sites, and of these Madison was first and Columbus second. In the same hour the board accepted the Madison site and settled this all-important question.

The contest for the location of this hospital was spirited and each site had a large group of active partisans made up of the best citizens of the locality, as it was understood the state contemplated a large expenditure for a splendid institution which would make it a valuable asset for any community. Nevertheless the manner of selection by the board proved satisfactory to all parties and the conclusion was accepted without noteworthy criticism.

	Scale.	Columbus.	North Vernon.	Seymour.	Madison.	Charlestown.	New Albany.	Bedford.
1. Sanitation:								
a. Sewage disposal	10	8	8	9	10	7	6	7
b. Healthfulness	10	9	10	9	10	10	10	10
2. Water Supply:								
a. Quantity	10	8	9	8	10	9	9	9
b. Quality	10	8	8	8	9	8	7	7
c. Availability	5	5	3	5	3	4	4	5
3. Transportation:								
a. Rates	10	8	9	9	10	9	10	8
b. Accessibility	10	8	10	10	4	5	9	5
4. Building Materials:								
a. Brick and stone	6	3	3	2	5	4	5	6
b. Sand and gravel	4	4	2	3	3	2	2	3
5. General Adaptability:								
a. Building site	5	3	3	2	5	3	3	4
b. Farming and gardening	12	12	5	10	9	6	6	8
c. Scenic environment	8	5	6	3	8	3	6	7
Total	100	81	76	78	86	70	77	79

The site selected was at once purchased at a cost of $39,214.84 for 363 acres. The tract is in the form of an irregular parallelogram and occupies a part of a level plateau on a bluff, 450 feet above the river. To the south it overlooks the City of Madison and the beautiful valley of the Ohio River for a distance of 14 miles. The steep bluff in front and the ravines on either side are well covered with fine native trees. In the valley, at the foot of the bluff, six acres of land were secured for the water supply and this is connected by a narrow strip of land 32 rods wide with the tract on the top of the hill, and also runs to the river front, to furnish a right of way for water and sewerage lines, and wharfage if ever needed.

It is worthy of mention that when the organic act of this hospital was created Indiana had had four hospitals in service many years, which represented the four types of construction in most general use throughout the United States and foreign countries—the Kirkbride or corridor, the cottage, the block or pavilion, and the radiate plans. After having tried out these several plans by the test of actual experience during many years, it was the consensus of opinion of the best informed and most interested that the salient features of the cottage plan should be duplicated in the construction of the new institution. Hence this plan was stipulated in the organic act.

Work on the plans and specifications for a cottage hospital was begun by the medical adviser and architect in December, 1905, and completed, with the exception of a few minor details, on July 23, 1906.

In the work the medical adviser was given full latitude. He made sketches showing dimensions and floor plans for each structure from which the architect prepared preliminary drawings, which were submitted by building or groups of buildings to the commission and after consideration and approval they were put into permanent tracings by the architect. After all the drawings were completed they were arranged with relation to each other, the cottages being 80 to 100 feet apart, to a north and south axis, and with reference to the topography with the largest possible amount of southern exposure.

Meantime a complete topographical map of the building site was made by R. L. Sackett, of Purdue University, who later became the consulting engineer.

The plans when completed provided for a normal capacity of 1000 and a maximum capacity of 1250 patients, to be accommodated in 22 cottages, subdivided into 30 wards, one-half to constitute the department for men and the other one-half the department for women, ranging in capacity from 20 to 70 beds each, with an administration building for offices and officers' quarters; a service building for the kitchens, the congregate dining-rooms, the assembly hall, employees' quarters and dining-rooms, and necessary appurtenances; a power house; a store house; a laundry; an industrial building for a sewing room, a shoe shop and rooms wherein patients may be safely employed; a workshop for painters and carpenters; a pumping station; a water tower and a stable. It was decided to transmit the necessary steam for heating, water and electric current through underground tunnels for the several buildings and cottages.

Sealed bids for the construction work were received, opened and considered September 10, 1906, and a general contract was entered into on September 19, 1906. This contract aggregated

$1,172,217.30, and did not include the special hardware, which the board preferred to let by special contract for $8855.19.

The work of construction under the general contract was started on October 15, 1906, and reasonable progress was made with it during the ensuing eight or nine months, but under the inefficient direction of the general contractor, and in spite of the efforts of this board and its representatives, it lagged throughout the latter part of the summer and the autumn of 1907. The contractor's difficulties, financial and otherwise, increased and work practically ceased in the latter part of January, 1908. Then on March 12, 1908, the board by legal proceedings terminated the general contract and took possession of the premises. On May 28, 1908, the contract was relet and June 1, 1908, the work was again under way.

The loss to the state by reason of the failure of the first contractor was inconsiderable, except for the vexatious delay, as the surety company made good the financial loss by the payment of $65,000 for damages, which enabled the board to contract for three small buildings not included in the general contract.

The structures were all finally completed and accepted on July 10, 1910.

Meantime contracts had been made and filled on specifications prepared by the medical adviser for the entire equipment, including household furnishings, kitchen, laundry, cold storage equipments, office supplies and blank records and all other necessary supplies, except subsistence. This equipment was not only delivered, but was put in place in the various departments in minute detail, even to the marking of the linen, and the preparation of blank case records and all necessary blank forms.

It also included a complete telephone system with 40 stations, a Hahl automatic clock system, a night watchman's signal service and all necessary electric light fixtures. The total cost of the entire equipment was $123,216.98.

The organic act provided for the organization and management by a board of trustees of four members, two from each of the leading political parties, appointed by the Governor. Governor Thomas R. Marshall accordingly appointed the members, as follows: Ephraim Inman, Charles Cravens, George S. Pleasants and Samuel B. Sweet.

By election of this board of trustees Dr. Edward P. Busse was made medical superintendent.

On July 28, 1910, the Board of Commissioners by resolution delivered to the Governor the completed hospital fully equipped in all essential details. The Governor's proclamation was at once issued, the Board of Trustees was placed in charge and the institution was opened for the admission of patients on August 15, 1910.

The hospital was completed as originally planned with the exception of one cottage in either department especially arranged for epileptics, two small shops and the barn. The sites of the cottages were, however, made ready and the tunnels with all necessary service lines of water, hot and cold, steam and electric wiring in place. These omissions are now being supplied by the present management.

The 31 completed structures harmonize architecturally. The light-buff pressed brickwork of the structures, with its oolitic stone trimmings resting on light-brown pressed brick foundations, surmounted by overhanging roofs of red Spanish tile, contrasted with the blue sky of the Ohio River Valley, affords a color scheme as beautiful and soothing as that of an old Italian village.

All foundations are made of hard burnt paving block and laid in Portland cement, faced above grade with brown pressed vitrified brick. The stairs are all slate except in the administration building.

The total capacity is 1100 beds, divided equally into the two departments of 10 cottages each, varying from 30 to 70 beds each. In each department of 10 cottages are 15 wards of 20 to 70 beds, arranged for nine groups of patients—receiving, sick, infirm, convalescent, chronic, and working, suicidal and depressed, epileptic, active and violent. The two last named groups may each be graded in two cottages of two wards each, almost entirely single rooms. The single room capacity is now 40 per centum of the total, but will be reduced to 35 when the epileptic cottage is put into service.

All cottages are built on the house plan with day and night quarters entirely separated. Five cottages have two horizontal wards each, and the others one vertical ward each, with day quarters on the first and night quarters on the second floors. All day-rooms, whether on the first or second floor, are provided with two or more ample porches. The clothing and bath rooms are unusually large, the linen closets are numerous, and the toilet rooms were intentionally made small to prevent the congregating of patients therein. All porches and loggias have Welch quarry tile floors; the bath rooms, toilet rooms and sculleries, white vitreous tile; the dining rooms encaustic tiles and the large kitchen, white vitreous tiles. Elsewhere the floors are all $\frac{3}{4}$ x $1\frac{1}{2}$ inch white maple laid on pine. Every sitting room has an open grate, protected by a wire guard, and a neat brick mantel.

The hospital group in each department consists of two cottages, with 50 beds each, one for the sick and the other for the infirm and untidy. Between the cottages and connected with them by enclosed corridors is a structure with diet kitchen and dining room. The hospital cottage is well-equipped, with a good operating room and ample baths, and the sick rooms are large and well ventilated and lighted by southern exposure. Quarters and office are provided for a woman physician in the women's hospital and likewise for a man physician in the men's hospital.

The convalescents' cottage was built with special reference to homelike surroundings and is limited to 30 beds. It is contemplated to place it in charge of one nurse, where, with an open-door supervision, convalescents may be tried out under the conditions of the home, as near as possible, for a period of a month or two before leaving the hospital.

The service building is carefully worked out and it contains the general kitchen, two congregate dining halls, employees' dining hall, officers' dining room, and general reading room on the first floor, and on the second floor are the assembly hall with seating capacity for 700, and 106 single rooms for employees properly segregated.

The general kitchen is 60 feet wide and 160 feet long, with a white vitreous tile floor and white enameled walls and steel ceiling. This kitchen is one story high for 105 feet of its length and is covered by a long ventilating monitor, under which the steam cooking utensils are grouped. The cold store and bakery are located at the extreme corners and are detached by covered corridors. The cooking utensils are grouped in the center of the room and the range is center construction with down draft. No sinks or utensils of any kind are placed against the walls.

The dining halls each have a capacity of 400; the floors are encaustic tiles and the walls are enameled brick with slate base surmounted by pressed buff brick. The employees' and nurses' dining room has a seating capacity of 200 and is similarly built. The cold store and bakery are large and equipped with the latest improved apparatus.

The industrial building is a comfortable structure intended for the employment of patients. It has a sewing room, tailor shop, mattress room, shoe shop and the like.

The power house is centrally located and its equipment includes three batteries each of two B. & W. boilers of 228 h. p. each, or a total of 1368 h. p. The power plant consists of three electrical units of 100 kw. each. Otherwise all parts of the mechanical equipment are in duplicate. The current is direct, 220 volts, and is distributed on a three-wire system.

The electric wires, steam and water lines are carried through tunnels entirely underground to the various structures. These tunnels are made of paving block laid in cement, covered with cement and damp-proofing, floored with cement, are 7 feet high and vary from 4 to 6 feet wide. They grade to the power house for gravity steam returns and are made without reference to the surface, being at some points 20 feet underground. They are lighted by electricity and may be conveniently inspected at all hours. They run under no structures whatever, but each building is connected to the main tunnel by a spur tunnel 30 to 40 feet long and at the entrance to the building valves and cut-offs are set in, making it possible to completely and quickly detach any structure from the general service.

The sewer system collects all the sewage by vitrified and iron pipe lines which converge into a common closed basin at the top of the bluff, whence it is carried in a ten-inch cast-iron pipe with a fall of 450 feet in its length of 1600 feet into the Ohio River.

The water supply is abundant and of fine quality. It is taken from gang wells 135 feet deep located in the valley by an air lift and an electric screw pump and delivered into a basin near the pumping station, whence it is lifted by two heavy-duty steam pumping engines into a brick protected steel water tower, 125 feet high and 20 feet wide, and located 1600 feet away among the cottages on the building site. All the pumping apparatus is in duplicate.

The plumbing is all modern and the work is the open variety. With the exception of the enameled iron bath tubs the fixtures are solid porcelain throughout, and all are double trapped and back vented.

The heating system is a Warren-Webster low pressure steam vacuum process, chiefly indirect radiation with steam mains and returns carried through tunnel conduits heretofore described, and so arranged as to provide gravity returns to the power house. The hot air flues open in the wall seven feet above the floor, and the foul air ducts are set five inches above the baseboards and open directly into the attics surmounted by large louvres for gravity circulation.

The laundry is a very large one-story structure in the form of a Greek cross. The apparatus is complete, of the latest type, and in the main operated by electric current.

The cottages are fairly flooded with sunshine for many hours each day, and the 14 miles of winding Ohio River in the valley 450 feet below, with the rounded, wooded hills of Kentucky beyond, afford a view delightfully peaceful, and should bring rest to many a weary mind.

The cost of this hospital is set forth in the following summary:

Total funds available			$1,527,544.33
Disbursements for land		$39,214.84	
Permanent improvements:			
Contract construction	$1,268,124.36		
Construction at contract fixed charges	7,369.18		
Extra work	9,458.95		
Water supply	6,707.27		
Walks and grading	18,797.11		
Total permanent improvements		1,310,456.87	
Farm and grounds		9,462.68	
Equipment—personal property.		123,216.98	
Repairs to old structures		311.36	
Architect's and experts' fees	$21,207.06		
Supervision of works	7,431.19		
Commissioners' expense	5,472.27		
Office expense	3,409.92		
Total operating expenses		37,520.44	
Total cost			1,520,183.17
Balance returned to the state treasury			$7,361.16

Extra work added to contract price	$9,458.95
Credits deducted from contract price	27,339.31
Unexpended balance returned to state treasury	7,361.16

Per capita cost for 1100 patients of land and permanent improvements	$1,269.97
Per capita cost of equipment	112.01
Total cost of each patient's bed	$1,381.98

Capacity, or number of patients' beds	1100
Number of beds for nurses, attendants and employees	210

It is worthy of special mention that this large amount of construction was carried to completion with extra work outside of the contracts, as shown above, amounting only to $9458.95, and the deductions from the contract prices aggregated $27,339.31. It is also a source of satisfaction that when the work was completed as contemplated and all financial obligations had been discharged a balance of $7361.16 was unexpended and was returned to the state treasury, and that the examination of the records and accounts by the State Board of Accounts reported them correct in every detail.

This was the largest financial undertaking, save one, in the history of Indiana, and it was carried through to a successful end without public scandal or criticism of any kind and without even the suggestion of the wonted legislative investigation.

BOARD OF TRUSTEES.

Ephraim Inman, president	1910-in office
Samuel B. Sweet, vice-president	1910-1911
Charles Cravens, treasurer	1910-in office
George S. Pleasants, secretary	1910-1911
James W. Lilly, vice-president	1911-in office
Francis M. Griffith, secretary	1911-in office

MEDICAL SUPERINTENDENT.

Edward P. Busse, M. D.	1910-in office

ASSISTANT PHYSICIANS.

Harry L. Devine, M. D. 1910-1911
Alice N. Pickett, M. D. 1910-1911
James K. Pollock, M. D. 1911-1913
Aleck P. Harrison, M. D. .... 1911-in office
Thyra Josselyn, M. D. .... 1911-in office
Clyde C. Bitter, M. D. .... 1912-in office
Floyd F. Thompson, M. D. .... 1913-in office
Ralph M. Funkhouseer, M. D. .... 1913-in office
Minor Miller, M. D. .... 1913-in office

CLERK.

Walter F. Wanderlich .... 1910-in office

STOREKEEPERS.

George W. Miles 1910-1911
Patrick J. McInnerney .... 1911-in office

SECRETARIES.

Katherine E. Gosler 1910-1911
Elizabeth Lesh .... 1911-in office

BOOKKEEPER.

James Atwell .... 1912-in office

CHAPLAIN.

Joseph H. Barnard .... 1910-in office

APPENDIX A.

An Act Entitled an Act Providing for the Location and Erection of an Additional Hospital for the Insane and Providing for the Management and Maintenance Thereof.

Be it enacted by the General Assembly of the State of Indiana:

Section 1. *Southeastern Hospital for Insane—Commission—Appointment.*—That the Governor shall, within 60 days after the taking effect of this act, appoint four commissioners, not more than two of whom shall belong to the same political party, who, together with the Governor, who shall be, *ex-officio,* a member, are hereby constituted a board of commissioners to procure the location, employ an architect and superintend the preparation of the plans and specifications, and the letting of the contract for the erection, completion, furnishing and equipment of a hospital for the insane, which hospital shall be designated and called the Southeastern Hospital for the Insane, and shall be located and erected within one of the counties named in section 8 of this bill. Such commissioners, except the Governor, shall hold their office for a period of three years from the date of their appointment and until their successors are appointed and qualified, unless sooner released by order of the Governor. . . . .

SEC. 2. *Duties of Commissioners.*—It shall be the duty of such Board of Commissioners, after careful examination, to select and purchase, without delay, a suitable tract of real estate, not exceeding 360 acres, whereon to erect the necessary buildings for such hospital, such tract of real estate having ample water supply, facilities for drainage and sewerage, being in a healthful location and having ample and convenient railroad facilities. . . . . The Board of Commissioners shall, after selecting and acquiring the necessary real estate for the site of said hospital, cause plans and specifications to be prepared for any and all parts of the work contemplated by this act, including offices, buildings and such other structures as may, from time to time, be deemed necessary to the complete establishment and equipment of such hospital for the care, treatment and safekeeping of patients according to modern, advanced and practical methods, said hospital being constructed upon what is commonly known as the "cottage plan." . . . .

SEC. 5. *Superintendent of Construction—Estimates—Warrants.*—A competent and skilled superintendent of construction shall be selected by such Board of Commissioners, who shall remain on the hospital grounds and oversee and superintend the erection of said buildings and other work to be performed, and see that all work is well and faithfully done according to contract, and shall make monthly estimates of the work done under oath, which estimates, when endorsed by the architect and approved by said Board of Commissioners, in such manner as they may prescribe, shall be filed with the Auditor of the state, who shall thereupon draw his warrant upon the Treasurer of the state, less 10 per centum thereon, which amount of 10 per centum shall remain unpaid until the work is fully completed and accepted by said Board of Commissioners, when the Auditor shall draw his warrant therefor. The board shall have power to suspend or remove such superintendent of construction and appoint a successor at any time. And such superintendent of construction shall execute a bond payable to the State of Indiana. . . . .

SEC. 6. *Contracts—When Void.*—Said board shall have the power to declare all contracts made under this act void when the work is not being done according to contract, or the materials furnished are not furnished in quality or quantity or in the time stipulated for in the contract, and shall, in such event, relet the work upon the same terms, except as to notice, as is provided in this act, and the substance of this section shall be set forth in each contract.

SEC. 7. *Compensations.*—The Board of Commissioners, other than the Governor and the superintendent of construction, shall be allowed and paid each five dollars per day for all the time necessarily employed by them in the performance of the duties required by this act, together with all necessary travelling expenses, out of the funds hereinafter appropriated.

SEC. 8. *Southeastern District—Admission to Hospital.*—The counties of Monroe, Brown, Bartholomew, Lawrence, Jackson, Jennings, Ripley, Dearborn, Ohio, Switzerland, Jefferson, Scott, Clark, Floyd and Washington are hereby constituted and designated as the Southeastern District, and all persons resident in said district adjudged insane and eligible to admission to an insane hospital shall be admitted to and cared for by the hospital herein provided for, and when said Southeastern Hospital for the Insane shall be completed, organized and ready for the reception of patients, the Governor shall issue his proclamation reciting such facts, and he shall thereupon order transferred from the Central Hospital for the Insane, to said Southeastern Hospital for the Insane, all inmates therein at such time who shall have been committed from any of the counties hereinbefore named in this section. . . . . The Governor shall have the power to require the superintendent of the said Southeastern Hospital for the Insane to remove from the Central Hospital for the Insane all inmates whose removal is provided for in this section, and the expense of such removal shall be paid, as by law provided, out of the funds hereafter appropriated for the maintenance of said Southeastern Hospital for the Insane: *Provided,* That the Governor of Indiana may transfer any county to or from said district, as public convenience may require.

SEC. 9. *Trustees—Appointment—Duties—Powers, etc.*—Upon or before the completion of the said Southeastern Hospital for the Insane the Governor shall appoint a board of three trustees for the management thereof in all respects as provided by the acts of the General Assembly of Indiana of 1897, page 157, in force March 5, 1897, so far as said act may be applicable, and the Governor shall, in making such appointments, fix the time when such trustees shall take office, and the said board of trustees so to be appointed shall qualify, organize, serve, control, conduct, manage and govern said Southeastern Hospital for the Insane under and pursuant to all laws hereafter in force in reference to the Northern, Eastern and Southern hospitals for the insane so far as the same may be applicable and pertinent: and said board of trustees shall have and enjoy the same tenure of office, pay, power, privileges and responsibilities as are now or may hereafter be conferred by law upon the boards of trustees of said last mentioned hospitals, all under and pursuant to the same rules and laws, so far as applicable and pertinent, and all laws and parts of laws not in conflict with this act heretofore or hereafter enacted for the government and control of said Northern, Eastern, Southern hospitals for the insane, so far as applicable, are extended to and declared to embrace and govern said Southeastern Hospital for the Insane.

SEC. 10. *Expert Adviser to Commissioners.*—The Board of Commissioners of said Southeastern Hospital for the Insane shall, from time to time, have power to employ, consult and pay an expert adviser, who shall be a physician who has had experience in a hospital for the insane, with reference to any or all parts of the work necessary to be done in the performance of their duties as contemplated by this act. Any such service shall be paid for out of any funds appropriated for carrying out the provisions of this act, upon the certificate of the said Board of Commissioners, filed with the Auditor of the state. . . . .

SEC. 11. *Appropriation—How Available.*—For the purpose of carrying out the provisions of this act there is hereby appropriated out of any funds in the state treasury not otherwise appropriated the sum of $560,000, or so much thereof as may be necessary, to be expended by the said Board of Commissioners as herein provided. Of this sum $60,000 shall be available November 1, 1905; $250,000 June 1, 1906; $250,000 January 1, 1907.

INDIANA HOSPITAL FOR INSANE CRIMINALS.[1]

MICHIGAN CITY, IND.

The Indiana Hospital for Insane Criminals, the most recent of the state institutions for the care of the insane, is a department of the state prison at Michigan City, and is under the control of the Board of Trustees and the warden of the prison, with a physician in charge.

The act of authorization approved March 5, 1909, carried an appropriation of $65,000 to cover building and equipment. It called for a capacity of not less than 145 beds; for fireproof construction, with the advantages of a hospital and the security of a prison.

Excavation was begun May 9, 1910; the building was occupied October, 1912; with the exception of the plumbing, the work was done entirely by prison labor.

Indiana made the first provision for her criminals in 1822, when the prison at Jeffersonville was opened. In 1848 the insane were first cared for in the Hospital for Insane at Indianapolis; but 60 years were allowed to pass before it was thought necessary to officially recognize and segregate the great intermediate group—the criminal insane.

In 1859 the Prison North at Michigan City was established; in 1897 the Prison South at Jeffersonville became the reformatory, and since then receives only indeterminate-sentence men over 16 and under 30 years of age. In the same year the Prison North became the state prison; it receives all life men of whatever age, and all indeterminate-sentence men over 30 years.

Those previously convicted, the incorrigible, and the insane at the reformatory may be transferred to the prison upon an order of the Governor.

If the insane were recognized among the prison population in the early years of these institutions, existing records fail to indicate that they received much attention. But in the annual report of the Northern Prison for 1872, 13 years after its establishment, the

[1] By J. W. Milligan, M. D.

physician says: "I must earnestly recommend the construction of a room or ward adjoining the hospital for the purpose of confining those who are temporarily insane as well as those feigning insanity."

The following year the warden in his report says: "It is very necessary that a suitable building should be erected for the confinement of prisoners who are more or less insane."

The warden in his report of 1892 says: "There are quite a number of insane convicts in the prison. Some are objects of absolute pity. None of them can be cared for here as they should be." The population of the prison was then 753.

A law of 1889 provides that girls from the girls' school and women from the women's prison, if insane, shall be transferred to the "Asylum for the Insane." The law of 1895 made similar provision for the men when it authorized the "transfer of insane persons from the state prisons to the insane asylums of the state." However, very few such transfers were made; the prisons were evidently slow to take action, and the hospitals certainly did not urge it; the fact that in some cases elopement soon followed the transfer no doubt acted as a deterrent.

In 1896 Dr. A. L. Spinning, of the Prison North, in his report says: "Owing to the limited facilities for caring for the insane patients, they are by necessity confined in very undesirable places awaiting a permit to transfer to an insane hospital."

And thus for year after year this sad and inexcusable condition existed; insane patients were confined in cells, misunderstood and uncared for. Annual reports, private letters, and verbal communications all indicate the same condition of pathetic neglect.

In 1897 a radical change was made in the correctional system of the state, for in that year the indeterminate sentence and parole law was enacted. The Prison South at Jeffersonville became the reformatory; the Prison North became the state prison.

The young men then at Michigan City were transferred to Jeffersonville; the men over-age at the reformatory were transferred to the prison; also at various dates since there have been transfers of "incorrigibles" and men over-age from the reformatory to the prison. All these facts have a very important bearing upon the character of the prison population and partly explain the rapid increase of the insane.

Another advance was at least advocated when the Legislature of 1899 provided for the establishment of the "Indiana Hospital for Criminal Insane" at Jeffersonville under the management of the reformatory and appropriated $25,000 therefor; the capacity to be 50 beds. However, nothing was done and the fund reverted to the State Treasury. The location was not considered proper, "and the circumstances were such that it was impossible to do the work in the time specified."

Warden George A. H. Shidler, in his report for 1900, states that the prison is caring for 20 insane and a nearly equal number of feeble-minded. He adds: "This department is a source of great concern to the management; we are not equipped for the care of insane men. . . . . I certainly recommend a hospital for insane criminals."

At this time an attendant of experience was in charge of the insane, though they were still confined in the cell house.

All through this period frequent reference is found in the annual reports to the need of better provision for the care of defectives, either in a separate institution or at least in a proper ward, which was finally opened in 1902 during the service of Warden James D. Reid; it was a modest ward, situated on the second floor of the general hospital of the prison.

Referring to this event Dr. L. H. Streaker in his report under date of October 31, 1902, says:

"At that time one of the most radical changes that has been made in connection with this institution for a number of years was inaugurated, when our insane—22 in number—were transferred from their cells to the hospital, where a large, well-ventilated and comfortable day room and dormitory had been prepared for them." This provided for all insane but two or three cases under observation.

In the spring of 1905 a yard for the exercise of patients was provided; and in October of that year an additional ward was opened, bringing the capacity up to 42.

Under existing conditions no further increase was made till the present hospital was opened.

During this interval the most urgent cases were cared for in the insane ward; the others in the cell houses, being given such employment and exercise as were possible.

The rate at which defectives were accumulating in this period is indicated by the following figures:

Dr. Streaker in his report under the date of October 31, 1904, with a prison population of 833, gives a total of 56 defectives (39 insane, 14 feeble-minded and 3 epileptic).

In October, 1906, the writer classed 112 as defective, about 12 per cent of the population (67 insane; 4 feeble-minded; 16 epileptic; 25 constitutionally inferior); 48 of these were received within the biennial period.

On September 30, 1908, the prison population was 1128. The defectives numbered 170 (88 insane; 3 feeble-minded; 23 epileptic; 56 constitutionally inferior).

By September, 1910, with a total population of 1096, the defectives numbered 190 (147 insane; 27 epileptic; 16 constitutionally inferior).

In his report for the year ending September 30, 1912, Dr. Paul E. Bowers (since April, 1911, physician to the prison) states that lunacy commissions had been held on 78 cases; 36 insane had been transferred from the reformatory; 18 had been committed by the courts; and 48 others were under observation, pending commissions in the near future.

Thus before the Hospital for Criminal Insane was ready to be occupied the prison already contained 180 patients for its 145 beds; these figures include very few belonging to the moron group.

So far as available data indicate, the situation at the Prison South corresponds to that of the Prison North up to 1897; at that date the transformation of the Jeffersonville institution into the reformatory, with its younger class of men, altered somewhat the character of its problem, though without decreasing its difficulty.

The act of authorization called for a building having a capacity of not less than 145 beds; the appropriation of $65,000 to cover equipment also.

The yard contains about four acres, being 300 by 600 feet, and is surrounded by a wall 24 feet high; the north wall of this yard is the south wall of the prison; 1200 lineal feet of new wall were built at a cost of some $10,000, leaving about $55,000 for building and equipment.

The building consists of a three-story center with two-story wings extending at an angle of 45 degrees from each day room;

the first and second floors are duplicates; each has a central dining room, with a day room to the right and left; from each day room leads a wide corridor with single rooms on either side, and at the end a dormitory of 18 beds; there are thus two wards on each floor. The third floor contains a dormitory, offices, operating room, dispensary and a modest hydrotherapy outfit. The present capacity is 172.

The building is red brick, with concrete block trimmings; the roof steel truss, reinforced concrete and tile; partitions brick or hollow tile; subfloors reinforced concrete; the day room floors and the third-story dormitory, hard maple. The side room floors are finished in cement; all other floors are terrazzo. With the exception of the side rooms and second-floor dormitories, the first and second floors are wainscoted throughout with terrazzo slabs—part of it in panel. All doors are built up, birch veneer, mahogany finish, brass trimmings, perfectly plain. The windows are protected by substantial basket window guards. The bathrooms and lavatories contain the usual standard porcelain equipment; in addition one-half of the side rooms have porcelain toilet seats.

The building is electric-lighted, and heated by forced indirect radiation. The furniture is plain, substantial, antique oak made by the reformatory at Jeffersonville.

The plans and specifications were worked out by Freyermuth & Maurer, of South Bend, from the original drafts prepared by the institution.

The appropriation was secured by Warden James D. Reid; after his death, September 2, 1910, the building was carried to completion under the direction of Warden E. J. Fogarty.

The practical results and economy obtained are due in no small degree to the efficient supervision of Mr. A. C. Clark, for many years superintendent of construction of the prison.

The location of the hospital at the prison has never had the unqualified approval of the Board of State Charities. This board took the ground that it should be removed from prison influence and be either a separate institution or located at one of the hospitals for insane.

But a separate institution was financially out of the question; none of the hospitals were anxious for the addition, though perhaps one might have consented. The need was urgent; the prison could do the work at greatly reduced cost to the state, and stood ready to undertake it.

That the state will need to provide a separate institution for criminal defectives in the not distant future is evident; and in that event broad acres must be secured and other advantages sought.

Under the administration of Warden E. J. Fogarty, the hospital was opened October 19, 1912, Dr. Paul E. Bowers, physician to the prison, being the physician in charge.

By a readjustment of duties, the writer on April 1, 1913, was assigned to the Hospital for Insane; Dr. Bowers continuing his efficient service in the prison. This relieved the pressure of medical work, and also a possible embarrassment growing out of the fact that heretofore the preliminary proceedings for commitment and the recommendation for discharge were vested in the same individual.

The force consists of one supervisor; seven day attendants; five night attendants.

Maintenance is derived from the prison appropriation. The food is prepared in the kitchen of the prison hospital and delivered through a subway. Heat, light, laundering and repairs are likewise derived from the prison.

So far occupation has been fairly abundant; housework is an unfailing source of employment; an acre devoted to gardening has been of especial value; grading the grounds and preparing walks and playgrounds, the care of lawns and flowers, all have been entered into with zest.

Baseball is the favorite out-of-doors recreation and has an enthusiastic following. Sunday afternoon concerts by the prison band; an occasional moving picture entertainment; the usual indoor games; books, magazines, a piano and stringed instruments; a vocal music class; a limited amount of drawing and fancy work, afford partial relief from monotony.

The Legislature of 1915 appropriated $10,000 for the purchase of equipment and material for the manufacture of such simple articles as will best furnish work to those whom it is possible to thus employ. A request for an industrial building and a larger garden was denied.

Patients are committed to the hospital:

1. From the prison or reformatory upon an order of the Governor, after a properly appointed lunacy commission has found the prisoner insane.

2. Upon an order of any court of competent jurisdiction, a special plea of insanity made at the time of trial having been sustained.

In either event the commitment is indefinite as to time; discharge is contingent upon recovery, and is not influenced by expiration of sentence; time passed in the hospital counts on the sentence, however.

Of the 205 men admitted up to September 30, 1914, 35 were committed by the courts; 124 were committed from the prison; 46 were committed from the reformatory (of those from the prison 18 had been transferred from the reformatory prior to being declared insane).

Of these, 64 were charged with crimes of violence (murder, assault, or manslaughter); 25 with sexual crimes (rape, sodomy, incest); 41 with burglary, robbery or arson; 70 with larceny, embezzlement or forgery; 5 with bigamy, wife desertion, obstructing railway track.

There were: white, 155; colored, 50.

Sec. 16½ of the act of 1909 which governed commitment by the courts was by the Supreme Court held unconstitutional, in that it provided only for "the trial of any *male* person accused of felony . . . . ." This defect was corrected by the law of 1913.

In order to adjust matters 20 men who had been committed by the courts before the amendment of 1913 were, upon order of the Governor, returned to their respective counties (August 7, 1913).

As compared with the ordinary hospitals for insane, perhaps the most striking difference is the large number of cases of dementia præcox, especially of the paranoid type; persecutory delusions abound; acute psychoses, either manic or depressive, are rare; general paresis is not frequent (six cases in 205 admissions). The ethical standard is low. Unfortunately the number of recoveries is small.

In a modest way hydrotheraphy is used with excellent results. The Wassermann or Noguchi tests were applied in 1914 to 165 men; 44 of these showed positive reaction.

So far as it has been possible to trace the family history, mental or nervous defects appear in an exceedingly large per cent of cases; complete figures are not at this time available.

In the daily routine no especial difficulties are encountered other than those common to middle and back wards; nor are measures incompatible with the highest hospital standards necessary.

INDIANA SCHOOL FOR FEEBLE-MINDED YOUTH.[1]

Fort Wayne, Ind.

The Indiana School for Feeble-minded Youth was established by the Indiana Legislature in the year 1879, and the children were housed along with the sailors' and soldiers' orphans at Knightstown, Ind. By the end of 1886, 175 children had been received. In 1887 the Legislature gave the Indiana School for Feeble-minded Youth an independent existence, appropriating $10,000 to purchase land located near Fort Wayne and $40,000 to begin the erection of buildings thereon. With the $10,000 appropriated for the purchase of land the Board of Trustees secured 57 acres one and a half miles northeast of the City of Fort Wayne. The first building was completed in 1890 and 300 children were removed from Richmond, where they had been temporarily housed in a building erected for a hospital for the insane, after the building at Knightstown had been destroyed by fire. In the year 1893 some farm land was rented about a mile and a half northeast of the institution; in 1895 the sum of $20,000 for farm land and $10,000 for buildings was granted by the Legislature. With this amount 255 acres of land were purchased, which was the beginning of the farm colony, which now is composed of 564 acres. About 30 acres are in garden, 25 acres in orchard and small fruits and the remainder in pasture and general farm crops. There is a dairy herd of 75 cows, 30 head of horses, 25 colts and 150 hogs. On this farm is a brick building for boys, with a capacity for 180 inmates.

On the home grounds the original buildings planned and constructed consist of a school house, administration building, with chapel and dining room, attached to which is a wing for a group of

[1] By Dr. George S. Bliss, superintendent.

220 boys on the east, and 290 girls on the west; one hospital building, one power plant and laundry, and one industrial building. Many buildings have been added since to the original group; a custodial cottage for girls was finished in May, 1900, with capacity for 180. In this building are housed a group of girls who are unable to attend school or do very much constructive industrial work. The next large building was finished in August, 1902; it provides for 135 feeble-minded adult women, to be admitted between the ages of 16 and 45 years. The capacity of this building was increased by the construction of another building in connection with it of about the same capacity, for the same class of inmates, in 1911. The cottage for the custodial grade of boys, which accommodates 180 inmates, was finished July 1, 1907. This present year there have been erected the center part and east wing of a large hospital building at a cost of $110,000, which will care for 100 patients, with extra rooms for nurses and other help. This will be occupied about July 1, 1915.

The buildings of various description on the main institution grounds are 24 in number, valued at $663,000; at colony farm, 25 in number, valued at $75,000.

The children are housed under mental grade and classification in cottages ranging from 180 to 280 in capacity. Each cottage has a matron in charge, with sufficient attendants and other help. Each cottage has a separate dining room and kitchen.

The school term extends for nine months of the year and is under the direction of a principal and a staff of 14 teachers. The schools are graded similarly to the public schools, but the work is necessarily very slow and few of the children advance above the sixth grade.

Children are developed especially along the lines of manual training, greatly excelling the public schools in this respect. Besides the regular school development, 12 purely industrial teachers work with the children in different departments of the institution, making baskets, rugs, shoes, mattresses, boys' clothing, girls' clothing, baking, etc.

Special attention is given to music. There is a girls' orchestra and a boys' band; several large classes among the boys and girls are doing chorus work, and a number of girls take piano lessons.

The population as of September 30, 1913, was, boys, 545; girls, 472; adult females, 235; total, 1252.

SUPERINTENDENT.

George S. Bliss, M. D.

RESIDENT PHYSICIAN.

Thomas L. Taylor, M. D.

ASSISTANT PHYSICIAN.

Nellie Hanaway, M. D.

W. C. Boren, D. D. S., dental interne.
Melvin Druckemiller, chief clerk.
Edith C. Bell, principal school department.

INDIANA VILLAGE FOR EPILEPTICS.[1]

NEW CASTLE, IND.

On March 6, 1905, the General Assembly of the State of Indiana approved an act for the establishment of an institution for "the scientific treatment, education, employment and custody of epileptic residents of Indiana," to be known as the Indiana Village for Epileptics.

The act provided for the appointment by the Governor of a commission to purchase not less than 1000 acres of land, the subsequent appointment of a superintendent, the procuring of building plans, the form of commitment, etc., and appropriated the sum of $150,000 for carrying out the provisions of the act.

The commission completed the task of selection and purchase of the land in the early spring of 1906. The site selected consists of 1250 acres of diversified land located three miles north of New Castle, Henry County, Ind. The tract includes the valley of the Blue River one mile in width and the wooded blue grass hills on either side of the valley.

[1] By Dr. W. C. Van Nuys, superintendent.

The members of the Board of Trustees were appointed and assumed office March 17, 1906. Dr. W. C. Van Nuys was appointed superintendent and assumed his duties May 9, 1906.

The plan of development as worked out contemplated the utilization of the Blue River Valley for the separation of the sexes, and the erection of three groups of buildings for patients on each side of the valley as follows:

1. A group for adults of the better class. 2. A group for children of the better class. 3. A group for low grade adults and children.

The plan contemplates the further classification of each group in small, plain, simply constructed buildings, most of them one-story, the construction of school and industrial buildings in the various groups and the construction of certain general buildings, such as administration building, chapel, power house, store room, cold storage, bakery, etc., in a separate group centrally located.

Up to the present time progress has been made as follows:

1. A temporary frame building erected. 2. Eight old houses remodeled for residences for superintendent, steward, farmer, gardener, and three farm employees. 3. Two cottages erected for secretary and bookkeeper. 4. An adequate water supply provided, including deep wells, electric pumps, 100-foot water tower located on highest elevation and bricked in, and between three and four miles of 6-inch water mains extending to vicinity of all buildings constructed or proposed. 5. Electric light and power lines to sites of all buildings constructed or proposed. 6. Private telephone lines with switch-board connecting office with all parts of premises. 7. Reinforced concrete and brick "service building," comprising storeroom, cold storage, bakery and ice manufacturing plant, centrally located on a 15 car siding. 8. A start has been made in four of the six contemplated groups of buildings for patients. Ten buildings for patients are completed and occupied. 9. Five buildings, including power house, are in course of construction. These buildings should be ready for occupancy June 1, 1915, and will increase the capacity about 100. 10. Three large modern barns have been constructed for dairy, horses and stock cattle. 11. Numerous minor improvements have been made; old barns and sheds have been repaired, lawns graded and roads made, 16

miles of wire fence erected, shade and shrubbery, fruit trees and small fruits planted.

Appropriations available October 1, 1915, will provide for the construction of two cottages for 50 boys; $21,350 for the improvement of the farm, repair of old buildings etc.; and $111,900 for beginning one of the groups for females.

The institution has grown quite slowly to its present capacity of 234 patients, but is in position now to expand more rapidly. No buildings for females have been constructed.

It is not expected that the ultimate population will be in excess of 1500, but the plan of separate groups and independent units in these groups will admit of this number being doubled without serious inconvenience.

So far no indoor industries have been established. The patients engage in all sorts of outdoor work and live in the open air so far as possible. It is hoped to have industrial buildings in the near future and the institution is in need of special hospital facilities denied it by the last General Assembly.

THE CARE OF THE INSANE IN IOWA.

No provision existed in Iowa for the care of the insane prior to the establishment of the Mt. Pleasant State Hospital. Some who were troublesome or dangerous to be at large were confined in common jails, while others remained at large, a terror to their friends and neighbors and exposed to hardships and ill-treatment.

The first state hospital for the insane was opened at Mt. Pleasant, Iowa, March 6, 1861, and on the 30th day of the next November had 140 patients. The state then had a population of 750,000.

The second state hospital was opened at Independence, Iowa, in 1873; the third at Clarinda about 1888, and the fourth and last at Cherokee in August, 1902. The name of the town where the institution is located preceding the words "State Hospital," constitutes the legal name of each hospital, as, Mt. Pleasant State Hospital.

In addition to the above, a department for the criminal insane has been established in connection with the reformatory at Anamosa in 1888. In 1876 the state established the Iowa Institution for Feeble-minded Children at Glenwood, Iowa; and in 1906 the State Hospital for Inebriates at Knoxville.[1] This last is an institution for the care of narcotic and alcoholic cases, and has a capacity of 225 beds.

State hospitals for the insane in Iowa are not distinct legal entities, but are agencies of the state without separate corporate existence. Each one is carried on by its own officers and employees with a superintendent, who must be a physician, at the head.

Prior to July, 1898, each hospital was under the control of its own board of managers, sometimes called commissioners and sometimes called trustees, but at the time named they passed under the Board of Control of State Institutions, which now supervises and directs their management, the construction of buildings and the purchase of machinery and supplies.

All patients received in state hospitals are examined and committed by the Commissioners of Insanity. There are no voluntary patients. It is not necessary that all commitments of the Com-

[1] The committee has been unable to obtain a history of this institution.

missioners of Insanity be made to state hospitals; they may be made to private institutions properly equipped, or to county homes in cases not requiring hospital care, as, for example, cases of senile dementia.

When patients, in the opinion of the superintendent, are cured they are discharged by him as cured, but most of those released are paroled or discharged as improved or unimproved, or are transferred to county homes.

Patients are paroled when their condition warrants a trial outside the institution, and many are discharged while on parole. Those transferred to county homes are such as are not likely to be benefited by further hospital treatment. All patients not cured are released or transferred only on the order of the Board of Control.

Periodical appropriations for the support of patients are not required, but there is a standing appropriation of $14 per month for each patient in the state hospitals at Mt. Pleasant and Clarinda, and $15 per month for each patient in the Independence and Cherokee hospitals. These sums are paid monthly from the state treasury, but each county is required to refund this sum to the state for each patient having a legal settlement in the county, and the county is authorized to collect it from the patient or his responsible relative. About one-twelfth of the patients have no known legal settlement in the state and are supported by the state. In addition to the per capita allowance, each hospital has a farm, the smallest containing 860 acres, all of which farms are cultivated largely by patients and yield bountifully in farm and garden products. The per capita allowance and products of farms and gardens pay the salaries of the officers and employees, and for food supplies, fuel and other ordinary expenses of carrying on the hospitals, including ordinary repairs.

Insane in Private and County Institutions.—About one-fourth of the insane of the state who require custodial care are in private and county institutions. Those in county homes are almost wholly supported by the counties; those in private institutions are supported by themselves or relatives or friends. Both of these classes of institutions are subject to inspection by the Board of Control, and patients not properly cared for are moved by it from such institutions to state hospitals. In practice, most of the requirements of the Board of Control are met and there are few removals to state hospitals.

There have been few radical changes in the laws relating to the commitment and treatment of the insane since 1870. The most important are the creation of the Board of Control and the provision relating to the inspection of county and private institutions and removal in case of lack of proper facilities, abuse or lack of proper care.

It is believed that the system of care now in vogue is equal to that of other states except as to voluntary commitments and provisions for care and observation before commitment in psychopathic hospitals. There are no provisions for such commitments to and care in state institutions. Admissions to state hospitals are made only on formal commitments by boards of commissioners of insanity.

Private institutions for the care of the insane are authorized to receive and restrain patients on the certificate of two reputable physicians, at least one of whom shall be a resident of the state, and many insane patients are so received and treated by such institutions. The right of such institutions to restrain a patient so received against his will has never been adjudicated in this state.

The effect of a finding by a board of commissioners of insanity that a person is insane and his commitment to a hospital for treatment creates a presumption of insanity and of a lack of contractual ability, and this presumption continues until the patient is discharged as cured or he is found to be sane by a judicial tribunal authorized to act. The law of the state on this matter is neither full nor clear.

Classes Committed.—All insane persons not idiots, with a legal residence in the state, are entitled to admission. Persons found without a legal settlement must be cared for in a state hospital until their legal residence can be ascertained.

Legal Procedure for Commitment.—Each county has a Board of three Commissioners of Insanity and whenever the district court is held in two places, one such board at each place, consisting of the clerk of the district court, or his deputy, one physician in actual practice and of good professional standing, one lawyer in actual practice and of good standing, to be appointed by the judge of the district court for terms of two years. The clerk of the board must sign and issue all notices, appointments, warrants, etc., and file and preserve in his office all papers connected with any inquest by the commissioners.

Application to the Commissioners of Insanity for admission to the hospital must be made in the form of information, verified by affidavit, alleging that the person is believed to be insane. The commissioners may examine the informant and other witnesses under oath and may require that the person be brought before them. Any citizen of the county or relative may appear and resist application and employ counsel. The commissioners must appoint some regular practising physician of the county to make a personal examination of the person, who must obtain from the relatives or from others answers to prescribed interrogatories, to be attached to his certificate. If the commissioners find the person is not insane they must order his immediate discharge, but if insane and a fit subject for custody and treatment they must order his commitment to the hospital in the district in which the county is situated.

The Commissioners of Insanity, with the consent of the Board of Supervisors of any county having insane persons and no proper facilities for their care and treatment, may, with the consent of the Board of Control, provide for their care at the expense of the county at any convenient private or county institution.

No person may be confined in any private institution except upon certificates of a Board of Commissioners of Insanity of some county in the state, or two reputable physicians, at least one of whom must be a *bona fide* resident of the state.

Appeal from Commitment.—On a statement in writing, verified by affidavits to a judge of the district court of the county in which the hospital is situated, or of the county of his legal settlement, the judge must appoint a commission of not more than three persons, one a physician and another a lawyer. They must forthwith report to the judge the result of their examination and accompany it by a statement of the case, made and signed by the superintendent. If the judge finds the person not insane he must order his discharge; otherwise he must authorize his continued detention. The applicant must pay the costs if the judge finds that the application was without probable grounds. A commission of inquiry may not be repeated oftener than once in six months.

Costs of Commitment.—The expenses of arrest, care, investigation and commitment of an insane person without legal settlement are paid by the county in which the person is found. If he has a legal settlement in another county the expenses are to be paid by that county. If the person has no legal settlement within the state, the expenses are paid by the state.

MT. PLEASANT STATE HOSPITAL.[1]

Mt. Pleasant, Iowa.

At the opening of the Fifth General Assembly of the State of Iowa in 1855 Governor Grimes in his message strongly urged the erection of a state hospital for the insane.

The following is an extract from his message:

> The General Assembly cannot be too urgently called upon to take immediate steps to establish state charitable institutions. According to the most reliable information there are more than 100 pauper insane persons in the state; one-half of these are confined in common jails and are thus placed beyond a reasonable hope of recovery. The others are remaining at large, a terror to their friends and neighbors and by exposure to exciting causes rendering their diseases hopelessly incurable. Every dictate of humanity and every principle of sound policy demands that the state should make immediate provision for the care and treatment of this unfortunate class of fellow-citizens.

A commission was accordingly selected by the Legislature, consisting of Governor Grimes, Edward Johnston and Dr. Charles A. Clark. These men had business experience, and were honest, conscientious and zealous in the discharge of the duty assigned them. Governor Grimes was succeeded by Governor Lowe and he in turn by Governor Kirkwood as an *ex-officio* member. This was the pioneer work of the state in public charities.

The 6th section of the act establishing the hospital provided that the cost of the building should not exceed $50,000, "but it is advised that the plan determined upon by the board should be one to admit of future enlargement."

The commission purchased 173 acres of land adjoining the City of Mt. Pleasant on the southeast, the ground itself being well adapted to the use proposed, being part prairie and part undulating woodland. The commission seems to have had but little idea of a water supply requisite for the wants of even 300 patients or of the necessity of providing for the removal of the sewage; in fact they thought that an ordinary well in front of the building 10 feet in

[1] The material for this history of this institution prior to 1898 has been extracted from the Bulletin of State Institutions, Volume III, pp. 305-316; the material subsequent to that date has been furnished by C. F. Applegate, M. D., superintendent.

diameter and 50 or 60 feet deep, with some large cisterns in the rear of the building to catch roof water, would afford an ample supply of water. Had they been conversant with the needs of such an institution, by the addition of a few hundred dollars they could have purchased a farm west of the town and adjacent to the track of the C. B. & Q. R. R., where there was an abundant supply of pure drinking water and where a full supply for other wants could have been obtained from Big Creek, only a half mile distant. The selection of this site would have saved the state an expenditure of $50,000 in the item of water supply.

The commission entered upon its duties and visited Boston and other cities in the East and conferred with Drs. Ray, Bell and Kirkbride. Their visit convinced them that the sum of $50,000 was entirely inadequate for a building such as the wants of the state demanded. They determined to erect a substantial building, with a capacity for 300 or 350 patients, which it was estimated would cost $300,000 or $350,000, and to rely on the generosity of the Legislature and the people of the state to carry through the project. Alvin Saunders, member of the Senate, and Samuel McFarland, member of the House, were responsible for the passage of this measure and the location of the institution at Mt. Pleasant.

Saunders afterwards became Governor of Nebraska and Colonel McFarland fell at the head of his regiment at Prairie Grove in 1862.

When the commission decided upon the plan for a building that would accommodate 300 inmates at a cost of $300,000 or $400,000 a hue and cry went up from all parts of the state at the elaborate plan adopted and the required outlay of state funds.

At the next session of the General Assembly contentions arose over the large appropriations required to carry on the work; a stringency in monetary affairs had opened up; banks by the score were breaking; there was a financial depression and a crisis such as that of 1836 and 1837. There were violent contentions in the Legislature; investigating committees were the order of the day. It required strong men to stem the storm, but Grimes, Saunders and McFarland were the men to meet it.

It was a bold undertaking and perilous to the party in power to attempt the building of such a structure as the commissioners adopted with the meager appropriations made by the Seventh

General Assembly. The opposite political party took advantage of this dilemma and hurled against the party the bitterest kind of denunciation.

In their embarrassed condition for funds the Legislature passed an act in 1855 to appropriate all funds derived from the sale of the saline lands for this purpose. This act was, however, repealed in 1857 and no funds were derived from this source.

The commissioners selected Henry Winslow, from the State of Maine, as superintendent of the building. He had been engaged in like work in the East, and entered upon his duties in October, 1855, and remained in charge of the work until the opening in 1861, when he was selected steward by the Board of Trustees. As the work on the building was not yet completed he also remained in charge of it in connection with his duties as steward.

The first meeting of the Board of Trustees appointed by the Legislature met December 1, 1858, and formed a temporary organization by electing Samuel McFarland, president, and J. M. Shaffer, secretary.

The hospital being in an unfinished condition and unfit for the reception of patients, nothing was done except recommending that the commissioners make a loan of $50,000 to carry on the work and to put it, as soon as possible, in a condition for use.

March 2, 1859, the board met and decided that it was inexpedient to elect a superintendent at that time.

Again on the 6th of July, 1860, the following trustees met: Samuel McFarland, Harpin Riggs, G. W. Kinkaid, John B. Lash, Maturin L. Fisher, D. L. McGugin, E. L. Elbert, and permanently organized with Fisher as president and McFarland as secretary.

The work of the building was not sufficiently advanced to justify the board in electing the first superintendent until a meeting in September, 1860. There were many aspirants for the position. The board was unanimous in offering it to Dr. McGugin, of Keokuk, on account of his distinguished position in the profession, but he declined to accept because his whole time was occupied in his college work and general practice and furthermore, as he stated, he was well advanced in years and had no special training for duties pertaining to the superintendency of such an institution.

Dr. R. J. Patterson was then elected head of the institution and entered upon his duties in March, 1861. The salary of the superintendent was then fixed at $1600 per year with residence in the hospital.

Dr. Dewey, of Iowa City, was elected first assistant and ably and faithfully discharged his duties in that capacity until he resigned.

The formal opening of the institution was in March, 1861, when the board and superintendent announced the institution ready to admit patients.

The cry against the extravagance of the state in providing such a capacious structure was met in 1865 by the urgent appeal of the superintendent and trustees for more room; that the capacity of the building was overtaxed; that the number of patients had reached 400 and that 350 were the outside limit.

Again in the sixth biennial report the number had increased to 500 and the residents of other states and territories had been removed or orders had been issued for their removal. The overcrowded condition had become a serious embarrassment to the authorities. The harmless and incurable were ordered back to their respective counties as fast as the counties could in any way provide for their care.

In 1865 Dr. Patterson, who had served the institution in a very acceptable manner for nearly five years, tendered his resignation to take effect October 1. The Board of Trustees at their quarterly meeting in September elected Dr. Mark Ranney as his successor. Dr. Ranney appeared and qualified as superintendent October 1, 1865.

Dr. Dewey resigned his position about this time and Dr. H. M. Bassett, who before this time had been second assistant, was made first assistant.

In 1873 Dr. Ranney resigned in order to take charge of the State Hospital for the Insane at Madison, Wis. He vacated his position July 4, 1873, and Dr. H. M. Bassett was made his successor. In the spring of 1875 the trustees became convinced that matters were not running smoothly under the administration of Dr. Bassett, charges of mismanagement having been made in various quarters. In March, 1875, the trustees met and an investigation was ordered which resulted in the following findings:

The board having completed their investigations into the affairs, general condition and management of the hospital, find no gross abuses. Yet they find many violations of the rules adopted for the government of the hospital and inexcusable negligence in many instances on the part of the employees.

After this action of the board Dr. Bassett promptly tendered his resignation, as did likewise his assistants. The failure of Dr. Bassett was solely on account of his lack of executive ability; he had labored honestly and faithfully, but could not control the work of his subordinates.

About this time Dr. Ranney, who had resigned his position at Madison on account of some friction between himself and his Board of Trustees, was in Chicago arranging for a visit abroad. A member of the board from this hospital was deputed to visit him and offer him his old position, which he accepted on the condition that Dr. Bassett should remain as his assistant. He at once re-entered his work here in March, 1875.

By this change order was soon restored and the institution placed in good working order and continued so until his death, which occurred in February, 1882, from acute pneumonia.

After the death of Dr. Ranney Dr. Bassett again became temporary superintendent. At a special meeting of the board July, 1882, Dr. H. A. Gilman, assistant physician in the Jacksonville Institution for the Insane, was elected superintendent and soon after entered upon his duties.

Like his predecessor, Dr. Ranney, he had had a long training under eminently careful and experienced guides for this special work.

Dr. Bassett remained the ever faithful assistant up to the time of his death in July, 1887.

Dr. Max Witte, afterward superintendent of the Clarinda Hospital, succeeded Dr. Bassett as first assistant.

Dr. Gilman remained as head of the institution until October 8, 1898, when his death occurred suddenly from cerebral hemorrhage.

After purchasing the original plat of ground for the hospital, 173 acres, the commissioners purchased a roadway to the hospital grounds 100 feet wide. This road was on a line a little east of the original building. It became apparent to the trustees that the land lying between the hospital grounds and the main highway would in all probability soon be divided up into lots and be sold for dwelling purposes and perhaps small houses and outbuildings would be erected and would thus obstruct the front view of the building. Hence they determined, if possible, to secure this ground for decorative purposes.

After one year's consideration of the subject the board, at its annual meeting in 1869, made a purchase of this property, consisting of 12 acres, for $2700.

The following spring Mr. Cleveland, of Chicago, a man with much experience in designing such improvements, was employed to make a survey of these grounds. He presented a design which was adopted and the improvements in drives and walks and ornamentation which have been made from time to time since have been made substantially in accordance with this design.

In May, 1861, the trustees concluded to sink an artesian well on the premises. At a depth of about 1100 feet they obtained a fair supply of water, but it was not of good quality.

The only pure water for use was rain water from the roof collected in cisterns and this amount would suffice only for a few months during the rainy portion of the year.

In 1866 Mr. Chesbrough, an hydraulic engineer of standing in Chicago, was consulted in regard to obtaining a supply of water by a system of reservoirs. This engineer submitted plans and estimates for draining the creek east of the hospital building and pumping water into a reservoir on the north. His plans and suggestions were adopted by the board.

After the system of reservoirs was completed the superintendent and trustees congratulated themselves that the water question had been solved. The reservoir in front of the building, 200 feet in diameter at top, 160 at bottom, was filled during a freshet and retained water with but little leakage.

The dam in the branch running east of the building afforded an outlet for a large water shed, dry in summer, but affording a large amount of water in spring and autumn. A large amount of earth was removed from the bottom and a substantial wall with stone abutments was thrown across the branch and a boiler house erected. From this the reservoir in front could be kept filled by a surplus from the dam and reservoirs below. Thus a good supply of water existed constantly for fire protection.

The county infirmary on the ground adjacent to the hospital grew apace with the population of the county. In order to find an outlet for their sewage they drained it into a branch on their farm which opened into the main branch and consequently into the basin. Besides this the water-shed for miles along the branch became thickly settled; the drainage from houses, barn yards and stock yards with the drainage from the county house polluted the reservoir water and rendered it wholly unfit for drinking purposes. In consequence typhoid fever and other diseases were prevalent from impure drinking water.

After years of trial with the reservoir system, a company contracted with the City of Mt. Pleasant for a water supply from Big Creek. At a point one and one-half miles from the city a dam was made across the creek and water pumped into a tank in the city and pressure thus obtained for fire and culinary purposes. The hospital agreed and contracted for a supply of water from this source. A few dry summers made the supply short; besides it was often so full of vegetable matter and dust that it was wholly unfit for use in the buildings. An extensive filter was constructed at the hospital, which obviated in a measure this difficulty.

The hospital farm as now constituted is a very valuable tract of land; although a high price was paid for a portion of it, yet as a whole it is now worth twice its original cost. The surface is sufficiently diversified to make it attractive, and being partly rich prairie land and partly broken woodland, it affords fine blue grass pasturage for the milk cattle and fertile land for roots and cereals.

The pressing importance of more room for the insane of the state was met in 1883 by the appropriation of $100,000 to add a wing on the east of the building with a capacity for 200 male patients, and in 1885 the same amount to complete a wing to the west to accommodate the females. These two wings doubled the capacity of the institution and enabled the superintendent to keep up a better classification of patients. They were built under the direction of Dr. Gilman and the work was done in a very substantial manner.

During the efficient management of the institution by Drs. Ranney and Gilman many substantial changes were made and many defects were corrected; although lacking in some respects the convenience of a modern hospital, it is still a substantial and commodious building, meeting the wants of the state in this regard.

During the year 1898 the Board of Control of State Institutions of Iowa was given full charge of all of the state institutions.

Dr. Gilman died in the fall of 1898, and Dr. Frank C. Hoyt, former superintendent of the Clarinda State Hospital, Clarinda, Iowa, was appointed his successor.

At the same time Dr. Max E. Witte, the first assistant physician of the Mt. Pleasant State Hospital, was given charge of the Clarinda State Hospital. This change was made because Dr. Hoyt had proved very efficient in organization, and the Mt. Pleasant State Hospital was in a run-down and disorganized condition. Dr. Hoyt continued in charge of the institution for about two years and six months, when he died.

Dr. C. F. Applegate, first assistant at the Clarinda State Hospital, was placed in charge of the Mt. Pleasant State Hospital in June, 1901.

Considerable money has been appropriated for improvements, additional buildings and for enlargement of the farm during the 12 years subsequent to 1901. Most of the wards of the institution have been thoroughly overhauled, much painting has been done, new ceilings have been placed on most of the wards and many new floors have been installed. Barns that were near the building have been moved to some distance and reconstructed and a new laundry, cow barn, sheds, piggeries, etc., have been built.

A new psychopathic hospital complete for women has been constructed at a cost of about $90,000, fully equipped, and has been in use during the past four years.

A new addition to the tuberculosis hospital has recently been completed and will soon be occupied. The basement of the main building throughout has been cemented, all steam corridors have been thoroughly cleaned and cement floors placed in them. A new general kitchen and a new bakery have been built, and there are other changes of importance in the main building. A poultry plant, the largest of any state institution in this country, has been in operation for several years.

The farm, which originally consisted of 500 acres, has been enlarged by the purchase of adjoining land, until there are now about 1000 acres. The garden, which originally consisted of about 20 acres, has been increased to 60 acres. Vineyards, cherry orchards, peach orchards and a large apple orchard have been planted, and some of the trees now bear fruit.

Almost 3000 lineal feet of tunnel have been constructed, carrying all the water pipes, steam and return pipes, electric wiring, telephone wires, etc., and connecting the new building to the main building and engine room. The front lawns and grounds about the building have been changed and greatly improved.

In the past few years a large dairy herd has been raised on the hospital farm, and this institution now has one of the finest dairy herds of the Middle West.

The Thirty-fifth General Assembly of Iowa appropriated $90,000 for the building of a new psychopathic hospital for men. Appropriations are now being asked for an employees' home, the superintendent's residence and additional land.

This is the oldest state institution of Iowa, except the prison at Fort Madison. While the institution is old, it is in fairly good repair and in architecture and general arrangement the main building is very much like the institutions that are being built to-day; in fact this institution was greatly in advance of the times when it was planned and constructed, as there has not been much change in the general architecture of main buildings during the past 60 years. All additional buildings will be on the cottage plan. The main criticism of this main building is that it is too large, and there are not sufficient cottages.

SUPERINTENDENTS.

Dr. R. J. Patterson	1861-1865	Dr. H. A. Gilman.......	1882-1898
Dr. Mark Ranney.......	1865-1873	Dr. Frank C. Hoyt......	1898-1901
Dr. H. M. Bassett.......	1873-1875	Dr. C. F. Applegate (in office)	1901-
Dr. Mark Ranney.......	1875-1882		

ASSISTANT PHYSICIANS.

Dr. Dewey	1861-1865	Dr. C. F. Davis.........	in office
Dr. H. M. Bassett......	1865-1873 1875-1887	Dr. P. M. Murdock.....	in office
		Dr. J. Hermanies.......	in office
Dr. Max Witte.........	1887-1901	Dr. Ella Blackburn.....	in office
Dr. Frank T. Stevens...	1898-1910	Dr. Amelia Dickinson...	in office
Dr. T. E. Roe..........	in office		

INDEPENDENCE STATE HOSPITAL.[1]

INDEPENDENCE, IOWA.

An act providing for the erection of a second state hospital for the insane was passed by the Iowa Legislature April 6, 1868. This bill was introduced by Senator W. G. Donnon, of Buchanan County. The act designated E. G. Morgan, Maturin L. Fisher and Albert Clark a Board of Commissioners to locate the institution and erect the buildings. It required that a site comprising not less than 320 acres of land be obtained within two miles of the City of Independence and without cost to the state. The sum of $125,000 was appropriated for the erection of buildings.

It is said that this action to locate the hospital at Independence was severely criticised by many residents of the city and vicinity, who feared that insane patients would prove undesirable and constitute a menace to the community. Nevertheless sufficient funds for the purchase of the required location were subscribed by the citizens.

The plans and specifications for the construction of the hospital were prepared by S. V. Shipman, of Madison, Wis. George Josselyn, of Mt. Pleasant, was appointed superintendent of construction.

Albert Clark, of the commissioners, soon died and the vacancy was filled by the appointment of George W. Bemis, of Independence in 1869.

In 1870 the Legislature appropriated $165,000 in order to continue the construction of the hospital and also about that time elected seven trustees to take charge of the institution when the commissioners of construction should have completed their work. The first meeting of the trustees was held July 10, 1872, at Independence.

On October 3, 1872, Dr. Albert Reynolds was appointed superintendent of the hospital.

The hospital was opened for the reception of patients May 1, 1873. The plan adopted provided for a central building five stories high to serve the administrative and domestic departments. Upon each side of this central building were wings three stories high,

[1] Prepared by W. P. Crumbacker, M. D., superintendent.

each of which comprised four sections of corridors or wards. This arrangement provided twelve wards in the north wing for male patients and an equal number in the south wing for female patients. The estimated capacity of the completed building was 600. When the hospital was opened two sections only of the north wing had been constructed, which afforded accommodations for 150 patients. The hospital was built piece-meal and was not completed according to the original plan until 1883. The building was faced with sandstone, giving it an imposing appearance. The basement walls were of prairie granite. The total cost of construction of the first building was about $800,000.

In 1883 an appropriation of $25,000 was made for the erection of a substantial two-story brick detached cottage, known as Farmer's Lodge, which provided accommodation for 100 able-bodied working males.

In 1886 the Legislature appropriated $40,000 for the construction of another two-story brick detached cottage, known as Grove Hall, to provide for 100 chronic infirm male patients.

In 1894 the sum of $40,000 was appropriated for the erection of a two-story detached cottage, known as "Sunnyside Villa," to accommodate 100 chronic infirm female patients.

In 1907 an appropriation of $125,000 was made for the construction of another detached cottage. This appropriation provided a psychopathic hospital with 134 beds; 67 for males and an equal number for females. It comprises a basement above grade and two stories, with a center or administration section of three stories. The extreme dimensions are 259 feet by 125 feet; the whole building is of concrete and brick, fireproof construction. It is faced with straw-colored pressed brick and has polished trimmings of Bedford stone. The hospital is provided with an operating room, complete in its appointments; a hydrotherapeutic outfit; a cabinet for administering electric light baths and extensive electrotherapeutic devices.

There are about 1200 patients in the hospital and the monthly pay roll comprises nearly 200 names. The farm consists of 1360 acres. The total value of the buildings, land and other appurtenances is estimated at $1,130,000.

The hospital has had three superintendents. Albert Reynolds, M. D., occupied the position from the 1st of February, 1873, until his resignation, November 1, 1881.

During his administration the duties and powers of the superintendent were fixed by statute and were substantially as follows: He was the chief executive officer of the hospital, and had entire control of the medical, moral and dietetic treatment of the patients. It was his duty to see that the several officers and employees of the institution faithfully and diligently discharged their respective duties. He had authority to employ attendants, nurses, servants and such other persons as he might deem necessary for the efficient and economical administration of the hospital and had authority at any time to discharge any of them from service. He was also required to personally superintend the farm, grounds and all the property of the hospital.

The second superintendent was Gershom H. Hill, M. D., who had been first assistant physician for many years. He filled the position from December, 1881, until his resignation, July, 1902.

Dr. W. P. Crumbacker, the third superintendent, has occupied the position since the 1st of July, 1902.

The management of the hospital passed from the Board of Trustees to the Board of Control of State Institutions by legislative enactment July 1, 1898.

The Thirty-fourth General Assembly granted an appropriation of $40,000 for the construction of a home for nurses. An additional allowance of $17,000 for this purpose was made by the Thirty-fifth General Assembly. The building erected from this grant has been finished and is now occupied. It is a brick structure of three stories, with a commodious basement and slate roof. The construction is fireproof. The extreme length is 130 feet and the greatest depth is 73 feet. It is intended to accommodate 92 employees. There are 52 single rooms and 20 rooms for married couples. The floors throughout the three stories are made of fine white stone and cement terrazzo of beautiful design. This work marks a new and improved era in the management of Iowa institutions.

About nine hours each week are given to the meetings of the medical staff, which are attended by all of the physicians connected with the hospital. The meetings are held in the psychopathic hospital and all patients are brought before the staff. Physicians and advanced medical students who are not connected with the hospital are frequently in attendance. Outside patients are sometimes examined by the staff at these meetings, generally on the recommendation of their physician, who may accompany them.

In the psychopathic department an average of about 15 patients a day are treated with hydrotherapy and massage.

The routine examination of each patient admitted to the institution includes: Blood count, consisting of the estimation of the hemoglobin; counting the red and white blood cells; differential count, including classification of the polymorphonuclears by Arneth's method. Urinalysis, including reaction, specific gravity, albumin, sugar, indican and microscopical examinations. Spinal fluid: The proteins are estimated by Heller's contact test and by boiling in acetic acid. The euglobulins are tested by the Noguchi method. The amount of pyrocatechin is estimated by adding different amounts of the spinal fluid to one cc. of Fehling's solution.

The complement fixation test is performed by the Wassermann-Noguchi modification.

Other examinations, such as staining slides, bacteriological examinations by culture, preparation of vaccines and other miscellaneous tests are employed when indicated either in diagnosis or treatment. Autopsies are made on each cadaver when permission can be obtained. This includes macroscopic and microscopic examinations.

TRUSTEES.

Name	Term
Rev. John M. Boggs[1]	1872-1872
George W. Bemis	1872-1874
T. W. Fawcett	1872-1874
Prudence A. Appelman	1872-1876
Charles C. Parker, M. D.	1872-1876
Maturin L. Fisher	1872-1876
Erastus G. Morgan	1872-1884
John G. House, M. D.[1]	1872-1880
Stephen E. Robinson, M. D.	1876-1880
David Hammer	1878-1882
Lewis G. Smith	1878-1890
Jed Lake	1880-1888
Jane C. McKinney	1880-1884
Albert Reynolds, M. D.	1882-1890
John L. Whitley, M. D.	1884-1891
Frederic S. Thomas, M. D.	1884-1888
R. A. Dunkelberg, M. D.	1888-1892
William E. Rosemond	1888-1896

[1] Died in office.

Charles W. Fillmore	1890-1898
Almon G. Case	1890-1892
Edward Hornibrook, M. D.	1891-1896
Isaac R. Kirk	1892-1898
Frank E. Whitley, M. D.	1892-1898
Alexander T. McDonald	1896-1898

SUPERINTENDENTS.

Albert Reynolds, M. D.	1873-1881
Gershom H. Hill, M. D.	1881-1902
W. P. Crumbacker, M. D.	1902-in office

ASSISTANT PHYSICIANS.

Willis Butterfield	1873-15 months
Gershom H. Hill	1874-7 years
Henry G. Brainard	1878-8 years
Charles H. Penfield	1881-4 years
Sarah A. Pangburn (Kime)	1882-2 years
E. Amelia Sherman	1884-3 years
Edwin C. Bliss	1885-2 years
Hoel Tyler	1886-1 year
Henry S. Williams	1887-1½ years
Edward B. Thompson	1887-3 years
M. Nelson Voldeng	1887-8 years
E. E. Whitehorn	1888-1¼ years
John C. Doolittle	1889-16 years
Horace W. Burnard	1889-5 years
Jacob W. Wells	1891-4 years
George Boody	1895-7 years
Albert M. Barrett	1895-6 years
M. Charles Macklin	1895-3 years
Arthur S. Hamilton	1897-7 years
Susanna P. Boyle	1898-6 years
Joseph C. Ohlmacher	1902-7 years
Lavinia F. McPhee (Green)	1902-5 years
Cornelia N. Bos	1904-1 year
Charles E. Ingbert	1905-2 years
Samuel C. Lindsay	1905-present
George Donohoe	1905-5 years
Harry A. Lindsay	1907-present
Cora B. Murdock	1908-present
Oliver P. Bigelow	1909-present
Robert C. Butz	1911-present
James B. Rogers	1913-present
P. B. Batty	1914-present

CLARINDA STATE HOSPITAL.[1]

CLARINDA, IOWA.

An act of the Twentieth General Assembly of the State of Iowa, chapter 201, authorized the appropriation of $150,000 for the purpose of establishing an additional hospital for the insane. The act went into effect April 23, 1884, and provided that the Governor should select three commissioners, with power to locate the site for the hospital somewhere in Southwestern Iowa.

The act provided that not less than 320 acres of land should be purchased in the name of the state, so selected as to insure an abundant supply of good, pure water and to be susceptible of proper and efficient drainage. It was also provided that no gratuity or donation should be offered or received from any place as an inducement for its location; that the commissioners should, as soon as the location was fixed, secure and adopt plans and specifications and estimates for the buildings to be erected. All buildings to be fireproof, the exterior plain and of brick, to be built on the cottage plan; the board to invite bids after publication for 30 days in Des Moines newspapers; the contract to be let to the lowest bidder complying with the requirements of the commissioners. They were to employ a competent architect and superintendent of construction, appoint a secretary and keep accurate minutes of their doings.

The Governor appointed as commissioners the following: E. J. Hartshorn, of Palo Alto County; J. D. M. Hamilton, of Lee County, and George W. Bemis, of Buchanan County. These gentlemen met at Des Moines on May 21, 1884, and organized. George W. Bemis was elected president of the board, E. J. Hartshorn treasurer and J. D. M. Hamilton secretary.

On the 16th day of July, 1884, the commissioners met again at Des Moines for the purpose of deciding upon the site of the new hospital. They had already visited and carefully inspected every site that was being offered as a location. After two full days of

[1] Compiled from "History and Contract of the Hospital at Clarinda," by T. E. Clark, Bulletin of Iowa State Institutions, Vol. II, No. 4, and from subsequent reports of the superintendent.

deliberation these gentlemen, by a majority vote, selected Clarinda as the place combining in the fullest degree the requirements of the statute under which they acted.

Mr. Bemis resigned his position after Clarinda had been chosen as the site of the hospital and thereby progress was impeded until August, when Governor Sherman appointed George B. Van Saun, of Cedar Falls, to the vacancy thus created. On August 29 the new board convened at Clarinda and reorganized, with Mr. Van Saun as president.

In October, 1884, the commissioners purchased 513 acres of land one-half mile north of Clarinda. Upon this charming site, commanding a beautiful view of the Nodaway Valley, the hospital was built. The site is well drained and there is an abundant supply of pure water. The cost of the land was $29,425. The Pfiefer Cut Stone Company bid $10,788 for the stone work; the Dearborn Foundry Company's bid on the iron work was $22,100; G. W. Parker's bid for roofing and cornice was $3100. These bids were accepted. The Chicago, Burlington & Quincy Railroad Company, at its own expense, laid a switch from its St. Joseph branch line, just east of the hospital, down to the hospital.

The firm of Foster & Liebbe, of Des Moines, was engaged to design and supervise the entire structure. These men determined in the outset to enlighten the commissioners and themselves as well in the latest and best methods of hospital building. To this end they suggested an extensive tour of this country. Upon their return the outline plans were projected, submitted, criticised, remodeled and a plan was adopted.

The plan adopted is somewhat in violation of the strict letter of the act creating the hospital and is what is known as the "Corridor Connected Pavilion" plan, consisting first of a central administration building containing the official and executive departments of the institution, connecting by a rear corridor to the hospital system to the right, left and rear. At the right is the female wing, at the left the male wing and at the rear are the maintenance and operative sections. Like most of the earlier state institutions, the appropriations were so limited that only a part of the institution as designed could be erected during any biennial period. Instead of attempting to lay the entire foundation and then waiting for additional appropriations for the superstructures and so attempting the whole group at one and the same time, the wiser policy was pursued of first erecting the administration building and one wing. These were finished in advance, with temporary arrangements for heating and culinary work. Thus earlier accommodations were provided for patients sadly needing relief from the poorhouses of counties, which were worse than prisons.

On the 4th day of July, 1885, the corner-stone was laid by the Iowa Grand Lodge of Masons. The Governor was present with many other distinguished men of the state.

By December, 1885, the central building and supervisor's department were under roof and one wing nearly so.

In 1886 an appropriation of $103,000 was secured with which to carry forward the work.

The hospital was first opened for occupation December 15, 1888, with 222 male patients received from Independence, Mt. Pleasant and Mercy hospitals.

The commissioners filed their final report and were dissolved by an act of the Twenty-second General Assembly, which at the same time created a Board of five Trustees. The first board consisted of E. J. Hartshorn, president; L. B. Raymond, secretary; J. H. Dunlap, J. D. M. Hamilton and Edward H. Hunter. These officers came into power March 14, 1888, assuming the duties and powers of the commission dissolved by the act aforesaid. The board elected L. E. Darrow treasurer. The board also elected P. W. Lewellen, M. D., of Clarinda, as the first superintendent, who selected Dr. J. M. Aiken, of Clarinda, assistant physician, M. T. Butterfield, steward, and Mrs. Alice W. Lewellen, matron.

With occupation came activity. Patients were set to work, grading, sodding, tree planting and farming.

Additional appropriations were made from session to session and in like fragmentary manner wings and wards were added year by year, until in 1897 the hospital stood complete. The first building erected was the administration building with its connecting corridors, the supervisors' section and the east wing. Next the kitchen and help's departments, then the west wing and cold storage buildings. After this the permanent boiler house and east infirmary wards and at last the west infirmary wards.

It is difficult to give an intelligent pen picture of this ample structure. Its total frontage is 1128 feet; its total depth 840 feet, with a length of extended walls of one mile and a quarter and covering many miles of floor space. It provides comfortable apartments for 1000 persons.

The style of the buildings is what is called modern Gothic, most appropriate for the material used in its construction, brick and stone with steep slated roofs and such variety of outline and form that from all points of view there is harmony with contrast, a light and shade that ever pleases the eye. The height of the buildings is generally three stories, though the administration building is four.

The structure is fireproof, being composed of brick, stone, steel, plaster, tile and cement. The hospital is especially noted for its light, secured by a judicious separating and spacing of its wings and sections. The shade of one wing does not darken the windows in the adjacent wing.

No pains, especially in the newer and later wards, have been spared as regards the sanitary features.

Thousands of air flues and ducts facilitate a constant circulation of pure air and by these means carry out all impure air, the latter being accelerated by numerous electric fans.

The structure is amply warmed in the winter season by low pressure steam, all from the boiler house at the rear, where many large boilers afford all needed steam both for heat and power.

The buildings are lighted by electricity which is generated in the dynamo room at the rear.

Good, wholesome water is obtained by a steam-driven deep-well pump and a chain of storage cisterns, besides numerous soft water cisterns.

There are infirmary wards with circular bay dormitories, large open fire places and toilet arrangements.

Various industries have been a prominent feature in the economy of this hospital. Thus there has been continually in operation for a number of years a department for the manufacture of clothing. Here all clothing worn by the patients, both men and women, is made, with the exception of white dress shirts for the men and hose and hats. Cloth and material are bought in large quantities by the bolt and are cut by a tailoress and made into clothing under her supervision by several assistants and a number of patients. Clothing not sufficiently worn to be condemned is repaired and put in a suitable condition for further use. A second very satisfactory industrial department is the shoe shop, where all the footwear for both men and women is manufactured under the direction and supervision of a shoemaker, who is assisted by patients who have a liking and aptitude for that class of work. Another industry is that of wood working, where furniture of various kinds is made and repaired. This is located in a separate building, and here under the supervision of a foreman some 12 to 25 convalescing or mildly disordered patients may be seen every week day busily engaged in planing, scraping, matching and manufacturing all sorts of wooden articles and useful pieces of furniture. A simple, modest equipment of machinery is installed in this place and is used to good advantage.

In connection with this industrial building is a broom-making department, where all the brooms needed for the hospital are manufactured. The only thing bought is the twine wire and occasionally broom handles, which, however, are used over and over again until practically worn out. Broom corn is raised on the farm and usually a two-years' supply is laid in stock.

A mattress making department is also connected with this building, where in a separate room all the new mattresses used in the institution are made. Mattress hair is bought and also a good quality of material for the cover, which is made up in the sewing room and afterwards filled by patients, who become quite expert in the making of mattresses and who work under the supervision of the foreman of the industrial building. Soiled or worn mattresses in which the hair has become packed are taken apart, thoroughly renovated by steam, dried, thoroughly picked and the hair used over again. Part of the time a tin shop is operated in connection with the industrial building, although it is located in a different building, and the needed repairs to the tinware of the institution are made, but the manufacture of new tinware has not been attempted to any considerable extent.

In the amusement hall chapel services are held each Sabbath and frequent plays performed for the benefit of the inmates. Performances are put upon the stage by the talent of the institution; the medical staff, below the superintendent, frequently participating and the attendants nearly always taking some part. There are frequent dances in this hall to exhilarate and enliven the many patients who engage in the amusement. The hospital band has for years been the pride of the hospital and of the town as well.

Dr. P. W. Lewellen was the first superintendent. On December 31, 1892, he resigned his position. Dr. Frank C. Hoyt was his successor. The board brought him from St. Joseph, Mo., where he had found wide experience in the hospitals of that state. He resigned his position on September 30, 1898, in order to take up a cherished project in Chicago, and the board selected Dr. Max E. Witte, of Mt. Pleasant, as his successor. Since October 1, 1898, Dr. Witte has filled the place to the entire satisfaction of the state.

On the 1st of July, 1898, the Clarinda State Hospital was put under the charge of the Board of Control of State Institutions.

The institution at that time had a capacity and population of 811 patients, and this number was rapidly increasing from year to year so that an increase in capacity became necessary. This has since been furnished by the erection of two large fireproof cottages; one for men (South View Cottage), with a capacity of 104, and another for women, with a capacity of 100. These cottages have served their purpose well, are of sightly appearance and pleasing construction, and conveniently arranged so that they meet the needs of a certain class of patients in an admirable manner; besides this, the state acquired land about three-fourths of a mile distant from the institution, where a fireproof cottage (Willowdale), with a capacity of 40 patients, has been constructed and is maintained and operated much on the plan of "Graycroft" at Utica, N. Y. For convenience, greater comfort and efficiency, many improvements and alterations have been made in the main building in the way of installation of more modern machinery for the purpose of lighting, ventilating and more efficient heating of the institution, besides a plant for the manufacture of artificial ice and refrigeration for all necessary cold storage needs.

Various little industries were early installed at this institution and have been maintained with pleasure and benefit to patients as well as economy in the administration of the institution.

Profitable and pleasant employment and recreation are provided as largely as possible for all patients who can thus be benefited; and this being above everything else an agricultural state, most of the male patients find helpful employment about the farm, gardens, green-house and the various stables. This is not only primarily a matter of paramount importance as a diversion for the patients, but often proves remedial; besides its economical value is not inconsiderable. The institution supplies all its needs in garden vegetables, with the exception perhaps of potatoes, of which article additional purchases are often necessary. It produces all the milk, fresh pork and lard consumed at the institution, besides a share of the poultry required.

The farm land belonging to the State Hospital at Clarinda, in 1898, consisted of some 500 acres. This has been increased to 860 acres by purchase; and barns, stables and other means have been added to ensure a more successful administration of hospital affairs. The grounds in the immediate vicinity of the hospital buildings have been beautified according to a consistent and artistic plan, so that the surroundings are more pleasing and beautiful than ever before and bid to be more so in the future.

Patients are committed to the hospital without previous consultation of hospital authorities. Upon entrance all patients, irrespective of conditions, are confined to bed for a few days at least until physicians and nurses can be more familiar with the patient. They are also, within the first few days of their admission, carefully examined as to their physical and mental or nervous disorders or anything abnormal which presents itself. Where the history accompanying the patient is defective it is endeavored to obtain further information from friends and correspondents and others who may have knowledge pertaining to the patient's previous life. The history of each individual patient is kept up and memoranda made at stated intervals and as much oftener as changes in the patient's condition may render it desirable.

Patients are classified according to condition. The acute are cared for in specially equipped wards by nurses who are selected for the requirements of the ward for disturbed and acute cases. The sick are maintained in a regular hospital ward for the sick employees. The infirm are kept on special wards and those on the men's side are in charge of women nurses. The tubercular patients are cared for in special rooms on certain wards. An appropriation has been asked for the erection of a regular tuberculosis pavilion and also for a special building with a capacity of 200 for new and disturbed patients of both sexes. There are maintained for each sex special wards for the care of epileptic patients.

The training school for nurses was organized in the early 90's and has been maintained ever since. A three-years' course of eight months of theoretical and practical instruction, which includes general and surgical nursing as well as that peculiar to mental disorders, is maintained and satisfactory work and successful passing of a searching examination is rewarded with a diploma as graduate nurse. This diploma is accepted by the State Board of Health and permits the holder to come up for examination, although it is usually advised that a short service in a hospital with practical obstetrics be taken.

The general spirit of the institution is to have the asylum idea as much in the background as possible and to supply surroundings and influences as much like those at home as can be made. In this connection a farm cottage with a capacity of 50 patients is maintained, distant three-fourths of a mile from the main structure.

TRUSTEES.

E. J. Hartshorn.
L. B. Raymond.
J. H. Dunlap.
J. D. M. Hamilton.
M. N. Spencer.
Rev. T. McK Stuart.
T. E. Clark.
W. W. Morrow.
Ed. H. Hunter.

SUPERINTENDENTS.

Dr. P. W. Lewellen 1888-1892
Dr. F. C. Hoyt 1893-1898
Dr. Max E. Witte ....1898-in office

ASSISTANT PHYSICIANS.

Dr. J. M. Aiken........	1888-1889	Dr. Anne Burnet........	1895-1901
Dr. P. J. Ibaugh........	1889-1891	Dr. A. F. Gundry.......	1895-1898
Dr. T. E. Powers.......	1891-1893	Dr. A. D. Wade........	1897-1898
Dr. H. E. Markham....	1892-1895	Dr. B. F. Gilmor.......	1898-1899
Dr. C. A. Drew.........	1893-1895	Dr. J. W. Wherry......	1899-
Dr. C. F. Applegate.....	1895-1901	Dr. F. A. Ely..........	1899-

Dr. George Boody.
Dr. M. C. Macklin.
Dr. E. A. Saylor.
Dr. Roy Moon.
Dr. W. A. Bryan.
Dr. W. D. Ranyon.
Dr. J. C. Ohlmacher.
Dr. C. D. Harlan.
Dr. F. R. Sparks.
Dr. S. R. Klein.
Dr. R. D. Smith.
Dr. Pauline M. Leader.

STEWARDS.

M. T. Butterfield.......	1888-1890	E. D. Cullison..........	1892-1898
K. L. Clock............	1890-1891	E. R. Bailey............	1899-

C. H. Amick.[1]

MATRONS.

Mrs. Alice Lewellen	1888-1889 1892-1892	Mrs. M. A. Wilson......	1893-1893
		Miss C. Martin.........	1893-1894
A. M. Cresswell........	1889-1892	Kate Rumsey	1894-1896
Agnes Martine	1892-1892	Lizzie Webb	1896-

Anna E. Blair.[1]

[1] Date of service not obtained.

CHEROKEE STATE HOSPITAL.

CHEROKEE, IOWA.

The biennial reports submitted to Governor Boies, of Iowa, in 1894, presented an alarming condition of affairs. The state hospitals at Independence, Mt. Pleasant and Clarinda, with a capacity of about 2100, had 2252 patients. Large numbers of insane persons had also been sent back to the counties for lack of room in the state institutions.

The number of insane in the state outside of the hospitals was variously estimated at from 1500 to 2000. The superintendents of all three of the state hospitals strongly recommended a continuance of state care.

The question of building a new hospital was not a new one; the matter had been under discussion for some time. In 1892 the State Medical Society, in session at Des Moines, strongly advocated the building of a new hospital, and at Burlington, in the following year, had passed a resolution by a unanimous vote that neither county poorhouses nor county asylums are proper places for the care and treatment of the insane, and that another hospital for the insane should be located the next year in the northwestern quarter of the state, to be made ready for use as soon as practicable.

[1] The material for this sketch has been furnished by Dr. M. Nelson Voldeng, the superintendent.

Governor Boies in his biennial message took issue with the generally expressed opinion in favor of state care of the insane, and, while he recognized the lamentable condition of the insane in the county poorhouses and the need of different accommodations and different care, he believed that it might be given nearly as well and much cheaper in county asylums than in state hospitals. In a lengthy discussion of the question he advocated a system of county care like that authorized by the laws of Wisconsin and estimated that the state would save $228,000 each year by adopting it.

The question was discussed pro and con and a bill was finally introduced in the Senate providing for the location of a state hospital for the insane in Northwestern Iowa and the appointment of three commissioners by the Governor, with the consent of the Senate, to purchase a site for the new hospital of not less than 320 acres; to contract for additional land in the vicinity; to secure a tract of 640 acres and to select plans for the hospital, providing that the location of the hospital be approved by a joint convention of the House and Senate. Pending the consideration of this bill two resolutions had been introduced relating to the same matter—one a concurrent resolution providing that the three superintendents of the state asylums and the chairman of the visiting committee be a committee to visit points competing for the location in Northwestern Iowa, to report to the General Assembly and especially to report as to water supply, drainage, railway facilities, etc. This resolution was passed unanimously. The other resolution provided for a commission to inspect the county asylum system of Wisconsin and to report to the next General Assembly. This resolution did not emerge from the committee to which it had been referred.

The committee appointed under the first resolution visited the towns of Fort Dodge, Storm Lake, Cherokee, LeMars and Sheldon and made an exhaustive report on each town to the General Assembly. On March 20, 1894, the bill providing for a new asylum passed the Senate with only one dissenting vote. It afterwards passed the House with only one dissenting vote and became a law by publication March 28, 1894. On the evening of March 29, 1894, the Senate and the House met in joint convention for the purpose of selecting a site for the hospital for the insane in Northwestern Iowa according to the law just passed by the General Assembly.

After an exciting evening Cherokee received a majority of the votes on the fourteenth ballot and was declared the site of the new hospital.

During the same session an appropriation of $12,000 for the purchase of land for the site and $200,000 to begin the work was made. It was also provided that the superintendents of the three state hospitals, together with the three commissioners appointed by the Governor, should constitute the building commissioners of the hospital. Edward Wright, of Des Moines, William G. Kent, of Fort Madison, and Jed Lake, of Independence, were accordingly appointed commissioners to act in conjunction with the superintendents of the three hospitals as building commissioners.

The commissioners purchased 360 acres of land for the sum of $11,500 and contracted for 240 acres more for $12,500, subject to the approval of the succeeding General Assembly; all lying in a body to the west of the City of Cherokee and just without its corporate limits.

Subsequently appropriations were made by the Legislature to complete the payment upon the land and in addition appropriations were made aggregating $100,000 a year for the succeeding four years for the erection of buildings. An excellent building was erected in consequence of this appropriation with stone foundation, brick superstructure and stone trimmings. The building was fireproof.

For some reason the building after it was completed stood idle for some years, but was finally opened August 15, 1902.

From August 15 to August 26, 1902, eight patients were admitted. On the latter date 306 patients were received from the Independence State Hospital—172 men and 134 women. On August 28 the hospital received by transfer from the Clarinda State Hospital 252 patients—136 men and 116 women.

Since 1902 there has been a steady increase in population until the institution has become a little city in itself with 1022 patients —588 men and 434 women—and nearly 200 employees.

With the increase in population has come the need of more land and more buildings. Since the opening of the institution the following buildings have been erected:

Three well towers, laboratory, industrial building, addition to coal shed, addition to laundry, fire station, hog house, poultry house, dairy barn, carriage barn, draft horse barn, root cave, built of solid concrete for 8000 bushels of vegetables, ice house, two implement houses, wagon shed, granary, corn crib, three pavilions, sheep barn and greenhouse.

A farm cottage, to accommodate 150 men, has been built at a cost of $65,000; also a psychopathic hospital, at a cost of $125,000, to accommodate 120 men and 120 women. The buildings are fire-proof throughout, with reinforced concrete floors and tile roof.

The psychopathic hospital is splendidly equipped with the most modern hydrotherapy equipment and a complete operating room. The percentage of recoveries has been greater since the installment of this apparatus three years ago.

The following treatments are given: Wet sheet packs, continuous baths, shower baths, electric baths, soapsuds shampoo, salt glow, olive oil rubs, alcohol rubs.

The number of tubercular patients appears to be on the increase and a separate building, which has been greatly needed, is now in process of construction. This building will accommodate 80 patients and will cost $50,000. The rooms are built around courts, which are glass covered and in which will be fountains, palms and birds the entire year. This building represents a new departure in arrangement as well as construction.

The buildings at present are valued at $1,300,000. The state farm of 1000 acres is valued at $200,000. With each succeeding year the fertility of the farm and garden has been improved. All portions of land in need of tile drainage have been thoroughly drained; there is an orchard of 30 acres with all kinds of large and small fruit.

Much work has been done in beautifying the grounds, such as grading, road building, tree and shrubbery planting and the construction of cement walks and gutters. All the farm fences, many of them old and dilapidated, have been replaced by new ones made of good material and well constructed.

A training school for nurses has been in successful operation since the opening of the institution. The importance of this training school to the welfare of the patients is very evident. With each succeeding year some important additions have been made to the clinical experience of the nurses. Opportunity has been given members of the senior class to be present at autopsies and to listen to demonstrations by the pathologist. They have also received practical training in the care and arrangement of the operating room incident to operative work. The training school offers a course for trained attendants and trained nurses; two full years for the former and three years for the latter. Private nursing in the city and surrounding county has been encouraged among the graduates whenever one could be spared without injury to the institution.

The superintendent of the hospital is of the opinion that suitable employment, conducted systematically, is one of the greatest agents for the treatment of mental disorders. Patients are impressed with the idea that their employment is for their own benefit and greater interest is manifested. A life of activity and contentment is substituted for one of monotony and discontent. Every industry in the institution is at present represented by the patients. Occupation has undoubtedly contributed to their improvement as well as their comfort. It is not uncommon for 400 men patients to be willingly occupied with various employments. This work is of course all purely voluntary.

An art teacher instructs and directs the women in all kinds of fine hand work, such as embroidery of various styles, Mexican drawnwork, Swedish work, all forms of knitting, tatting, crocheting and lace making.

The hospital has a library of over 2000 well-selected books. It is remarkable the amount of reading done by the better class of patients, both chronic and convalescent. The interest manifested in the current events as recorded in the daily papers or monthly magazines is always keen.

The beneficial and even curative effect of pleasant diversion has prompted the superintendent to furnish a variety of entertainments, such as theatricals, concerts, fancy dress parties, sociables, where all sorts of games are played, stereopticon and moving picture exhibitions, and to prepare special programs for the holiday season. The music for the weekly dance, so eagerly looked forward to by the patients, is furnished by the hospital orchestra. During the winter months the orchestra gives concerts in the amusement hall and throughout the summer season the hospital band furnishes two weekly open-air concerts on the campus.

Games of ball, tennis, croquet and quoits are enjoyed during the summer months and, when the weather is not suitable for outdoor recreation, billiards, pool, chess, checkers, crokinole and various games are enjoyed.

Sunday morning chapel services, conducted by the pastors of the city, are always well attended. The spiritual welfare of the patients, both Protestant and Catholic, has been well cared for by the clergy of the city and many clergymen from over the district have made visits to members of their respective churches. Mass has been celebrated at stated intervals during each year for the benefit of the Catholic patients.

Thanksgiving, Christmas and New Year services have each year been conducted by ministers from Cherokee, the hospital choir and orchestra furnishing appropriate music.

OFFICERS JANUARY 1, 1914.

Dr. M. N. Voldeng .... Superintendent.
Dr. T. L. Long .... First assistant.
Dr. W. A. Bryan .... Second assistant.
Dr. F. B. E. Miller .... Third assistant.
Dr. Rose A. Russell .... Fourth assistant.
Dr. Lena A. Beach .... Woman physician.
Andrew Rae .... Steward.
Ella McNiven .... Matron.
W. S. Young .... Chief engineer.
Henry Stocking .... Gardener and florist.

ASSISTANT PHYSICIANS.

(Since Opening of Hospital.)

Dr. C. C. Willhite.
Dr. Charles F. Sanborn.
Dr. W. S. Osborn.
Dr. B. R. McAllaster.
Dr. W. Huckin.
Dr. F. E. McClure.
Dr. Goodrich Snow.
Dr. H. D. Earl.
Dr. E. P. Benedict.
Dr. C. H. Dragoo.
Dr. E. W. Martin.
Dr. T. B. Throckmorton.
Dr. Earl Caddick.
Dr. G. J. Stone.

THE REFORMATORY.[1]

ANAMOSA, IOWA.

The department for the insane of the Reformatory, at Anamosa, Iowa, was established about 1888, when the institution was a penitentiary. It was designated as the reformatory in 1907.

The building of the department for the criminal insane is three stories in height, with a row of small cells, 7 x 7 x 4½ feet, against the outer walls north and south, and facing a broad corridor or ward room. The cells are supposably ventilated by air ducts in the outer walls, but are without the means for forced ventilation essential for well-built hospitals according to modern engineering, architecture and sanitation. They have absolutely no sanitary appliances, reliance being placed upon the hideous old "cell bucket" at night. The inmates are kept out of these cells during the daytime, but sleep in them at night.

The yard attached to this building is used for recreation and exercise. An endeavor is being made to secure the means with which to build a wall, enclosing the triangular space next to the railway and to the west of the building, in order to start garden work with the inmates. The whole institution is located in the heart of the town of Anamosa, so that there is no suitable campus for other out-door treatment.

This institution takes care (such as it is) of all the insane criminals in the state while under sentence, or while their trials are in temporary arrest due to the development or discovery of insanity during trial. On expiration of sentence, if the prisoner-patient is still insane, he is transferred by authority of the Board of Control of State Institutions to one of the state hospitals, where, for the first time, he comes under the care of a skilled alienist and his assistants. The poor fellow whose trial has been arrested by the trial judge and a trial for insanity substituted therefor, and who has been committed to this department "until sane," may have a life sentence to serve under prison conditions without having been convicted of crime and without the aid of scientific treatment. The care afforded is only that which an

[1] By Charles C. McClaughry, warden.

ordinary physician and his "hospital steward" may be able to render with the aid of keepers who have had no special training as nurses and who, from the circumstances of the case, regard these patients as prisoners first. It is therefore simply custodial care.

There are 63 patients in this department at present. There are no accommodations for women who might be insane criminals. In the women's department of this institution there is now a woman who may be insane and is under observation. If she proves to be insane there must be a commutation of her sentence so that she may be sent to one of the state hospitals for treatment.

Since the establishment of the department for criminal insane the medical officers who have had charge of this department while acting as physicians to the reformatory have been:

Dr. L. J. Adair 1888-1896
Dr. Dwight Sigsworth .... 1896-1896 (died)
Dr. H. W. Sigsworth 1896-1896
Dr. Wm. T. McKay 1896-1898
Dr. S. Druett 1898-1910
Dr. T. C. Gorman 1910-1914
Dr. John Dale Paul .... 1914-to date

THE IOWA INSTITUTION FOR FEEBLE-MINDED CHILDREN.

Glenwood, Iowa.

The Iowa Institution for Feeble-minded Children is located at Glenwood, the county seat of Mills County, Iowa, on the main line of the Chicago, Burlington & Quincy Railroad. It is surrounded by the wooded hills of the Missouri River Valley and is in the center of a beautiful and productive country. The institution is situated on a commanding elevation, three-quarters of a mile from the business portion of the town, and overlooks the city and surrounding country.

The institution was organized April 26, 1876, under an act passed by the Sixteenth General Assembly. The first superintendent was Dr. O. W. Archibald, of Glenwood, who served from 1876 to 1882. The second superintendent was Dr. F. M. Powell, who served from 1882 until 1903, and the third and present superintendent is Dr. George Mogridge. The act creating the institution set aside for its use about 12 acres of land, on which was a small brick building that had been occupied until 1874 as a western branch of the Soldiers' Orphans' Home.

The first pupils were received September 4, 1876. During the first year there were admitted and cared for 87 children. The number has gradually increased until there are at present nearly 1500 under care. Necessary buildings have been added from time to time and additions made to the land.

The institution has its own system of water works, electric light plant, cold storage and artificial ice manufacturing plant, stores, shops, brickyard, printing office, fire department, bakery and dairy; it also has a well-organized school system, a band and an orchestra.

The farm, garden and orchards fill an important part in the economy of the institution, as well as providing avenues for industrial teaching.

The purpose of the institution is to provide special methods of training for that class of children deficient in mind or marked by such peculiarities as to deprive them of ordinary benefits and privileges. Such methods of training and discipline are adopted as tend to make each child approach as nearly as possible the movements and actions of normal people. It also provides a home for those who are susceptible of mental culture. The latter are provided with such training as may tend to correct their habits and create an interest in their own welfare.

In the school department lessons are imparted in the simple elements of instruction taught in the common schools as well as in the rudiments of such industries as are suited to the capacity of the pupils. Girls learn plain and fancy sewing and general housework, while the boys are detailed to work on the farm, in the garden, shoeshop, carpenter shop and to assist in the various departments of the institution.

The patients are supported by the state, the support fund being $12 per capita per month. Clothing supplied patients is charged to the county of their residence. The products of the farm, orchard and garden, together with receipts from sales, are added to the support fund.

The status of the population January 1, 1915, was: Males, 745; females, 726; total, 1471. Number of officers and employees, 215. Total acreage, 1015.18. Valuation of lands, buildings and all equipment, $1,061,179.78.

"THE RETREAT."

Des Moines, Iowa.

"The Retreat" is said to be the only private institution in Iowa which is recognized by the Board of Control of State Institutions as a hospital caring for patients whose minds are affected. The Retreat is not licensed, nor is there any sanitarium in Iowa which has any legal authority for detaining insane persons except in accordance with the authority given by a certificate signed by two physicians.

The superintendent is Dr. G. H. Hill.

THE CARE OF THE INSANE IN KANSAS.[1]

The first legislative assembly of Kansas, which met in 1855, enacted a law providing for the appointment of a guardian for any idiot, lunatic or person of unsound mind and incapable of managing his affairs. This act was re-enacted in 1859, with the addition of the clause, " or habitual drunkard," between the words, " unsound mind " and the next clause. This act was for the protection of the property rights of the individual suffering from insanity. There was apparently no provision for the care and treatment of the indigent insane of the state prior to the establishment of the Osawatomie State Hospital in 1863. The Legislature of 1875 provided for the establishment of a second state hospital, which is now known as the Topeka State Hospital. In 1899 a third asylum was established at Parsons; in 1903 this was made a state hospital for epileptics, both sane and insane. The Legislature of 1909 authorized the establishment of an additional hospital for the insane, which has been located at Larned, and is known as the Larned State Hospital. In addition to the above, the Legislature of 1881 established the State Home for Feeble-minded, which is located at Winfield; the Hospital for Criminal Insane was established in 1911 on the grounds of the state prison at Lansing.

In 1865 the Osawatomie State Hospital was placed under the management of three trustees, appointed by the Governor. In 1873 the Osawatomie State Hospital, together with the School for the Deaf and the School for the Blind, was placed under the management of one Board of Trustees, consisting of six members, appointed by the Governor. They were paid three dollars per day and mileage and appointed all officers and employees. The same act created a visiting committee of three citizens, to be appointed by the Governor for a term of three years, to visit at least twice in each year all of the state institutions. Their pay was three dollars per day and mileage.

[1] Compiled from material furnished by H. C. Bowman, president of the Board of Control.

The Legislature of 1875 changed the first-mentioned Board of Trustees to five members, not more than two of whom were to be from any one county and none from a county where an institution was located.

By 1899 six more state institutions had been erected and placed in charge of this Board of Trustees, namely: Topeka State Hospital, State Industrial School for Boys, State Home for Feeble-minded, State Orphans' Home, Industrial School for Girls, and State Hospital for Epileptics. The salary of the members was fixed, in 1899, at $1200 per annum and expenses. This was raised, first to $1700, then to $2000 per annum, until finally the Board of Control bill fixed the salaries of the three members of the board at $2500 per annum and provided for an office force.

The Legislature of 1901 enacted what was called "the Code of Charities and Corrections of the State of Kansas." The first part of the act was in reference to the management and control of the state institutions under charge of the Board of Trustees. This act continued in force until 1905, when the Board of Control of State Charitable Institutions was created and assumed the power previously held by the Board of Trustees.

The Board of Control of State Charitable Institutions consists of three members, appointed by the Governor for a term of four years. The board appoints the superintendents of the different institutions and the superintendents employ and discharge all employees under civil service rules. The board lets the contracts and supervises the erection of all buildings. All supplies for the institutions are purchased semi-annually by the board, and things not so purchased are bought monthly by the superintendents on estimates furnished by the board. In addition to the management of the state institutions, the State Board of Control has the supervision of the private insane institutions, children's associations and institutions, and in addition all private institutions of the state of a charitable nature which receive state aid.

In 1874 the Legislature forbade the Osawatomie Asylum from collecting any money from any county for the care and maintenance of patients after March 1, 1874. In 1875 the Legislature placed the expense of keeping and maintaining the indigent insane of the state in the insane asylums upon the state. Since the acts of 1874 and 1875 the state has not collected from the counties, but has collected from the estates of patients or relatives where means existed from which such collections could be made. Patients are classified as either private or county patients. Private patients not only pay for their care and maintenance, but also for their clothing. While the law classifies the patients into private and county patients, there is in fact another class that may be called reimbursing patients.

In the act creating the Osawatomie State Hospital in 1863 nothing was said as to the manner of admission of patients. From the opening of the institution in 1866 until 1870 patients were admitted by special arrangement with each county after the patient had been adjudged incompetent under the guardianship act of 1855, which has been already noted. If the patient had a sufficient estate to maintain him the guardian gave a bond to the state, and if the patient did not have a sufficient estate, then the county commissioner signed an agreement to pay for the care and maintenance of the patient at the hospital.

The Legislature of 1870 enacted additional provisions, setting forth two ways for the admission of patients. First, after an adjudication under the above-mentioned guardianship act, which provided for a jury of six persons, one of whom had to be a physician in regular practice and good standing. The probate court then determined the question of maintenance and made application for admission of the patient to the Osawatomie Asylum. If the superintendent notified the probate judge that the patient could be received, the judge then issued a precept in lunacy and a warrant in lunacy; in the warrant it was specified whether the patient would be maintained out of his private estate or whether the county of his residence would maintain him. The second way of admission, as provided by the Legislature of 1870, was without an inquest in lunacy, and simply upon a physician's certificate certifying that the physician believed the patient to be insane, and a bond signed by individuals promising to pay for the care and maintenance of the patient, which bond had to be approved by the probate judge. It will thus be seen that Kansas, as early as 1870, went farther than any other state has ever gone in reference to the admission of patients to insane institutions without any adjudication of insanity. Some states have provided for voluntary commitments, but the act of 1870 provided that patients could be involuntarily placed in the state asylums at private expense without an adjudication of insanity, and this law was not changed until 1901.

Since the act of 1901 patients are admitted to the state hospitals only after they have been adjudged insane, there being no provision at the present time for voluntary commitments to the state insane hospitals. The commitment to the state insane hospital makes the patient incompetent to testify in court as a witness or to handle his estate.

Authority to discharge patients from the state insane hospitals is vested in the State Board of Control, but may be and is delegated by the board to the superintendents, under such regulations as the board sees fit to adopt. Paroles are also granted. A paroled patient can be returned to the state hospital from which he was paroled without an application for his readmission. Patients discharged as "improved" or "unimproved," who have not been discharged as restored by the probate court, can be readmitted upon a new application, made to the State Board of Control on the original papers, together with a certificate from a physician showing the present mental condition of the patient. When a patient is discharged as cured the superintendent sends notice to that effect to the probate court, and it is the duty of the judge of said court to enter upon his docket an order restoring the patient to all his rights as a citizen and removing the guardian, if a guardian has been appointed. If the patient has been discharged as not yet restored to sound mind, the probate judge of the county in which the patient was adjudged insane may hear evidence tending to show that such patient has been restored to reason, and if satisfied as to his recovery, may make and enter a similar order, and thereafter the patient is not liable to be again committed to any hospital or insane asylum without a new inquest. No formal action is necessary when he is discharged from a state hospital as cured.

The State Board of Control is in one sense a state lunacy commission and passes upon the papers to see whether the person has been legally adjudged insane and also whether he is eligible for admission to the state insane hospitals. If everything is right and the person is a fit patient for the state hospitals, the board sends the probate judge an order of admission and forwards all the papers to the state hospital to which the patient has been ordered admitted. The probate judge then issues a lunacy precept to the guardian of the patient or to a friend or to the sheriff, commanding him to take the patient without any unnecessary delay to the state hospital, and the probate judge also issues a lunacy warrant to the superintendent, stating whether the patient is to be maintained as a private patient or at the expense of the state. At the time of giving the order of admission the State Board passes upon the financial statement and notifies the probate court whether the patient will be received as a private patient or as a county patient, and if as a private patient, then a bond is also required. As above mentioned, the county furnishes all of the clothing required at the time of admission of county patients.

Classes Committed.—All insane persons except idiots and epileptics are committed.

Legal Procedure.—Any reputable citizen of the town or township may file a sworn statement with the probate judge of the county that the person named is insane and unsafe to be at large; that the welfare of himself and others requires his restraint or commitment to some hospital. The statement must be accompanied by the names of two witnesses. If the person has not been examined by a physician, the judge may appoint a qualified physician to make an examination.

Inquests in lunacy must be by jury or commission at the discretion of the court. Inquests must be by jury when demanded by the person alleged to be insane or by any person acting in his behalf. The court must appoint competent counsel for the person.

When no jury is demanded or trial by jury is not expedient the probate judge must appoint a commission of two qualified physicians in regular practice to make a personal examination and a sworn report of their findings. The commission has power to administer oaths and take sworn testimony. Inquests may be in open court or in chambers or at the house of the person alleged to be insane. The presence of the accused is indispensable.

A jury of four persons, one of whom must be a physician in regular practice for three years and of good standing, must be impaneled when a case is tried by jury. The person must be present, represented by counsel and may challenge jurors. The verdict must be signed by all members of the jury and contain a brief statement of medical treatment in the case, signed by the physician or physicians upon the jury. If the person is adjudged insane and a fit person to be sent to a hospital the court must order his commitment. If not satisfied with the findings the probate judge may set them aside and dismiss the proceedings or order another inquest.

Insane persons must be committed to private hospitals in the same manner as to a state hospital. The probate judge in selecting a private asylum must be governed by the wishes of the friends and relatives of the person. No county can recover for the care of an insane person in a private hospital unless he has been refused admission at one of the state hospitals for want of room.

Insane persons not resident may not be detained in any private institution unless committed in accordance with the laws of the state or territory of which they are residents or with the laws of this state.

Appeal from Commitment.—Appeals may be made to the district court and the question must be decided by the probate court, after inquiry, with or without a jury. Such inquiry may not be held oftener than once in six months.

Cost of Commitment.—In case of county patients the costs must be paid from the county treasury, but in case of private patients the costs must be paid by the guardian of the insane out of his estate. When a person is found to be sane the court may require that the costs be paid by the person who filed the statement.

OSAWATOMIE STATE HOSPITAL.

Osawatomie, Kans.

The Osawatomie State Hospital was opened for the reception of patients in 1866. A previous Legislature had appropriated $3000 for a building. At that time ten persons had been adjudged insane in Kansas. They were placed in a little two-story frame building, which is still preserved.

The institution has grown until in 1911 there was an investment of about $1,000,000 in land and buildings, and more than 1300 patients under care.

The buildings are as follows: The main building; administration building in front, on each side one wing for male and one wing for female patients, and in the rear, shops, power plant, etc. The two wings of the main building accommodate about 600 patients. There are two detached buildings for chronic cases, one for men and one for women. These buildings accommodate 300 patients each. There is a detached infirmary building accommodating 100 patients. Here all surgical cases are cared for, as well as patients bedfast for a considerable period of time. Two tuberculosis pavilions have been recently erected, one for men and one for women. They will accommodate about 50 patients. Still later improvements consist of a separate cottage for female nurses and a new commissary building with cold storage equipment.

No records are available as to the names of the medical officers who have served at this institution prior to 1911. At that time they were:

L. L. Uhls, M. D. ....Superintendent.
J. Van Nuys, M. D. ....Assistant superintendent.
L. R. Sellers, M. D. ....Assistant physician.
H. H. Hill, M. D. ....Assistant physician.
H. L. Goss, M. D. ....Assistant physician.

The officers in 1914 were:

F. A. Carmichael, M. D. .....Superintendent.
C. R. Hepler, M. D. ....First assistant physician.
P. B. Newcomb, M. D. ....Clinical director.
F. B. Kramer, M. D. ....Pathologist.
M. V. Church, M. D. ....Assistant physician.

The officers in 1916 were:

F. A. Carmichael, M. D.........Superintendent.
Philip B. Newcomb, M. D.......First assistant physician and clinical director.
J. J. Harrington, M. D..........Second assistant physician.
B. F. Frazier, M. D.............Third assistant physician.

TOPEKA STATE HOSPITAL.[1]

Topeka, Kans.

In 1875 the Legislature of the State of Kansas provided for the establishment of an institution for the insane at Topeka by an act appropriating $25,000 to build an asylum. The same act fixed the location of the institution as follows:

> Said asylum shall be located at some convenient, eligible and healthy point within two miles of the Capitol Building in the City of Topeka. The ground selected for said asylum shall contain not less than 80 acres, and the title of said ground or tract of land must be clear and unencumbered and vested in fee simple in the State of Kansas, without any cost to the state, and the same shall be tillable land and accessible to an abundance of water.

In a subsequent section the character of the buildings was specifically indicated as follows:

> Said Board of Commissioners shall cause to be prepared complete plans and specifications, for the erection of an insane asylum, as contemplated by the second section of this act, which plans and specifications shall be prepared for, and the building, or buildings, shall be constructed upon what is known as the segregate or cottage system, that is, with one main central building, and other buildings grouped around the same; each building, except the main central hospital building, to be two stories high and of sufficient capacity to accommodate 40 patients each; and in number sufficient to accommodate 300 persons in the aggregate, exclusive of officers and employees; and the said buildings, except the main central hospital building, shall not cost to exceed $25,000 each.

A person unacquainted with conditions in Kansas would be astonished, after reading the act of the Legislature authorizing the establishment of the Topeka Hospital, to observe the disregard of the specific instruction of the law in the building of the institution.

The two-story cottages, with a limitation of 40 beds capacity, and segregated, have been changed to a group of six modified Kirkbride buildings, three stories high, each with a capacity of 140 patients, and erected at an approximate cost of $75,000 for

[1] Compiled from material furnished by T. C. Biddle, M. D., superintendent.

each building; these again have been supplemented by one large custodial building for male patients, with a capacity of 435 beds, erected at an initial cost of $150,000.

In fact, until the time of the erection of the recent enlargement of the institution, that is, during the past five years, the law has not been complied with as to the character of the buildings erected. These later buildings have been cottages conformable to the statutory provisions.

Again it will be observed that the original act provided that the institution should "accommodate 300 persons in the aggregate."

This provision as to the capacity of the institution in the original law has been increased to a present capacity of 1400 beds, plus a reception hospital now nearing completion, which will provide 140 additional beds, or a total of 1540 beds. Other enlargements are contemplated in the plans for the completion of the institution, which will add not less than 210 beds, thus furnishing an institution with a capacity of 1750 patients when completed.

The excuse for the unfortunate disregard of the statute in the construction of the institution has been based on the necessity of providing a greater amount of room for the care of the insane than was contemplated in the original act, and also on economic considerations.

Following the instruction of the Legislature, with the modifications above described, the commissioners proceeded with the erection of two buildings, which were ready for occupation in the spring of 1879, at which time Dr. B. D. Eastman, then superintendent of the asylum at Worcester, Mass., resigned his position at Worcester, and came to Topeka to assume the superintendency of the new institution. He became superintendent of the Topeka Asylum April 1, 1879, and at once actively engaged in necessary preparatory work for the opening of the asylum, the first patient, Ernest A. Henzel, of Nemaha County, being admitted June 1, 1879. Since then 7438 cases have been admitted and 1391 were resident January 1, 1912.

Dr. Eastman's superintendency of the institution was long and conspicuously successful, though on two occasions, for political reasons solely, his tenure of office was broken for short periods. Following each absence he returned to the superintendency and did not finally sever his connection with the institution until July,

1897, when, for a third time, he was relieved from his charge because of a change in the political administration of the state.

Thus, for fifteen years, during the developmental period of the asylum, the state received the benefit of the services of this eminently efficient and honorable man. Dr. Eastman was first relieved from duty for the reasons above stated July 1, 1883, and was absent until March, 1885, during which time Dr. A. P. Tenney was the medical superintendent. Dr. Eastman was again superseded July 1, 1893, when Dr. J. H. McCasey was installed as his successor. Dr. McCasey remained in charge until February, 1895, at which time Dr. Eastman was for a third time returned to the superintendency and continued as such until July 1, 1897, when he was superseded by Dr. C. H. Wetmore, who was superintendent until October 1, 1898. Following Dr. Wetmore's resignation, Dr. L. D. McKinley was acting superintendent until April 1, 1899, at which time Dr. T. C. Biddle, the present superintendent, was installed, and has remained continuously in service as medical superintendent.

The act of Legislature establishing the insane asylum at Topeka, Kans., provided that three members of the State Board of Trustees of Charitable Institutions should be appointed to act as commissioners of the Topeka asylum.

The Board of Trustees of State Charitable Institutions at that time was composed as follows: Edward Knowles, president; C. E. Faulkner, secretary; A. T. Sharpe, treasurer; J. L. Wever and Thomas T. Taylor.

From these Edwin Knowles, Thomas T. Taylor and J. L. Wever were selected to be commissioners for the Topeka asylum.

On the 9th day of May, 1877, the first contracts were let for the erection of the buildings.

Upon the organization and opening of the asylum, the special commissioners retired and the asylum passed under the supervision of the State Board of Charities, the personnel of which board was frequently changed during the following years. The board, composed of five members, continued as a Central Board of Administration of the Charitable Institutions without change of title until the Legislature of 1905 enacted the "Board of Control" law.

This provided that the board should be composed of three members only, and its authority was enlarged and made more specific —the law conforming in its essential features to the board of administration laws of other states, which have adopted the policy of a single Board of Control.

On July 1, 1905, when the Board of Charities was discontinued and the Board of Control took charge of the institution, the board was composed as follows: E. B. Schermerhorn, president; S. G. Elliott, treasurer; H. C. Bowman. Since that date the board has continued without change in its personnel, except the resignation of Mr. Schermerhorn in April, 1911, and the appointment of Charles D. Shukers to fill the vacancy.

By act of Legislature in 1901 the official name of the institution was changed from the Topeka Insane Asylum to the Topeka State Hospital.

The growth of the institution has been coincident with the increasing demand for additional room for the care of the insane of the state and has corresponded to the state's growth in population until it has attained its present capacity.

Approximately, $1,200,000 have been specifically appropriated by the several Legislatures for the erection of buildings and equipment. The reception hospital for the treatment of acute and curable cases, the most important addition to the equipment of the hospital, is at this time approaching completion. This building is built after the most approved and modern plans of similar buildings and is thoroughly equipped with surgical, electrical and hydrotherapeutic appliances, and also has a clinical laboratory. Its cost will be $120,000 when completed and furnished.

The Topeka State Hospital is situated two miles west of the Capitol Building of the state, on a tract of land containing 420 acres. The site is unusually attractive and its natural advantages have been improved by liberal landscape-gardening and planting, until very few insane hospitals in the country are favored with a more favorable or attractive environment.

The following is a list of superintendents, physicians and assistant physicians in the service of this institution, with the length of service of each, from the period of opening June 1, 1879, to 1914:

SUPERINTENDENTS.

B. D. Eastman.......... 1879-1883
A. P. Tenny............ 1883-1885
B. D. Eastman.......... 1885-1893
J. H. McCasey.......... 1893-1894
B. D. Eastman.......... 1895-1897
C. H. Wetmore......... 1897-1899
T. C. Biddle........... 1899-

ASSISTANT SUPERINTENDENTS.

W. S. Lindsay.......... 1879-1885
L. F. Wentworth........ 1885-1892
E. B. Thompson........ 1893-1893
Anna M. Kniberg...... 1893-1895
H. S. Willard.......... 1895-1897
T. W. Scott............ 1898-1899
C. W. Myers............ 1899-1904
W. C. Van Nuys........ 1904-1906
J. C. Bennett............ 1906-1908
J. H. Cooper............ 1908-

ASSISTANT PHYSICIANS.

John Punton 1884-1887
Fred O. Jackman....... 1887-1891
G. A. Wall.............. 1887-1889
Geo. L. Beers........... 1889-1893
Geo. L. Limmer........ 1891-1893
M. M. Cloud........... 1894-1895
H. D. Brothers.......... 1894-1895
J. E. McCraig.......... 1895-1896
H. T. McLaughlin....... 1895-1897
L. V. Duncan........... 1896-1896
J. L. Moorhead......... 1896-1897
P. F. Wellman.......... 1897-1898
D. H. Smith............ 1897-1899
L. D. McKinley......... 1898-1898
C. C. Stivers........... 1898-1899
E. W. Minney.......... 1899-1901
J. S. Scott.............. 1899-1902
J. F. McNaughton...... 1901-1904
W. C. Van Nuys........ 1902-1904
J. C. Bennett........... 1904-1906
J. H. Cooper............ 1905-1908
R. A. Taylor............ 1906-1907
F. C. Cave.............. 1907-1907
J. M. Becker............ 1907-1907
T. P. Scott............. 1907-
G. W. Hochrein......... 1908-1909
R. A. Taylor............ 1909-1910
Maggie L. McCrea...... 1909-1912
R. A. Young........... 1910-1910
L. E. Haughey......... 1910-1911
G. E. Hesner (second assistant) 1911-
L. C. Bishop (third assistant) 1912-
Maud S. DeLand (fourth assistant) 1912-

STATE HOSPITAL FOR EPILEPTICS.[1]

PARSONS, KANS.

For several years prior to 1899 the two state asylums for the insane in Kansas had been crowded with patients and many for whom application for admission had been made could not be admitted because of lack of room. The indigent insane who could not be received into the state institutions were cared for by the counties in jails, almshouses and private asylums, and each Legislature was called upon to appropriate a considerable sum to reimburse the counties for their support. This being an expensive and unsatisfactory arrangement, the Legislature of 1899 appropriated $100,000 for the purpose of establishing a third asylum for the insane. The bill provided for a committee of nine, to be made up of members of the Senate and House of Representatives, to select a site and acquire not less than 640 acres of land for the new institution. It further provided that the location should be decided upon not later than June 30, 1899, and that the Board of Trustees of State Charitable Institutions should then proceed to have erected an insane asylum built upon the segregate or cottage system. An active campaign was at once started in a number of cities and towns in different parts of the state to secure the new institution. The greatest rivalry existed between the cities of Clay Center in the north-central section and Parsons in the extreme southeast corner of the state. The contest was decided in favor of the latter place and the committee contracted for a section of land in the immediate vicinity of Parsons. Before title to the land could be acquired, however, some of the citizens of Clay Center secured an injunction against the location and erection of the institution at Parsons. This litigation completely tied the hands of the Board of Trustees for about 18 months. The question was finally passed upon by the Supreme Court of the state and a decision favorable to the Parsons location was handed down. The board having decided upon a building plan for the institution with an ultimate capacity of 800, awarded a contract for the first group of buildings in the spring of 1902, and actual construction work

[1] Prepared by Dr. M. L. Jones, superintendent.

was started a short time thereafter. The building plan provided for a male and a female department of equal capacity, each to comprise the same number of buildings, similarly arranged. Three types of buildings for patients were designed, each building to be an individual unit or complete household, with day or sitting rooms, bed rooms and dormitories, a kitchen and a dining room.

The largest building planned, of which there was to be one in each department, was to accommodate 115 custodial patients. A second type of building, four for men and four for women, was to be an unscreened, open-door cottage, with a capacity of 36. The third type was a smaller open cottage for the housing of 16 to 20 patients. The plans called for eight such buildings for each sex. The long period of litigation over the location enabled the Board of Trustees to give an unusual amount of study to questions pertaining to the organization and development of the new institution. In their work in connection with the state hospitals for the insane the board had been impressed with the urgent need of some special care for epileptics. There were at the time about 200 epileptics in the two state hospitals for the insane. These patients were all classed as insane and had been so committed, although many of them showed only a mild form of mental reduction, which is often found associated with chronic epilepsy. Such patients, as is usually the case with epileptics confined in institutions for the insane, were somewhat discriminated against in such matters as the wards to which they were assigned, the privileges allowed them, etc. Under such conditions they were a disturbing element and a source of annoyance to the other patients with whom they were associated. There were also a considerable number of epileptics in the county poorhouses and some of the more dangerous types were held for extended periods in jails. Being thoroughly aroused to the deplorable condition of these unfortunates and realizing that there were throughout the state a large number of sane and noncommitted epileptics in need of special care, the board, largely through the influence of its president, Mr. Henry J. Allen, determined to make an effort to have the new institution changed into a hospital or colony for epileptics. The idea of such a change had been borne in mind when the original plans were drawn, and the buildings were designed accordingly. A bill providing for this transformation was presented to and passed by the Legislature of 1903. Section 1 of this act reads as follows:

> The Parsons State Hospital, the erection of which was provided for by chapter 13 of the session laws of 1899 and chapter 20 of the session laws of 1901, shall be devoted to securing the humane, curative, scientific and economical care and treatment of epileptics and insane epileptics, and shall be governed and controlled by the Board of Trustees of State Charities and Corrections.

The first contract included a central power and heating plant and five cottages for patients. Long-time contracts were also made with local companies for a supply of natural gas for all fuel purposes and for water and electricity to meet the requirements of the institution. It was decided to receive only male patients at first, so all of the cottages were erected in the men's group. They consisted of a custodial building for the more demented and mentally disturbed, two open-door cottages for the chronic middle class, and two small cottages to accommodate 18 patients each, for those in better mental condition. All buildings were to be two-story, with basement, and of the slow burning type. By midsummer of 1903, the construction work being well advanced, it was thought to be time for the selection of a superintendent. Dr. M. L. Perry, pathologist of the Georgia State Hospital for the Insane, was appointed to this position and took charge in July of that year. There was an urgent demand from all parts of the state that the institution be opened for patients at the earliest date possible. Work was concentrated on the completion of the custodial building and the two smaller cottages, one of which was fitted up as a temporary administration building. The work of equipping and furnishing the cottages and organizing a force of employees was in progress even before the buildings were completed, and the institution was opened for the reception of patients October 19, 1903. On that day there were transferred from the two insane hospitals 110 men. On account of the overcrowded condition of the hospitals for the insane and the demand for state care for the insane who had been previously refused admission to the hospitals and were still county charges, it was determined that all epileptics confined in the state institutions for the insane should be transferred to the epileptic colony as rapidly as room could be provided for them. This policy was pursued and after the erection of a duplicate group of cottages in the female department in the next year the epileptic insane women were transferred. Since 1904, therefore, there has been in this state a complete separation of the epileptic and non-epileptic insane. Kansas was one of the first states to carry out this policy. No one connected with these institutions has since doubted the wisdom of this course.

Dr. T. C. Biddle, superintendent, State Hospital, Topeka, in a paper discussing the merit of the Kansas plan of complete separation of the epileptic from the ordinary insane, says: "It has been my privilege to observe the influence of the epileptic in the same hospital, both before and after removal. I am sure no superintendent will wonder when I testify that no other innovation has brought so much relief and comfort to our hospital population. ....I consider most important the demonstrated fact that the so-called insane epileptics are greatly benefited by such removal. My personal experience is to me quite conclusive as to the benefit of separation. Several of the cases that were transferred from the Topeka Hospital to Parsons were, while at Topeka, disorderly and a very disturbing influence in the hospital. It has been reported to me that these persons, in the environment of the epileptic colony, are quiet, orderly and well behaved." That the epileptics themselves indorse the plan is shown by the fact that of those originally transferred, although brought from well-established, excellently equipped, and admirably conducted institutions, surrounded by beautiful and well-kept lawns, and placed in another of meagre equipment, with more or less barren grounds bestrewn with debris from recent construction, not one expressed a desire to return to his former environment. Their satisfaction resulted largely from better classification and the greater amount of liberty and outdoor life permissible under colony methods.

The act creating the hospital vested in the Board of Trustees authority to make such rules and regulations as were deemed necessary for the admission of epileptics, sane or insane, for their care and treatment and their transfer or discharge. The rules relating to these matters which were formulated at the opening of the institution are with a very few alterations still in force. By these rules any resident of the state who is afflicted with epilepsy (excepting only low-grade imbeciles and idiots) is admitted upon application submitted in regular form. It has been thought wise to refuse admission to low-grade epileptic imbeciles and idiots on account of the deterring influence the presence of such types would have on applications for the admission of the really sane and those only slightly reduced in mind. Such low-grade patients as are not received at Parsons are cared for in the State Home for Feeble-minded. All applications for admission are made through the office of the probate judge of the county of which the patient is a resident, the judge certifying to the residence and the financial condition of the applicant. Those in poor or moderate circumstances receive board, care and medical attention free, but for those whose financial condition will justify it a charge is made just sufficient to reimburse the state for the amount expended on them by the institution. This rule is given a very liberal interpretation, only a small percentage of patients being required to pay. All application papers contain a blank to be filled out by the family or attending physician, giving a rather comprehensive medical history of the case, particularly as regards the development and course of the epilepsy. If the patient is insane a regular commitment in lunacy is required, the same as that in use for the ordinary insane. Sane epileptics are admitted on voluntary commitment, the patient signing the application if of legal age and if a minor the parent or guardian signing for him. The following form of application is used:

I hereby make application for admission as a patient to the State Hospital for Epileptics at Parsons, Kans., and if admitted I promise to obey faithfully all rules and regulations of the hospital.

I fully understand and agree that the rules and regulations of the hospital are to govern my habits, diet, medical treatment, exercise and employment.

I fully understand and agree that, in case I wilfully or persistently violate the rules and regulations of the hospital, I lay myself liable to be dismissed at any time.

I fully understand that the nature of epilepsy is such that continuous treatment for a period of two or three years is required to effect a cure or permanent improvement, and it is my intention to remain a patient in the State Hospital for at least that length of time, or until discharged under the rules and regulations of the hospital or by order of the State Board of Control.

(Signed) ....

Post-office ...., ...County, Kansas.

Date ....19..

For the first several years that the hospital was in operation the management had no legal authority to hold a patient so committed against his will for any length of time. Such an arrangement was not found to be entirely satisfactory, as patients who, under normal conditions, were entirely willing to remain in the hospital might, while temporarily disturbed in mind as a result of epileptic attacks, demand their release when not capable of taking care of themselves. Several instances of this kind occurred. To meet such a contingency the passage of the following act was secured, since when there has been no further difficulty in connection with voluntary commitments.

Chapter 234, Session Laws 1909.—All persons admitted to said hospital as sane epileptics under the provisions of section 2, chapter 384, of the session laws of 1903, shall, until paroled or discharged, be under the custody and control of the superintendent of said hospital, and the superintendent may restrain any such patient when he deems it necessary for the welfare of the patient and the proper conduct of the institution. Any patient admitted as a sane epileptic who is of legal age, or the parent or guardian of any such patient, if a minor, may at any time obtain the discharge of such patient from the institution by giving ten days' notice in writing to the superintendent of the desire to obtain such discharge.

It has been the desire of the management to avoid the adoption of any other measures compromising or restricting the purely voluntary character of the commitment in all cases not insane. This has seemed to be a wise course to pursue, as many sane epileptics and also the parents of children of normal mentality who have only recently developed epilepsy will not consider an application for admission to an institution that binds the patient to stay against his own or his parents' will. It is just such patients for whom most can be done by institutional care and who are the most desirable and at the same time the most difficult to obtain.

During the first few months following the opening of the hospital the superintendent did all medical work in addition to his other duties of an administrative and executive character, but in January, 1904, Dr. A. L. Skoog was appointed assistant physician. He served the institution faithfully and efficiently in this capacity and later as assistant superintendent until he resigned in 1906. The female department was opened in the latter part of 1904. This rendered the services of another physician necessary and Dr. F. F. Malone was appointed assistant physician in August,

1905. Dr. Malone was an exceptionally able man in his profession and the institution sustained a decided loss when he resigned in January, 1906. The vacancy thus occasioned was filled by the appointment in January, 1906, of Dr. O. S. Hubbard. He was promoted later in 1906 to the position of assistant superintendent, at which time Dr. H. P. Mahan was appointed assistant physician. They are both still in the service, there having been no other change in the medical staff.

The method of treatment is largely custodial, due to the fact that the great preponderance of patients received are chronic cases for whom there is little or no hope of recovery. Only 2 per cent of the admissions have been epileptic less than one year. All patients are given a thorough mental and physical examination directly after coming to the institution and are then assigned to a cottage, where they will be associated with others of a similar type. Classification is recognized as one of the most important features of colony life, and the comparatively small cottages at the Parsons colony have made it possible to classify patients in a much more satisfactory manner than is found feasible where larger buildings or units are used. Individual patients are given special medication to meet indications, but in a general way the treatment of most cases is along hygienic and dietetic lines, with a judicious administration of sedatives. Employment is a valuable adjuvant to the medical treatment of epilepsy and all patients at the hospital in good physical condition are required to do some work. They assist with the housework and are employed in the laundry, dairy, about the lawns, in the garden and on the farm. Farming and gardening are carried on rather extensively, about 400 acres being devoted to those industries.

In 1906 a school was organized and is conducted for eight months each year. There being no suitable building for this purpose, a school room has been improvised by dividing the day or sitting room of one of the women's cottages and using a part of it. Twenty-five regular pupils are thus accommodated. In addition to these pupils of usual school age there are also classes of adults who are given instruction in manual work. About one-half the time in school is devoted to ordinary grade work and the remainder to manual training. Under the latter is included instruction in sewing, various kinds of fancy work, mat and rug weaving, basketry, bead work, lace making, wood carving and elementary sloyd work. A school building has been and is at present one of the needs of the institution.

In 1909 an administration building was erected at a cost of $70,000. This building stands at the head of the main entrance drive and contains, in addition to the offices, living apartments for officers and employees and a commodious assembly room seating 600.

The institution at present (1914) comprises a total of 20 buildings and has a capacity of 515 and a population of 510. Since the beginning 1290 patients have been under treatment. There are 90 officers and employees connected with the hospital. The annual budget amounts to approximately $35,000 for salaries and wages and $70,000 for care and maintenance. The per capita cost reckoned on the total amount expended for salaries, wages, care and maintenance and ordinary repairs, less fees collected from private patients, sale of products, etc., and turned into the state treasury, divided by the daily average number of patients actually in the institution, amounts to $195.09 per annum.

The management has been, since 1905, under the State Board of Control. The following is a list of trustees and board members connected with the hospital since its organization:

TRUSTEES.

Henry J. Allen	1903-1905	G. W. Kanavel	1903-1905
F. B. Denman	1903-1905	C. A. McNeil	1903-1905
R. Vincent	1903-1905		

MEMBERS OF STATE BOARD OF CONTROL.

E. B. Schermerhorn	1905-1912	H. C. Bowman	1905-
S. G. Elliott	1905-1913	W. E. Brooks	1913-
C. D. Shukers	1912-1913	Stance Myers	1913-

LARNED STATE HOSPITAL.

LARNED, KANS.

This hospital was established by an act of the Legislature in 1913 and located in the western part of the state, because all the other state institutions in Kansas for the care of the insane were in the eastern portion. Owing to the crowded condition which existed in the older institutions it was deemed advisable to make the location at a point where it would relieve other institutions and at the same time supply treatment for patients in the immediate vicinity.

In May, 1914, but a single cottage had been erected, which was complete in itself, having a dining-room, kitchen and cold storage facilities.

The patients under treatment, now numbering 40, have been selected from other institutions.

The buildings are modern and fireproof. It is intended to build one cottage each year to relieve the congestion in the other institutions, and eventually to build an administration building and psychopathic hospital and other necessary buildings; after which time the hospital will receive patients of all classes from all counties of the state.

The farm consists of about 1000 acres of bottom land, which is placed under irrigation.

The only medical officer at present on duty is Dr. B. F. Hawks, superintendent. The institution is under the control of the State Board of Control of Kansas.

HOSPITAL FOR THE DANGEROUS INSANE.

LANSING, KAN.

Provision for the criminal insane and for insane criminals is made in connection with the State Penitentiary. There are at present accommodations for 41 criminal insane—that is, insane persons under criminal charge who have been declared dangerous—and for 22 insane criminals. There are no wards of special construction for the accommodation of these men. They are under the care of the keeper during the day and of a night officer at night. These officers are assisted by prisoners, one of whom as night watch patrols the ward at night, and two of whom act as attendants upon the inmates during the day, looking after their cells, their clothing and the like. Four men confined in the psychopathic ward as insane persons are well enough to attend to the dining room and wait on the table.

The food is prepared in the general kitchen, and luxuries are supplied from the hospital kitchen of the penitentiary three times a week.

Four of the insane criminals accommodated in the psychopathic ward are well enough to work in the shops attached to the penitentiary.

The title of the institution is "The Hospital for the Dangerous Insane," and under the law any insane person confined in any state hospital who becomes dangerous or violent may be sent to the institution. Such patients, however, thus committed, must be brought before a district court judge or a probate court judge and examined by two reputable physicians. Counsel is also allowed for them by the state.

Two persons usually occupy a room, except in cases of extreme violence, when it becomes necessary for an individual to be placed singly in a cell. There are no special facilities for care and treatment.

STATE HOME FOR FEEBLE-MINDED.[1]

WINFIELD, KANS.

The Legislature of 1881 located this Home temporarily in the first State University building, Lawrence, Kans., and provided that the trustees cause suitable accommodations to be arranged for the comfort, maintenance and education of such pupils as may be admitted. The Legislature of 1885 located the Home permanently at Winfield, but said nothing about the maintenance of the pupils.

The law provided that the board "shall admit into said asylum all idiotic and imbecile youths who have been residents of the

[1] By F. C. Cave, M. D., superintendent.

State of Kansas six months and are not over 15 years of age and who are incapable of instruction in the common schools," and that "the object of this institution is to train and educate those received so as to render them more comfortable, happy and better fitted to care for and support themselves," and that "persons afflicted with contagious, infectious or loathsome disease, whose presence might endanger the health, morals or safety of the inmates of any institution, shall not be admitted to any institution." The foregoing statement and the change of name to the Kansas Home for Feeble-minded Youth are self-explanatory and indicate plainly and fully that the purpose of the institution is to board and school the feeble-minded youth of Kansas who are under the age of 15 years, and pupils over 15 years of age if its capacity will allow the reception of others.

The institution consists of three large buildings, each capable of housing 200 inmates. The general arrangement of each is practically the same throughout the institution—large dormitories, play rooms, bathrooms, halls, etc., each floor being designed to take care of 50 patients. There are at present 540 inmates (1915).

A school of letters is maintained up to the fifth grade; also a manual training department, largely for girls, where sewing, basketry, weaving, wood-work, clay modeling, etc., are taught. Children are employed in different pursuits as far as possible on the farm, in the laundry, engine room, carpenter shop, bakery, kitchens, household work, etc.

The institution possesses 430 acres of land, a good dairy, pigs, chickens, sheep, etc. It is maintained wholly by the state. The per capita cost is $160 per annum.

The present superintendent is Dr. F. C. Cave.

THE CARE OF THE INSANE IN KENTUCKY.

Kentucky was one of the first of the states to make provision for its insane in a special hospital, the Eastern Lunatic Asylum at Lexington having been opened on May 1, 1824. Prior to that time Kentucky provided for her insane paupers by the appointment of one or more individuals to take care of them upon terms fixed at the discretion of the judge before whom the case was tried. As late as 1842 the laws of Kentucky allowed the quiet and peaceful insane to be maintained at their homes out of the public treasury. Until 1844 the Lunatic Asylum was maintained with the idea that madmen were dangerous and must be confined, and that all that could be done for them was to keep them in custody. This system of care, or rather lack of care, was changed for the better in 1844, when Dr. J. K. Allen became superintendent.

In 1854 the state established a second institution, now the Western State Hospital, Hopkinsville; and in 1869, a third asylum, now known as Central State Hospital, Lakeland, designed at first as a "State House of Reform for Juvenile Delinquents," but converted into an asylum for the insane in 1873.

There is in addition an institution for feeble-minded children, which was established in 1861 at Frankfort. These institutions were at first under the control of separate boards of commissioners. In 1906 they were placed under a single board of control, known as the Kentucky State Board of Control for Charitable Institutions.[1]

Board of Control.—The Board of Control consists of four members, appointed by the Governor, by and with the advice of the Senate, for four years. In order that the board may be free from political control, it is provided that it shall be non-partisan in character. Each commissioner is required to take the oath of office required of other state officers and to execute a bond to the Commonwealth of Kentucky in the sum of $25,000 for the faith-

[1] For list of members of Board of Control, see p. 470.

ful discharge of his duties. Such bond must be approved by the Governor and filed in the office of the Secretary of State.

The Governor, when the Senate is not in session, may make removals of the members of the board for causes to be given in writing, and may fill vacancies in the board subject to the approval of the Senate when it convenes, and in any case of removal the Governor shall submit the facts and reasons for the Senate's approval and the Senate shall have power to reinstate such persons removed. The Board of Control elects one of its members president and each member receives as compensation for his services $2500 per year and necessary traveling expenses in the discharge of his duties.

The board elects a secretary, who holds his office at the pleasure of the board and receives $150 per month and his necessary traveling expenses. The board also elects a treasurer for each institution, whose salary is not to exceed $500 per year and who is required to give bond, to be approved by the Board of Control, for the faithful performance of his duties, such bond being renewed once each year. The Board of Control is provided with an office at the Capitol and at least one member of the board and the secretary remain in Frankfort when not attending a board meeting at one of the institutions.

The Board of Control holds regular meetings at each institution under its control once each month and oftener if necessary and makes a thorough examination of the affairs, management, property, clothing, food, supplies, condition of buildings and grounds, and the conduct of every official and employee of said institutions.

The board must keep a complete record of such examinations, together with such rules and regulations as may be established. The board also maintains a vigilant inspection of such institutions and ascertains that all money appropriated for their aid has been judiciously and economically expended and whether the objects of the institutions have been properly accomplished and the laws in reference to the same fully complied with.

The treasurer, under order of the board, receives from the treasurer of the state all moneys appropriated for the use of the institution and receipts to him therefor. The treasurer receives and pays out all moneys due and belonging to the institution. He makes to the board a monthly report of the financial condition of the institution, with a detailed statement of the income and expenditures for the month, and keeps true and complete books of all the financial transactions.

The Board of Control has power to appoint a medical superintendent, a first, second and third assistant superintendent, each of whom shall be a skilled and competent physician who has practiced medicine under the laws of the state; and a steward. Their term of office shall be four years and they are subject to removal for cause by the board. But one so removed can have an appeal to the Governor, who, upon hearing the case, may reinstate him. There is one woman physician in each asylum for the insane in the commonwealth which receives women patients. She receives the same salary and has the same rights as male physicians and is assigned to duty upon wards for women. The Board of Control keeps a record of its proceedings which, with the books of the secretary and other officials and books and papers of other institutions, is open for examination and inspection.

Commissioners or other officers shall not sell to the institutions herein mentioned or make any contracts with them in which they are interested.

The State Board of Control has full power at all times to look into and examine the condition of the several institutions of the state mentioned, financially or otherwise, to inquire and examine into the government and management of their inmates, the official conduct of the officers and employees and the condition of the buildings, grounds and other property connected therewith, and into all other matters pertaining to their usefulness and good management.

The Board of Control has power also to expend in its discretion any surplus standing to the credit of an institution from time to time in carrying out the purposes for which it was created, and in so doing may use such surplus upon any of the institutions under its control without reference to the fact that such surplus may have arisen from some other institution.

The Board of Control may also require that the institutions be reimbursed from the estates of such persons as are able to pay at the rate of $150 per year.

The Board of Control may purchase supplies for all the institutions collectively or may purchase for each institution separately, but when the supplies purchased aggregate sums exceeding $1000 it must advertise for such supplies and award the contract to the lowest bidder.

The salary of each superintendent shall be $2000 per year; of each first assistant physician $1250; of each second assistant physician $1000; and of each third assistant physician $800 per year; of each steward $1100; and of each receiver $600[1] per year. The medical superintendent has general management, supervision and control of patients and devotes his entire time to them. He keeps an accident book, a case book, a restraint book, and records all material facts in these books. Mechanical restraint is not applied in any case without the direction of and under the supervision of one of the physicians nor is the restraining apparatus kept in the wards when not in use.

It is the duty of the superintendent of each asylum to appoint a receiver or storekeeper who is to have custody of all supplies and stores and to inspect and distribute them to every department.

Separate asylum or hospital districts are assigned to the three institutions for the insane in Kentucky. The superintendent of each institution purchases incidental or emergency supplies for the institution, subject to the approval of the Board of Control, to whom he renders a monthly itemized statement giving the facts and circumstances of each expenditure.

If a patient is found insane and is committed to the State Hospital, the circuit court or county court judge must notify the hospital to send a person to accompany him to the hospital.

We are told that in all institutions of the state all forms of restraint have been abolished and that patients are not placed in solitary confinement by night or day.

Training schools for nurses have been established at the Central State Hospital and the Western State Hospital and a third school is being organized at the Eastern State Hospital.

In connection with the Central and Western State hospitals buildings have been erected for the care of tuberculous patients, and a similar building is proposed for the Eastern State Hospital.

In Kentucky no separate provision is made for the care of the criminal insane. They are not cared for properly in prisons and

[1] The receiver performs the duties of a store-keeper.

it is not thought to be safe to place them in ordinary institutions for the insane.

Many of the insane of the chronic class are still inmates of county almshouses. To arrange for the proper care of such persons an additional hospital for at least 1000 patients is required.

The existence of pellagra has given rise to a suggestion on the part of the Board of Control that a separate hospital be built for the care of pellagra patients. In the Central State Hospital 28 cases of pellagra were found during the three years from July 1, 1910, to 1913; seven patients had the disease when admitted to the institution, and the remaining 21 patients apparently developed it at the institution.

Classes Committed.—All insane persons except idiots, epileptics and the harmless incurable are admitted.

Legal Procedure.—Inquests must be held by the circuit court of the county. If no circuit court is in session the inquest may be held by a judge of a circuit court or the presiding judge of the county court.

The personal presence of the person charged with being of unsound mind is required, unless it shall appear by the oath or affidavit of two regular practicing physicians that they have personally examined him and find him to be insane and that his condition is such that it would be unsafe to bring him into court.

The case must be heard before a jury. If the judge is satisfied with the inquest, judgment must be entered accordingly, or he may order the inquest set aside and order a new inquest.

Whenever it appears from an affidavit filed that a person found of unsound mind has been restored to his proper senses, or that the inquest was false or fraudulent, the court must direct that the facts be inquired into by a jury in open court and make all necessary orders or decrees in the premises.

Cost of Commitment.—The expense is paid by the state.

EASTERN STATE HOSPITAL.[1]

LEXINGTON, KY.

The Eastern State Hospital, first called Eastern Lunatic Asylum, was opened as a state institution May 1, 1824. Its history dates back to 1816, when, at the hands of benevolent citizens, the most active of whom was Andrew McCalla, the Fayette Hospital was incorporated. The corner-stone of the building was laid June 30, 1817, and a brass plate was laid in the corner-stone with this inscription: "The first erected west of the Appalachian Mountains." The asylum at Williamsburg, Va., was established in 1773, the first state asylum, while that in Kentucky was the second. As early as 1751 a department for the insane had been established in the Pennsylvania Hospital, but it was not until 1841 that a public hospital was established in Pennsylvania.

Among the early physicians to asylums, Dr. Samuel Theobald, for several years attending physician to the Eastern Kentucky Asylum at Lexington, was notable. About 1830 he published an account not only of his institution but also of the care of the insane in Kentucky prior to the establishment of the asylum for the insane.[2]

Dr. Theobald says that in the early days Kentucky, like most of her sister states, provided for her insane paupers by the appointment of one or more individuals to take care of them upon terms fixed at the discretion of the judge before whom the case was presented. For this purpose the state paid $15,500 in 1822 and $18,000 the following year.

The disadvantages of the existing system were so apparent and the needs of better provision so great that in 1821 Governor Adair said in his message to the Legislature that the old system of supporting the insane had proved to be wholly inadequate to the purpose of restoration to mental soundness. He therefore proposed that the state establish an asylum for the insane, giving as an

[1] Taken from "A Sketch of Psychiatry in the Southern States," by T. O. Powell, M. D. Transactions of the American Medico-Psychological Asso., Vol. IV., pp. 96-98.

[2] Transylvania Journal of Medicine, 1829-1830.

additional reason that "if only one out of 20 of those unfortunate beings, laboring under the most dreadful of all maladies, should be restored, will it not be a cause of great congratulation to a humane and generous public?" Governor Adair also urged as one reason for establishing a state insane asylum that "it would prove highly beneficial to the medical school of Transylvania University, which would in time repay the obligation by useful discoveries in the treatment of mental maladies." In 1822, in consequence of this appeal, the Legislature of Kentucky, for "humane and politic" motives, decided upon the establishment of an asylum for the insane. The sum of $10,000 was appropriated for the purpose of carrying the act into effect. The commissioners appointed in accordance with the act proceeded promptly to the selection of an advantageous site containing about 17 acres and having thereon a spring of never-failing water. The tract selected had also a large and handsome brick edifice which had been constructed about the year 1817 by an association of individuals as a private hospital, called the Fayette Hospital, "for the diseased of every character," but the company had failed in this humane intention and the building remained unfinished and unoccupied.

Having purchased this property, the commission proceeded immediately to have the building finished and such additional improvements made as were then deemed adequate to the object in view.

On May 1, 1824, the house was opened for the reception of patients. A curious and interesting circumstance is that the first patient was a colored woman named Charity, aged 21, who had never been able to walk or talk, nor had she ever partaken of solid food.

The commission of 10 deputed to carry into operation the act relating to the asylum "were required scrupulously and carefully to examine the case of every subject brought to the asylum, distinguishing by all means in their power between such persons as might be sick or imbecile only, and such as were actually insane or of unsound mind, admitting only the latter. Also carefully to distinguish maniacs, or persons who are dangerous, from such as are quiet and peaceable, making orders for their confinement or otherwise. The first day of May ensuing the passage of the act was fixed as the period at which all laws committing persons of unsound mind to the care of committees and charging the treasury of the state therewith should cease, and that thereafter the care and safe-keeping of all such persons should be confided to the lunatic asylum." The commission was further invested with full power to discharge restored patients.

It was further enacted that no person should be supported at the asylum at the public charge who had an estate for his support. Andrew Stainton was made superintendent and Dr. James C. Cross was appointed resident or house physician. The medical faculty of Transylvania University, then a famous medical school, in a spirit of humanity and liberality which reflects much honor on them, tendered their services gratuitously as consulting physicians. In a short time Dr. Cross resigned. He was succeeded by Dr. William L. Thompson, who also had a short service. Dr. Theobald became attending physician in January, 1826, and served several years.

The laws of Kentucky in 1842 still allowed the quiet and peaceful to be maintained at their homes out of the public treasury. There was also considerable prejudice against hospital establishments so that few except the worst cases among paupers or the wealthier class were sent to the asylum. The asylum was primarily intended for the insane poor alone, but for some years prior to 1842 had received other patients from Kentucky and other states at the cost of $2.50 per week. Dr. Bush was physician to Lexington Asylum in 1841 and his report, according to Dr. Jarvis, showed great improvement in the care of the insane, and the Legislature was inclined to grant desired appropriations. It is interesting to note that tickets of admission to the asylum were issued to the members of the medical class of Transylvania University. The faculty of the medical school had the hospital in charge until 1844. It was a mad-house for the safekeeping of lunatics rather than an asylum for their care.

From May 1, 1824, to October 1, 1871, the whole number admitted was 3492—males, 2195; females, 1297. Of these 1200 were reported recovered, 1196 reported as having died, 354 removed, 146 as escaped, and there were remaining 536—males, 289; females, 247; showing the proportion of females to males to be rapidly increasing.

For 20 years, or until 1844, the institution was managed with the idea that madmen as a class were dangerous to a community and must be confined, and that all that could be done was to safely keep patients from harming others or themselves.

With the coming of Dr. J. R. Allen in 1844 there was a decided change for the better and the reign of moral treatment began. He remained in charge until 1855, when he was succeeded by Dr. W. S. Chipley, who held the place for 15 years. Dr. George Bryant, Dr. R. C. Chenault, Dr. W. D. Bullard, Dr. F. H. Clark and Dr. Edwin M. Wiley all had short terms, and upon January, 1896, Dr. W. E. Scott was appointed superintendent. At this time the farm consisted of 250 acres of land, and there were in the asylum 791 persons, of whom 128 were colored. He was succeeded by Dr. J. S. Redwine, of Jackson, who served until July, 1908. Dr. R. L. Williams served but a single year. He was followed by Dr. C. A. Nevitt, then first assistant physician, who served during the remainder of the unexpired term. In October, 1912, he was succeeded by Dr. Joseph A. Goodson, the present superintendent.

At present the Eastern State Hospital has grown until there are 1300 patients; the buildings are commodious and sanitary. The buildings first erected in 1817 are still in use, and, although the architectural design followed the old idea of a place of confinement only, they have been remodelled until the quarters are most cheerful.

There is a hospital separate and distinct from the rest of the institution for bedridden cases, and separate tubercular quarters are under construction.

The committee has been unable to obtain details of the subsequent history of this institution. In 1914 the capacity of the hospital was 1345 beds.

WESTERN STATE HOSPITAL.[1]

Hopkinsville, Ky.

The Western Lunatic Asylum of the State of Kentucky was established in 1854 and opened to receive its first patient September 18 of the same year. The name of this institution has been changed three times since its establishment, each change being made with a view of getting farther away from the term insanity.

This institution was the second one to be erected in the State of Kentucky, and after its establishment the first Board of Managers made the following statement concerning it:

> It is an enduring monument of the humanity and liberality of the citizens as represented in the Legislature. No state of this Union has a building better adapted for the purpose, and, while there are some larger, it may be questioned whether there is one constructed on a better plan or in a more substantial manner. The magnificent portico fronting the public highway, with its six lofty columns and its graceful entablature, is in a highest degree ornamental. The ascent to the front entrance is by a fine flight of stone steps, which form a graceful relief to the elevated platform of the portico. The entire front is 375 feet, with two wings extending back at right angles 190 feet.

This statement was made by the Board of Managers 64 years ago, and, while there have been many improvements in architecture, no institution has surpassed in magnificence and beauty the colonial architecture of this building; the succession of additions following out in perfect detail the original plan has developed the architectural unit into a perfect structure, accommodating 1200 patients in a most healthful and hygienic manner. In addition to the four wings that have been added to the main building, there have been erected two buildings for colored males and two for colored females, also two cottages for white females and a colony has been established for the care of tubercular patients. This colony is a unit by itself, being composed of two center buildings surrounded by small open tent-houses, and is located several hundred yards from the main building.

The institution was placed in the western part of the state in order to accommodate the counties in that district and for the purpose of reducing the expense of transportation and relieving

[1] By H. P. Sights, M. D., superintendent.

the congestion of the Eastern Lunatic Asylum, now the Eastern State Hospital. The first superintendent of the institution was Dr. Samuel Annan, a competent and successful physician, whose management was a credit to the state. The institution was maintained by a per capita allowance of $140 per annum, together with an appropriation from the Legislature to cover any deficit. The site of the institution is located about two miles east of the City of Hopkinsville, in a beautiful valley surrounded by hills with picturesque outcroppings of limestone formation, covered with a luxuriant growth of blue grass. The original 370 acres have been increased to 727 by the purchase of two adjoining farms. The main enclosure occupied by the buildings, drives, groves and playgrounds comprises about 35 acres, adjoining which are an apple orchard of 35 acres, a large modern dairy accommodating 100 cows, and a well selected garden of 40 acres.

This institution accommodates all classes of insane, including the criminal and epileptic and dangerous idiots. All the wards are arranged as large hallways, with individual rooms on the sides as well as one or two small dormitories, and a day room with bay windows. Each ward has its own dining room; the diet is supplied from a central kitchen. All windows and doors are screened against flies and mosquitoes. The absence of iron bars to the windows is an attractive feature. Iron sash, with 8 x 10-inch glass, serves as a protection against escape and does not mar the appearance of the building. Some of the wards are supplied with large day porches, giving patients the opportunity of fresh air under all conditions of the weather. The baths and toilet rooms have terrazzo floors, with modern plumbing and shower and tub baths.

The original building cost $375,000 and accommodated 350 patients. To-day the estimated cost of the institution is $980,000.

In 1852 there was a demand for another state institution, as the Eastern Asylum, at Lexington, could not accommodate the demands made upon it, and the number of insane in the county jails and under the care of relatives or friends was increasing. Accordingly the Legislature provided for the erection of an asylum to be located somewhere in the western part of the state; and an act was passed providing for the appointment, by the Governor, of a Board of Managers to select the location and secure plans for its erection. This board consisted of five members, whose duties were to for-

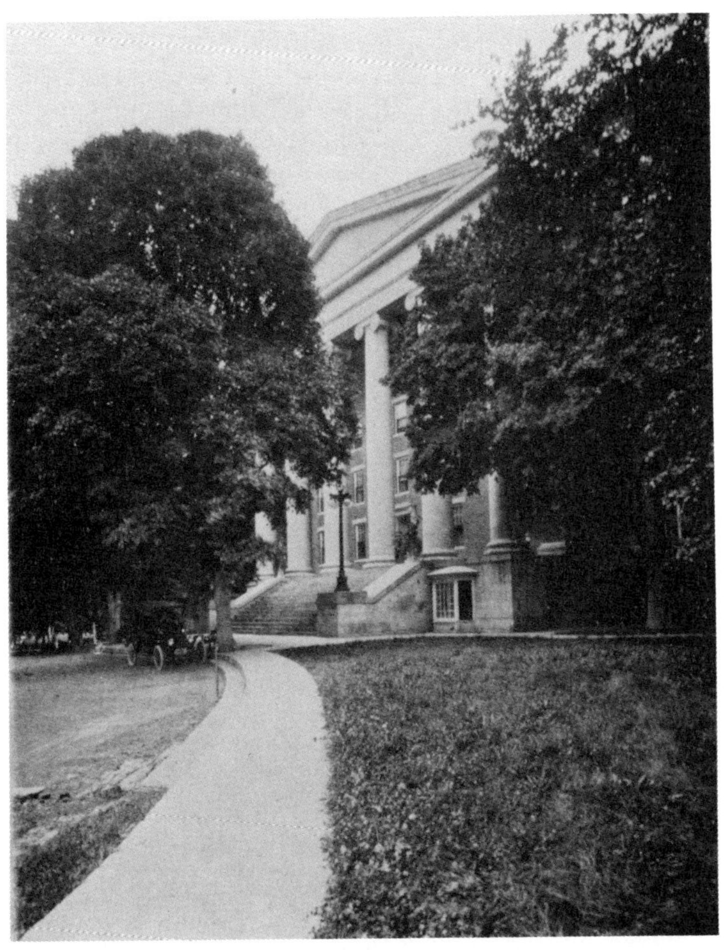

WESTERN KENTUCKY HOSPITAL, HOPKINSVILLE, KY.

mulate suitable by-laws for the government and regulation of the asylum; they were vested with the powers of appointment and removal of the superintendent, assistant physician, steward and matron, and were authorized to receive into the asylum all classes of insane patients, with the exception of idiots, unless dangerous.

This Board of Managers was evidently guided by the recommendations made by a committee appointed at a meeting of the Association of Medical Superintendents of American Institutions for the Insane, held in Philadelphia May 21, 1850. The Kirkbride style of building was then outlined and adopted and the recommendations of the above-mentioned committee were accurately and strictly followed in building this institution.

The first Board of Managers was composed of John P. Campbell, George Poindexter, C. M. Collins and Edward R. Clark. Dr. Samuel Annan, the first superintendent, opened the building to receive patients September 18, 1854, and at the end of his term there was a population of 180; he resigned in 1858 and was succeeded by Dr. Francis Montgomery, his first assistant being Dr. William Freeland. Dr. Montgomery was superintendent from 1858 to 1862. It was during his administration, on November 30, 1861, that the building was destroyed by fire, leaving only the massive walls.

The conflagration was started by a spark out of a chimney, about midday; a strong wind was blowing, and there was evidently a very poor equipment available for protection against fire, which no doubt was the leading cause of the complete destruction of the buildings. Fortunately only one patient was lost by the fire, and this resulted from the fact that he locked himself in his room; many eloped.

This completely disorganized the work and every available space in Hopkinsville was utilized for the care of the outcasts. The work of rebuilding was pushed, but required two years for completion. There was one great good that came out of this disaster, namely, the development of a spirit of interest and guardianship in the citizens of Hopkinsville that lasts until to-day, as a blessing to the institution.

In 1863 Dr. James Rodman was appointed superintendent, his first assistant being Dr. O. H. Perty. Dr. Rodman was superintendent for 26 years. His first assistant in 1867 was Dr. Hugh F.

McNary, who was later appointed superintendent of Central Asylum, Louisville, Ky.

In 1869 Dr. B. W. Stone was made first assistant and remained as such for 14 years. Dr. James Rodman continued his work with enthusiasm and success; he demonstrated remarkable ability as an executive and psychiatrist, and his high moral character gave the institution a high standing. He prudently and faithfully managed the affairs of the institution for the best benefit of the unfortunates under his care; and while he never abolished restraints, he exacted kind treatment of patients and prohibited any form of cruelty. He believed in furnishing the inmates entertainment and employment of some kind. The institution is a monument to his good taste in laying out the parks, planting trees and building driveways. His additions to the institution carried out the Kirkbride plan, with the exception of some detached cottages.

No internal dissension occurred during his administration. He was truly an able and great superintendent.

He was born at New Castle, Henry County, Ky., March 6, 1829, a member of a distinguished Kentucky family. He received a classical education and read medicine with his brother, Dr. Hugh Rodman, of Frankfort, and in 1849 graduated from the medical department of the University of Louisville.

After receiving his diploma he came to Hopkinsville and practiced his profession for three years, and then returned to Henry County and remained for some time; he later went to Frankfort, where he received the appointment to the Feeble-minded Institution; he superintended the erection of that institution, and after three years was selected for the superintendency of the Western Lunatic Asylum, where he began the best work of his life. Through his energies and progressive ideas he developed the institution into one of the leading asylums of the South.

In 1873 an act was passed by the Legislature requiring the appointment of a commission of nine members, to be selected locally, by the Governor, to govern the institution, but without power to appoint any official of the institution.

Dr. Rodman resigned in 1883; Dr. Barton W. Stone succeeded him, with Dr. B. F. Eager as first assistant; Dr. Wallace second assistant. Dr. Stone was considered one of the most competent superintendents in the state, and his administration was a successful one in every respect. He left marks of his wise policies and progressive management.

He and his assistants were removed by Governor Bradley in 1896 and Dr. Ben F. Letcher was appointed to succeed him; Dr. Miller of Owensboro, Ky., first assistant; Dr. Katherine Houser, second, and Dr. Frank Stanley, third.

Dr. Letcher resigned April 18, 1897, and Dr. T. W. Gardiner was appointed to fill out the unexpired term as superintendent; Dr. H. P. Sights, first assistant, and Dr. Cora Brown, second assistant. In July, 1900, Governor Beckham appointed Dr. E. B. McCormack to succeed Dr. Gardiner; Dr. Walter Lackey, first assistant; Dr. J. W. Stephens, second, and Dr. Florence Meder, third. Dr. McCormack was born November 18, 1854, at Masonville, Ky., and graduated from the Hospital College of Medicine, Louisville, Ky., in 1881. He practised in Owensboro and later returned there, after leaving the hospital in 1902.

Dr. W. W. Ray, of Springfield, Ky., was appointed to succeed Dr. McCormack; Dr. Ray resigned in 1904 and was succeeded by Dr. Milton Board, February 4, 1904, who resigned April, 1906, to qualify as a member of the State Board of Control, which had just been created in place of the commissioners by the Legislature. Dr. Board was born at Hardinsburg, Ky., October 4, 1870. He graduated in medicine at the University of Louisville, March 13, 1893. His administration as superintendent of the Western Hospital for the Insane was characterized by executive ability and progressive policies.

Dr. J. W. Stevens, of Elkton, Ky., succeeded him as superintendent from 1906 to 1908, when a bi-partisan board was created by the Legislature, consisting of two Republicans and two Democrats.

Dr. T. W. Gardiner was appointed by the board to succeed Dr. Stevens. He was born in Daviess County, October 9, 1848. He graduated at the Louisville Medical College in 1872; was interne at Louisville City Hospital in 1872, and was appointed first assistant physician at Central Asylum for the Insane, now Central State Hospital, April 1, 1873, serving three years, after which he located at Madisonville, Ky., where he practised medicine until April 1, 1897, when he was appointed superintendent of the Western State Hospital by Governor W. O. Bradley. July 1, 1900, he returned to Madisonville, Ky., and resumed the practice of medicine, and, as stated above, was appointed superintendent by the State Board of Control July 1, 1908. June 1, 1910, he was appointed a member of the Board of Control by Governor A. E. Wilson, and on January 1, 1911, was reappointed. Dr. Gardiner's record as superintendent is an enviable one; his economical administration and executive management are to be complimented. It was through him that the Governor and the Board of Control attempted at this institution to do away with all restraints. This was practically accomplished during his administration. This policy proved not only possible but was followed by a great improvement in the control of the patients.

July 1, 1910, Dr. H. P. Sights was appointed superintendent, with Dr. D. A. Campbell, first assistant; Dr. W. E. Render, second assistant; Dr. Roy Robinson, third assistant. In December, 1912, Dr. U. G. Davis was appointed third assistant and pathologist for the institution. In October, 1910, a training school was established for the instruction of nurses. November, 1910, moving picture shows were introduced as an innovation in the treatment of patients. In 1911 regular staff meetings were inaugurated, at which all patients received were examined both physically and mentally, properly classified and treatment agreed upon. The recognition of the prevalence of tuberculosis in the institution suggested the isolation of all patients suffering from this malady. In 1911 the Sunny Side Colony was established for the open air treatment and isolation of tubercular patients. This colony was located about one-fourth of a mile from the main building, consisting of male and female departments, each having a central plant surrounded by small tent houses constructed similar to the Nordack shack. This colony cost about $15,000 and accommodates 60 patients.

Three and a half years' experience proves this to be a most beneficial policy, it being the first colony established for the isolation of the insane tubercular cases in the state. This colony also takes care of the pellagra cases. In 1912 a laboratory was established for the purpose of the study of pellagra and hook worm.

In 1912 the Legislature changed the name of this institution from the Western Lunatic Asylum to Western State Hospital.

The history of the institution would not be complete without a description of the present condition, size and equipments. The cost of the present plant is $980,000; it is supported by a farm of

727 acres, having a dairy barn of the most modern type, accommodating 100 cows and managed under the best sanitary regulations. The arrangement of the buildings consists of a main building with two wings, comprising four 100-foot extensions at right angles to each, four stories in height, accommodating 800 patients. Six cottages and a colony in addition accommodate 400.

The main building is equipped with a hydrotherapeutic apparatus, shower, tub and continuous baths. Terrazzo floors in toilets and baths. The whole plant is newly equipped with modern plumbing; the electric lighting is constructed with underground cables in conduits. Electric and hydrotherapeutic treatment is furnished.

Dr. H. P. Sights, the present superintendent, was born October 28, 1863, in Henderson County, Ky. He received his medical education from the medical department of the University of Louisville, graduating in March, 1894, and then practised for two years at Henderson, Ky. He graduated from the Polyclinic, New York City, 1896. July 1, 1897, he was appointed first assistant at Western Kentucky Insane Asylum. In July, 1900, he located in Paducah, Ky., and practiced there for 10 years, and in July, 1910, was appointed superintendent of the Western Kentucky Insane Asylum.

The management of the Western State Hospital and the remaining three hospitals in the state, as has been already noted, are under a bi-partisan Board of Control, comprised of two Republicans and two Democrats, and a secretary. They visit the institution once a month, audit accounts, inspect the general condition of the institution and assist the superintendent by their advice and counsel and direct the general financial and social condition of the institution.

The following is a list of the superintendents and physicians of the Western State Hospital from 1854 to 1915:

SUPERINTENDENTS.

S. Annan, M. D. 1854-1857
Frank Montgomery, M. D. 1858-1862
James Rodman, M. D.... 1863-1884
Barton W. Stone, M. D.. 1884-1895
Benjamin F. Letcher.... 1896-1897
Thomas W. Gardiner, M. D. 1897-1900
E. C. McCormack, M. D. 1900-1902
W. W. Ray, M. D...... 1902-1904
Milton Board, M. D..... 1904-1906
J. W. Stevens, M. D..... 1906-1908
Thomas W. Gardiner, M. D. 1908-1910
H. P. Sights, M. D. (in office) 1910-

FIRST ASSISTANT PHYSICIANS.

William Freeland, M. D. 1858-1859
C. F. Hart, M. D........ 1861-1862
C. H. Perry, M. D....... -1866
Hugh F. McNary, M. D.. 1867-1868
Barton W. Stone, M. D... 1869-1884
B. F. Eager, M. D....... 1885-1895
F. A. Miller, M. D....... 1896-1897
H. P. Sights, M. D...... 1897-1900
Walter Lackey, M. D.... 1901-1903
A. Bailey, M. D......... 1904-1905
J. M. Ferguson, M. D.... 1906-1907
D. A. Campbell, M. D.... 1908-1912
H. G. Sanders, M. D..... 1913-1916

SECOND ASSISTANT PHYSICIANS.

B. F. Eugine, M. D...... 1879-1885
Howe Wallace, M. D..... 1886-1896
Katherine Houser, M. D. 1896-1897
Cora Brown, M. D...... 1898-1900
J. W. Stephens, M. D.... 1901-1903
J. M. Ferguson, M. D.... 1904-1905
Minnie Dunlap, M. D.... 1906-1907
W. E. Render, M. D..... 1908-1912
Roy F. Robinson, M. D... 1913-

THIRD ASSISTANT PHYSICIANS AND DRUGGIST.

W. F. Rodman, M. D... 1883-1884
A. F. Stanley, M. D..... 1896-1900
Florence Meder, M. D... 1901-1905
Minnie Dunlap, M. D.... 1906-1907
Roy F. Robinson, M. D... 1908-1912
U. G. Davis, M. D....... 1912-

SUPERNUMERARY.

L. B. Trigg, M. D........ 1912-

CENTRAL STATE HOSPITAL.[1]

LAKELAND, KY.

The Central State Hospital, formerly the Central Kentucky Asylum for the Insane, is located at Lakeland, Ky., about 11 miles east of Louisville, and is accessible by the Louisville & Nashville and Louisville & Interurban railroads, both of which pass near the institution.

The institution originated by an act of the Legislature of 1869, which appropriated $75,000 for the purchase of buildings and grounds and $10,000 to defray the necessary incidental expenses of the support and management of a "State House of Reform for Juvenile Delinquents"; it was conducted as such an institution until the year 1873. By reason of the inability of the Eastern and Western asylums to accommodate all of the insane of the state, the Legislature of 1873 converted the institution into an asylum for the insane, and designated it the "Central Kentucky Asylum for the Insane."

The farm on which the institution is located contained at that time 240 acres of land, with but few buildings, but the estate has been increased from time to time until it now contains 580 acres of land, improved with large and commodious buildings sufficient to care for 1400 patients. The first patient admitted to the institution was received by Dr. Thomas W. Gardiner, then an assistant physician, now a member of the Kentucky State Board of Control for Charitable Institutions.

The architecture is of the style in vogue at that time, consisting of an "administration building" centrally located, with three-story wings extending from either side, containing wards of the old type, consisting of long halls or corridors, with bed rooms or small dormitories on both sides. This type of building prevailed, with the addition of a new wing now and then, until 1890, when the first "open ward" building was constructed, the same being only two stories high, and consisting of five wards and a general dining-room, with a capacity of 225 patients. This is now known as the "Pusey Building," being named for Dr. H. K. Pusey, at that time

[1] Prepared by W. E. Gardner, M. D., superintendent, 1912.

superintendent; since that time this type of building has gained favor and was the first approach to the "cottage system," now so popular.

In 1900 an "industrial and amusement building" was completed, which now contains the sewing room, billiard room, dance hall and chapel. On the second floor of this building there is an open ward for female patients, one of the prettiest in the institution.

There are other isolated cottages of the "closed ward" type about the grounds of the institution, having capacities of from 50 to 200 patients. Some have individual dining-rooms, others have a single dining-room for several wards.

There has just been completed a "tuberculosis shack," with a capacity of 24 patients, at a cost of $10,000, the same being of wood and concrete and having broad and extensive porches, with all modern facilities for the proper care of tuberculosis cases. This is the first building for the isolation of tuberculosis, and will take care of all tubercular patients at this time.

This institution has its own heating, lighting and power plant, a new and modernly equipped laundry, a cold storage and ice plant, and is now being connected with a main from the Louisville Water Company, for which an appropriation of $65,000 was made by the last Legislature.

The institution is supported by a per capita allowance of $150 per year, the same having been fixed by the Legislature in 1894, but which is now inadequate. It is hoped to increase this allowance to $180, so that many contemplated improvements can be made.

The institution was under the supervision of a local Board of Commissioners, consisting of nine members, appointed by the Governor, until April, 1906, when by an act of the Legislature it was placed in common with all other institutions of like character in the state under the control of a central board, known as the "Kentucky State Board of Control for Charitable Institutions." This board is now bi-partisan and consists of four members, appointed by the Governor.

MEDICAL SUPERINTENDENTS.

C. C. Forbes, M. D...... 1873-1879
R. H. Gale, M. D........ 1879-1884
H. K. Pusey, M. D....... 1884-1888
W. J. Byrne, M. D....... 1888-1891
H. K. Pusey, M. D....... 1891-1896
H. F. McNary, M. D..... 1896-
L. E. Goslee, M. D....... 1897-1900
J. G. Furnish, M. D..... 1900-1904
M. H. Yeaman, M. D.... 1904-1907
Louis H. Mulligan, M. D. 1907-1910
W. E. Gardner, M. D... 1910-1914
F. L. Peddicord, M. D. (in office) 1914-

ASSISTANT PHYSICIANS.

Thomas W. Gardiner, M. D. 1873-1876
A. W. Bartlett, M. D.... 1874-1875
James Irwin Keller, M. D. 1876-1880
G. T. Erwin, M. D....... 1880-1884
F. T. Riley, M. D........ 1882-1884
F. H. Clarke, M. D...... 1884-1886
W. C. Dugan, M. D...... 1884-1887
W. F. Boggess, M. D.... 1886-1889
W. B. Pusey, M. D...... 1887-1887
W. H. Rogers, M. D..... { 1887-1888, 1895-1896 }
F. T. Burgloui, M. D.... 1887-1887
E. H. Jones, M. D....... 1888-1891
Moses Collins, M. D..... 1889-1892
Silas Evans, M. D....... 1891-1892
S. W. Halloway, M. D... 1891-1892
J. Young Brown, M. D.. 1892-1896
Eugene A. Smith, M. D.. 1892-1894
J. Morgan Sims, M. D... 1892-1896
Edward M. Green, M. D. 1894-1895
L. E. Goslee, M. D....... 1896-1897
W. R. Hefflin, M. D..... 1896-1900
M. M. Lively, M. D..... 1897-1900
B. F. Porter, M. D...... 1896-1900
J. W. Hill, Jr., M. D..... 1900-1904
M. H. Yeaman, M. D.... 1900-1904
Louise Ballard Trigg, M. D. 1901-1908
J. W. Stephens, M. D... 1904-1907
W. E. Gardner, M. D.... 1904-1910
John K. Wood, M. D.... 1907-1908
Florence Meder, M. D. (in office) 1908-
T. J. Crice, M. D........ 1910-1912
A. J. Davidson, M. D. (in office) 1910-
H. B. Pryor, M. D....... 1910-1912
F. L. Peddicord, M. D... 1912-1914
W. E. Remeer, M. D. (in office) 1914-

BOARD OF COMMISSIONERS.

Presidents.

B. K. White............ 1873-1874
S. J. Hobbs............ 1874-1880
S. L. Garr.............. { 1880-1884, 1892-1894 }
Albert G. Herr......... 1884-1887
Richard J. Brown....... 1887-1888
John C. Sherley......... 1888-1889
William Hughes 1889-1892
T. P. Satterwhite....... 1894-1904
W. H. Newman......... 1904-1906

Commissioners.

J. W. Goslee............ 1873-1875
W. W. Hill............. 1873-1874
S. J. Hobbs............. { 1873-1874, 1888-1894 }
William Terry .... { 1873-1880, 1880- }
William Hughes .... { 1873-1880, 1892-1894 }

Name	Years
L. P. Weatherby	1873-1874
J. C. Sherley	1873-1876
S. L. Garr	1873-1880; 1887-1892
R. K. White	1874-1881
Hamilton Ormsley	1874-1881
J. M. Holloway	1874-1880; 1888-1892
Col. E. D. Hobbs	1876-1880
J. W. Walker	1876-1881
Thomas R. Walker	1877-1880
James Bridgeford	1880-1881; 1882-1884
Andy Barnett	1880-1884
G. W. Owens	1880-1881; 1882-1884
A. G. Herr	1880-1881; 1882-1884; 1887-1892
Logan C. Murray	1880-1881
Chas. Bremaker	1880-1894; 1896-1902
Thomas Burns	1881-
Wesley Whipps	1881-1887
J. M. Robinson	1882-1888
C. B. Blackburn	1882-1884
John E. Green	1884-1888
R. J. Brown	1884-1887; 1888-1892
W. H. Wathen	1884-1887; 1892-1896
John G. Roach	1884-1888; 1892-
E. D. Standiford	1884-1887
E. H. Chase	1887-
R. S. Veech	1888-1892
Hancock Taylor	1889-1892
H. H. Grant	1892-1898
T. P. Satterwhite	1892-1894
W. P. D. Bush	1892-1894
R. Lee Suter	1893-1898
Thomas R. Gordon	1894-1896; 1900-1902
R. W. Brown	1894-1903
Geo. H. Alexander	1894-1899; 1903-
W. C. Dugan	1894-1900
M. A. Houston	1894-1896
I. W. Bernheim	1896-1901
R. H. Dorr	1896-
J. W. McGee	1897-1900
E. C. Bohne	1898-1901
John J. Barrett	1898-1904
John S. Morris	1900-1906
C. W. Long	1900-1905
Chas. F. Taylor	1901-1904
J. R. Allen	1902-1904
M. S. Tyler	1902-1904
J. W. Guest	1901-1906
M. K. Allen	1904-1906
B. W. Smock	1904-1906
W. C. Van Der Espt	1904-1906
Matt O'Doherty	1904-1906
Chas. P. Dehler	1904-1906
J. M. Fetter	1905-

BOARD OF CONTROL.

Name	Years
Percy Haly, president	1906-1908
Milton H. Board, M. D.	1906-1908
R. G. Phillips	1906-1908

BI-PARTISAN BOARD OF CONTROL.

Name	Years
Albert Scott, president	1908-1911
Percy Haly	1908-1909
Judge A. J. G Wells	1908-1911
Stanley Milward	1908-1909
Thos. W. Gardiner (reappointed 1914 for four years)	1910-
Judge Garrett S. Wall (reappointed 1913 for four years)	1910-
Thomas A. Hall	1912-
J. Norton Fitch	1912-

INSTITUTION FOR FEEBLE-MINDED CHILDREN.

FRANKFORT, KY.

Sixty-two years ago the State of Kentucky signalized her intention of taking care of her feeble-minded children by erecting a magnificent building near the site upon which the present buildings stand. The contract was awarded to John Haly in 1860, who completed the building and had it ready for occupancy in 1861, Dr. James Rodman becoming the first superintendent on May 3, of that year. In 1889, during Dr. J. Q. A. Stewart's administration, the buildings were destroyed by fire. New buildings were erected in 1889 and seven years after and during Dr. Huff's administration, on September 1, 1896, the second structure was burned to the ground. The present buildings were erected in 1896 and 1897 and were occupied in the early part of 1898, showing that the State of Kentucky has lost neither time nor opportunity in her endeavor to care for these unfortunate children.

Another evidence of the state's determination along this line is the fact that in selecting a location for this structure she chose one of the most picturesque spots in all the commonwealth. Nature seems to have almost outstripped herself in her endeavor to make these surroundings both healthful and attractive. The front lawn is a gradual slope of 30 acres, covered by pure blue grass and grand old forest trees. A more beautiful or better adapted location could not be selected in this state.

The following superintendents have served the institution since it was instituted in 1861:

Dr. James Rodman was first superintendent. Mr. Abbott, who was not a physician, succeeded him and served three years. He was succeeded by Dr. E. H. Black, who served 10 years. Then Dr. J. Q. A. Stewart, who served 16 years. At the close of his term he bought the state property known as the Kentucky Military Institute, located six miles south of Frankfort. At the close of his term as superintendent the population was 142, and of this number he took about 30, who were pay patients, to his place, called the Stewart Home. He was succeeded in 1895 by Dr. J. T. Berry, who gave the population at that time as 114. Dr. Berry served two years. He was succeeded by Dr. James Huff, who served two years. He was in turn succeeded by Dr. Long, who served for one year, and he by Dr. Ely, who served six months. Then came Dr. C. K. Wallace, he being succeeded by Dr. Yeaman, who only served one month. Dr. C. C. Owens served four years, being succeeded by Dr. W. E. Gardner, who served one month. Dr. J. W. Hill then was appointed and served four years, being succeeded by Dr. James H. Mulligan for two months. Dr. A. Bailey then followed and served two years, he being succeeded in 1908 by Dr. W. L. Nuttall, who served 11 months. Dr. C. A. Nevitt served only three months. Dr. D. J. Healey succeeded him and served seven months. Dr. G. W. Arms was then made superintendent and served three years, he being succeeded by Dr. H. C. Kehoe in May, 1913, who is the present superintendent.

The population has grown largely since 1908. At that time there were but 167 pupils. At the present time, February 10, 1914, the population is 318 patients.

The present Board of Control for Charitable Institutions has made many improvements during its administration.

In 1908 it erected the new building now being used as the male department.

In 1911 it erected the kitchen, bakery and grocery supply department, which is one of the most up-to-date buildings connected with any institution in the state.

Dr. J. Q. A. Stewart established during his term the training system now being used in this institution, which has been largely augmented since his time. There is now a literary department, a domestic science and art department, a manual training department and a broom making establishment.

THE CARE OF THE INSANE IN LOUISIANA.

The East Louisiana Hospital for the Insane was established at Jackson, La., in 1847, and opened for the reception of patients in November, 1848. Prior to the opening of this hospital insane persons were cared for in separate wards in the Charity Hospital at New Orleans, but it is doubtful whether the care received by them was more than merely custodial in character.

Certain it is that many insane persons must have been incarcerated in jails or were allowed to wander at large. The history of the care of the insane in a majority of the states prior to the establishment of asylums presents such a uniformity of neglect and ill-treatment that it is safe to assume in the absence of definite knowledge that the care meted out to these unfortunates in Louisiana was of the scantiest.

In 1904 the state established a second institution, the Louisiana Hospital for Insane, at Pineville. This institution was at first designed for the care of negroes exclusively, but was later changed to a general asylum, and its wards opened for the treatment of whites and negroes in equal proportion.

The inspection of public charitable and correctional institutions and private insane asylums in Louisiana is a duty of the State Board of Charities and Corrections, consisting of six members, five appointed by the Governor for a term of six years, the Governor being chairman ex-officio. The members of this board serve without compensation. In addition there is a Board of Administrators for each state hospital, consisting of nine members, eight appointed by the Governor for a term of four years, the Governor being a member ex-officio.

The cost of maintenance of patients in state hospitals in Louisiana is a charge against the state.

An act approved July 1, 1910, provided for a ward for the criminal insane in the East Louisiana Hospital for the Insane at Jackson.

Classes Committed.—Indigent insane persons residents of the state.

Legal Procedure.—On written complaint or information of any respectable citizen to the judge of the district court that any lunatic ought to be sent to one of the state hospitals the judge must order him before him and summon two licensed and reputable physicians, one of whom must be coroner of the parish and the other the physician of the person, neither to be related by affinity or consanguinity, or have any interest in his estate. The judge and the two physicians constitute a commission to inquire whether the person is insane and a suitable subject for a hospital and must summon witnesses who know the person. The physicians in the presence of the judge must satisfy themselves and the judge as to the mental condition of the suspected person. If the two physicians do not agree the judge determines the issue. (The recorder of the city court of New Orleans may, however, commit insane persons.)

Cost of commitment is paid out of the parish treasury.

EAST LOUISIANA HOSPITAL FOR THE INSANE.

Jackson, La.

We learn from Dr. T. O. Powell[1] that for years as many as 60 patients were cared for in separate wards in the Charity Hospital at New Orleans.

In the report of that hospital to the Senate and House of Representatives of Louisiana in 1845 it was strongly urged that provision be made for the insane then confined in the hospital. It was also recommended that the place chosen for the site of the proposed asylum be removed from the city, where the " advantages derived from rural beauty and profound solitude can be obtained." Such appeals had their effect and on March 5, 1847, the Governor approved an act to establish an insane asylum in the State of Louisiana. According to this act a board of five administrators was appointed to provide buildings and accommodations for the insane at Jackson. No more than $10,000 per annum was allowed for the support of the institution. The asylum was ready for

[1] " A Sketch of Psychiatry in the Southern States." Transactions of the American Medico-Psychological Association, Vol. IV, page 118.

occupancy about the middle of November, 1848, when 85 patients were removed from the hospital in New Orleans to Jackson.

In the first report of the Board of Administrators, dated January, 1848, we read: "The land on which the asylum is located is within convenient distance of the business part of the pretty village of Jackson, and at all times of easy access to the same, but separated from the noise and bustle of the village by a valley and small stream, which render it sufficiently secluded to protect the patients from the annoying gaze of the idle and curious." There were about 150 acres of land owned by the asylum, 100 well timbered, and the balance enclosed for the use of the patients.

The buildings of the asylum consisted of two wings, each 94 feet in length and 48 feet in depth, and three stories in height. Among the accessories to the buildings were three large cypress cisterns lined with sheet lead, containing in the aggregate about 18,000 gallons of water. Two of these cisterns were situated in the third story and received rain water, and the third was supplied from a large well by means of a force pump worked by horse power.

A supplemental act was passed in March, 1848, appropriating $20,000 for the completion of the building then under contract.

In the second biennial report of the Board of Administrators it is stated that the men and women who were able to perform some manual labor had some occupation assigned to them; some of the men worked from six to seven hours a day in the brick yard,[1] while the women were employed in making and mending clothes, sheets, towels and in various kinds of needle work.

The management of the Louisiana Insane Asylum was committed to a Board of Administrators in 1855. This board consisted of eight persons and the members were appointed for a period of four years. The Governor was ex-officio president of the board. The members were required to visit the institution at frequent intervals, not less than monthly, and report the condition and management to the president of the board. The Board of Administrators had power to make all rules and regulations for

[1] In this report it is stated that "about 150,000 bricks have been burnt for the construction of some proposed additional buildings, which, when completed, are designed for the accommodation of persons from the adjoining states whose situation, unfortunately, demands the aid of such an institution."

their own government not contrary to law, and to make all necessary contracts, provided that no member of any board should in any manner be connected with the making of a contract. It was also made the duty of the board to elect the superintendent, who was to be the chief physician and executive officer of the institution. He and his family were to reside on the premises, but he was forbidden to practice his profession beyond that limit. The superintendent was appointed during good behavior and could only be removed for cause. He was to name to the board suitable physicians to act as his assistants, also a steward and matron, all of whom could be removed by the board on the recommendation of the superintendent.

At the regular meeting of the board two of its members were appointed a visiting committee to visit the hospital at least once a week to ascertain the manner in which the regulations were complied with and to report at each monthly meeting on the condition of the hospital. The Board of Administrators was required to present an annual report to the Legislature.

Dr. Preston Pond was the first physician of the institution and James King its first superintendent. This dual arrangement seems to have been done away with in 1857, when Dr. J. D. Barkdull became superintendent.

From the beginning the institution received idiotic and feebleminded youths and criminals as well as the insane. Up to 1858 there had been more than 600 admissions, the average number for several years having been over 100. In that year the annual appropriation of the Legislature for the support of the institution was about $20,000, and there were in the asylum 124 patients; of these nine males and three females were pay patients. Among the state patients were eight free patients of color. Two-thirds at least of the patients were of foreign birth, principally Irish and German, brought from the City of New Orleans.

Dr. J. D. Barkdull was succeeded as superintendent by Dr. J. W. Jones, who seems to have served during the period of reconstruction, when, because of the injunction against the State Treasury, it became necessary at times for the superintendent to raise funds upon his private security. At one time so great was the distress that the officers were tempted to throw open the gates and let the patients go forth to beg their daily bread. It was mainly through the efforts of Dr. Jones that such a calamity was averted. In this connection the report of 1875 is of interest, there being at that time 162 patients under treatment.

The report discloses a sad condition of affairs in the asylum. There was a lack of accommodations and a consequent overcrowding; the buildings were in a dilapidated, tumble-down condition. The water pipes were worn out and leaking to such an extent as to render portions of the building practically uninhabitable. The plastering was falling off and the floors were beginning to rot, the cellar floor in places being but a quagmire. The heating apparatus was defective or burnt out. The windows were without grating and the balconies without guards, while painting and glazing were required for the whole building. There were no suitable kitchens or laundry buildings. The water closets could not be used, and the sills of the bathroom were so much decayed that they threatened to fall and break down with them the water-tanks, thus endangering the lives of patients. Much of the furniture was unserviceable, and there seems to have been a lack of all the conveniences of a well-regulated hospital. The building occupied by the more disturbed patients was without the means of proper ventilation or heating, and the only protection against cold was found in the clothing and blankets furnished.

Appropriations for the support of the asylum were made in depreciated state paper, and the salaries of the officers and attendants remained unpaid. The credit of the institution was exhausted, and the report ended with the following statement: "Unless the proper aid is soon extended the closing or rather the opening of the doors and the turning loose of the whole insane population must be the next step in its history. The end is now reached, and *untold* and *unspeakable suffering* must and will follow unless your honorable body grants immediate relief to these unfortunates by a special and temporary appropriation."

In 1876 the institution was in debt some $40,000. The following year the Legislature appropriated $25,000 for necessary expenses; and in 1878 $40,000—$25,000 for current expenses and the remainder for repairs, clothing and furniture.

On April 29, 1878, there were 204 patients under treatment. At that time there were in the City Asylum, New Orleans, 150 insane patients, and in the Retreat, New Orleans, 75 patients. There were at large and in jails waiting admission to the asylum about 100 insane persons, and a number were under care in asylums in adjoining states. The superintendent, Dr. Jones, estimated the number of insane in the state at 1000. He also reported that the few negro patients under treatment were put in the same wards with the whites.

In 1879 225,000 bricks were made by patients' labor, at a cost of less than $2 per thousand; these bricks were to be used in erection of additional buildings, for which purpose an appropriation of $20,000 was asked from the Legislature.

The demands for admissions which could not be met resulted in the detention of many patients in the jails and in the City Asylum in New Orleans. There were admitted during the year 50 patients; discharged recovered, 11; died, 27; remained at close of year, 210.

At the opening of the biennial period 1883-1884 there were in the asylum 244 patients. Admitted during period, 244; total under treatment, 721; discharged recovered, 59; improved, 14; unimproved, 11; not insane, 1; died, 164; total, 249.

The closing of the City Asylum at New Orleans resulted in the reception on one day of 129 patients from that institution. In consequence the asylum became so crowded that the superintendent was compelled to put two and three into rooms originally intended for but one person. The superintendent reported that a large number of the patients were employed during the year, and that in the brickyard connected with the institution 2,200,000 bricks had been made. At that time the wards were devoid of any arrangements for lighting other than candles.

It has not been possible to obtain details of the subsequent history of the institution.

Dr. Jones was succeeded as superintendent by Dr. A. Gayden, who in turn was succeeded in 1897 by Dr. George A. B. Hayes.

In 1905 Dr. Hayes was succeeded by the present superintendent, Dr. Clarence Pierson. The capacity of the institution in 1914 was 1450 beds. The appropriation for maintenance for the year 1914 was $254,000. The number of admissions, 310, and the per capita cost per day 43 cents. At present there are five new buildings in course of construction.

[1] The first purchase of land for the East Louisiana Hospital for the Insane was made in 1847 by the Board of Administrators from L. S. Lyon. This was a tract known as the "Old Ronaldson Tract," embracing 31¼ acres, originally purchased from the Louisiana College for $1000. The first plans were drawn by C. N. Gibbons at a cost of $100, and a contract was let to A. N. Thompson for $7665 for the erection of what is now known as the left wing.

The hospital was ready for occupancy about the middle of November, 1848, and on November 21 85 patients were removed from the asylum at New Orleans to Jackson. At that time the buildings for patients, attendants and resident officers consisted of the new brick building and three frame houses which had been found on the premises when the land was purchased by the board. In November, 1854, plans and specifications for the present center building, prepared by F. F. Noon, architect, were accepted by the board, and contracts for the construction of the building were let to C. N. Gibbons for all the wood work and to Elfreth Hazard for all the brick work of the building.

The salary of the superintendent was placed at $800 a year, not including maintenance, board and lodging, etc., for himself and family, and the salary of the visiting physician at $600 a year. Mr. William D. Collins was the first superintendent. He was succeeded in August, 1849, by Mr. James King. At the opening of the hospital Dr. W. H. Selby was appointed physician. He was succeeded by Dr. James Pond. In 1855 Dr. G. Meyberry was elected the first resident superintendent and physician. Dr. Meyberry was succeeded in 1857 by Dr. J. D. Barkdull, and upon the death of Dr. Barkdull in 1865 Mr. James King was again made superintendent. In 1868 the board appointed Dr. L. A. Burgess superintendent. Dr. Burgess was succeeded in 1874 by Dr. J. W. Jones.

In 1878 the number of patients in the hospital had increased to 204. In 1888 there were 467 inmates; in 1897 this number had increased to 871, and in 1905 to 1342. The present population is 1610 patients.

[1] The following details were furnished subsequent to the printing of the preceding history.

SUPERINTENDENTS AND PHYSICIANS.

Dr. W. H. Selby	1848-	Dr. L. A. Burgess	1868-1874
Dr. Preston Pond	1848-1855	Dr. J. W. Jones	1874-1888
Mr. Wm. D. Collins	1848-1849	Dr. L. G. Perkins	1888-1891
Mr. James King	1849-1855	Dr. A. Gayden	1891-1897
Dr. G. Meyberry	1855-1857	Dr. Geo. A. B. Hayes	1897-1905
Dr. J. D. Barkdull	1857-1865	Dr. Clarence Pierson (in office)	1905-
Mr. James King	1865-1868		

ASSISTANT PHYSICIANS SINCE 1897.

Thos. Reagan	1897-	L. F. Lake	1908-1909
J. W. Lea	1897-	Henry Daspit	1908-1909
J. W. Sanders		J. K. Griffith	1909-1910
W. E. Kittridge	1902-1903	O. P. Daly	1910-1914
E. M. Hummell	1902-1905	C. J. McGrane	1911-1911
W. Lassiter	1903-1905	C. S. Miller	1911-1914
R. C. Kemp		A. S. Cooper	1911-
T. J. Finley	1905-	C. S. Holbrook	1914-
C. Pierson	1905-	W. F. Scott	1914-1914
L. Kaffie	1905-1908	R. P. Truitt	1914-
E. M. Hummel	1905-1907	T. W. Evans	1915-
S. L. Thetford	1907-1911		

LOUISIANA HOSPITAL FOR INSANE.

PINEVILLE, LA.

The Louisiana Hospital for the Insane, Pineville, La., was established by an act of the General Assembly in 1904 and was originally designed for the exclusive care of negro patients. Its name was changed, however, from the Insane Asylum for the Colored People of the State of Louisiana to that of the Louisiana Hospital for the Insane, and its wards opened for the treatment of whites and negroes in equal proportion.

The buildings were completed and opened for the reception of patients in January, 1906, when 91 patients were transferred from the Insane Asylum at Jackson.

The establishment of this institution was undertaken because of the overcrowded condition of the asylum at Jackson, then the only institution in Louisiana, in consequence of which there was a large waiting list of patients in the jails of the state.

Dr. George A. B. Hayes, who had been formerly superintendent of the Insane Asylum at Jackson, was elected as superintendent and came to supervise the completion of the building, September 1, 1905.

The institution is located in a pine forest on gently sloping land which has good natural drainage. At the time of its opening there were four well-equipped dormitories, thoroughly well ventilated and heated, with galleries extending the whole length of the buildings. The kitchen and bakery were already completed and each of them had facilities for serving several hundred more patients than could be accommodated in the dormitories. There were two dining-rooms, one for the white patients and the other for the colored. The attendants' dining-room, owing to the lack of an administration building, was divided and converted into offices and a pharmacy, a reception room for visitors, a sewing room and a clothing storeroom. Additions were also made to the patients' dining-room, thereby furnishing a dining-room for the employees.

The building is heated by electricity and the water supply, although not ample, is sufficient for present needs.

The greatest improvement which took place during the biennial period folowing the opening of the hospital consisted in the installation of a new 150 horse-power boiler to furnish steam for the institution. It also became necessary in consequence of an accident to one of the wells which supplied water to the hospital to have a pipe line laid to connect with the water system of the City of Alexandria, and also to bore an artesian well, which, at the depth of 1000 feet, gave a magnificent flow of 125,000 gallons per day of pure, sweet water. Additional land was also procured and new dormitories were erected upon the river bank at some distance from the old building. These were three-story brick dormitories, with sitting rooms, bath rooms and closets, furnishing accommodations for 165 male patients.

This hospital is located within 10 miles of the center of the state, on the banks of the Red River, one mile distant from Alexandria, where seven railroads center. It is consequently much more accessible than the institution at Jackson, which is in the extreme eastern part of the state and difficult of access to patients, who have to be transported by two, three and sometimes four lines of railway, in order to reach it.

At the time of the establishment of the institution at Jackson patients were transported by carriage road, a distance of 13 miles from the nearest landing on the river, in order to reach the institution.

In 1912 the number of patients had increased to 617, by reason of the erection of rooms for additional patients in the gallery of the dormitories already built.

Under careful attention to the physical condition of patients there has been a great diminution in the number of deaths. From April, 1906, to 1908 there were 138 deaths; from April, 1908, to April, 1910, there were 140; from April, 1910, to 1912 there were 82 deaths, notwithstanding an increase of 212 patients during that period.

At that date there were between 30 and 40 cases of pellagra in the institution.

In the report for 1912 it is stated that 80 per cent of the work done in the institution is provided by the negro inmates, who work in the field and garden and at cutting wood; while the laundry work for over 700 people is done by the negro women. The white patients do sewing and mending, otherwise practically nothing. It is also stated that only about 30 per cent of the white male patients are available for profitable work.

Negroes are received under the same circumstances, are given the same treatment and shown the same consideration as white patients. They are domiciled in separate buildings. The white and colored patients are about evenly divided as to numbers.

The original buildings were four in number, with a capacity of 105 patients each. In 1909 another building was opened with a capacity of 160 patients. The buildings were of brick, three stories in height, and had rooms for individual patients. They were not fireproof. Since that time two modern brick cottages, practically fireproof, have been erected and are ready for occupancy. They will accommodate 160 patients each. No separate building exists for the chronic insane.

During the last biennial period extensive repairs and improvements have been made; shower baths have been installed in all male wards, screens and electric fans installed in the dining room, and the kitchen screened. Two dormitories of pressed brick have been erected for patients; large barns built; and, in addition, two cottages for patients completed.

The hospital owns 2061 acres of poor pine woods land, 500 acres of which are cultivated. All forms of vegetables and farm products are raised, but the land is so devoid of fertility that fertilizers need to be constantly employed.

Wood, which has been obtained from this tract without additional cost to the state, has saved the hospital in the matter of fuel about $40,000.

The hospital at the close of the biennial period ending March 31, 1912, had 697 patients under treatment. It is divided into four departments, two departments for white men and women, respectively, and two departments for colored men and women.

Dr. George A. B. Hayes resigned as superintendent January 7, 1909; he was succeeded by Dr. John N. Thomas, who is still in office.

SUPERINTENDENTS.

Dr. George A. B. Hayes 1905-1909
Dr. John N. Thomas ....1909-in office

ASSISTANT PHYSICIANS.

Dr. W. Lassiter.
Dr. W. W. Pugh.
Dr. Leopold Kaffie.
Dr. G. A. Ozenne.
Dr. E. M. Hummell.
Dr. H. L. Fougerousse.
Dr. G. B. Adams.
Dr. F. W. Quin.

MATRONS.

Mrs. G. A. B. Hayes.
Mrs. John N. Thomas.

CLERKS.

G. L. Hayes.
J. D. Weast.

THE CARE OF THE INSANE IN MAINE.

Prior to 1820 Maine was an integral part of Massachusetts, having been acquired by the latter in 1691. The early history of the care of the insane in Maine is, therefore, identical with that of Massachusetts, and is treated at length in the chapter pertaining to the latter state.

In 1820, however, Maine became a separate state, and as such assumed her own distinct laws.

Prior to 1839 the several towns in Maine provided in various indifferent ways for such insane persons as were in indigent circumstances. Dangerous lunatics were simply chained in the common prisons without means of care or relief. This deplorable state of affairs was first called to the attention of the Legislature by Governor Jonathan G. Hunton in 1830. Nothing was done, however, and the question seems to have rested until 1833, when a committee of the Thirteenth Legislature submitted a report, of which the following is an abstract, on "sundry petitions praying for the establishment of a state hospital and also for an insane hospital":

> Your committee have taken view of this subject, which humanity forbids them to pass over in silence. It is ascertained that there are between 200 and 300 insane persons in this state, many of them exposed to much suffering, offering a picture of misery. Some are in the county jails, which can afford but poor accommodations for wretched maniacs; others are taken care of by their friends, while many are left to wander wherever their distracted minds might lead them. Their privations and misery are great, and have a direct tendency to augment their derangement and their sufferings. It is the opinion of your committee that there is no class of people whose situation calls so loudly on the state for legislative aid as the insane; none that have, when rightfully viewed, such strong demands on the charity and compassion of the Christian, the philanthropist or the statesman, as those of our fellow beings who have lost their reason; while the liberality of the state and of individuals have been extended to many other institutions and to many different objects, nothing has been done for that class of persons who, on account of the loss of their reason, are necessarily shut out of society; and shall we shut them out of our compassion? Is it an argument that a Christian community should with-

draw its compassion for the insane, because they have lost their reason, without which man is of all creatures the most wretched? Ought we not rather to do by them as we would wish to be done by, did we know it was to be our lot to be in a similar condition? Does it comport with civilization and the Christian religion to let the insane suffer for the want of that attention and assistance which is in our power to confer upon them? How often is our sensibility shocked, our hearts pained and even our humanity put to the blush, when we see the poor maniac wandering without where to lay his head. It is not, however, merely to provide a refuge for the insane that a hospital is necessary. Many of those who are deranged might be restored to sanity and health by skillful treatment and kind attention, in a close retirement from those scenes which excite attention and disturb and agitate the mind, and be restored to society and usefulness. It needs no argument to prove that a well-regulated hospital is the only suitable place for the successful treatment of insane patients; the fact having been demonstrated in numerous instances in this and many of the enlightened nations of Europe.

The report of the committee bore fruit, for on March 8, 1834, the Legislature appropriated the sum of $20,000 for the purpose of an insane asylum, provided that a like sum be raised by individual donations within one year. Before the time limit was reached Reuel Williams, of Augusta, and Benjamin Brown, of Vassalboro, each agreed to contribute $10,000 for the purpose. With this foundation the Maine Insane Asylum at Augusta was commenced, and with the aid of a state appropriation of $29,500, in 1838, and $28,000 in 1840, was finally completed and opened for the reception of the first patient on the 14th of October of the latter year.

The Eastern Maine Insane Asylum, now known as the Bangor State Hospital, at Bangor, was created by an act of the Legislature of March 5, 1889.

The third state institution is the Maine School for Feeble-minded, established at West Pownal in 1908.

On July 1, 1911, by act of the Legislature, the Board of Trustees which formerly conducted the two insane hospitals of the state was done away with, and a new board organized, called the Board of Hospital Trustees; this board to have the management of the insane hospitals at Augusta and at Bangor, and of the School for Feeble-minded at West Pownal.

Up to January 1, 1910, the towns committing a patient were held responsible for the support of said patient, but in cases where the relatives could not reimburse the town, the state, by an act passed in 1856, agreed to pay the town $1 per week as partial support; later this was raised to $1.50 per week. Since the first of January, 1910, the state has assumed the care of all patients unable to pay for their own support. This act resulted in the transfer to the insane hospitals of all the insane in almshouses.

R. S. 1871, Chapter 137, Section 1, provides that "When any person is indicted for a criminal offense, or is committed to jail on a charge thereof by a trial justice or judge of a police or municipal court, any judge of the court before which he is to be tried, when a plea of insanity is made in court, or he is notified that it will be made, may, in vacation or term time, order such person into the care of the superintendent of the insane hospital, that the truth or falsity of the plea of insanity may be ascertained." This was one of the earliest so-called observation laws enacted in this country.

Chapter 217, laws of 1909, amendment to R. S., Chapter 144 (1903), provided for the temporary absence of a patient from a hospital for a period not to exceed six months.

Commitment.—All insane who are legal residents of a town are entitled to admission to the state hospitals for the insane.

Legal Procedure.—Parents and guardians of insane minors must within 30 days after an attack of insanity, without legal examination, send them to one of the hospitals or to some other hospital for the insane.

Insane persons not thus sent are subject to examination. The municipal officers of towns constitute a board of examiners and on complaint in writing of any blood relative, husband or wife of an alleged insane person, or of any justice of the peace, must immediately inquire into his condition, appoint a time and place for a hearing and notify the person. They must take the necessary testimony, and if they think such a person insane and that his comfort and safety or that of others will thereby be promoted, they must forthwith send him to one of the insane hospitals with a certificate of insanity and direct the superintendent to receive and detain him until he is restored or discharged.

To establish the fact of insanity, evidence from two reputable physicians under oath is required, together with a certificate signed by the physicians and filed with the board, the evidence and certificate being based upon due inquiry and personal examination.

The judge of probate has power to examine insane persons, and upon complaint in writing of any blood relation, husband or wife or of any justice of the peace, accompanied by the certificate of some reputable physician, may appoint a time and place for hearing the case. He has power to summon witnesses, and if the person is found insane, must forthwith send him to one of the hospitals for the insane. The registrar must keep a record of the doings and furnish a copy to any interested person. The municipal officers or the judge of probate first taking jurisdiction have exclusive jurisdiction until the complaint is finally disposed of. In case of a refusal to commit after notice and hearing, no other complaint is possible within 30 days after the decision is recorded, and only after application to each of said tribunals.

Appeal from Commitment.—Persons liable for the support of a patient who has been in a hospital for six months and who has not been committed by the supreme judicial court and not afflicted with homicidal insanity, may apply to the municipal officers for his release, if they think him unreasonably detained. If the application is unsuccessful it may not be renewed until the expiration of another six months. When the committee of visitors become satisfied that an inmate, other than one charged with or convicted of crime and committed by order of court, is unnecessarily detained, they must apply for a writ of *habeas corpus,* and if the judge is satisfied that the inmate is not a proper subject for custody and treatment he must discharge the inmate.

Cost of Commitment.—The town is liable for the expense of examination and commitment, but may recover the amount from the person, if he is able to pay, or from persons liable for his support, or from the town of his settlement. If he has no legal settlement the expenses must be refunded by the state.

AUGUSTA STATE HOSPITAL.[1]

Augusta, Me.

The attention of the Legislature was first called to the need of care of the insane in 1830 by Governor Jonathan G. Hunton; but nothing definite was done until 1834, when Governor Dunlap urged that systematic and suitable provision be made by the state for the relief of her insane.

On the 8th of March, 1834, the Legislature appropriated $20,000 for the purpose, upon condition that a like sum should be raised by individual donations within one year. Before the time limit was reached Reuel Williams, of Augusta, and Benjamin Brown, of Vassalboro, each agreed to contribute $10,000 for the purpose. Mr. Brown proposed to convey to the state as a site 200 acres of land lying on the Kennebec River in Vassalboro, and consented to a sale of the estate if it was deemed advisable to build elsewhere. The Legislature accepted the land and sold it for $4000 and the present more eligible site was selected in Augusta, on the eastern bank of the Kennebec River, nearly opposite the state house, for which $3000 was paid. Reuel Williams, who was appointed a commissioner to erect the hospital, sent John B. Lord, of Hallowell, to examine similar institutions, and the general plan of the asylum at Worcester, Mass., was adopted. During 1836 contracts were made and materials collected, but in March, 1837, Mr. Williams resigned the office of commissioner and John H. Hartwell was appointed, under whose supervision the work was carried on for another year. In March, 1838, a further appropriation of $29,500 was made to complete the exterior, and Charles Keene was appointed in place of Mr. Hartwell. In 1840 a further appropriation of $28,000 was made to complete the wings, and on the 14th of October a room was occupied by the first patient.

Dr. Cyrus Knapp, of Winthrop, was appointed superintendent and physician; Dr. Chauncey Booth, junior assistant; Henry Winslow, steward, and Mrs. Catherine Winslow, matron. In 1846-7 appropriations of $29,400 were made to erect a new wing, which was completed during 1848 and provided for 75 additional male patients.

[1] From material furnished by Dr. Henry M. Miller, former superintendent, and Dr. Forrest C. Tyson, superintendent.

Dr. Knapp resigned early in 1841 and was succeeded in August by Dr. Isaac Ray, of Eastport, the author of the "Medical Jurisprudence of Insanity," the first edition of which had recently appeared and given him deserved reputation. During his residence at Augusta he rewrote the work and published a second edition, which became an authority in Europe and America. He was succeeded, March 19, 1845, by Dr. James Bates, formerly a member of Congress from Norridgewock. He remained until after the fire of December 4, 1850, in which 27 patients and one attendant lost their lives. Dr. Henry M. Harlow, who became an assistant to Dr. Bates in June, 1845, was made superintendent June 17, 1851. During that and the following year $49,000 was appropriated to rebuild and improve the buildings and to heat them by steam.

By 1854 facilities were ample for 250 patients.

Dr. Harlow's resignation was accepted on the 18th of April, 1883, and Dr. Bigelow T. Sanborn, who had been his assistant for more than 16 years, was appointed his successor.

When the hospital was opened in 1840 two classes of patients were received: (a) Patients sent by the towns. (b) Reimbursing patients. For the admission of patients sent by towns a written request for such admission, signed by the overseers of the poor, was required. For the reception of other patients, a good and sufficient bond for the payment of the expenses, including board, etc., was required.

The Revised Statutes of 1841, Chapter 178, Section 13, provided for commitment of an insane person "so furiously mad that the public safety requires his immediate restraint" by any two justices of the peace, one of them being of the quorum, on complaint under oath and a hearing before them, who shall, on adjudging the facts so as to be, by a joint warrant under their hands and seals, commit such person within 60 days to the house of correction for the county, or to the insane hospital, there to be detained till he becomes of sound mind, or be otherwise delivered by due course of law."

The law as to the support of patients was as follows: The person so committed shall be kept therein at his own expense if he have sufficient property, otherwise, at the expense of the persons or town that would have been chargeable for his maintenance, if he had not been committed; and if he have no settlement in the town, at the expense of the state; and he may be delivered up to any friend or to the overseers of the poor of the town where he has a settlement.

The Revised Statutes of 1841 provided for the commitment to the insane hospital of an insane person under indictment for crime if found to be insane.

In 1842 a computation showed that there were over 600 insane in the state and much was written by Dr. Isaac Ray, the superintendent, urging the importance of the commitment of these cases. It was obligatory on the part of the overseers of the poor to send insane paupers to the insane hospital, but there was no way to exercise this compulsory power over the town. One potent cause for the non-commitment of these patients was that the majority of the relatives were unable to pay the necessary cost of maintenance of $2 per week.

In 1846 the trustees called attention to the necessity of having some definite and uniform mode of determining the question of insanity, and suggested that a formal hearing before a competent tribunal prior to admission into the hospital be held.

As the result of agitation for a formal hearing an act was passed in 1847 providing that the municipal officer of the towns shall constitute a board of examiners and, on complaint in writing of any relative or justice of the peace of their town, they shall immediately inquire into the condition of any insane person therein; call before them all testimony necessary for a full understanding of the case; and if they think such person is insane and that his comfort and safety or that of others interested will thereby be promoted, they shall forthwith send him to the hospital, with a certificate, stating the fact of his insanity. If he be a person unable to pay for his support, they may certify such fact in writing to the superintendent; and if the superintendent is satisfied that such certificate is true, the treasurer of the hospital may charge to the state $1 per week for his board.

The hospital has been the recipient of various bequests since the original gifts of Reuel Williams and Benjamin Brown in 1834. In 1842 Bryce McLellan left a legacy of $500, the interest of which was to be expended in the purchase of books for the use of the inmates. In 1848 Benjamin Vaughn left to the hospital the medical portion of his library, containing over 600 volumes. The library was again added to in 1855, when Col. John Black, of Ellsworth, left a legacy of $3000, the interest of which was to be used for the purpose of forming a library for the benefit of the inmates. In 1882 $1000 was bequeathed by Mrs. Sempronia A. Orne, late of Malden, in the State of Massachusetts, "to be appropriated to the benefit of the patients." In 1886 $50,000 was bequeathed by Abner Coburn, "to be used for purposes not provided for by the state." Interest on the fund was used as an amusement fund. In 1897 $1000 was bequeathed by Joseph H. Williams, of Augusta, to the State of Maine on condition that a sum of money, not less than $40, be appropriated—and paid annually—to be expended for articles of art or used for the diversion of patients in Maine Insane Hospital. In 1905 $1000 was bequeathed by Mrs. Ellen A. (Williams) Gilman, daughter of one of the founders of the hospital, the interest to be expended for amusements, recreation and diversions. In 1911 $2000—twenty shares in the First National Bank, Portland, drawing interest at 7 per cent—was donated by ex-Governor Frederick Robie, for over 20 years president of the Board of Trustees, the interest to be used in the purchase of books for patients in the hospital.

On December 4, 1850, a disastrous fire destroyed two wings of the hospital and caused the death of 27 male patients and one male attendant. The trustees made record of the occurrence in their report for 1851 as follows:

> The two south wings and most of the main building of the Insane Hospital have been burnt. This noble edifice, the pride of our state, consecrated by public and private munificence to the most noble purposes of humanity, has been destroyed by fire, and, melancholy to relate, 27 of the inmates perished in the conflagration. One of the attendants, H. D. Jones, while nobly exerting himself to rescue the patients, shared the same fate.
>
> This catastrophe occurred between 3 and 4 o'clock on the morning of the 4th of December last. The fire originated in the hot air chamber under the old south wing, and spread with great rapidity. The flues leading from the hot air chamber, affording a direct communication, very quickly filled the galleries with smoke, gas and heat incompatible with human life, rendering it probable that those who perished were suffocated before the fire reached them.

As soon as the fire was discovered, every effort was made for the rescue of the inmates; and the progress of the fire was checked before it reached the north wing, consequently the female patients were all safely removed.

The libraries, books and papers belonging to the hospital were safely removed; also part of the furniture, though much injured and broken by hasty removal.

The officers without much difficulty succeeded in procuring good temporary accommodations for the inmates in private dwellings, in the Augusta House, and, for some of the most furious, in the county jail, under the immediate supervision of the attendants, until they could be removed by their friends or otherwise provided for.

The trustees held a meeting as soon after the fire as practicable—saw the patients who had not been removed—found them comfortable, quiet and well provided for, under the immediate supervision and care of the officers and attendants of the hospital.

On February 24, 1887, two straw barns with their contents were destroyed by fire; and on July 22, 1904, the piggery was burned; on October 12, 1906, the laundry building was burned and the carpenter shop adjoining damaged.

Previous to 1903 there was no provision of law for the segregation of the criminal insane of the state. Criminals and persons accused of crimes pleading insanity were sent to the Insane Hospital and were not restrained apart from the other patients.

At the legislative session of 1903 that body created a criminal department for the insane at the state prison and set aside a portion of one of the wings for their care, the supervision of which was placed in the hands of a commission composed of the superintendent of the Maine Insane Hospital, the warden of the state prison and the prison physician. The Legislature also authorized that all of the insane criminals that had hitherto been cared for at the insane hospital be returned to that department, and that all becoming insane in the various jails of the state before final sentence was passed be ordered to that department by the Governor and council for supervision.

The statutes also provided that when a person became insane in the prison he should be transferred to that department, to remain so long as insanity continued.

The Legislature of 1907 passed an act providing for the transfer of persons from the insane department of the state prison to the building for the criminal insane, connected with the Maine Insane Hospital, at Augusta. This building, known as the Criminal Departmentt of the Maine Insane Hospital, was completed and occupied early in 1909. The building is located upon what is known as the Arsenal grounds of the hospital, and was constructed at a cost of a little over $40,000. It accommodates 30 patients. A law passed by the Legislature of 1911 provided for the removal of time-expired patients to the other department of the hospital when such removal was deemed expedient.

The trustees in their report for 1904 called attention to the real estate and buildings on Widow's Island, located near Vinal Haven, about 12 miles from the City of Rockland. These buildings were erected by the United States at an expense of about $75,000 in 1885 for the quarantine and treatment of the sick with yellow fever. When the growth of scientific knowledge as to yellow fever had rendered the buildings unnecessary, the national government presented the property to the State of Maine, with the proviso that it be used for some well-defined public good. The executive department of the state in November, 1904, called the attention of the trustees of the two insane hospitals to the question of using these buildings as a summer home for the curable inmates of the institutions.

Early in December the trustees accordingly visited this island and made a careful examination of the real estate and buildings thereon. While the general feeling of the board was unfavorable to the use of the property as a sanitarium for the insane, still the trustees present were greatly pleased with the general appearance of the large buildings, as well as with the thorough workmanship and fine material used in their construction; and all were of the opinion that, so far as the buildings themselves were concerned, they fully met the requirements of a proper summer home by the ocean for a judiciously selected company of insane.

It was estimated that the rooms of the building would accommodate 75 patients, and that an expenditure of $6000 would fully equip it for occupancy. While the trustees were not prepared to advise the immediate use of this property, they considered the question of sufficient importance to bring it directly to the attention of the next Legislature, in order that the whole subject might be fully investigated, with the idea of occupying this valuable real estate, if the best interests of the insane could be promoted.

The report of the trustees for 1905 announced the opening of the summer colony and the acceptance by the State of Maine, by the unanimous vote of the last Legislature, of the gift from the United States of Widow's Island and the buildings thereon; also an appropriation of $6000 made from the state funds that had been economically expended under the direction of the Board of Trustees. During the months of July, August and September the buildings and the grounds were occupied and used by a selected number of patients from both insane hospitals.

The new annex was visited several times by the trustees, and from careful personal observation and the reports of the physicians and attendants they were able to say that the sanitary influences and advantages of this department have exceeded their expectations.

The name, Widow's Island, had no particular significance and was changed to Chase Island, in honor of Edward E. Chase, who obtained an acceptance of this valuable gift by the Legislature of the State of Maine in 1905.

Every summer since 1905 patients have been sent to the Summer Hospital at Chase Island. For six weeks, commencing about the middle of June, approximately 65 women patients proportionately selected from the two hospitals are sent to this resort and at the expiration of their visit the same number of male patients are sent for the same length of time.

This unique summer colony has proven a most successful experiment. The outing not only aids patients during convalescence, but stimulates and enthuses the working patients, who have come to look forward to this break in their monotony of daily hospital life with all the expectancy of those who are more fortunate in being able to choose the time and place for a summer vacation.

During the year 1913 much work about the institution has been done. A new dining room has been prepared for the use of patients occupying the Burleigh Pavilion and Annex. The third and last building in the Stone group for women has been thoroughly renovated, the old wooden interior being replaced by steel and concrete construction and the open dormitory style adopted. In this building are modern facilities for caring for the acute and disturbed cases. Owing to some difficulty with the old Board of Trustees and the committee of the Legislature at the last session, the appropriation was not placed in the hands of the trustees, but given directly to the Governor and Council. This building will be occupied by January 1, 1915, the retiring committee wishing it completed before the present Legislature convenes. Many other improvements in the building have been instituted. The entire engineering plant, which includes heat, light and power, has been carefully investigated by a consulting engineer and plans drawn for a complete renovation of this department. Efforts have been made to make more efficient existing conditions and changes have been made carefully and after thorough investigation.

DIRECTORS AND TRUSTEES.

Name	Years
Benjamin Brown	1840-1843
Reuel Williams	1840-1846 1847-1857
Rev. William C. Larrabee	1840-1841
James McKeen, M. D.	1841-1842
Amos Nourse, M. D.	1842-1844
Edward Kent	1843-1846
Levi J. Hain, M. D.	1843-1845
John H. Hartwell	1843-1845
Josiah Prescott	1843-1844
Moses Mason	1844-1845
Edward S. James	1844-1847
Edward Swan	1845-1848
Cornelius Holland	1845-1847
John Hubbard	1845-1850
Charles Millett, M. D.	1846-1849
Isaac Reed	1846-1852
Ebenezer Knowlton	1847-1853
Gilman L. Bennett	1848-1887
William Oakes	1849-1855
Robert H. Gardiner	1850-1887
George Downes	1852-1858
Rev. Rubard Woodhull	1853-1869
Joseph Barrett	1855-1869

TRUSTEES.

Name	Years
Moses Sweat	1857-1860
Archibald Talbot	1857-1864
Alexander Burbank, M. D.	1858-1867
John Benson	1860-1863
William Swazey	1860-1863
George A. Frost[1]	1863-1872
George C. Comstock	1863-1869
John T. Gilman, M. D.[2]	1864-1881
Moses R. Ludwig	1864-1870
A. G. Wakefield[1]	1869-1877
Ezra L. Pattangall[1]	1869-1879
N. P. Monroe, M. D.	1870-1873
Wm. B. Lapham, M. D.[1]	1871-
H. A. Shorey[2]	1873-1879
E. W. Woodbury	1873-1879
John W. Chase	1873-1879
Fred. E. Richards	1877-1879
J. S. Cushing, M. D.[1]	1877-1879 1880-1883
R. S. Morrison[1]	1879-1880
John Ware[2]	1879-1880
Dr. A. J. Fuller	1879-1880
Dr. A. P. Snow	1879-1880
W. D. Hayden	1879-1880
J. H. Manley[2]	1880-1888
Dr. Silvester Oakes[1]	1880-1885
Dr. Charles W. Johnson	1880-1883
Mrs. C. A. Quinby	1880-1883
J. T. Hinkley	1883-1885
W. O. Bowen[2]	1883-1889
Mrs. E. J. Torsey	1883-1892

[1] President. [2] Secretary.

Name	Years
James Weymouth[1]	1884-1889
Dr. Elbridge A. Thompson[2]	1885-1891
Dr. Jeremiah W. Dearborn	1885-1889
George E. Weeks	1888-1893
Frederick Robie, M. D.[1]	1889-1911
Leyndon Oak[2]	1889-1895
William H. Hunt	1891-1894
Mrs. J. R. Smith	1892-1907
Judson S. Clark	1893-1899
A. F. Crockett	1894-1897
Charles S. Pearl	1895-1902
P. O. Vickery	1897-1902
R. B. Sheperd[2]	1899-1900
Thomas White	1899-1913
H. T. Powers[2]	1899-1905
Sidney M. Bird	1901-1907
Charles E. Field[2]	1902-1911
George E. Macomber[1]	1902-1911
Edward E. Chase	1905-1911
Mrs. Frederick Cony[2]	1907-1914
Alonzo R. Nickerson	1907-1911
Dr. Seth C. Gordon[1]	1911-1914
Raymond Fellows	1911-1911
Frank W. Burnham	1911-1914
Young A. Thurston	1911-1914
Albert O. Marcelle	1911-1914
Meander Dennett	1911-1914
Oliver L. Hall	1913-1914
Fred. A. Chandler, M. D.	1913-1914
Fred. R. Smith	1913-1914
Hartley C. Baxter	1914-
Howard L. Keyser	1914-
Willis E. Parsons	1914-
Albert J. Stearns	1914-
Elizabeth Burbank Plummer	1914-
Alexander C. Hagerty, M. D.	1914-
Charles W. Clifford	1914-
Oliver L. Hall	1914-

SUPERINTENDENTS.

Name	Term
Dr. Cyrus Knapp	October, 1840, to Mar., 1841
Dr. Isaac Ray	August, 1841, to Feb., 1845
Dr. James Bates	March, 1845, to Feb., 1851
Dr. Henry M. Harlow	Feb., 1851, to April, 1883
Dr. Bigelow T. Sanborn[3]	April, 1883, to April, 1910
Dr. Henry W. Miller	June, 1910, to Jan., 1914
Dr. Forrest C. Tyson	March, 1914, in office

ASSISTANT PHYSICIANS.

Name	Years
Chauncey Booth, Jr.	1840-1843
Edward R. Chapin	1843-1843
Horatio S. Smith	1844-1844
Henry M. Harlow	1845-1850
Jerome C. Smith	1854-1856
Paul Merrill	1856-1859
John Hart Prentias	1859-1859
John Blackmer	1859-1860
Richard L. Cook	1860-1862
Thomas H. Emery	1863-1865
Samuel S. Emery	1863-1865
James D. Nutting	1865-1866
Bigelow T. Sanborn	1866-1883
Maria A. Merservey	1873-1874
E. C. Neal	1874-1880
Horace B. Hill	1881-1908
O. C. S. Davies	1883-1890
Mary Chandler Donell	1887-1891
P. H. S. Vaughn	1890-1901
Geo. D. Rowe	1890-1893
Emma Virginia Baker	1891-1900
D. B. Crediford	1893-1895
Daniel W. Hayes	1897-1898
Byron W. McKeen	1898-1899
H. L. Horsman	1899-1909
Gertrude E. Heath	1900-1908

[1] President. [2] Secretary. [3] Died in office.

Dr. Henry K. Stimson..	1900-1904	M. W. H. Pitman, M. D..	1909-1911
Dr. J. B. McDonald.....	1905-1907	Annette Bennett, M. D...	1909-1911
Dr. B. F. Hayden.......	1905-1905	John C. Lindsay, M. D...	1911-1912
Dr. John L. Davis.......	1906-1907	Marie C. Strom, M. D...	1911-1913
Karl B. Sturgis, M. D...	1907-	Stephen Vosburg, M. D.	1912-
Harris C. Barrows, M. D.	1907-1908	Joseph H. Toomey, M. D.	1912-1914
Carl J. Hedin, M. D.....	1908-1912	Anita Alvera Wilson, M. D.	1913-1914
Herbert W. Hall, M. D...	1908-1909	Arthur C. Wright, M. D.	1914-
H. W. Abbott, M. D.....	1908-1908	Harris Bass, M. D.......	1914-
Roland L. McKay, M. D.	1908-1909	Frank E. Rowe, M. D....	1914-
Herbert W. Hall, M. D..	1909-		

STEWARD-TREASURERS.

Henry Winslow	1840-1842	Corydon B. Lakin.......	1874-1882
Joshua S. Turner.......	1842-1853	R. W. Soule...........	1882-1885
Theodore C. Allen......	1853-1864	John W. Chase..........	1885-1890
Jefferson Parsons	1864-1870	Manning S. Campbell...	1890-1913
William E. Leighton.....	1870-1874	Fred. W. Wright, M. D...	1913-

BANGOR STATE HOSPITAL.[1]

BANGOR, ME.

For a number of years prior to 1889 there was a growing feeling in the eastern part of Maine that a new insane hospital should be established at a point more accessible to this region than was the Maine Insane Hospital at Augusta. Residents of Aroostook, Washington, Hancock and Penobscot counties were forced to make a long and expensive journey, both for the commitment of patients and for visiting relatives in the hospital at the capital.

As the eastern section of the state developed and the population increased this need became more urgent; therefore, in 1889, a statement of facts was presented to the State Legislature with a resolve introduced in the Senate by E. C. Ryder, of Bangor, a member of the Committee on Insane Hospitals, in part as follows:

The present insane asylum is insufficient to accommodate the constantly increasing number of insane. Large numbers of patients cannot be successfully treated in one institution, as has been recognized by our sister states, many of which have several insane asylums. The location of the present institution is convenient for Western and Central Maine, but puts a heavy burden upon those having the care and support of patients from the northern and eastern portion of the state. Bangor being a railroad center, easily accessible from the north and east, furnishes all the advantages required for a location of such an institution.

"*Resolved,* That the Governor, with the advice and consent of the Council, shall appoint a board of three commissioners, whose duty it shall be to select an eligible site at or near the city of Bangor, in the county of Penobscot, for an insane hospital, to be known as the Eastern Maine Insane Hospital; and to procure a good and sufficient title and conveyance of said site to the state; and cause plans and specifications to be made for suitable buildings according to the most recent approved methods for such an institution; all the acts of said commissioners shall be subject to the approval of the Governor and Council.

"Said commissioners shall receive in full compensation for their services $3 per day while employed, and all necessary expenses incurred while so employed. And the sum of $25,000 or so much thereof as is necessary, is hereby appropriated to carry out the provisions of this resolve, to be paid by the State Treasurer."

Through the earnest efforts of Mr. Ryder, ably seconded by Ezra L. Pattingill, a former trustee of the Maine Insane Hospital,

[1] From material furnished by Dr. Frederick L. Hills, superintendent.

this resolution passed both houses and was approved by Governor Edwin C. Burleigh, March 5, 1889. In compliance with the provisions of this resolve, Gov. Edwin C. Burleigh appointed as commissioners Col. Joseph W. Porter, chairman; Col. Jaspar Hutchins and Col. Daniel A. Robinson, M. D.

This commission, after a long and careful inspection of sites in Bangor and towns in its vicinity, selected a site in the City of Bangor adjacent to the Water Works.

This site comprised three estates, in all containing 105 acres, bounded southerly on State Street and the Penobscot River; easterly on the Hogan road; northerly on Mt. Hope Avenue, and westerly on land belonging to the estate of the late Thomas N. Egery.

The commissioners availed themselves of the advice and assistance of Dr. Bigelow T. Sanborn, superintendent of the Maine Insane Hospital at Augusta.

Dr. Sanborn inspected the various sites suggested to the commissioners and most cordially approved the selection.

George M. Coombs, of Lewiston, architect, was selected to assist in the preparation of plans. Mr. Coombs had much experience in this particular work. The commissioners and Mr. Coombs visited hospitals in Washington, D. C., Pennsylvania, New Jersey and Massachusetts.

A joint special committee was appointed by the Legislature to consider a resolve for an appropriation for the Eastern Maine Hospital at Bangor. This special committee adopted a resolution that a commission of three be appointed by the Governor to take immediate steps to erect a building on the site selected at Bangor, to be known as the Eastern Hospital Commission, and that the sum of $200,000 be appropriated during the years 1891-92 for the erection of the Eastern Maine Insane Hospital.

This resolve failed of passage owing to strong opposition arising in both houses of the Legislature. In 1893 another effort was made to obtain from the Legislature an appropriation for the construction of the hospital.

Finally, however, in the same year, at the 67th session of the Legislature, a resolve in favor of the Eastern Maine Insane Hospital was introduced with accompanying statement of facts. This resolve passed both houses of the Legislature and was signed by

Governor Henry B. Cleaves, who appointed the following commission to carry out its provisions: Albion E. Little, Portland, chairman; Samuel Campbell, Sidney M. Bird and as an advisory member, the superintendent of the Maine Insane Hospital.

The resolution provided that their reasonable expenses be paid while they are engaged on the commission and that they also receive reasonable compensation. They were directed to take immediate steps to erect, not later than January 1, 1897, upon the site at Bangor already purchased by the state for the purpose, fireproof buildings for the accommodation of the insane of the state, after plans to be selected by them, subject to the approval of the Governor and Council. For that purpose the sum of $75,000 was appropriated, to be expended during the year 1896. They were authorized to lay any drain or sewer that might be necessary from the site to the Penobscot River, and enter therein below the dam; and for that purpose might cross any land, highways or railroads.

The commissioners began their work immediately after their appointment by a careful study of the site which had been purchased by the former commission appointed for that purpose. As a result the commissioners were unanimous in their decision to build the hospital at the very top of the hill.

The decision rendered necessary a great amount of grading and bids were immediately asked for the removal of the required amount of earth and ledge. The lowest bid received being from W. N. Sawyer, of Bangor, a contract was made with him and work at once begun upon the lot.

The commissioners then turned their attention to consideration of architectural designs and style of construction.

For this purpose the commissioners with Dr. B. T. Sanborn, advisory member, visited a great number of modern-built hospitals for the care of the insane. They conferred with superintendents of many years' experience, as well as trustees and commissioners, and after due deliberation decided to build the hospital on what is known as the pavilion plan.

To select an architect the commissioners decided to institute a competition, which was accordingly done and resulted in the selection of John Clavin Stevens, of Portland.

As soon as possible after the selection of the architect working plans and specifications were prepared in order to obtain bids from the various contractors. Owing to the length of time this work would occupy, however, it was deemed advisable to contract for the foundation separately, and as W. N. Sawyer's bid was the lowest one received, it was accepted and work upon this portion of the building commenced in October, 1895.

During the winter of 1895 and 1896 operations continued and 40,375 cubic feet of earth on the lot and 23,628 cubic feet of ledge were removed, making a broad and level plateau on which the buildings were to stand.

A portion of the stone taken from the excavation has been used in the construction of the buildings, and as foundation for permanent macadamized roads from the buildings to the city streets, a length of 4000 feet.

A description of the plans as adopted is as follows: The general plan of the buildings is after what is known as the pavilion plan, viz.: Separate buildings connected by corridors giving passage for the transportation of food from the kitchen and clothing from the laundry to the various wards, and also passage for water and steam pipes.

The plant consists of a central or administration building, kitchen, laundry and power house, on a central axis which runs from north to south. On the east and west are situated the various wards.

The boiler house, which is in the extreme rear, has been placed at that point in order to provide for proper pitch of the return pipes, the level of the boiler room floor being 32 feet below the main floor and 23 feet below the kitchen floor. The boiler house is of ample size to accommodate a plant capable of caring for 1000 patients.

Opening off the boiler room is a coal pit, arranged so that the coal teams can be driven to the top and the coal dropped through scuttles in the roof.

Just south of the boiler room is the laundry building, which contains in the basement a room for dynamos and engines, also a large store room, which can be utilized for additional engine room should occasion demand.

On the first floor is a wash room and ironing room for the laundry, with ample room for all machinery. Opening off the wash room are two large rooms for the reception of the soiled linen and for the sorting of the clothes after being washed.

The second floor is devoted to sleeping rooms for the laundry help and a large sewing room for general repair of clothing and making up of linen. Ample toilet accommodations are provided for both sexes.

South of the laundry building is the kitchen department, the basement story being devoted to a store-room for provisions, etc. The first floor contains a scullery room for the storage of flour, bread room, bake room, and a large store-room with two large refrigerators.

The connecting corridor from the central building swings around the kitchen, so that cars containing soiled clothes can be carried directly to the wash room; it also gives access to the kitchen.

These buildings are built of the local stone found on the lot, with brick trimmings and flat gravel roofs. Provision has been made everywhere for the admission of as much sunlight as possible and for ample ventilation. In the arrangement, economy in the operation of the domestic departments has been considered the most important item, and throughout the buildings have been built large enough to provide for all appliances and machinery to care for a complete hospital, so that future extensions to the buildings themselves will not be necessary.

The total length of these buildings is 235 feet and the total width 110 feet. Eighty-five feet south of the kitchen department is the central or administration building, which is 52 feet wide and 125 feet long, its length being upon the north and south axis, making a total length of 445 feet. The walls of this building to the level of the first story windows are built of the same material as the kitchen department. Above this point the walls are built of brick, laid in gray mortar with trimmings of pink granite from the quarries at Redstone. The roof is hipped and slated, with various gables and dormers necessary for lighting the upper story. In the basement a dining-room is provided for the help, and various rooms which can be used as sleeping rooms.

On the main floor in the first story is a large entrance hall with open fireplace, reception rooms, superintendent's office, toilet rooms, etc. Opening from this office is a large fireproof brick vault for the reception of important papers, books and documents. Just back of these rooms is a connecting corridor which runs to the wards on either side. Back of this corridor a large dining-room for the officers; the dispensary and sleeping rooms for the housekeeper and her assistants, and necessary toilet rooms. On the second floor the front portion of the building is devoted to the living rooms of the superintendent and his family, and officers. The back portion of this story is devoted to a chapel or amusement hall, fitted with stage, dressing rooms and gallery. This room is extended into the roof, making a large hall 50 by 72 feet.

The other two stories in the front portion of the building are devoted to sleeping rooms, 14 in all. On each floor are bath rooms and toilet rooms. The entrance front of this building, while not elaborate, is pleasing, the small amount of ornamentation being confined to the large entrance arch.

The wards on either side provide for the accommodation of 33 patients on each floor, and as the building is three stories high, each building will thus accommodate about 100.

The corridors in these buildings are wide and thoroughly lighted, so that they can be used as day rooms or sitting rooms for the patients in addition to the rooms provided for that purpose. Each ward is so arranged that for the purpose of classification it may be divided temporarily into two wards, and as the toilet rooms are provided in projecting wings at either end of the building, when so divided each ward will have separate toilet facilities.

A large dining-room is provided for each ward, accessible from both sides when the ward is divided, but the room is of such size that all the patients on the floor can be amply provided for at the same time if necessary.

Care has been taken to provide for an ample amount of sunshine, and the rooms are so arranged that each and every room will command a fine and extensive view of the surrounding country.

The buildings are entirely fireproof in construction, with walls and partitions of brick and terra cotta and floors of steel and concrete. The finish of all the buildings is of North Carolina pine.

For the transmission of food from the kitchen to the various dining rooms, corridors in the basement give access to all the wards and cars are provided with closed receptacles for carrying the food, and with electric lifts running directly to each dining room.

A thorough system of heating and ventilation is installed, from plans made by Prof. S. H. Woodbridge, of the Massachusetts Institute of Technology.

While the greatest possible care has been taken to provide substantial and fireproof buildings, economy has been the watchword of the commissioners throughout, and every effort has been made to keep the cost at the lowest point consistent with good workmanship.

When the plans were finally ready proposals were asked for the construction of the buildings from various contractors by advertisements in the daily papers throughout the state. The bid of M. C. Foster & Son, which included the iron and steel construction, was found to be the lowest, and a contract was made with them for $60,775. For fireproof floors the bid of the Columbian Fireproofing Company for the sum of $8934 was accepted.

Later on an additional contract, amounting to $556.90, was made with M. C. Foster & Son for work connected with the coal pit, and a contract for $2900 made with Megquier & Jones Co., of Portland, for the iron and roofing of the coal pit.

An estimate giving a full account of necessary items to complete the buildings for the reception of patients is as follows:

To complete building for laundry, kitchen and boilers	$12,700
To complete central or administration buildings	16,600
To build two ward buildings, at $71,650	143,300
For heating and ventilation	22,000
For electric work, dynamos, etc.	9,500
For plumbing, drains and sewers	14,500
For main sewer and grading	3,000
Total	$221,600

Bills were introduced into the Legislature in 1897 appropriating sufficient money to complete the work, but all these bills failed of passage. An attempt was again made to obtain the necessary appropriations during the sixty-ninth Legislature, 1899, when a sufficient sum was appropriated to complete the hospital. The same Legislature passed an act placing the Maine Insane Hospital at Bangor under the management of the Board of Trustees.

This act provided that the government of the Maine Insane Hospital should be vested in a committee of seven trustees, one of whom should be a woman, to be appointed and commissioned by the Governor, with the advice and consent of the Council, but for not longer than three years under any one appointment.

The trustees of the Maine Insane Hospital were authorized to organize and prepare it for the reception of patients, to appoint a superintendent, treasurer, steward and other necessary officers, whose salaries they were to fix, and to perform such other acts as might be necessary to properly care and provide for patients therein. The action of said trustees was subject to the approval of the Governor and Council.[1]

The full Board of Trustees made a visit to the new hospital June 6, 1900, and, after a thorough examination of it, returned home, satisfied that the building in design and architectural construction would fully meet the expectations and needs of the state. The board made a second visit November 27, 1900, and were pleased with the progress and splendid character of the work. The $225,000 appropriated by the last Legislature to be expended during 1899 and 1900 had been entirely exhausted and nearly $40,000 additional had been advanced by Gov. Powers to be used for completing the buildings.

There appeared to be an earnest wish that Dr. G. W. Foster, a native and former resident of Bangor, should receive the appointment of superintendent of the new hospital. The trustees had already received numerous communications, strongly recommending him for the position. As there was urgent need of the advice of a superintendent in completing the equipment of the institution and settling many details incident to its occupancy, the trustees concluded that the time had come for making the appointment and accordingly unanimously recommended to the executive department of the state "the name of G. W. Foster, M. D., of Washington, D. C., who has had a long and successful experience in hospital work, and comes strongly recommended."

The hospital was completed and opened for the reception of patients July 1, 1901.

[1] This act repealed July 1, 1911. See "The Care of the Insane in Maine."

The first patient was admitted to the hospital June 26, 1901. Two others had been admitted when, on the first day of July, a detail of 70 female patients was received from the hospital at Augusta, followed upon the 6th by 75 males from the same institution. There have been 66 other admissions (prior to November 30, the limit of the hospital year) which have come from this section of the state, making the entire number under treatment during the period of five months, 214.

By appointment of the trustees, Dr. P. H. S. Vaughn, who had for some years rendered efficient service in charge of the male wards at the Augusta Hospital, became assistant superintendent, and Dr. B. F. Howard, of Bangor, assistant physician. Dr. Howard also performs the duties of clinical pathologist. C. F. Perry, of Augusta, became the steward, and Mrs. Adelaide C. Brown, matron. Walter S. Bolton, who acted as engineer before the opening of the hospital, continued in that position.

The hospital site contains 120 acres. Opposite its south front winds the Penobscot, 150 feet below, showing glimpses of its surface through an extent of several miles. Beyond the river to the south a range of blue mountains extend east and west as far as the eye can reach; while to the north a wide sweep of variegated country is bounded upon the horizon by the Charleston hills and distant Katahdin. To the west the City of Bangor is in full view, its nearer margin not half a mile away; while in the opposite direction is a mountainous region that suggests the Alleghanies in Virginia.

The training school for nurses was organized in 1901, and the first class graduated in 1903. The instruction given follows the course outlined by the committee of the American Medico-Psychological Association.

The hospital farm was enlarged by the purchase of 50 acres additional in 1905 and a second purchase of 50 acres in 1909. The farm now contains 250 acres, of which about 100 acres are under cultivation.

In 1907 an appropriation was made for an additional building for women patients, providing accommodations for 150 patients and 19 nurses. On the first floor is the dining-room, seating 150 patients. In 1907 an appropriation of $30,000 was made for the construction and equipment of a hospital for the tubercular insane of the state in connection with the Eastern Maine Insane Hospital. This building was opened for the reception of patients in the spring of 1910. It consists of two wards for men and women, each ward accommodating 24 patients, each having its own dining-room opening into a common kitchen. The wards have screened verandas, free ventilation by windows and transoms, so that patients can obtain a maximum amount of pure air and sunlight. In connection with each ward is a nurses' room, two rooms for isolation of patients critically ill, baths, lockers and lavatories. This hospital was built on the southern side of a pine-covered hill and is sheltered from the prevailing winds.

In 1909 an appropriation of $175,000 was obtained for a new wing to accommodate 150 male patients and a bathing pavilion equipped with shower baths and dressing room. This was completed and occupied in January, 1911. In 1912 the population of the hospital was 525 patients, with a capacity of approximately 600.

The nursing staff consists of 31 women nurses, six of whom are on night duty and four on the male wards. The ratio of women nurses to women patients is 1 to 11. There are 25 male attendants, six of whom are on night duty, and the ratio of men nurses to men patients is 1 to 12.

The hospital has a well-equipped laboratory and employs a pathologist.

The dental needs of the patients are provided for by a visiting dentist, who comes to the hospital one day of each week.

Staff meetings are held four mornings of each week and all new patients are presented for examination after the case histories have been prepared by the ward physicians.

During the last six years the so-called non-restraint system has been enforced, in that no restraining devices have been employed other than baths and wet packs. Chemical restraint is not employed. The hospital is equipped with a hydrotherapeutic outfit, apparatus for electrical treatment, and in the new male wing, continuous baths.

The name of the hospital was changed on July 1, 1913, to Bangor State Hospital.

The population of the hospital December 1, 1914, was 612. There has been no recent material addition to the plant of the hospital, with the exception of the installation in 1913 of a cold storage plant and the construction of a storehouse.

SUPERINTENDENTS.

Dr. George W. Foster...	1900-1904	Dr. H. W. Mitchell......	1907-1910
Dr. P. H. S. Vaughn....	1904-1907	Dr. Frederick L. Hills..	1910-

ASSISTANT SUPERINTENDENTS.

Dr. P. H. S. Vaughn...	1901-1904	Dr. Forrest C. Tyson....	1907-1914
Dr. Burt F. Howard....	1904-1907	Dr. Pearl T. Haskell....	1914-

FIRST ASSISTANT PHYSICIANS.

Dr. Burt F. Howard....	1901-1904	Dr. James W. Crane....	1909-
Dr. Ezra B. Skolfield...	1904-1906	Dr. Harriet E. Chalmers	1910-1911
Dr. Harry L. Johnson...	1904-	Dr. Fred. H. Freeman..	1911-1912
Dr. Forrest C. Tyson...	1906-1907	Dr. James A. Barrett...	1912-1913
Dr. Mary Paulsell Mitchell	1907-1910	Dr. James A. Powers...	1913-
		Dr. Lester F. Norris....	1913-

INTERNES.

Dr. LeRoy A. Luce.....	1906-	Dr. Donald J. MacLean.	1912-
Dr. Louis W. Parady...	1907-	Dr. Louis O. S. Wallace.	1914-
Dr. James W. Crane....	1908-		

PATHOLOGIST.

Dr. Herbert W. Thompson....................1910-

MAINE SCHOOL FOR FEEBLE-MINDED.

WEST POWNAL, ME.

The Maine School for Feeble-minded was established in 1908. As a location for the school the state bought at West Pownal eight or nine farms, having a total area of about 1200 acres. On the central part of this tract of land the institution is now being developed.

According to the present plan of development of the institution, the dormitories will be placed in a slightly irregular semicircle, with the proposed administration building and amusement hall in the center. At present there are two brick buildings, located 260 feet apart and accommodating 70 girls each. There is also a brick building for women attendants, located in the same semicircle, and about 250 feet outside the dormitories; this building will accommodate 21 persons.

There are two farm colonies; one located three-fifths of a mile from the main institution, and the other one mile distant in the opposite direction. These colonies have wooden dormitories, accommodating 50 persons each.

The institution is a custodial institution as well as a school for the feeble-minded. All classes of feeble-minded are received from the age of six years and upwards.

The Montessori system is used as far as it is applicable to the class of inmates. Grade work, industrial and manual training work are taught by the most practical methods suited to the mentality of the inmates.

The present capacity of the institution is 273 persons.

The superintendent is Dr. Carl J. Hedin.

THE CARE OF THE INSANE IN MARYLAND.

In the year 1773 the General Assembly of Maryland authorized the establishment of poorhouses in certain counties in the state, amongst which were St. Mary's, Harford, Anne Arundel and Baltimore. These poorhouses, which were in charge of the trustees of the poor, were divided into two parts: almshouses for the sick and disabled, and workhouses for those persons who were deemed able to work and were spoken of as "beggars, dissolute, disorderly and vicious." This latter class undoubtedly included many insane, since there was little discrimination at that period between the insane and the disorderly.

The first legislation affecting the insane was a law passed on December 27, 1791, authorizing the justices of the peace to levy a sum for the support of "two lunatics," Mary Brown and Eleanor Love. The petition regarding them runs as follows:

WHEREAS, It has been represented to this General Assembly by the petition of Thomas Brown, of Prince George's County, that his wife, Mary Brown, and her daughter, Eleanor Love, are now and have been for some time past in a state of lunacy and that he is unable to care for them; therefore,

Be it enacted by the General Assembly of Maryland, That the justices of Prince George's County be and they are hereby empowered at their meeting and annually thereafter to levy on the assessable property of said county such sum not exceeding forty pounds of current money, as they may think necessary, for the support, maintenance and safekeeping of Mary Brown and Eleanor Love during their state of lunacy and to apply the same as they may think best for the purposes aforesaid.

Two years later another act, dated December 28, 1793, provided for the support of Rebecca Fowler, on petition of her mother, Juliana Fowler, who set forth that "her daughter Rebecca has convulsion fits, is blind and that she has in a great measure been deprived of the use of her senses, and that she, her mother, is no longer able to take care of her, but desires to keep her out of the almshouse." The sum of twenty pounds a year, required for that purpose, was duly appropriated.

In another petition of about the same date an appeal was made by a father and mother, who stated that up to that time they had supported four helpless imbecile children, "unable to walk, to dress or to feed themselves," and as they themselves were advancing in years, they asked that the "trustees of the poor be permitted to pay a pension for the care of Solomon, aged 30, Sarah and Mary (twins), aged 28, and Eliza, aged 26, the sum not to exceed $30 a year for each."

The records all make it evident that the friends of the insane had a strong feeling against sending them to the county almshouses. The reason given for asking state aid in many instances is the wish to keep an insane relative at home, it being generally thought that those who were feeble, helpless and deranged were better cared for out of the almshouse than in it.

The first act providing for a state institution for the insane was passed on January 20, 1797. It reads as follows:

AN ACT

To Encourage the Establishing of a Hospital for the Relief of Indigent Sick Persons and for the Reception and Care of Lunatics.

Whereas, There are frequently in many parts of this state poor distempered persons who languish, being in pain and misery under various disorders of body and mind and who cannot have the benefit of regular advice, attendance, lodging, diet and medicine but at an expense which they are unable to defray, and therefore, often suffer for want thereof; and

Whereas, It is represented to this General Assembly that there is a charitable disposition in divers inhabitants of this state to contribute largely towards establishing a common state hospital in or near the City of Baltimore, properly disposed and appointed, where such afflicted persons may be comfortably subsisted and where their health may be regularly attended to; therefore, for the encouragement of so beneficial an undertaking:

Be it enacted by the General Assembly of Maryland, That the Treasurer of the Western Shore of Maryland shall and he is hereby directed to pay to the Mayor of the City of Baltimore, or to his order, out of any unappropriated money that may be in the treasury, the sum of $8000 to be applied to the establishment of said hospital upon bond being given with good and sufficient surety for the faithful application of said money to the founding, building and furnishing said hospital according to the one intent and meaning of this law.

The "charitable disposition to contribute largely" refers especially to a gift made by Jeremiah Yellott, of Baltimore, of seven acres of land, which he proposed to give to the State of Maryland on condition that the Legislature granted the means necessary for the purposes of a "lunatic and general asylum." The sum of $8000 appropriated by the Legislature, however, was not sufficient and the City of Baltimore, together with some of its citizens, contributed an additional sum of $18,000, making $26,000 in all, with which a building was begun on a plan believed to meet the wants of the time. It was not completed, however, and, after a short time, fell into neglect until the year 1808, when the City of Baltimore granted a lease of it, for a period of 15 years, to Dr. James Smythe and Dr. Colin Mackenzie, to be used by them in the care of the insane as well as of general patients and to be known as the Maryland Hospital, they undertaking on their part to put the premises into good condition. In order to complete the buildings already begun and construct an addition which was needed to ensure proper accommodations for the patients, a large sum of money was required. To provide this the Legislature again granted $18,000 and in 1816 it made a further appropriation of $30,000 accompanied with the privilege of raising $20,000 by lottery. In addition to this Dr. Smythe and Dr. Mackenzie contributed $60,000 out of what are described as "their profits and private resources," and in 1815 they applied for an extension of their lease for another 10 years in order that they might reimburse themselves for their outlay. The whole amount expended was, therefore, $154,000, the hospital, on its completion, accommodating about 40 insane and 150 general patients.

At this time an agitation in behalf of the insane developed in the state which terminated in an act of the Assembly, passed in 1827, reasserting the rights of the state to the Maryland Hospital, on the ground that the land had been purchased and the buildings erected, in part at least, from funds contributed by the state. An ordinance was passed by the Mayor and Council of Baltimore City which deeded the property to the state, and the state passed an act of incorporation which vested the title of the property, with all rights of the state, in a president and Board of Visitors, appointed from different counties, subject to the lease of the hospital and premises held at that time by Dr. John P. Mackenzie, a son of Dr. Colin Mackenzie, who died in 1827, and successor to him and to Dr. James Smythe, who died some years earlier. The Board of Visitors organized and began to investigate the affairs of the hospital. In so doing they ascertained that no lease had ever been executed to Dr. John P. Mackenzie and that he held the property only by virtue of an ordinance of the corporation of Baltimore, passed and approved March 16, 1821, which gave him charge of the property contingent upon his compliance with certain conditions. In a subsequent report of the Board of Visitors, June 29, 1829, it was stated that Dr. Mackenzie had no lease of the property or any legal title to its possession. In the same report it was also declared that an examination showed the west wing of the property to be so much out of repair as not to be habitable, while the terms of the original lease to Drs. Mackenzie and Smythe required them to keep the buildings in repair. The visitors further spoke in terms of disapprobation of the treatment of insane patients. The hospital had become essentially a private institution and the public were not, in the opinion of the committee, well taken care of.

In an abstract of the public documents of the Board of Visitors of the Maryland Hospital, under date of May 19, 1828, printed in the documents of the Maryland Assembly for that year, are to be found the first rules and regulations established by the visitors upon their organization as a board. There is, in addition, a series of resolutions submitted by one of the visitors which were adopted. The most important of these is in section 4, as follows:

It shall be the duty of the standing committee to inquire forthwith into the competency and ability of the steward, the number and ability of the matron and servants, the sufficiency and quality of the mattresses, beds and bedding, and furniture; and also to inquire into the state of repair and general condition of the hospital and other buildings thereunto pertaining and of the government and regulation thereof.

At a later date this committee reported that:

1. They found that Dr. Colin Mackenzie and Dr. James Smythe leased the property originally upon the 24th of June, 1808, for a period of 15 years, and that a supplementary ordinance in 1814 gave an extension of 10 years to the original terms of the lease upon certain conditions, which, in the opinion of the committee, had not been complied with. Also that no new lease had ever been executed after the expiration of the first period of 15 years, and that upon the death of Dr. Colin Mackenzie no lease had ever been executed to Dr. John P. Mackenzie, his son, although the latter had taken possession of the property.

2. That by a resolution of the Mayor and City Council, approved February 4, 1828, the right and title of the Maryland or City Hospital had been deeded to the State of Maryland and that this right and title had in turn been transferred to the president and Board of Visitors of the Maryland Hospital.

Upon a subsequent page of the same public documents of the Legislature a report of the standing committee is printed by order of the Senate in 1829. It is evidently a report made in compliance with the resolution adopted at a meeting of the Board of Visitors on May 19, 1828. The main statements are as follows:

1. The committee believes the steward and matron to be intelligent and good-tempered and (*as far as they know how*) they discharge their trusts, but nothing has occurred to impress the committee that they possess the degree of method, order, invention or energy which are important in such an institution. The committee recommends that the hospital be placed under the care and control of the Sisters of Charity (for its domestic purposes), whose fitness has been manifested in the Baltimore Infirmary.

2. That the number of attendants are 16, of whom 11 are females and 5 males. Of the former there are 1 seamstress, 4 nurses, 1 waiter, 1 cook, 1 dairy maid, 1 chamber maid, 1 washer-woman; of the latter are 3 cell-keepers, 1 gate-keeper and 1 baker.

The committee believes that the number is not numerous enough for the lunatics, who require not only attendance to clean and change them, but, in the opinion of the committee, the kind and amiable attention of intelligent nurses, who will linger in their cells and return from time to time to relieve them from the solitude of dungeon confinement and, on proper occasions, to walk with them in the open air and to endeavor to excite some of the feelings and ideas which belong to human nature.

The number of patients is at present 57 *in toto,* of whom 28 are mariners and 29 lunatics, of which last number 21 are males and 8 females.

3. That the bedding, beds and furniture the committee found in the rooms of these so-called boarders are pretty good; beds generally have not hair mattresses, which, in the opinion of your committee, ought to be in use. Few of the lunatics have either beds or bedsteads and this your committee has been told is necessary for their comfort, as straw is substituted from the facility with which it can be changed, but your committee is sorry to add that from the report of its steward and also from the strong smell of the straw in the cells, it does not appear that the change of this article is as frequent as it should be for the comfort and benefit of the lunatics.

4. The committee then states that the old wing has fallen into complete ruin and will soon fall into a state of total dilapidation. It recommends a complete separation of the sexes and a better classification to separate the noisy and vociferous from the calm and gentle. The committee complains of a lack of neatness about the hospital.

5. That there are two resident physicians and six students in the hospital, but their powers and duties are not defined. There is a lack of conveniences for warm bathing. The committee complains of a lack of skilled medical and surgical care. It recommends in conclusion that they render the institution a public one as soon as practicable.

In the same documents is contained a memorial from Dr. John P. Mackenzie to the Legislature, in answer to the report of this committee, in which he denies the truth of the statements as to any lack of convenience for the patients or any other of the arrangements of the hospital, and lauds the work of the steward and his wife.

The Legislature, after finding that the position of the state was not a strong one, owing to the fact that it had not asserted its rights until some years after the expiration of the original contract, and that equity, at any rate, was upon the side of Dr. Mackenzie, whose family had spent considerable money in the erection of buildings, finally decided not to investigate any of the allegations of the committee as to the title of the property or the mode of conducting the institution, but to wait until the expiration of the lease for the additional term of 10 years. The Board of Visitors maintained its organization and legal control of the property, but did not assume charge until the 1st of January, 1834.

From the year 1834 the number of patients steadily increased, especially in the insane department, so that it became necessary to apply to the Legislature for means to provide increased accommodation. The sum of $30,000 was granted, and in the act making this appropriation it was provided that the institution should hereafter be devoted exclusively to the care of the insane; also that one-half of it should be reserved for the use of insane patients from the different counties, the said counties having the privilege of sending them at a cost of $100 a year for each patient.

The hospital buildings having become greatly overcrowded, the Legislature of 1852 appointed a commission to select a site for the institution. A property known as Spring Grove, near Catonsville, Baltimore County, was selected and work was begun on the new buildings in 1853. After many delays, due chiefly to the Civil War, the new hospital was opened for the reception of patients on October 7, 1872. It is now known as Spring Grove State Hospital and has a capacity of 750 patients.

The second state hospital for the care of the insane in Maryland is the Springfield State Hospital, Sykesville, which was authorized by an act of the Legislature in 1894. At that time over 1000 insane persons were confined and improperly cared for in the almshouses and jails of the counties of the state. On March 8, 1898, the first group of buildings of the new hospital was opened for the reception of patients. On October 1, 1913, the population of this hospital was 1344 patients.

On April 11, 1910, the Legislature of Maryland created a third hospital for the care of the insane under the name of "The Hospital for the Negro Insane of Maryland." An appropriation of $100,000 was provided for the purchase of lands and the erection of buildings. This hospital is for the care of the negro insane exclusively, and is located at Crownsville, Anne Arundel County.

The Eastern Shore State Hospital, located at Cambridge, is the fourth state institution for the care of the insane in Maryland, and was authorized by the General Assembly of 1912. On December 11, 1913, 24 patients were admitted to be cared for in temporary quarters, pending the erection of buildings that are now in process of construction. When completed the institution will accommodate 200 patients.

Indigent insane persons from the City of Baltimore are also cared for in a department of the Baltimore City Almshouse at Bay View, near the City of Baltimore. On the 1st of January, 1910, there were 438 patients at this institution, but with the opening of the Eastern Shore Hospital at Cambridge, a majority of the city patients at Bay View will be transferred to the various state hospitals. The State of Maryland has also an arrangement with the Sisters of Charity, proprietors of Mt. Hope Retreat,[1] whereby state patients are cared for by that institution at a rate of $150 per year per capita.

In 1888 the state established at Owings Mills the Rosewood State Training School for Feeble-minded. This institution has a capacity of 700 beds.

In Maryland the investigation of the system of state aid to institutions and the inspection of institutions receiving state aid devolves upon the Board of State Aid and Charities. This board consists of seven members, appointed by the Governor, who serve without compensation. In addition the supervision of all institutions in which insane are detained is in the hands of the Lunacy Commission. This is a body of five members, appointed by the Governor, and of which the Attorney General is ex-officio a member. They serve without compensation, and two of them must be physicians, each a graduate of some legally authorized medical college with at least five years' actual practice of medicine

[1] See history of Mt. Hope Retreat in this volume.

just preceding the appointment; one of these must have had at least two years' experience in the treatment of the insane.

In addition each state hospital is under the immediate control of individual boards of managers, as is indicated in detail in the individual histories of these institutions.

By an act approved April 8, 1910, the Lunacy Commission has power to appoint a board of five uncompensated visitors for each county asylum and almshouse where insane are confined, to serve at its pleasure.

Classes Committed.—All insane persons are entitled to admission to the state hospitals.

Legal Procedure in Commitment.—The County Commissioners and Supervisors of Charities in the City of Baltimore must cause indigent insane persons who have no relatives to be sent upon the written certificate of two qualified physicians to the almshouse of the county or city or to the hospital.

If demanded by alleged insane person or his relatives or friends or on the request of the county authorities or the Supervisors of Charities in Baltimore, the circuit court or the criminal court in Baltimore must convene a jury to inquire into the insanity of the person. If the authorities are not satisfied that he is insane, the state's attorney of the county or City of Baltimore must be notified and bring the question before the circuit court or the criminal court of Baltimore for determination.

No person may be committed or confined except upon written certificate of two qualified physicians made within one week after examination of the person, stating his insanity and giving the reason for the opinion.

Voluntary patients who make application in writing may be received, provided that the expense be borne by the person applying or by his relatives or friends. No voluntary patient may be detained for more than three days after having given notice of desire to leave the institution.

Appeal from Commitment.—The Lunacy Commission, when it believes a person confined in any institution to be not insane, may bring the matter to the attention of the state's attorney, who must apply to the proper tribunal for a writ of *habeas corpus*. After inquiry the court must discharge the person if found sane.

Cost of Commitment.—The cost of commitment is a charge upon the county from which the patient is sent.

SPRING GROVE STATE HOSPITAL.[1]

CATONSVILLE, MD.

The Maryland Hospital for the Insane is the third oldest hospital for the treatment of the insane in the United States; one in Pennsylvania and one in Virginia preceding it by a few years.

Although organized as a hospital in 1797, the nucleus for the institution was inaugurated in 1794 by a few gentlemen, at the head of whom was a Captain Yellott, a well-known citizen of Baltimore Town, who had observed the suffering, misery and lack of medical treatment among the numerous seamen arriving at the port of the growing town of Baltimore. These gentlemen accordingly erected a retreat for the relief and benefit of such persons, where they could obtain shelter and receive appropriate treatment for their bodily ailments.

This enterprise suffered various vicissitudes during its career, and its success was far from flattering. In 1797 a number of influential and philanthropic gentlemen, appreciating the great need of a hospital for the increasing sick and insane, now that Baltimore had been incorporated as a city, started a subscription and organized as a society to encourage the establishment of a hospital, where the pauper sick and mariners could be treated, and for the reception of such insane persons as were considered of a dangerous character and required restriction. These gentlemen determined to seek aid from the state, and their appeal was successful before the General Assembly of 1798, which appropriated $8000 to be paid to the Mayor and City Council of Baltimore, and to be spent by them for the building of a hospital for the pauper sick and insane of the state, and seafaring persons. The Legislature appropriated $3000 additional in November, 1798, and to this was added £600 sterling by the City of Baltimore.

A month after the action of the General Assembly the City Council appointed a commission, consisting of the Mayor and Messrs. Jeremiah Yellott, Richard Lawson and Alexander McKim, to purchase a suitable piece of ground in fee simple and erect thereon a hospital building. Negotiations were made for property

[1] Compiled from "History Maryland Hospital for the Insane," 1897, and from reports of the Spring Grove State Hospital.

occupied by the Retreat under the direction of Captain Yellott, which purchase was consummated on May 18, 1798, and the building commenced—the hospital to be known as the Public Hospital of Baltimore. The City Council assumed immediate control of its operations, and requested the Mayor and Commissioner of Health to employ such physicians and other employees as were necessary for its successful management, and to formulate rules and regulations for its government.

The hospital was formally opened and occupied in the latter part of 1798 by a few insane patients, a number of indigent sick and some mariners. From this time up to 1808 the city seemed to exercise exclusive control of the management and direction of the hospital, the state remaining dormant in reference to it, although not relinquishing any claim upon the institution.

In 1808 two eminent and enterprising physicians, Colin Mackenzie and James Smythe, recognizing the great need of increased hospital facilities from the rapid gain in the population of the city, made a proposition to the City Council to lease the hospital for a term of 15 years, which was accepted by the Council and approved by the Mayor, with the provision that the hospital was to be enlarged and better accommodations provided; and furthermore, it should be maintained for the treatment of the indigent sick and insane according to the charter of the organizers, and that full medical control should be vested in the above-named physicians and that they should receive any benefits accruing therefrom. In order to carry on the work on a large scale in accordance with their benevolent ideas, they obtained permission from the Legislature to raise a sum of money, not exceeding $40,000, by lottery. The scheme proved a most successful one, and a sum was raised sufficient to place the hospital in a position to receive an increased number of patients.

The hospital, under the skillful supervision of these active gentlemen, entered upon a successful career of marked usefulness. The General Assembly, appreciating their efforts, directed the Treasurer of the Western Shore, in 1811, to pay them the sum of $18,000 for certain necessary repairs and improvements to the hospital, and for the welfare of patients under their jurisdiction. Drs. Mackenzie and Smythe again besought the City Council of Baltimore in 1814 for a second lease of 10 years, which was duly granted by that body, provided, during the term of the original lease specified improvements should be made, which consisted of the addition of a center building and east wing, and who furthermore enjoined that separate apartments should be provided for the insane patients, who up to this time had been in the same building with those suffering from somatic diseases.

During 1814 the hospital was called into service for the reception of many soldiers, wounded at the memorable battle of North Point, so familiar to all Marylanders. The two physicians in charge again called upon the liberality of the General Assembly in 1816 for help to build an addition to their hospital building. The Legislature of the same year authorized them to borrow a sum of money for their requirements, which amount was to be divided into six installments and to be available at certain stated periods, the state assuming to pay the loan with interest three years after each loan was severally made. Accordingly the erection of a handsome and commodious building was commenced, which, in connection with those already constructed, would afford accommodations for about 75 patients. An act was also passed by the same Legislature incorporating the Maryland Hospital, the control and government of said hospital to be vested in a president and Board of Visitors, subject to the lease of Drs. Mackenzie and Smythe. The entire cost of the hospital up to this date can be estimated to have been between $154,000 and $170,000, and its possessions to have consisted of several acres of valuable property, with improved grounds; a center building, which was utilized as an administration building; and two wings—the west, known as the Lunatic Asylum, and containing the insane; and the east one, which was reserved for the treatment of general diseases.

In 1819 Dr. Smythe died and the management of the institution devolved upon Dr. Mackenzie, who continued to direct its course. The doctor, in view of his advancing years, prayed the City Council, in the event of his death, to transfer the lease of the hospital for the unexpired term of years to his son, Dr. John P. Mackenzie. An ordinance to that effect was passed by the Council, with the proviso that a Board of Visitors should be appointed, who should have general supervision of the property, and, in conjunction with the physicians in charge, shape the policy of the institution and see that the agreement between the Council and the physician was properly conformed with. This board was duly appointed, but, whether from lack of interest in the hospital or perfect confidence in the ability of Dr. Mackenzie and his son, the entire charge of affairs was left to them, and thus continued until 1827, when Dr. Colin Mackenzie passed away, to the profound regret of everyone connected with the hospital. The hospital accordingly passed to the control of Dr. John P. Mackenzie by the ordinance of 1821.

The hospital, dating from the lease of Doctors Mackenzie and Smythe, had practically become a private enterprise. The city, however, in February, 1828, in anticipation of the expiration of the jurisdiction of Dr. Mackenzie, authorized the Mayor to turn over to the state any title it might have in the City or Public Hospital or any part or portion thereof. This ordinance, on the part of the city, seemed to awaken the General Assembly to immediate action. Accordingly, in March, 1828, this body asserted its ownership to the hospital and passed an act incorporating the Maryland Hospital, and at the same time appointed a president and Board of Visitors, who were empowered to act for the state on all matters pertaining to the hospital. The board, consisting of one member from each county and several representatives from Baltimore City, was organized, and Dr. Richard S. Steuart elected president.

Immediately upon its organization the board appointed a committee to thoroughly investigate the condition of the hospital. The committee, after a thorough examination, reported that the institution was greatly in need of repairs in every department; its rules and regulations were loose and lax and not properly enforced, and the medical and surgical treatment not up to the standard of a well-managed hospital. The board, therefore, requested that Dr. John P. Mackenzie should turn the control and management of the hospital into their hands. This he refused to do unless certain monetary consideration be given him for the unexpired period of his lease. The board did not feel justified in such a course, and no further steps were taken looking to an agreement between the board and the physician-in-charge.

From 1828 to the 1st of January, 1834—time of the expiration of Dr. Mackenzie's lease—the relation of the board to the hospital did not change. Although holding regular stated meetings, and conscientiously inspecting the building and patients, their control was merely nominal, the authority and direction emanating from

Dr. Mackenzie. There were 57 patients in the hospital at this time, of whom 29 were mariners, for the support of whom the government paid, and 28 insane patients.

In 1833 the Board of Visitors prepared a memorial and presented the same to the General Assembly, requesting that a substantial appropriation should be granted the hospital to add many needed repairs and provide for the maintenance of the patients upon the expiration of Dr. Mackenzie's lease. The General Assembly complied with their request and appropriated a sum for the purpose stated, which, although not as large as desired, yet enabled the board to improve the hospital to some extent. On the 1st of January, 1834, the property passed to the Board of Visitors, acting for the state, and became strictly a state institution. Upon assuming jurisdiction the board considered it for the best interest and welfare of the hospital that a change in the management be made; consequently, an arrangement was made with the Sisters of Charity to act as nurses and one of their number to be matron and stewardess, with general supervision. The board also engaged the gratuitous services of Doctors J. I. Cohen, Wright, William Fisher, Richard Sexton, John Fonerden and John P. Mackenzie to act as physicians, and Doctors Geo. Gibson, H. W. Baxley, Jamieson and Gittings to take charge of the surgical department. These gentlemen gave their valuable services to the hospital for one year, but the duties became arduous and they were compelled to resign. Dr. William Stokes, a graduate of the University of Maryland, was appointed to perform the duties of resident physician under the direct supervision of the president of the board. The hospital, under the management of Dr. Stokes, was satisfactorily conducted, but in 1836, after one year of service, he resigned for private reasons, and Dr. William Fisher, an eminent and highly accomplished physician, was selected to fill the vacancy.

In 1836 the board purchased the lot of ground north of the building extending to Monument Street. This parcel of land was afterwards connected with the original tract by the closing of the old Joppa road, and was regarded as a valuable addition to the hospital in the event of the erection of any new buildings in the future. The General Assembly of the same year appropriated $15,000 for repairs to the building and the purchase of new furniture to properly equip the wards.

When the organization of the hospital was perfected in 1797 it was with the idea that the institution should afford suitable accommodations for the insane and the indigent sick of every description.

The board, recognizing the danger of allowing patients with contagious diseases to mingle with and be treated under the same roof as the insane and those suffering from general diseases, applied to the Legislature in 1834, and were granted permission to exclude all cases of contagious diseases from the hospital.

The care of the insane had been much neglected, and the board determined to ask the General Assembly in 1839 to make sufficient appropriation to enable them to accomplish their honorable and humane design of placing the hospital in a position to treat the insane in a more enlightened manner, and to place the hospital on a par with similar institutions in sister states. The board also strongly recommended that the hospital should be confined absolutely to the care and treatment of the insane, the improvements being made wholly with this idea in view. The board proposed to demolish the original building and to construct upon the land and the lot just beyond such buildings as the architecture pertaining to the modern treatment of the insane demanded. The General Assembly, in answer to their appeal, passed the following resolution:

Resolved by the General Assembly of Maryland, That the Treasurer of the Western Shore be and is hereby authorized and directed to pay to the president and visitors of the Maryland Hospital, or their order, the sum of $30,000, in six annual payments, from and after the passage of this resolution, to be by them applied for the benefit and improvement of said hospital, distinct reference being made to making the improvements to its exclusive use as a lunatic asylum.

The act goes on to state that one-half of the institution shall be appropriated to the accommodation of pauper insane from the state, and they shall be treated at the expense of the counties sending such insane, at a fixed price per annum.

The required improvements as contemplated were immediately carried out. The number of patients in the hospital upon completion of the new buildings was 50—32 males and 18 females—all of whom were insane.

The nursing in the hospital since the organization of the board had been performed by the Sisters of Charity, who had rendered excellent and faithful services to the patients entrusted to their care; however, after mature and careful consideration, the board decided that it was best for the welfare of the hospital that the Sisters should sever their connection with the institution, although fully cognizant of their faithful duty and assistance to the state in its work of charity. In the place of the Sisters a matron was immediately employed and a corps of competent nurses engaged.

Dr. William Fisher resigned his position in 1846 as resident physician, and Dr. John Fonerden, professor of obstetrics in the Washington College, Baltimore, was elected to fill the vacancy. Dr. Fisher had, during his services as the administrative officer, directed the affairs of the institution in the most satisfactory manner, and his executive ability had shown him to be a man well fitted for the position he held.

The number of insane had rapidly increased and it was with difficulty that suitable provisions could be made for the admission of new cases. The board urged the General Assembly to take some action in reference to the advisability of additional accommodations being provided for this class of patients. The hospital contained 133 patients; a large number in excess of the comfortable capacity of the building.

During the session of 1848 the General Assembly passed several acts pertaining to the hospital, the most important of which was a resolution requesting that Governor Thomas take steps to have an estimate formulated of the cost of the construction of additional accommodations for the insane. The Governor was asked to report the same at the first meeting of the Legislature following the present one.

The Governor sent the following message to the session of 1849:

By resolution No. 92 the Governor was requested to have full estimates made of the cost of additional buildings to the Maryland Hospital suitable for the accommodation of the insane persons in the penitentiary and the almshouse of Baltimore City and for the use of the insane poor of the state, and report the same to the next succeeding meeting of the Legislature.

Pursuant to this resolution, plans and estimates prepared with care and approval of the president of the hospital have been procured and are herewith submitted.

The plan, it will be perceived, contemplates the erection of two wings, extending south 250 feet each from either end of the present building, and is designed, as directed by the resolution, to accommodate 250 additional patients. The cost of the buildings, if warmed and ventilated by air furnaces, is estimated at $74,519, and if steam be substituted for the air furnaces the increased expense will carry the whole cost to $81,519.

Although the hospital is now filled to its utmost capacity, there are not far from 200 insane patients in the state, 123 of whom are in the Baltimore almshouse and 8 in the penitentiary, without means of proper treatment for the mitigation or cure of the awful malady with which they are afflicted.

However urgent may be the demand of humanity in behalf of this unfortunate class of persons, and however clear the obligation of society to provide for their wants, in view, nevertheless, of the proximity of the hospital and the City of Baltimore, and the limited extent of its ground, it is questionable whether, instead of enlarging the present building, it would not be wiser and better to dispose of the establishment and employ the proceeds, with such appropriations as the Legislature may choose to make, in the purchase of a sufficient quantity of land and the erection of an asylum upon a most modern and approved plan, adapted in all its arrangements for the comfortable accommodation, treatment and care of insane patients, and of style and character worthy of the munificence of the state.

No action was taken by the General Assembly during the session of 1849 upon the report of the Governor. The Board of Visitors again, in a report to the Legislature of 1852, urged the Assembly to consider the absolute necessity of additional accommodations for the insane, and in the same report declared that it was not expedient to enlarge the present buildings or make any additions thereto, but recommended that property outside the city be purchased and buildings erected thereon.

The General Assembly at the same session, now fully realizing that some suitable facilities must be furnished for the increased number of indigent insane, appointed a commission, consisting of Dr. Richard S. Steuart, Benjamin C. Howard, Richard Potts, Washington Duvall and D. H. C. Humphreys, to select a proper and convenient site for the erection of a new hospital.

The commission, after a thorough and exhaustive search, selected as a site the property known as Spring Grove, near Catonsville, Baltimore County. The tract of land contained 136 acres, overlooking the City of Baltimore and the surrounding counties, and was a most beautiful and appropriate spot for the erection of buildings for the treatment of the insane.

The property was paid for by private subscription, through the beneficence of many influential gentlemen of Baltimore and by aid from the General Assembly. The work upon the new hospital was begun in 1853 and proceeded without interruption until 1861, when the war interfered with any attempt to continue construction of the buildings. At this time the north wing was nearly ready for occupation, the center building raised to the second floor and the foundations of the south wing laid.

It is a noteworthy fact that the hospital again opened its doors for the shelter of wounded soldiers; for many of the wounded during this turbulent period of our history were cared for in its unfinished halls.

The General Assemblies of 1856, 1859 and 1860 made liberal appropriations to carry on the construction of the buildings. In 1862 the Legislature deemed it best for the interest and progress of the hospital to make a change in the commission, and consequently appointed J. S. Berry, Alexander Randall, Dr. John Whitridge, J. Reese and A. G. Waters to succeed the former commission in office. These gentlemen, after careful deliberation, decided, in consequence of the high price of labor and material, to abandon any idea of continuing the construction of the buildings. They therefore ordered the incomplete and exposed portions of the buildings to be properly protected from the action of the weather and a watchman appointed to guard the property from depredations.

The hospital remained in this condition until 1864, when, by a vigorous appeal from the commission, the General Assembly granted a sum sufficient to enable them to begin construction again.

In 1868 an act was passed by the General Assembly reinstating the original commission to power, and they were instructed to complete the institution as soon as practicable. Funds were sadly needed to carry on the work of completing the institution, and the Board of Visitors obtained permission to sell the hospital on Monument Street and to apply the sum resulting from such sale to that purpose. The property was accordingly sold to Mr. Johns Hopkins for $133,000, the release of the property being subject to the removal of the patients to the new hospital. On this site now stands The Johns Hopkins Hospital.

The commission in 1872 reported the building in a condition to receive patients, and on the 7th of October in the same year 112 patients were transferred from their old quarters to the present hospital at Spring Grove. The commission had expended all the money available, and in anticipation of further aid from the General Assembly had contracted a debt of $330,000, which the Legislature in 1872 provided for by an appropriation covering the full amount. This sum was insufficient to defray all the expenditures, and in 1874 the Assembly was petitioned to grant an additional sum of $53,153.08; but the members of that body, their patience having become exhausted, refused to extend to the hospital any further aid. The president and board decided that in order to carry on the operations of the hospital it would be necessary to place a mortgage of $150,000 on the property.

The original hospital continued under the direction of the same Board of Visitors until 1864, when a change was made in the board and it was reorganized, with Dr. William Fisher, former resident physician, as president; Dr. Stephen Collins, secretary, and Mr. Enoch Pratt, treasurer, Dr. John Fonerden remaining as superintendent under the new board and Dr. Taneyhill, assistant superintendent.

In 1868 Dr. Wm. F. Steuart was appointed resident physician, his wife acting as matron.

On the 6th of May of the following year Dr. John Fonerden, the superintendent, died, and Dr. William F. Steuart was unanimously elected superintendent, and Dr. James Steuart, assistant.

The General Assembly of 1876 passed an act authorizing the Governor to appoint a new Board of Managers, and the Governor named the following gentlemen to constitute the board: C. W. Chancellor, M. D.; ex-Governor A. W. Bradford, Barnes Compton, Henry D. Fernandis, Thomas R. Brown, John W. McCoy, Francis White, James McSherry, and L. W. Gunther.

Dr. C. W. Chancellor was elected president of the board and Dr. J. S. Conrad was appointed superintendent in the place of Dr. Wm. F. Steuart, resigned.

When the new board took charge of the hospital it contained 281 patients, among whom were many suffering from alcoholism and the effects of the excessive use of narcotics, but not insane. This class of patients was compelled to be thrown with the ordinary insane and acted as a disorganizing and disturbing element, and the board very wisely refused to receive such patients in the future and confined the hospital to the treatment of the insane.

The hospital was originally built to accommodate 325 patients, and, in consequence of the many admissions, it was only a question of a short time before the hospital would contain its full capacity. The president, in his annual report, called attention to this fact, and warned that body that additional accommodations would be required in the near future. Since then nearly every annual report reiterated the same request, but it was not until 1896 that such provisions were provided. At that date there were 747 insane persons supported by the state.

Dr. John S. Conrad resigned the position of medical superintendent on the 14th of March, 1878, and Dr. Richard Gundry, of Ohio, was appointed to fill the vacancy.

When the management of the hospital passed into Dr. Gundry's hands many of the patients were subject to mechanical restraint in all of its various forms; many were secluded, and few enjoyed any extended liberty. This mode of treatment he immediately dispensed with, although not without considerable opposition.

Instead of the straight-jacket, muffs and dark rooms, he prescribed in their place sunshine, fresh air and freedom. This was one of the few hospitals at that time which discarded restraint entirely; and to this date non-restraint continues to be one of the cardinal rules of the institution.

Among the many valuable and useful improvements made during Dr. Gundry's administration can be mentioned the fence surrounding the grounds of the hospital and the erection of lodge houses. He beautified the lawns and grounds, most of the work being performed by the patients, for he was a firm believer in the employment of all the patients who were able to work.

It was at his suggestion that a general refectory was built, which was in a condition to be occupied at the time of his death.

Dr. C. W. Chancellor, who was appointed president upon the reorganization of the board in 1876, resigned in 1880 and was succeeded by Col. Henry Taylor, who acceptably and faithfully filled the president's chair until his death in 1886. Dr. J. Pembroke Thom was chosen in his place and continued in service until 1890, and was followed by Mr. Wilmot Johnson.

Dr. Gundry died on the 23d of April, 1891, after a prolonged illness. He was succeeded by Dr. George H. Rohé, who was Commissioner of Health of Baltimore at that time.

Dr. Rohé during his term of office, which extended nearly five years, added many improvements to the hospital and inaugurated many changes in the regime. The construction of the present sewerage system under his directions marked an era in the sanitary improvements of the hospital. A pavilion for old and demented men and an additional ward for colored women were erected by his advice.

Dr. Rohé resigned in April, 1896, to accept the superintendency of the construction of Maryland Hospital No. 2 at Sykesville, Md., now known as Springfield State Hospital. He was succeeded by Dr. J. Percy Wade, who had been an assistant physician.

Spring Grove State Hospital is constructed upon the wing system, which was the popular and advanced mode of building at the date of its construction. The center is utilized as an administration building and the two wings contain the male and female patients. It commands a beautiful view of Baltimore, the Patapsco River and the surrounding country. The hospital is lighted by electricity and its water supply is abundant and pure. There are 763 patients upon the rolls; part are supported by the City of Baltimore, part by the counties and a few by their friends. The state also makes an annual appropriation for its maintenance.

In 1898 Dr. J. Clement Clark, who had been assistant physician for two years, resigned to accept the superintendency of the Springfield State Hospital. Dr. R. Edward Garrett, resident physician at Bay View Asylum, was appointed to fill the vacancy.

In the same year an industrial shop for male patients, with a capacity of 40 men, in which the various industries were to be housed, was erected, especial attention being given to the manufacture of willow baskets and willow work from willows grown on the hospital grounds.

In 1911 an appropriation of $80,000 was available from the sale of Maryland bonds. This amount was used in the remodeling and improvement of the kitchen of the hospital, which was badly needed, and also for the erection of a building for the purpose of a female industrial shop. One whole floor of the building, which adjoins the female department, is devoted to industries for the female patients, and can accommodate from 100 to 150. This building is constructed of stone, is fireproof, and cost about $80,000. The shop includes a department for sewing and mending, looms for carpets, machines for making stockings, and classes in raffia and fancy work. These comfortable quarters have been a great factor in interesting the female patients in this very important part of institutional work. The building was completed and occupied in 1912.

In 1913 the hospital purchased about 60 acres of land, on which was a very roomy cottage, located about one mile from the main building. In this building were installed new plumbing, a new heating plant and new dining-room; the entire building was remodeled and now accommodates 40 male patients for farm work. This colony has been in operation for six months and has been very successful. The patients are given all the liberty possible, and most of them appreciate the change from the main building. These farm colonies are maintained at a low per capita cost and are a great benefit to the convalescent and mildly demented cases.

The hospital now has under construction a psychopathic building. One wing will provide accommodations for about 60 female patients, together with the necessary nurses and medical staff. It will contain the modern equipment for caring for acute cases and will serve as a reception ward. The other wing when completed will provide accommodations for an equal number of male patients.

The hospital has in the last four years purchased over 130 acres of land for farming purposes, more than doubling the former acreage. On one of the pieces of property was an excellent stone quarry, which furnished all the stone used in the construction of the female industrial building, and also of the psychopathic building now being erected.

The hospital has had a variety of names. Until 1807 it was known as "The Public Hospital"; from 1808 to 1814 it was called the "City Hospital"; in the acts of the Legislature of 1808, 1811, 1813 and 1815 it was called the "Hospital in the Vicinity of Baltimore"; in 1816 it was called "The Maryland Hospital"; in 1828 it was called "The Maryland or City Hospital"; Resolutions No. 65, 1838, provided for the exclusive use of the institution as a *lunatic asylum*. For this reason, to the name "The Maryland Hospital," the words "for the Insane," were added. In consequence of the act of 1852 for the erection of a new hospital near Catonsville, the name was changed to "The Maryland Hospital for the Insane at Baltimore."

In 1912 the Legislature changed the name of the hospital from the "Maryland Hospital for the Insane" to "Spring Grove State Hospital."

PRESIDENT AND BOARD OF VISITORS FROM MARCH 14, 1828, TO JANUARY, 1870.

Dr. Richard S. Steuart..1828; 1868
Dr. Wm. Fisher..............1864-
Dr. James Thomas 1828-
Dr. John T. Rees 1828-
Dr. Gustavus Warfield 1828-
Dr. Octavius Taney 1828-
John G. Chapman 1828-
Wm. F. Johnson 1828-
Dr. Samuel F. Kemp 1828-
Dr. Henry Hiland 1828-
Dr. Joseph E. Muse 1828-
John C. Herbert 1828-
Dr. Robert Goldsborough 1828-
Dr. John S. Martin 1828-
Dr. Wm. Tyler 1828-
Dr. William Whitely 1828-
Dr. John C. Dorsey 1828-
Dr. George E. Mitchell 1828-
Dr. Henry Howard 1828-
Dr. James Montgomery 1828-
Brice W. Howard 1828-
Alexander Fridge 1828-
George Hoffman 1828-
Upton S. Heath 1828-
Dr. Joshua I. Cohen..........1828-
Charles Howard 1828-
J. I. Donaldson...............1828-
John Scott 1828-
David Keener 1828-
Hugh McElderry 1828-
William Hubbard 1828-
Evan T. Ellicott 1828-
Dr. P. Macauley 1843-
Dr. R. P. Hoffman 1843-
Joseph King 1843-
John H. B. Latrobe...........1836-
Dr. Thos. Edmondson........1843-
George W. Brown............1845-
George W. Dobbin...........1845-
Dr. Stephen Collins...........1845-
Thomas Wilson 1846-
James H. McHenry..........1849-
Johns Hopkins 1852-
Francis T. King 1852-
Wm. G. Harrison 1857-
Enoch Pratt 1857-
Wm. E. Mayhew 1858-
Dr. John M. Broome 1858-
Dr. B. F. Houston 1858-
Dr. Thos. J. Franklin 1858-
Daniel R. Magruder 1858-
Walter Mitchell 1858-
Dr. John W. Dashiell 1858-
Edw. Lloyd, Jr. 1859-
Dr. Henry H. Mitchell 1858-
Wm. B. Hill 1858-
Dr. Wm. H. De Courcy 1858-
Dr. Geo. M. Upshur 1858-
Dr. Thos. Sim 1858-
Dr. Joshua Wilson 1858-
Dr. Andrew Stafford 1858-
J. Philip Roman 1858-
Dr. J. L. Warfield 1858-
Edw. Lloyd 1859-
Allen B. Davis 1859-
Dr. Jas. Muse................1860-
Dr. A. A. Biggs 1860-
John G. Stone 1860-
Geo. A. Pearre 1864-
Basil D. Hall 1864-
Wm. Kennedy 1864-
J. J. Dalrymple 1864-
Robt. W. Todd 1864-
Wm. L. Jones 1864-
Thos. A. Millar 1864-
Dr. Thos. K. Carroll 1864-
Gerard Hopkins 1864-
Edw. Wilkins 1864-
George P. Tiffany 1864-
John B. Hopper 1864-
Dr. Wm. Stewart 1864-
John Harper 1864-

Dr. J. T. B. McMartin 1864-
Wm. McKim 1864-
Archibald Sterling, Jr. 1864-
Thos. Kelso 1864-
John W. Randolph 1864-
Thos. M. Smith 1864-
James Hooper, Jr.............1864-
Dr. James H. Miles 1867-
Reverdy Johnson, Jr. 1867-
Henry Janney 1867-
John Brown 1868-
Henry F. Thompson, Jr. 1868-
Dr. Wm. H. Keener 1868-
J. K. Longwell 1868-
Dr. Cary B. Gamble 1868-
Dr. Francis M. Slemons 1868-
John R. Franklin 1869-
Dr. James A. Steuart 1869-
S. Teackle Wallis 1869-
F. Key Howard 1870-
Dr. N. R. Smith 1870-
Richard Sprigg Steuart, M. D. 1870-
George Wm. Brown 1870-
Francis T. King 1870-
Dr. Edmond Duvall 1871-
Dr. John H. Mitchell.........1871-
Daniel M. Henry.............1871-
William J. Ross..............1871-
Wilson R. Byrn 1871-
James L. McLane 1872-
Alexander Hardcastle, M. D. .1872-
Alan P. Smith, M. D. 1873-
William W. Taylor 1874-

BOARD OF MANAGERS JANUARY 1, 1876.

C. W. Chancellor, M. D.
Thomas R. Brown, M. D.
John W. McCoy.
Henry D. Fernandis.
Ex-Gov. A. W. Bradford.
Barnes Compton.
Francis White.
James McSherry.
L. W. Gunther.

ADDED FROM TIME TO TIME.

J. Pembroke Thom, M. D.
Col. Henry S. Taylor.
James A. Buchanan.
Chas. G. W. Macgill, M. D.
David Fowler.
Gilmor Meredith.
Wilmot Johnson.
John H. Fowler.
Andrew C. Trippe.
George H. Cairnes, M. D.
John A. Whitridge.
Daniel R. Randall.
John Wilson.
John S. Gibbs.
Wesley M. Oler.
E. Stanley Gary.
Lawrason Riggs.
Robert Taylor.
William H. Gorman.
Charles Goldsborough.
Arthur D. Foster.
George Warfield.
John Gill of R.
John W. Renehan.
J. Charles Macgill, M. D.
Thornton Rollins.
Henry Vinsinger.
Gordon T. Atkinson, M. D.
Cecil E. Ewing.
Richard F. Gundry, M. D.
Samuel E. Reinhard.
G. Clem Goodrich.

DATES OF APPOINTMENTS OF SUPERINTENDENTS.

In 1834, when the Board of Visitors took charge, Dr. Richard Sprigg Steuart, president of the board, performed the duties of superintendent.

June 7, 1854, Dr. John Fonerden, appointed medical superintendent.

May 1, 1868, Dr. R. S. Steuart, re-appointed medical superintendent.

July 7, 1876, Dr. John S. Conrad, appointed medical superintendent.

May 1, 1878, Dr. Richard Gundry, appointed superintendent.

June 2, 1891, Dr. Geo. H. Rohé, appointed superintendent.

April 15, 1896, Dr. J. Percy Wade, appointed superintendent.

In 1834, when the Board of Visitors took charge, the medical duties were performed by the voluntary attendance of Dr. George Gibson, Dr. John Mackenzie, Dr. J. I. Cohen, Dr. Rd. Sexton, Dr. John Fonerden, Dr. William Fisher, and Dr. Richard S. Steuart, the president.

A year later (1835) Dr. Stokes was appointed resident physician to serve in consultation with the president of the board, Dr. Richard Sprigg Steuart. Dr. Stokes resigned and Dr. Starr served several months. Dr. William Fisher was then appointed and he served until 1844. Since that time the following physicians have served as assistants from time to time to date:

John Fonerden, M. D.
James A. Steuart, M. D.
G. Lane Taneyhill, M. D.
William F. Steuart, M .D.
John S. Conrad, M. D.
R. G. B. Broome, M. D.
Sydney O. Heiskell, M. D.
Randolph Barksdale, M. D.
W. S. Smith, M. D.
B. A. Turner, M. D.
E. M. Shaeffer, M. D.
B. D. Evans, M. D.
William L. Robins, M. D.
J. Percy Wade, M. D.
M. D. Norris, M. D.
Fred. Caruthers, M. D.
J. H. Scally, M. D.
Warren L. Babcock, M. D.
F. M. Clarke, M. D.
F. A. Councell, M. D.
Geo. F. Galloway, M. D.
J. Clement Clark, M. D.
Arthur Hawkins, M. D.
Cornelius DeWeese, M. D.
Jesse C. Coggins, M. D.
Joseph K. Shriver, M. D.
W. Turner Wootton, M. D.
R. Edward Garrett, M. D.
Thornton W. Perkins, M. D.
Robert P. Winterode, M. D.
Frank C. Ferguson, M. D.
T. F. Tompkins, M. D.
Cooper R. Drewry, M. D.
Matthew Conlin, M. D.
William R. Foard, M. D.
Thomas A. Hurley, M. D.
J. J. O'Donnell, M. D.
Platt W. Covington, M. D.
Arthur L. Wright, M. D.
Edward G. Altvater, M. D.
John G. Runkel, M. D.

SPRINGFIELD STATE HOSPITAL.[1]

Sykesville, Md.

In 1893 the members of the Medical and Chirurgical Faculty of Maryland were made to realize by their philanthropic president, Dr. George H. Rohé, then superintendent of the Maryland Hospital for the Insane at Catonsville, the most urgent need for the erection of a second hospital to accommodate the indigent insane. The committee that had been appointed by the Faculty's president to investigate the conditions stated in its report that over 1000 insane were confined and improperly cared for in the almshouses and jails of the counties.

In 1894 John Hubner, then State Senator from Baltimore County, became interested in the project and introduced a bill in the State Legislature at Annapolis for the establishment of an additional hospital for the insane of Maryland. This bill was quickly passed, was approved by Frank Brown, then Governor of Maryland, and $100,000 were appropriated for the purchase of a site and the erection of buildings and maintenance. During the same year the following Board of Managers was appointed by the Governor: Frank Brown, Governor; Spencer C. Jones, State Treasurer; Marion DeKalb Smith, State Comptroller; John Hubner, John Mitchell, Henry O. Devries, J. Oliver Wadlow, Richard McSherry and Edward Lloyd. On account of being appointed to other duties, Henry O. Devries resigned and his vacancy was filled by Wm. H. Forsythe.

Almost a year was spent by the Board of Managers in search of an appropriate site for the new institution, and finally the estate known as Springfield, a picturesque old farm of over 700 acres, situated near the town of Sykesville, in Carroll County, was thought to possess the most desirable features.

On January 15, 1896, the Board of Managers by formal resolution purchased the above farm for $50,000. Dr. George H. Rohé, who had been selected superintendent of the new institution, took charge of the property on April 11, 1896, and at once made preparation to receive patients at the earliest practicable date.

[1] Material for history furnished by Dr. J. Clement Clark, superintendent, and Dr. H. D. Purdum, assistant physician.

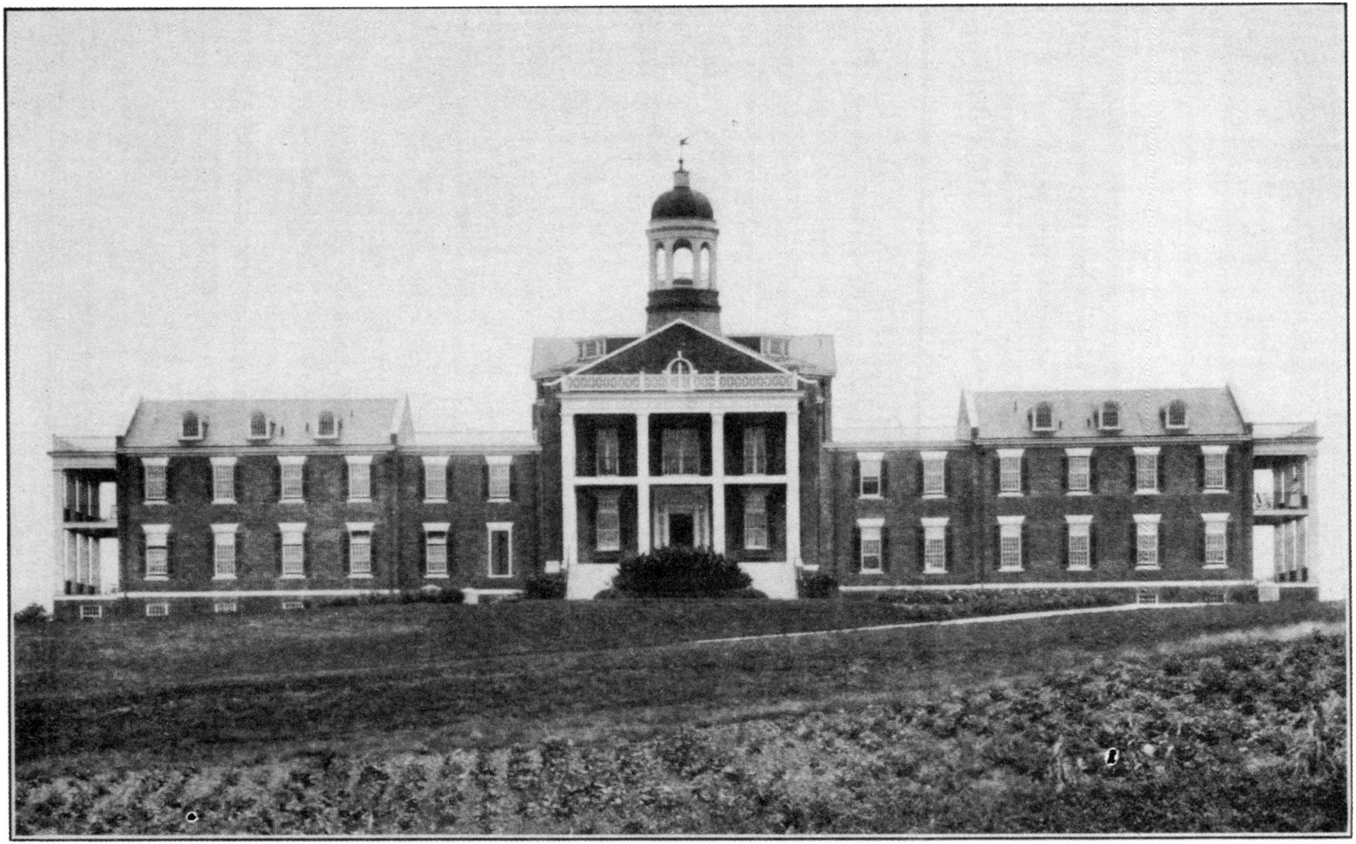

JOHN HUBNER PSYCHOPATHIC HOSPITAL.

The Board of Managers and the superintendent prepared and utilized several tenants' houses, already upon the place, for the temporary care of patients while the nucleus of the new hospital was under construction. On July 6, 1896, three months after the control of the property had been acquired, five patients were received from the Maryland Hospital for the Insane at Catonsville. During July 17 others were added and on the 16th of September one more was admitted, making a total of 23 under treatment at the close of the first fiscal year.

The plans for the new buildings called for a quadrangular group of detached cottages constructed of brick, one cottage to be used as a service building facing west and the others north, east and south respectively. While the patients were residing in the tenants' houses without barred windows or locked doors, awaiting the completion of the new buildings, they did so well that it prompted the superintendent and the Board of Managers to have the new cottages conpleted without barred windows or strong rooms and to adopt the open-door system.

On March 8, 1898, the first group of buildings was opened for occupancy; the population of the institution being at this time 98. After the patients had been removed into the new wards one of the farm houses, which had formerly been occupied and was in a fair state of preservation, was devoted to the care of 19 patients suffering from epileptic insanity.

Dr. Rohé died suddenly February 6, 1899, while in New Orleans, leaving the newly planned institution without a director. During his superintendency of three years he had assisted in selecting the location of the hospital and in formulating the plans for its construction.

The Board of Managers unanimously elected as superintendent Dr. J. Clement Clark, who had formerly been first assistant physician at the Maryland Hospital for the Insane at Catonsville.

During Dr. Rohé's administration no patient suffering from the acute forms of insanity was admitted, because it was thought that the open-door system would be impracticable for their care, but shortly after Dr. Clark was made superintendent he became of the opinion that this method of treatment could also be applied to acute cases as well. Upon the strength of this he received into the institution several such cases as a matter of experiment, and found that they responded admirably to the treatment.

The demand for admission to the institution became so great that in 1900 a group of buildings devoted to the care and treatment of both the chronic and acute female patients was erected and occupied. This group consisted of a service building and three cottages, constructed of brick and situated on an elevation three-quarters of a mile from the male group.

Owing to the isolation of the institution the superintendent was at a loss to know how to entertain the patients as well as the employees. Dances and other forms of amusement were provided, but did not fully meet the requirements, so in 1901 a dramatic club was organized and became a source of great pleasure to all. In 1902 Dr. Clark, having realized for some time that the mentally sick should be cared for by specially trained nurses, organized a training school. In the same year he also had music rendered in the general dining room of both groups during meal hours, and found it had a quieting effect upon the patients and prevented much loud talking and abuse. A baseball team was also organized, consisting of both male patients and attendants, and tennis courts were made for the women patients. During the same year a beautiful driveway, constructed of stone, connecting the two groups of buildings and extending as far as the entrance gate at the edge of the property, was completed. In building this driveway an immense amount of grading was necessary, all of which was done by the patients and a large stone and steel bridge built over the creek, which ran between the two groups of buildings.

In 1903, owing to the growing need for means of occupying the patients during the winter months, a new and up-to-date industrial building was completed. In this building brooms, shoes, clothing, mattresses, chairs, etc., are made. During the same year a new bakery, green-house and ice houses were built and long distance telephones installed in the offices of each group. In 1904, on account of the increasing number of patients, another cottage at the women's group was built, with a capacity of 85.

In 1905 all physicians within a convenient radius of the hospital were invited to attend the case readings and staff meetings at the hospital, with the idea of making them more familiar with the various types of insanity, so that they might introduce prophylactic measures to prevent its inception.

In the same year a new cottage was opened for male epileptics, with a capacity of 85 patients.

In 1906 a fifth cottage for women, a bungalow for 40 male consumptives and a general dining room and kitchen at the male group, with a capacity of over 600, were constructed and occupied.

In 1907 an extension was built from the main line of the Baltimore & Ohio Railroad to the institution for the hauling of coal, brick and merchandise, and during the same year an ice-plant was installed with a sufficient capacity to supply the institution during the hottest weather.

In 1911, owing to the large number of unoccupied chronic patients in the institution, a well-trained instructor was employed to stimulate their interest along industrial lines and to divert their thoughts from morbid channels into more wholesome ones. A large bright room in one of the new cottages, free from distracting influences, was set apart for this work. At first simple figure exercises, games and folk songs were employed and later basket making, embroidery, etc., were introduced. The results were so gratifying that early cases of dementia præcox were enrolled in the class and new features were added, such as afternoon tea parties, morning tramps through the woods and readings by different members of the class. Many patients who had formerly been idle and troublesome developed enough self-control to be employed in the general dining room, laundry and sewing room, and several cases of dementia præcox recovered sufficiently to return to their homes.

During 1912 a cottage for male patients, with a capacity of 200, and two cottages for female patients, with a capacity of 85 and 100 respectively, were completed and occupied. A large central power plant and laundry were also constructed in the same year at a cost of $75,000.

There are now 20 detached cottages, with 1425 patients, 7 physicians and 127 nurses and attendants. The last buildings erected are two isolation cottages for tuberculosis patients, each for 40 patients, and the John Hubner Psychopathic Reception Hospital. The erection of this hospital marks a definite era in the Maryland state hospital service. Through its agency a systematic and uniform scientific scheme of examination of all patients sent to the hospital has been established, developed and practically applied. Clinical inquiries into all factors to be considered in mental cases are now matters of daily routine. Careful records, properly indexed and classified, are kept of all patients, because such examinations and records have become valuable data in the study of many problems connected with the cure and prevention of insanity.

The problem of developing a plan which, without undue complication, would provide for the varied uses of this building was a perplexing one. It was necessary to care for both sexes, and it was highly desirable that the two departments, while entirely separate from one another, should be under one central control, and that the service to the various divisions be as simple as for a single ward. It was finally decided to adopt the shape of a Geneva cross, with the wards forming the four arms of the cross and the control at the crossing. This insured a complete separation of the principal divisions and gave a simple and highly centralized form of service and control. It had the further advantage of giving a maximum amount of exposure and ventilation to each division, and of assuring sunlight during some portion of the day in each of the wards, with ample sun porches for all, these porches being placed at each of the four terminals of the cross.

The basement contains dressing rooms, massage, hydriatic rooms and accessories, as well as the pharmacy, X-ray room, kitchen, pantries and storage rooms. By locating the first floor unusually high above ground it was possible to have large windows and, therefore, ample light in all portions of the basement.

The first floor is approached from the northern portico, and the north wing of this floor is given up to general admistrative purposes. Here one finds the waiting room, library, physicians' room, examining room and the offices of the administrative staff.

The three other wings of the first floor are practically duplicates of one another. As a person enters each of these wings from the central controlling octagon, he passes down a corridor, on either side of which are located the ward dining room, tub room and two private rooms, until the day room is reached. Communicating with each day room is a private room and a ward toilet; this latter also communicates with the main ward, which is beyond, and occupies the entire end of the wing. Each day room accommodates four beds, and each main ward cares for ten. Beyond the ward is a sun porch, a broad two-storied portico, very open in construction, and large enough to accommodate all the patients in the ward.

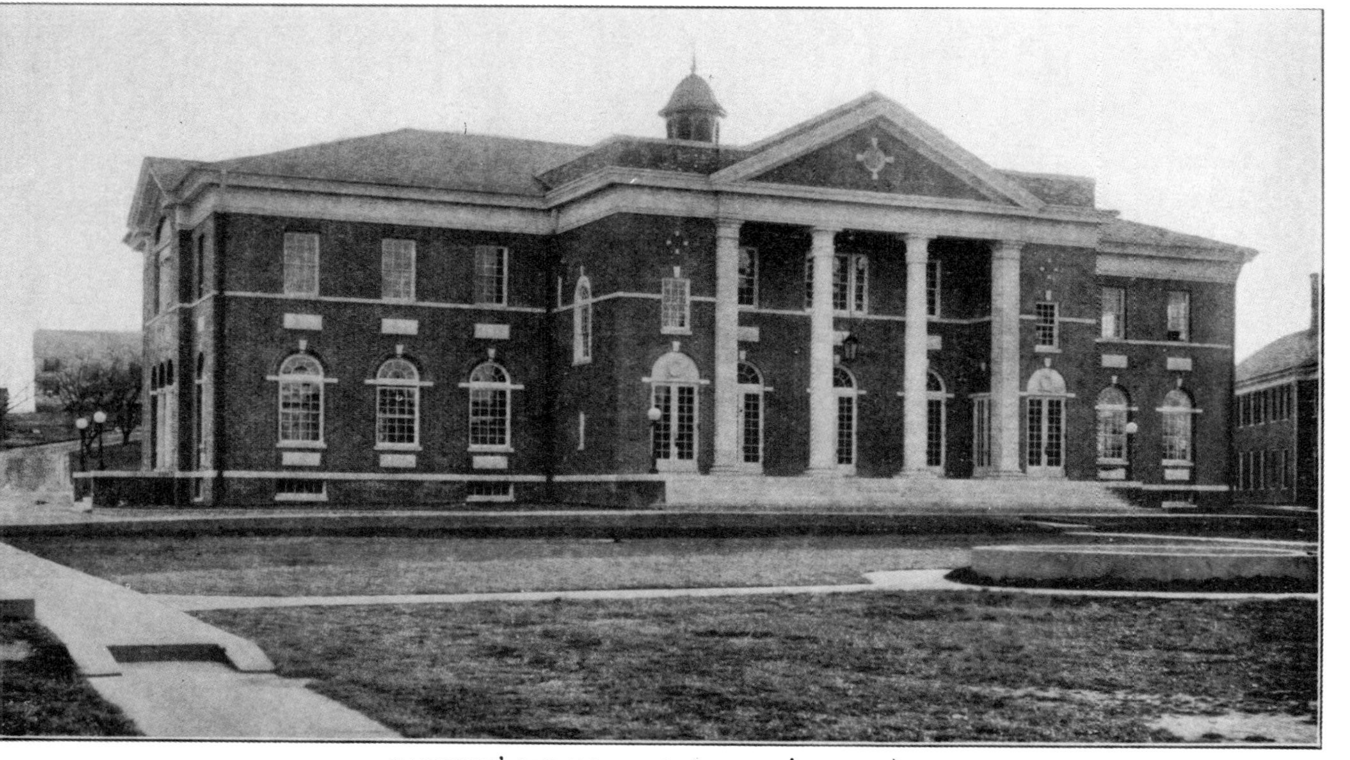

PATIENTS' DINING ROOM (WOMEN'S GROUP).

The second floor of the north wing contains quarters for the staff and the three other wings are duplicates of those on the first floor.

In the central octagon serving all these wings are the stairways, elevator and the diet kitchens. As all the corridors meet in the octagonal hall at the crossing it is possible for one person stationed at this point to have the entire building within immediate and positive control, he being in direct touch with the stairways, the elevator service and the hospital staff.

The third floor of the octagon continues up as a full story. Here the operating department is located, complete, with its elevator and stair service, anæsthetizing room, wash room, operating room, sterilizing room, recovery room, laboratory and surgeons' room. The attic space over the wings is not utilized; it performs a valuable service in protecting the second floor wards from undue heat during the summer months, and gives a fine well ventilated air space above these rooms.

The elevation of the building is of the Southern colonial type, very simple in design, and depending, for architectural effect, upon the refined and dignified treatment of wall surfaces, openings and porches rather than upon any meretricious elaboration of accents or ornaments. It occupies a commanding site on the hillside, midway between the men's and women's groups of the institution, and, with its fine mass and graceful surmounting cupola, forms a pleasing and satisfying addition to the general scheme.

The building is built of brick, each wing of which is 84⅓ feet long and 47½ feet wide, and it has a capacity of 75 beds.

BOARD OF MANAGERS.

Ex-Officio Members.

GOVERNORS.

Frank Brown	1894-1896	Austin L. Crothers......	1908-1912
Lloyd Lowndes	1896-1900	Phillips Lee Goldsborough	1912-1916
John Walter Smith......	1900-1904	Emerson C. Harrington.	1916-
Edwin Warfield	1904-1908		

TREASURERS.

Spencer C. Jones........	1894-1896	Murray Vandiver	1900-1916
Thomas J. Shryock......	1896-1900		

COMPTROLLERS.

Marion deKalb Smith...	1894-1896	Dr. Gordon T. Atkinson	1904-1908
Robert P. Graham......	1896-1898	Wm. B. Claggett........	1910-1911
Phillips Lee Goldsborough	1898-1900	Charles H. Stanley.....	1911-1912
Dr. Joshua W. Hering..	1900-1904 1908-1910	Emerson C. Harrington.	1912-1916

MEMBERS.

John Hubner	1894-	Charles Weber, Jr.	1896-1902
Henry O. Devries.......	1894-1894	Dr. Richard F. Gundry..	1898-1904
John H. Mitchell........	1894-1898	Frank Brown	1904-1910
William H. Forsythe...	1894-	C. Howard Lloyd.......	1907-1908
Richard M. McSherry...	1894-1895	Wm. S. Evans..........	1908-
J. Oliver Wadlow.......	1894-1912	C. Wilbur Miller........	1912-
Johnzie E. Beasman.....	1895-1896 1902-1914	W. Champ. Robinson....	1910-
Edward Lloyd	1896-1907	Thos. J. Shryock........	1914-

SUPERINTENDENTS.

Dr. George H. Rohé....	1896-1899	Dr. J. Clement Clark (in office)	1899-

RESIDENT PHYSICIANS.

Dr. Geo. H. Rohé, supt. (deceased).
Dr. J. Clement Clark, supt.[1]
Dr. John N. Morris.[1]
Dr. R. M. Bruns.
Dr. C. I. Hill.
Dr. Robert Reuling.
Dr. W. Henry Fisher.
Dr. J. A. Pfeiffer.
Dr. Vernon H. McKnight.
Dr. A. B. Eckerdt.
Dr. G. Ward Disbrow.
Dr. M. D. Smith.
Dr. J. W. Blackmer.
Dr. Louise D. Holmes.
Dr. Jessie M. Thornton.
Dr. Chas. J. Carey.
Dr. F. H. Brooks.
Dr. W. C. Stone.
Dr. Earl H. Snavely.
Dr. Aleck P. Harrison.
Dr. J. G. F. Smith.
Dr. H. D. Purdum.[1]
Dr. C. D. Hamilton.[1]
Dr. Henderson Irwin.
Dr. John L. Wethered.[1]
Dr. Hugh Clark.[1]
Dr. Mary Waters.
Dr. Maud M. Rees.[1]

[1] Present staff.

CROWNSVILLE STATE HOSPITAL.[1]

CROWNSVILLE, MD.

The hospital for the negro insane of Maryland, now known as the Crownsville State Hospital, was created by an act of the General Assembly on April 11, 1910, which made an appropriation of $100,000 for the purchase of land and the erection of buildings.

Sections of the act creating the hospital, Chapter 250, Laws of Maryland, 1910, provided that there should be established in the State of Maryland an institution for the detention and care of the negro insane of the state. It was expressly provided that the hospital should not be located in Baltimore City.

It was further provided that the Board of Managers of the hospital was to consist of the Governor, ex-officio; State Treasurer, Comptroller of the Treasury, and six other persons, to constitute a body corporate under the title of the "Hospital for the Negro Insane of Maryland," with the power to appoint the necessary officers and agents. The act named the following persons, who, together with the Governor, State Comptroller and State Treasurer, were to constitute the first Board of Managers of the hospital: Hugh H. Young and Thomas Parran, to serve from the date of the passage of the act until the first of May, 1912; John T. Daily and William L. Marbury, to serve until the first day of May, 1914; J. Harry Covington and Henry P. Mann, to serve until the first day of May, 1916.

It was provided that the Board of Managers should be divided into three classes, one-third of whom should go out of office every two years; and the Governor should have power, in case of any vacancy occurring, to appoint a person or persons to fill such vacancy or vacancies for the balance of term of said class.

It was further enacted by the General Assembly of Maryland "that the Board of Managers immediately proceed to the erection, construction and equipment of suitable buildings to care for such of the negro insane of the State of Maryland as may be sent to the said hospital from time to time, in accordance with the general provisions of the acts of the General Assembly of Maryland relative to the care and treatment of the insane of the state."

On December 13, 1910, the board by formal resolution pur-

[1] By Dr. Robert P. Winterode, superintendent.

chased the Boswell-Garrett-Hatch farm, located at Crownsville, Anne Arundel County, comprising 566 acres of land, with all improvements thereon, for the sum of $19,000. The title to the property having been examined by the Title Guarantee and Trust Company of Baltimore and found correct, the deed was transferred to the State of Maryland on May 22, 1911. The Board of Managers organizing on May 15, 1910, elected their respective officers and adopted by-laws.

At the meeting of the Board of Managers of May 23, 1910, Dr. Robert P. Winterode was appointed superintendent.

With the two-fold purpose in view of relieving the county homes of their charges at the earliest possible date, also of economizing in every way by utilizing the patients' labor to grade, cut poles and cross ties for the railway spur, excavate for the buildings, harvest the willow crop and commence the necessary farming operations, the idea of housing patients in temporary quarters suggested itself.

Active work was commenced immediately to convert the building formerly used as a willow plant into temporary quarters and prepare for the first transfer of patients.

After a month's work, everything being in readiness, the first allotment of 12 patients from Spring Grove State Hospital was received on March 13, 1911. The temporary character of the camp necessitated the reception of only quiet and good workers.

On March 18, 1911, four more were added, and on March 21, 1911, this number was increased to 21.

From this group three patients were selected to assist the cook and wait in dining rooms of patients and officers. Two were assigned to work with the farm manager. The remainder commenced harvesting the willow crop. Patients worked with vim and their enthusiasm increased in proportion to the results shown, and after six weeks the entire " holt " was cut, bundled and stripped for market.

The increasing demand for workers, combined with the excellent results so far obtained with the small colony, was sufficient to justify an increase in the population. The next quota of 16 patients was selected from Montevue Asylum at Frederick, and was transferred on July 21, 1911. These patients were assigned to work in the woods, cutting cross ties for the spur, also poles for the conveying of electric current for lighting the building.

As was to be expected, the work was crude and slow in the beginning, but with teaching, the type and quality of the work increased in efficiency until, when six weeks had elapsed, 750 cross ties were counted to their credit; also 20 poles, 35 feet long.

To accomplish this work required the felling of 200 or more trees and with inexperienced woodmen it was almost phenomenal that no accidents resulted. By this time the work on the farm had increased to such an extent as to occupy all of the labor and in order to assist in the excavating and construction of new buildings it was deemed expedient to increase the number. Accordingly on October 13, 1911, 32 patients were brought from Montevue Asylum, Frederick. This group included quite a number of epileptics and imbeciles of low grade; 80 per cent of the entire number had never been occupied. On October 21, 1911, two patients were transferred from Sylvan Retreat; on September 15, 1911, one patient was transferred from the county home in Talbot County; on June 2 another was transferred from Charles County. All these transfers were made without a single mishap.

The destruction of the construction camp by fire on the night of March 7, 1912, came at a time when the results of the first year's labor had just become apparent. To thus, in a few minutes, find themselves thrown back to the point of starting was a painful and discouraging experience to the officers of the hospital. The only available protection providing roof and shelter for the patients to be found was a mile and a half distant in barns, where, with meager facilities, the patients were made reasonably comfortable for the night. The buildings which afforded shelter for 10 days thereafter were shacks formerly used by the contractor while excavating for the foundation. With the necessary repairs, they were ready for occupancy in 24 hours.

Construction of more permanent quarters was commenced immediately, and at the expiration of 14 days the first dormitory was occupied. Meals were brought over from the shacks for a few days until the kitchen was cómpleted. In the absence of an immediate water supply, a temporary line of pipe was laid from the tank already constructed to supply water for building purposes.

This building, which has been converted into a farm colony, was the home of the patients during the construction of the first permanent building. A one-story layout comprised dormitories for quiet and disturbed cases, and there were separate rooms for isolation purposes, also dining rooms to accommodate 100 or more patients. Included in this building was a room fitted up with shower baths for patients, also clothes room and quarters for laundry help. The attendants occupied a separate building connected by a short passage-way. This included a dining room and bath and sleeping accommodations. The office, dining room and bedroom of the superintendent completed the layout.

As the demands for patients' labor on the new buildings were increasing daily and the present quarters had been taxed to their capacity, it was deemed advisable to add another dormitory to accommodate 50 additional patients.

On April 17, 1911, just one month and ten days after the fire, 19 men remaining at Spring Grove were transferred to the new hospital. On May 22, 18 Baltimore City patients were brought from Bay View. This number, on June 8, was increased by the transfer of 22 patients from Montevue. During the year new admissions were made from the counties, until the number under treatment at the close of the fiscal year 1912 reached 124. No more transfers were made until May 13, 1913, when 78 women and 18 men were brought from Montevue. The census of the population on September 30, 1913, was 255. Of this number 165 are men and 90 are women.

The first unit of the group, known as the Reception Building, on which work was commenced in October, 1912, was occupied on May 1, 1913. It consists of a central building of four stories and two wings with three stories, extending almost at right angles from the central portion. On the first floor are located hydrotherapy wards for both men and women. These sections, being equipped for prolonged baths, will afford modern facilities for treating patients. A large area of this space in each wing is occupied by the laundry, which is divided into two rooms, one being equipped for washing and the other for ironing. The washers, extractors and conveyor are operated by electricity with separate drum control, so that any one of them may be operated separately. The extractors are fitted with safety covers as a safeguard against accidents. The ironing is done by electric irons. Conduits for increased accommodations were also provided before laying the floor, so that additional facilities may be readily added. The remaining space of this floor is taken up with store rooms, dining rooms for both patients and attendants and heating plant. The second and third floors of the wings are devoted to day rooms and dormitories. The front of the first floor proper of the main building contains the administration offices, reception room for patients, clinical laboratory, pharmacy and offices for the staff. In the rear of this floor is a dining room for women, as well as a kitchen. The entire floor will be used for patients as soon as the central kitchen and administration buildings are completed, where accommodations for patients and officers have been provided. The second floor front of the main building is occupied by physicians. The two rooms in the rear are used temporarily for day room and sewing room. This entire space will later be converted into an infirmary. By these changes it will be possible to accommodate about 50 additional patients. The third floor of the central building is taken up with rooms for men and women nurses. The building is lighted by electricity and abundantly supplied with shower baths, toilets and washstands. The plumbing is modern in every detail.

The second building of the group, which is designated as the administration building, was completed in November, 1913. This building is of brick construction, three and one-half stories in height. On the first floor is a mortuary, post-mortem room, museum and storeroom. Offices of the staff and head nurse, laboratories, pharmacy, examination, reception and dining rooms for the officers occupy the first floor proper. Sleeping accommodations for the staff occupy the second floor. The third floor contains several rooms for employees.

Between the reception building and the administration building, and connected with both by covered corridors, is the third unit, known as the Central Kitchen Building. On the ground floor will be the bakery, storage rooms for flour, preparation rooms for vegetables, cold storage and two large industrial rooms. The first floor is taken up with a central kitchen, sculleries, separate dining rooms for attendants, also for men and women patients; the latter accommodating about 250 each. The second floor has two dormitories, each accommodating about 50 beds. The central portion of the building is utilized for a day room, also assembly hall for entertainments and religious services. The attic space is fitted up for sleeping quarters for help. The passage-ways connecting these buildings not only afford a means of easy access in unpleasant weather and at night, but, fully as important, serve as a cover for all pipes—heating and water supply—and conduits for electric wiring, which, in case of emergency, may be repaired without constantly digging and destroying property.

In the construction of buildings, operation of farm and preliminary construction work, patients' labor has been utilized in every possible way.

Work therapy, aside from a remunerative consideration, has proven a most valuable asset from a curative standpoint. Those patients capable of being developed along different lines have been trained in the industrial shop, where willow-craft work, rug weaving, lathe turning and broom making are carried on extensively.

The occupation of the women, though in different fields, has been given as much attention, with as encouraging results. All clothes worn by women, even the stockings, are made by them.

There is also excellent work done by the ward classes, such as rug making, knitting, crocheting, cross-stitch work and quilting.

The above does not include a large percentage of cases which are occupied in the laundry and general housework, and during the summer 30 or more work in the gardens.

The system of occupation has developed pari passu with the growth of the hospital.

BOARD OF MANAGERS.

The Governor, ex-officio.
State Treasurer, ex-officio.
Comptroller of the Treasury, ex-officio.

Harry. J. Hopkins.
William L. Marbury.
Henry P. Mann.
John T. Daily.
William P. Gundry.
Hugh H. Young, M. D.

SUPERINTENDENT.

Dr. Robert P. Winterode....................1910-in office

ASSISTANT PHYSICIANS.

Dr. A. M. Cross............................1913-1914
Dr. P. L. Keough...........................1913-1914
Dr. L. D. Barnes...........................1914-in office
Dr. Albert A. Nauman.......................1915-in office

PATHOLOGIST.

Dr. Nolan D. C. Lewis......................1915-in office

EASTERN SHORE STATE HOSPITAL.[1]

CAMBRIDGE, MD.

The Eastern Shore State Hospital for the Insane, located at Cambridge, Md., was authorized in the bond issue bill passed by the General Assembly of 1912. The Board of Managers, as given, was mentioned in the bill. The board at its first meeting elected Governor Goldsborough as president, J. Hooper Bosley, as secretary and treasurer, and Dr. Charles J. Carey, formerly assistant physician at the Springfield State Hospital, as the superintendent. The first duty of the board was to select a location. A committee consisting of the Governor, Comptroller and Senator Bosley visited numerous sites which had been proposed and finally recommended to the board one of three desirable farms in the immediate vicinity of Cambridge. The entire Board of Managers with the Lunacy Commission visited these farms and finally decided upon the Kirwan estate, located about a mile from Cambridge, on the banks of the beautiful Choptank River. This farm consists of about 250 acres, a part of which is wooded, the remainder being first-class farm land.

The board at its next meeting decided to have an architectural competition for plans for the building. Mr. Marshall, of the firm of Hornblower & Marshall, of Washington, D. C., was selected as the consulting architect. The rules of the American Institute of Architects governing such a competition were adopted, and, after the necessary forms were completed, six architects were invited to take part in the competition. A jury consisting of Dr. Hugh H. Young, president of the Lunacy Commission, and Messrs. M. B. Medary, Jr., and E. A. Crane, two well-known architects of Philadelphia, were asked to serve. The drawings were submitted sealed and opened in the presence of the jury; each set of drawings having a number and, accompanying the drawings, a sealed envelope with the number on the outside and the name of the firm on the inside, so that no member of the jury would know the name of the architect in the competition. After the drawings had been carefully studied by the jury and the awards made the jury submitted a statement in writing to the Board of Managers.

[1] Taken from the 28th report of the State Lunacy Commission.

At a later meeting the envelopes containing the names of the contestants were opened. The name of the successful architect was found to be the firm of Parker, Thomas & Rice, to whom the award was given. This firm immediately began the preparation of the working plans for the building; contracts were awarded and ground broken in November, 1913. Dr. Carey assumed his duties in July, and on December 11, 1913, 24 patients, who were from the Eastern Shore of Maryland, were transferred from Springfield State Hospital to the Eastern Shore State Hospital.

The two cottages on the property have been repaired and put in good condition. Sanitary plumbing and new heating equipment have also been installed, thus affording accommodations for the 24 patients, the superintendent and nurses.

Contracts were let for the buildings September, 1913, and building operations progressed steadily until the completion of the mess hall buildings, the laundry and the power house in March, 1915. The institution when fully completed will consist of 11 buildings, two mess hall buildings, six dormitories or cottages, a laundry building, power house, administration building and superintendent's house. The mess hall buildings are adjoining the kitchen building, with which they are connected by corridors, and contain serving rooms and three dining rooms. The kitchen, a detached building, is in the center between the two mess halls. The second stories of the mess halls contain, in addition to rooms for nurses and hospital employees, four large amusement or day rooms for patients, which in the present unfinished condition of the building are used as dormitories. The building is heated throughout by the hot-water expansion system, where the water is heated by the exhaust and live steam from the power plant through a system of converters or hot-water generators, the exhaust or waste steam being sufficient to heat the building except in very cold weather, when live steam must be added.

The kitchen is thoroughly modern in every respect. There is also an ice plant, of a capacity of two tons of ice per day, adjoining the kitchen; also a bakery and laundry. The power house is supplied with two large Edgemoor water-tube boilers, and the engine house has large electrical generators. The water supply is obtained from an 8-inch artesian well sunk to a depth of 415 feet, which supplies 180 gallons of water per minute. The mess halls are constructed of rough brick with tooled joints and are trimmed with Indiana sandstone. The second story is finished in stucco, with old English timber effect. The roof is of slate. The windows are protected with steel guards, the panels of which conform to the sizes of the lights and the sashes and are filled with copper wire screens. All floors throughout the building are of reinforced concrete. The finished floors of the first story are of Welsh tiles; the finished floors of the second story of Georgia pine. All interior walls throughout the building are finished with soft-glazed bricks of a brownish-gray color. All partitions are built from gypsum and plaster. The floors of the bathrooms, toilet rooms and laboratories are laid with terrazzo. Fire protection is provided by one Worthington fire pump of 500 gallons capacity per minute, the water supply being taken from a creek back of the power house. At present one of the dining room wings of the mess hall is fitted up for temporary offices.

On May 18, 1915, 203 patients, whose residence was upon the Eastern Shore of Maryland, were transferred from the different state hospitals.

BOARD OF MANAGERS.

Governor Phillips Lee Goldsborough..........1912-1916
Comptroller of Treasury E. C. Harrington......1912-1916
State Treasurer Murray Vandiver.............1912-1916
E. E. Goslin, of Caroline County[1].............1912-1916
Senator W. W. Beck, of Kent County..........1912-1916
Senator John F. Harper, of Queen Anne's Co....1912-1914
R. S. Dodson, of Talbot County...............1912-1914
Senator Jesse D. Price, of Wicomico County....1912-1918
Senator Louis W. Milbourne, of Somerset Co...1912-1914
John P. Moore, of Worcester County..........1912-1916
William T. Warburton, of Cecil County.........1912-1918
J. Hooper Bosley, of Dorchester County........1912-1918
Chas. F. Rich, of Queen Anne's County.........1914-
Frank Ross, of Talbot County................1914-
Robert Messenger, of Caroline County..........1914-

SUPERINTENDENT.

Dr. Charles J. Carey.

ASSISTANT PHYSICIAN.

Dr. Stacy T. Noland.

---

[1] Deceased.

MOUNT HOPE RETREAT.

Baltimore, Md.

In 1840 the Sisters of Charity, because of some dissatisfaction on the part of the Board of Directors, severed their connection with the Maryland Hospital, then situated upon North Broadway, Baltimore, where for several years they had been in charge of the insane inmates and where they had been eminently successful.

That they had the confidence of the patients and their friends was soon strikingly made manifest, for at the urgent solicitation of the parties most interested, the Sisters were induced to procure a home of their own, and 17 patients were at once placed in their care.

At first a small two-story brick house on Front Street, near Fayette, adjoining St. Vincent's Church, was obtained and Dr. Durkee was duly installed as medical attendant. This building soon proved insufficient and the Sisters were forced to seek more commodious accommodations. They finally purchased a lot improved by a frame building on the Harford Road, a short distance from the city limits, and called it Mount St. Vincent. This was arranged for the accommodation of patients, and the Sisters devoted themselves with renewed zeal and constantly increasing success to the good work they had undertaken. In 1842 Dr. William H. Stokes was invited to assume the medical charge of the new institution and his untiring energy, devotion and fidelity contributed greatly to its advancement and success. With the rapid growth of the institution, Mt. St. Vincent soon became overcrowded with patients, and the Sisters were compelled a second time to seek more ample quarters in order to meet the demand of those who appreciated their kindly care and attention.

In April, 1844, Mt. Hope College, situated in the vicinity of what is now North Avenue, Laurens, Park and Bolton streets, was purchased with its ample grounds from Mr. Treadwell by Rev. L. Deluol, who was then Superior of the order. On taking possession of this property the Sisters changed its name to Mt. Hope Institution. As it had been built as a college, it was found admirably adapted to the care of patients and the rooms and dormitories were very desirable. Several springs on the property afforded an ample supply of water, which was forced into the house by hydraulic rams.

After being repaired and enlarged this building, with its beautiful surroundings, situated at a convenient distance from the city, for many years formed a prominent feature among the institutions of Baltimore; its reputation soon became national, patients being received from all sections of the country. From time to time the structure was enlarged and extended to accommodate the unexpected influx of patients. The whole interior was remodelled, and all arrangements were made and appliances were introduced which the humane spirit of the age deemed essential for the successful treatment of mental disease.

But it was not to rest here. Within a few years Mt. Hope in its turn became crowded, and this fact, together with the extension of streets and the rapid encroachment of the city on the privacy of patients, necessitated another removal. After an examination of numerous sites, it was decided to purchase the property on the Reisterstown Road, extending back to the Liberty Road, known as the Meredith Tract. This location, about one mile from the present city limits, possessed many advantages.

The new hospital was designed by Long & Powell, architects, under the direction of Rev. F. Burlando, then Superior of the Sisters of Charity. The foundation stone was laid by him on July 2, 1859. The first wing was completed in 1860, and on the 8th of July four Sisters took possession of it; their number was soon increased to 12, and the patients were removed from Mt. Hope Institution as fast as accommodations could be provided. The new home was known henceforth as Mt. Hope Retreat and under this title was incorporated in March, 1870.

The site selected is upon a knoll 40 feet above the main road and about a quarter of a mile distant from it, being about 550 feet above tide water, and embraces 375 acres. The front of the building faces the southeast and the view from this presents a bold, undulating slope through orchards, meadows and fields to a brook which winds through the low lands, emerging at the extreme southern border of the grounds, about a mile distant. The main entrance is approached by a gateway of granite and iron through an avenue of trees and shrubbery, passing in front of the east wing.

The hospital consists of a main building and four extensive wings. The former is five stories high, with an attic surmounted by a dome 160 feet from the ground, which affords a magnificent view of the city, the bay and the surrounding country. In the center or main building are located the reception rooms, the parlor, the billiard room, the Sisters' apartments, chapel, special private rooms, the dormitories for patients and the sewing rooms. The wings are appropriated to the exclusive use of patients. There are numerous out-buildings, among which are the doctor's cottage on the north, a handsome two-story brick gate house, two large pavilions on the west, the laundry, the work-shop and the ice and engine house; while on the farm are stone cottages occupied by the manager, the gardener, the engineer, the watchman and others employed on the place. All told, nearly 1000 souls represent the modest family which 52 years ago formed the nucleus of Mt. Hope Retreat. To the southeast, about three-quarters of a mile from the main building, is a lake. In close proximity to this lake are picnic grounds on which stands another cottage fitted up as a kitchen for picnic parties, where may be prepared lunch or dinner as may be desired for the patients who frequently pass whole days on these grounds, and thus secure a desirable and delightful change from the monotony of "asylum" life.

The records show that 10,587 patients were treated between the opening of the modest asylum on Front Street in 1840 and 1892. The professional care of the inmates was for 45 years under the direction of Dr. Wm. H. Stokes, an able and beloved physician. In 1872 he called to his assistance Dr. I. D. Thompson, who zealously served in this capacity until his failing health compelled him to resign in 1881, when Dr. Charles G. Hill was selected to take his place. In 1888 Dr. Stokes resigned and Dr. Charles G. Hill was made his successor. Dr. Richard McSherry was appointed assistant physician and filled the position for a year. Dr. W. P. E. Wyse was appointed in his place, and served until he resigned to engage in private practice in 1891. Dr. F. J. Flannery, who in 1881 had been appointed second assistant physician, became first assistant physician, which position he still fills.

The annual report for the year 1892, while recorded as the 50th, was in reality for the 52d year of continuous existence. Since then there has been issued, each year, an annual report.

Dr. William H. Stokes, for 45 years the chief physician of the institution, died during the year 1893 at the age of 84 years. In 1888, by reason of the infirmities due to his long service and advanced age, he had been compelled to resign as chief physician. It was Dr. W. H. Stokes who, having seen the employment of non-restraint methods under the famous Connolly and other alienists of Europe, introduced them into Mt. Hope Retreat.

A new wing was added to the institution this year, its dimensions being 58 by 78 feet, three stories high, with a one-story wing containing the bakery, 25 by 40 feet, and a covered passage to the ice-house. This building contains a large kitchen, Sisters' dining room, serving room, linen room and elevators from the kitchen and cellar. The third floor, 55 by 58 feet in the clear, is devoted to the amusement and entertainment of the patients, there being an ample stage, well provided with movable scenery, and two dressing rooms.

In 1894 a new barn was added to the already extensive outbuildings of the Retreat and the facility of supplying fresh milk and cream for the use of the patients was enhanced. The new entertainment hall afforded not only the means for giving numerous theatricals, concerts, lectures, and dances, but also a suitable place for large classes of calisthenics, Swedish movement exercises, etc. While this new hall is of advantage at all times, it is indispensable during the long winter months when the patients are unable to get out of doors. The physical exercises and massage afforded form a valuable adjunct to the treatment.

The mortality for the year 1893 was 49, a very small percentage, the deaths recorded occurring principally among the old patients.

The training school for nurses reached its fourth year in 1895. During the year the classes were given weekly lectures by Drs. Hill and Flannery, at the same time they continued their courses under competent teachers who drilled them in bedside notes, the preparation of clinical charts and the chemical composition and preparation of foods. Hygienic laws were examined, together with the method and purposes of disinfection. All the nursing staff attended the lectures by the physicians and only graduates were exempted from the recitations.

Several important improvements were completed during the year. By increasing the steam power and enlarging the pipe capacity the storage reservoir is now amply supplied from the waters of an artificial lake, and the water supply is absolutely independent and unstinted. From this lake the winter harvest of ice is gathered and capacious storage houses are filled. The entire building was wired and electric lights installed, doing away with gas and other antiquated methods of lighting.

A new clinical laboratory, replete with every facility and appliance that science has devised for the investigation and diagnosis of disease, was built and equipped and is now in successful operation under the direction of a competent pathologist. By the aid of centrifuge and hæmatocrit, together with other mechanical and chemical adjuncts, examinations of blood, sputum, urine, stomach contents, etc., can now be made without delay and the diagnosis and treatment facilitated. This laboratory is not designed so much for investigation of diseased conditions found on postmortem examinations, as for the functional and organic disturbances of the living subject.

The report of the year 1896 shows a great increase in the population over previous years. The usual number per month averaged about 600. Owing to the success of the laboratory methods of treatment, a greater number of cures were effected and the discharges increased. The improvements made during this year were principally the completion of the new toilet rooms.

The laboratory has proved of great assistance, both in making the diagnosis and in suggesting the proper methods of treatment. Each new patient on entering is subjected to a thorough test as to the various secretions. A 24-hour analysis of the urine is made; blood is examined and the contents of the stomach, after the usual test meals, are likewise the subject of inspection and analysis.

During the year 1898 the laboratory was enlarged and many new instruments and appliances for diagnosis added.

Being chartered as a general hospital as well as an institution for the insane, many apply for treatment who are not confessedly insane, but suffering from some form of nervous or general disease or the drug habit, as well as a considerable number of inebriates who come and go as they feel the need of the protection and care of the institution. These, of course, are not under certificate, nor classified as insane, and come voluntarily.

Attention has been given of late to the possibilities and advantages of the cottage plan of housing and caring for the insane. Mt. Hope has this system practically under one roof, as there are 17 halls, each separate and distinct from the rest, governed by two Sisters and nurses and attendants. This subdivision allows each hall or family to maintain its own identity. The Sisters of Charity have entire control and charge of the institution and the physicians are not burdened with any clerical or administrative duties, and devote their entire attention to the examination and treatment of the patients.

The most important improvement during the year 1905 was the installation of a refrigerating plant and ice-making machine. The ice machine has a capacity of 500 pounds daily and the refrigerating plant takes care of the kitchen, bakery and storage rooms.

In 1906 the large parlors and waiting rooms were subdivided into smaller and more convenient rooms. This subdivision was forced upon the management by reason of the large and steady increase of patients seeking admission who wanted, when possible, the privacy of their own rooms.

In view of the fact that a certificate of graduation is required in many hospitals in this and other states, the usual course of lectures and instructions in the school for nurses was at this time made more systematic, and hereafter such as have completed their course and passed a satisfactory examination will be granted certificates setting forth their proficiency and graduation.

In 1907 a large amusement hall, with a capacity for seating 600, and with a well-equipped stage, was provided. Numerous plays have been given by the inmates as well as by outside talent. Two theatrical companies were organized, one from the women and the other from the men patients, who by constant drill and practice attained a surprising facility for the production of comedies and operas.

In 1908 the full equipment for making the Wassermann test was established.

During this year Sister Catharine, the beloved Sister Superior, who for 42 years had guided Mt. Hope, died. Sister Catharine left the hospital of the army in 1862 and returned to Mt. Hope. In 1867 she was made Superioress. During her administration

Mt. Hope grew from the one wing that was then completed to the magnificent building that stands to-day. Her successor was Sister M. Magdalene, who after years spent as a nurse both in old and new Mt. Hope was sent to St. Louis to take charge of old St. Vincent's. She remained there 19 years and during that time built the new St. Vincent's Retreat at Normand, a suburb of St. Louis, finally coming back to the scene of her early labors.

In 1911 the new chapel was built, it being a four-story brick building, the second and third stories being devoted to chapel purposes, and the first and fourth stories to new dining and sleeping quarters. The old chapel was converted into large dormitories. Large concrete and iron porches and fire escapes have been added to each wing, affording open air exercises to many patients who are unable to go to the grounds.

In 1912 a much-needed elevator of the most recent and improved design was installed. A new central power plant completed in 1913 consists of a boiler room 42 by 42 feet, with a height of 25 feet, equipped with three modern boilers of 150 horse power each, with sufficient space for the installation of a fourth boiler. There is a smokestack 125 feet high by 5 feet in diameter, a fuel bunker 22 by 43 feet, with a capacity of 300 tons of coal, and a pump room 10 by 36 feet, with modern pumps and duplicates of each, including feed-water heaters. The engine room is equipped with one direct-connected 50 kilowatt generator with proper switch-board and connections for supplying the entire building with light and power. The new cold storage, ice-making and brine room department is 19 by 34 feet, with a storage battery room of the same dimensions on the second floor. There is also a work-shop in this building. This structure has brick walls, reinforced concrete floor, stair and roof construction, finished floors of vitrified brick, cement and cement tile, the roof finished of slate and slag, and doors and windows of wood.

This plant is manufacturing electricity for lighting and power work, high pressure steam for kitchen and laundry purposes, hot water for the entire building, and brine for cold storage rooms and ice-making, in addition to heating the entire institution, including laundry and rooms for employees detached from the building proper.

In order to properly connect this power house with the institution it was found necessary to construct three tunnels, each 6 feet wide by 8 feet high, one of which is 50 feet, another 60 feet, and a third 200 feet long. These tunnels, in addition to their convenience for passage to and fro, carry the pipes for hot water supplies, high pressure steam supplies and returns, brine supplies, electric lines and heating mains and returns. The tops of the tunnels are covered with concrete slabs, reinforced, forming a pavement for outside travel in good weather.

The laundry building was also completely remodeled, the floor of the wash-room proper being built of reinforced concrete. The laundry has been equipped with three direct-connected washing machines, two direct-connected extractors, one starch cooker, one dry room tumbler, one continuous rapid dry room, one large mangle and 12 electric irons and boards, all of the latest and most modern types.

The number of patients remaining in Mt. Hope Retreat October 31, 1913, was: males, 264; females, 397; total, 661.

OFFICERS AND MEDICAL STAFF, JANUARY 1, 1914.

Sister M. Magdalene .... Sister superior.
Dr. Charles G. Hill .... Physician-in-chief.
Dr. Frank J. Flannery .... Resident physician.
Dr. C. B. Ensor .... Pathologist.

THE SHEPPARD AND ENOCH PRATT HOSPITAL.[1]

(FORMERLY THE SHEPPARD ASYLUM.)

TOWSON, MD.

Some time prior to the year 1853 Moses Sheppard, a member of the Society of Friends and long known as a successful merchant of Baltimore, made a will with the purpose in mind of endowing a hospital or asylum for the insane, to be established after his death.

Having informed his friend, Mr. David M. Perine, for many years registrar of wills of Baltimore, of his act, he was told by him that his will would be invalid as there would be no person or body corporate in existence at the time of his death to receive the property thus devised and to carry out the provisions of the will.

Upon the advice therefore of Mr. Perine a charter was drawn incorporating the trustees of the Sheppard Asylum. A bill was introduced into the Legislature of Maryland granting this charter, which was passed in May, 1853. In a letter dated May 20, 1853, to Mr. Philip Poultney, at Annapolis, Mr. Sheppard says: "The charter which I mention will be presented by a son of David M. Perine. As we only ask sanction to spend our own money to mitigate the suffering of the forlorn and wretched, I suppose there can be no objection to giving us the privilege to do so. It is very desirable that it pass at this session."

This is the first reference to his plans to establish a hospital for the insane which can be found in the correspondence of Moses Sheppard, with the exception of a brief allusion to the project in a letter to Dr. Nathan Shoemaker, dated March 19, 1853.[2]

[1] By Dr. E. N. Brush, superintendent.

19. 3 mo. 53.

[2] DR. SHOEMAKER: Thy letter of 2nd mo., 20th, was received and ought to have been answered sooner.—my fall has disturbed my nerves, and writing occasions a cramp in my hand. I also have a letter from Franklin, to which I have not responded, owing to the cause I have mentioned. Thee remarks that thee is afflicted with the Bronchitis;—we hear of old friends with new faces; and this I suppose is an old disease, with a new name. I have observed that the regular clergy are more subject to this disease, than any other class of public speakers. I have not heard of a Lawyer suffering from it. We have a new member in our gallery; whose exhortations are frequent and earnest; she generally speaks twice in a session, and speaks "as

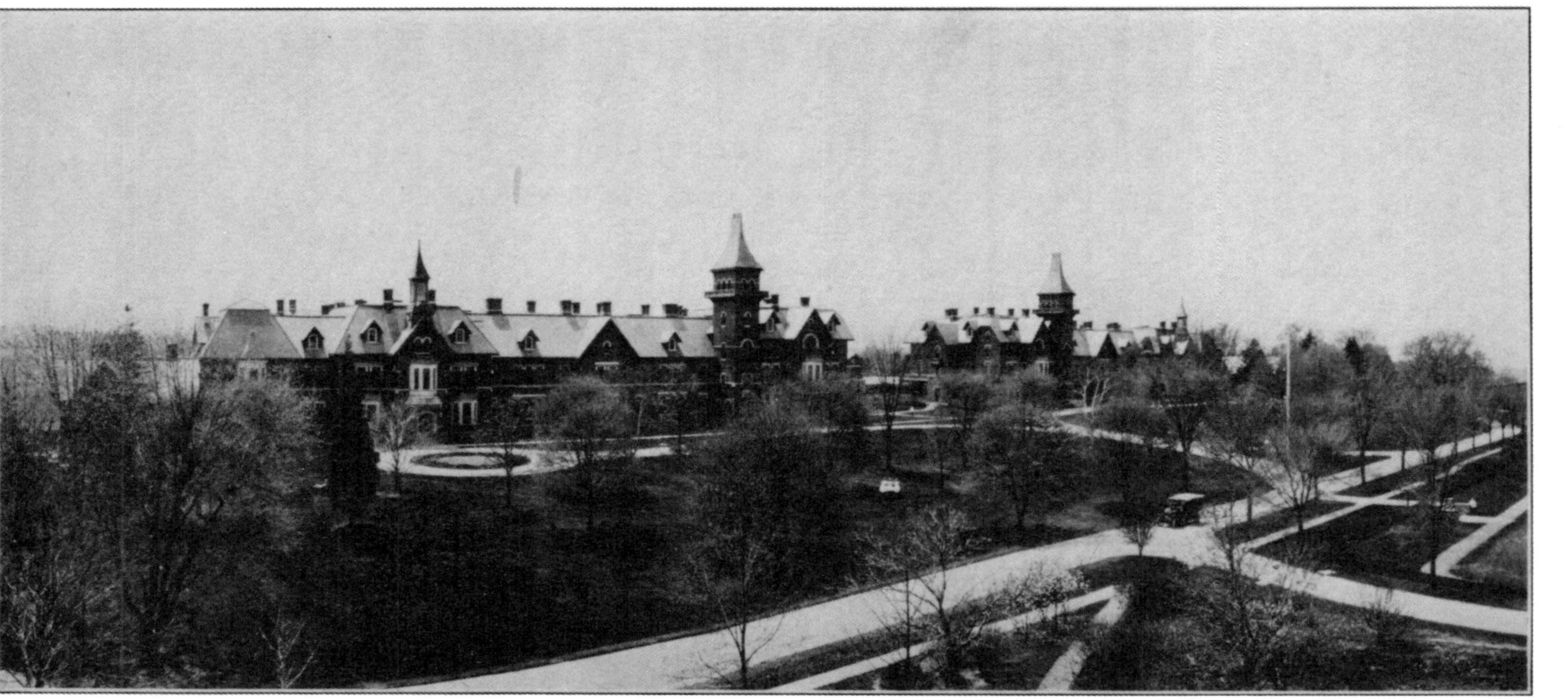

GENERAL VIEW, SHEPPARD AND ENOCH PRATT HOSPITAL, TOWSON.

The names of the first trustees as included in the bill granting the charter were Moses Sheppard, David M. Perine, William Riley, M. D., Archibald Stirling, Charles Howard, William M. Medcalf and Richard H. Townsend. The six gentlemen named in association with him were all chosen by Moses Sheppard, and he did not hesitate when, for reasons which are not disclosed in his correspondence, he desired to make changes in the personnel of the board to ask for the resignation of some members of the original board, the remaining members, in accordance with powers granted in the charter, filling the vacancies thus created, doubtless at Mr. Sheppard's suggestion.

No sooner were Moses Sheppard's benevolent intentions made public than he began to receive letters of advice and congratulation, as well as letters soliciting aid or contributions to various charitable institutions. A letter of congratulation from Dr. John M. Galt, medical superintendent Eastern Lunatic Asylum, Williamsburg, Va., is here reproduced in facsimile. See p. 560.

The first meeting of the board was held in Baltimore on June 23, 1853, at which time Moses Sheppard produced a copy of the charter incorporating the gentlemen named above as the trustees of the Sheppard Asylum.

Section second of the charter says: "The object and design of said corporation is hereby declared to be the founding and maintaining an asylum for the insane; the entire management of which shall be vested in the said trustees." At this meeting Moses Sheppard was elected president of the board and Richard H. Townsend, secretary. All of the trustees were present and each member of the board signed the minutes.

Meetings were held at various times to comply with the requirements of the charter, but there was no business to transact. The

---

one having authority, and not as a scribe." She visited ——— ———, and he has been much more depressed, since.—There is a strong movement here, to complete a juvenile house of reformation, and erect two Hospitals for the insane; one for white and one for black patients. My attention has long been directed to the case of the insane;—and I expect what I may leave, will take that direction, and not to individuals. It has been stated in England, that more of the Society of Friends become insane, in proportion, than of any other Society or class.—I don't know if it is so or not; but there are several here; and more of us half-crazy. I notice thy remarks on the future world, and coming judgment.—whatever was the original design of the creating power must and will be accomplished.

meeting held July 3, 1856, was the last session of the board attended by Moses Sheppard.

At a meeting held December 22, 1856, the following communication was received:

To the Trustees of the Sheppard Asylum.

GENTLEMEN: Please receive and accept my resignation of the presidency of the Board of Trustees of the Sheppard Asylum.

Respectfully,

BALTIMORE, 11 DECEMBER, 1856. MOSES SHEPPARD.

P. S.—I would respectfully suggest John Saurin Norris being placed in the situation I vacate.

The resignation of Mr. Sheppard was accepted and Mr. Norris, who had been elected a member of the board on July 2, 1856, was elected president.

At a meeting of the trustees held on February 21, 1857, the president announced the death of Moses Sheppard, which took place on February 1, 1857, in his 84th year.

Suitable resolutions were adopted and spread upon the minutes commemorative of the founder of the hospital and the appreciation of the trustees of his charitable intentions.

At a meeting of the trustees held April 22, 1858, an inventory of the estate of Moses Sheppard was presented, which showed the estate to amount at that time to $571,440.41, which at that period was a large sum of money, and a larger bequest than had ever been made to the care of the insane. At this meeting an advertisement for land was ordered and on June 3, 1858, the selection of a farm known as Mt. Airy, seven miles north of Baltimore, was confirmed and its purchase ordered. This farm lay between what is now known as the York Road on the east and a road which was an extension of Charles Street in Baltimore on the west, but there was no right of way to the Charles Street extension and accordingly on November 8, 1858, the purchase of additional land not to exceed 25 acres was ordered to obtain this right of way. With this additional land and a small purchase subsequently made the estate comprised a little over 375 acres.

On May 2, 1859, the president of the board was authorized to engage persons to make brick for the future buildings, suitable clay having been found on the farm.

A resolution was adopted at the meeting of the board on June 9, 1859, offering prizes of $300, $200 and $100 respectively for the

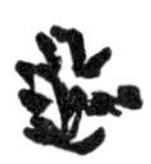

Williamsburg
Virginia
June 1st 1853

Dear Sir,

The accompanying Productions, — (the result of leisure moments, during my supervision of the Eastern Asylum, —) I take the liberty of sending, because I suppose that the subject of Insanity, possesses an interest with One, to whose expansive Benevolence, the most hapless of the Human race, are so deeply indebted.

There is no Temple raised to the Worship of The Most High, more pleasing in His sight, than an Asylum for these, His suffering Children:— and from this Refuge, as from a Holy Altar, the blessings of those "that are ready to perish", will ascend, and be received, with That Righteous Deed, into the Temple not made with hands, Eternal in the Heavens.

John M. Galt.

Moses Sheppard Esq.

first, second and third choice of plans to be presented for the buildings.

It was specified that the buildings were to accommodate 200 patients. There were to be a central building and two wings, to be of fireproof construction, warmed by flues and ventilated in the most perfect and complete manner; "*particular attention to be given to providing ample and suitable apartments, either within or without the principal structure, for exercise and employment of the patients in such occupation and amusements as may be conducive to their benefit.*"

Emphasis is placed upon this last direction in view of the awakening interest in exercise and diversional occupation which has been shown in many institutions within the last decade.

The trustees notified the competing architects that regard was to be had to durability, safety and utility rather than mere architectural display, and resolved that "while the trustees are not insensible to the deleterious effects produced upon patients by heavy, gloomy and unsightly structures, they will object to a redundancy of ornament on the one hand or a severe prison-like appearance on the other."

Moses Sheppard's wish was for buildings for "use, not for show," fireproof as far as possible.

The prizes for plans were awarded in the following order to Thomas and James Dixon, of Baltimore; to Samuel Sloan, of Philadelphia, and to Richard Upjohn & Co., of New York, in conjunction with Dr. D. Tilden Brown, medical superintendent of Bloomingdale Asylum. While the third prize was awarded to plans made under the advice of Dr. Brown, as will be subsequently seen, these formed the nucleus of the plans which, developed by Mr. Calvert Vaux, a well-known architect of New York, were finally adopted.

The plans awarded the first and second prizes, if drawings now in existence are any indication of their character, did not far depart from "a severe prison-like appearance."

In December, 1859, it was resolved to lay out a road to Charles Street and that appropriate trees and shrubbery be planted on the line of the roads. This very wise provision, which was carried out under the direction of Mr. J. Saurin Norris, who also saw that trees were planted generally about those portions of the estate subsequently to be used for building sites and recreation grounds, had provided when the buildings were finished, well-matured and suitably placed shade trees and ornamental shrubs which added materially to the appearance of the estate and have been a continuing source of pleasure to all.

No plans having been definitely accepted, on October 23, 1860, David M. Perine and William H. Graham were appointed, in conjunction with the president of the board, a Committee on Plans. On November 21, 1861, this committee reported in favor of plans suggested by Dr. D. Tilden Brown and drawn by Mr. Calvert Vaux. In December of the same year the president of the board was authorized to employ Mr. Vaux as architect and at the annual meeting on May 5, 1862, he reported his employment. At the same meeting an appropriation was made to pay the expenses of Dr. D. Tilden Brown to Europe for the purpose of "procuring information respecting the construction, equipment and organization" of institutions for the insane, that it might be availed of in preparing the asylum for its future uses and in subsequently administering the trust.

Dr. Brown made a report under date of April 30, 1863, which was presented at the annual meeting of the board in May of that year.[1]

On May 25, 1862, building operations were commenced and, with some delays incident to the difficulties of procuring iron beams because of the Civil War, the building was erected as fast as income available would permit.

This is not the place nor would it be of any profit to discuss the wisdom of the method suggested by Mr. Sheppard and pursued by the trustees, that is, building as fast as the income accumulated, rather than delaying operations until a sufficient income had accumulated to rapidly complete the buildings. One thing is evident: the slow method has resulted in structures which are remarkably well built, which show no evidences of insecure foundations or hastily built walls, and which, after 24 years of use, are in a state of excellent preservation, without being subject in that time to any extraordinary repair or renewal.

[1] Dr. Brown's report in full was published in The American Journal of Insanity, Vol. XX, October, 1863, p. 200.

The floors rest upon brick arches supported upon iron beams. The flooring is of Georgia pine, bought and placed under shelter for many months before being laid, resulting in tight joints throughout. The wood work, doors, window frames, etc., are of selected white pine treated in the same way.

The excellent character of the construction work in the buildings out of the material used is largely due to the persistent attention to details and the oversight exercised by J. Saurin Norris, president of the board from 1856 to 1882.

The hospital is composed of two buildings alike in plan and structure, extending upon an east and west axis and separated from each other by a space of 100 feet. One building is for men and one for women and each accommodate about 75 persons.

On January 28, 1891, at a meeting of the trustees it was unanimously resolved: "That the position of superintendent of the Sheppard Asylum be tendered to Dr. E. N. Brush, now assistant at the Pennsylvania Hospital for the Insane at Philadelphia." Dr. Brush accepted the appointment in a letter to the board dated February 9, 1891, subject to its approval of certain conditions and terms.

In September, 1891, he took up his residence at the asylum, having already aided in getting plumbing, electric lighting, etc., installed and in purchasing furniture and furnishings.

On November 25, 1891, the institution was declared open for the reception of patients. The first patients, two women and a man, were admitted on December 6, 1891, and the fiscal year of the hospital has been since that date from December 1 to November 30, inclusive.

The western building, now occupied by women, was finished first and opened for patients, men being placed on the first floor and women on the second, the plan of the building being such as to afford complete separation of the two floors and separate entrances for each sex. The eastern building was not opened until April, 1895, and the men patients transferred to it.

From the opening of the institution, bearing in mind the expressed wish of the founder, who declared it to be his "leading purpose to found an institution to carry forward and improve the ameliorated system of treatment of the insane, irrespective of expense," the hospital idea was kept always at the front.

In the first report the superintendent urged the reception of voluntary patients. He said "modern thought and modern practice in the care of the insane all point to the hospital idea, and if the general hospitals may receive without question or doubt any and all those who apply at their doors, it certainly seems in the line of progress to encourage the voluntary application of patients at the doors of these special hospitals."

This has been consistently followed up and the number of voluntary applicants has steadily increased until in the 24th year 72 per cent of the patients admitted came voluntarily.

In the first report reference was made to the extent of the work open to the institution and the desirability of increased endowment. The appeal appears to have met with prompt response, as in the second report it is stated that two ladies, residents of Baltimore, had made arrangements for legacies to the institution available at the death of the donors. The income of these legacies, which have been received, is to be used for the care of patients whose friends are unable to pay the cost of care and treatment.

In the third report Dr. Brush appealed for a well-equipped clinical and pathological laboratory to aid in carrying out the wish of Moses Sheppard to "carry forward and improve" the treatment of the insane. Laboratory work was undertaken and, as far as possible, with the resources available and the assistance obtainable, carried on from the very earliest days of the hospital's active work, and hopes were entertained of giving post-graduate work in psychiatry to young physicians who would come to the hospital as internes with that object in view. Near the close of the third fiscal year in the fall of 1894 Mr. George A. Pope, the president of the Board of Trustees, asked Dr. Brush, under the seal of confidence, to provide him with a written statement of what could be done with an increased endowment in promoting the original objects of the institution and advancing the knowledge and treatment of mental disorders. This statement was asked for by a gentleman who said that he had watched the course of the trustees and the conduct of the institution, and that in his opinion the trustees had more closely adhered to the wishes of the founder than any similar body of which he had knowledge.

The statement thus furnished referred to the charitable work which the hospital had already been able to accomplish under restrictions of its revenue caused by the naturally increased expenses due to the opening of the hospital.

It was pointed out that mental disorders were, even in cases which recovered, of somewhat prolonged duration, demanding a longer hospital residence than was incident to disorders treated in general hospitals, and that in many cases the cost of care and treatment was an exhaustive drain upon the resources of many families, often resulting in the pauperization of a whole family, and that in every community there were many cases whose relatives were unable to pay the charges in private institutions and yet who were not proper cases for state or municipal care.

The need of scientific study of all forms of mental disturbance, particularly an effort to determine their etiological factors, the introduction of more accurate and painstaking clinical observations, and the adoption of such laboratory and other methods of modern investigation as were found in the best general hospitals, in hospitals for mental disorders, were dwelt upon.

The fact that graduates of medical schools had no training in psychiatry and but inadequate instruction, it was stated, called for clinical instruction when possible and the introduction into the wards of young men as internes or clinical assistants who could be given a year or more of practical work in psychiatry. All these things, it was said, demanded enlarged resources, and to these, enlarged resources could be most effectively applied, and, when so applied, would be exactly in the line of the intentions of the founder.

On September 17, 1896, Mr. Enoch Pratt, the founder of the Enoch Pratt Free Library of Baltimore, president of the Farmers' and Planters' Bank, died and when his will was offered for probate it was found that he had made the trustees of the Sheppard and Enoch Pratt Hospital his residuary legatee. It was then stated by Mr. Pope that Mr. Pratt had asked for the statement referred to above.

The residuary estate, according to Mr. Pratt's will, was to pass to the trustees of the Sheppard Asylum upon the "condition and bargain" that at the first session of the Maryland Legislature following his death the trustees obtain from the Legislature an amendment of their charter changing their corporate title to "The Trustees of the Sheppard and Enoch Pratt Hospital."

The trustees, at a meeting on the 28th of December, 1896, resolved to accept the bequest of Mr. Pratt, and subsequently petitioned the General Assembly of the State of Maryland for an amendment changing their corporate title as required in his will.

Shortly after the opening of the session of the General Assembly in January, 1898, the first session following the death of Mr. Pratt, bills were simultaneously introduced into both houses providing for the desired change of corporate title. On January 28, 1898, the bill was unanimously passed in the Senate. Much opposition was made to its final passage in the House, instigated by persons named in the will who would receive the residuary estate if the trustees did not obtain the amendment to the charter making the change of name. This opposition was aided by some for sentimental reasons, the claim being made that Mr. Pratt was attempting to place his name on Mr. Sheppard's monument, and that the original benefactor would be lost sight of in the new title. These opponents knew little of Moses Sheppard's real character and were apparently ignorant of the fact that when the first charter was drawn he did not seek to have his name incorporated in the title of the corporation, and in writing to friends after the charter had been granted to the trustees of the Sheppard Asylum had said: "I thought I could proceed unnoticed, without a law," and again, "I want no such monument to my living fame."

The House of Delegates passed the same bill on February 24, 1898, by a vote of 65 to 20, and on March 2 the Governor affixed his signature and the measure became a law. On March 3, 1898, the trustees formally resolved to accept the amendment to the charter and the change of title therein involved and since that date have been legally known as The Trustees of the Sheppard and Enoch Pratt Hospital.

The question was carried to the Circuit Court of Baltimore by the interested persons named in the will and upon a decision being rendered in favor of the trustees later to the Court of Appeals, which affirmed the decision of the lower court in a unanimous opinion, which gave an interpretation of Mr. Pratt's will of a most satisfactory character.

The case was finally carried to the United States Supreme Court, but there dismissed on April 9, 1900, on the ground that no federal question was involved.

Mr. Pratt stated specifically in his will that he did "not wish to alter the operations and management in the working of the said asylum as now being carried on."

In commenting on the bequest, in the fifth annual report to the trustees the medical superintendent said:

Until the trustees shall officially signify their acceptance of the terms of the bequest and the Legislature shall make the necessary change in the corporate name of the board, it is too early to indicate the methods of carrying out Mr. Pratt's bequest. It is sufficient to say that the work lies all about you. The experience of five years in alleviating the care and anxiety of the friends and relatives of the helpless and dependent can but have given you a slight insight into the suffering and misery which cry aloud from hundreds of homes in this community and cry, alas, too often in vain. This insight must have increased your desire to do more in lifting the load, and can, I think, but cause a feeling of intense satisfaction that larger means have been placed at your disposal for this work.

After the action of the trustees in accepting the bequest, subject to the conditions named, the following, which outlines the policy which has since been pursued, and which indeed was adopted and carried out as far as possible from the first, is taken from the superintendent's sixth report:

The benefits to be derived from the mission of the Sheppard Asylum, under the broader and more comprehensive title of hospital, as I have said, cannot be estimated. The work is not for to-day, but for all time. The opportunities afforded by increased endowment are not solely, I conceive, to be spent in the medical treatment and fostering care of those who come hither. Moses Sheppard's desire was to carry forward and improve the ameliorated system of treatment of the insane.

He did not propose that his trustees should be content with saying we are doing as well as those who have preceded us, but that they should carry forward and improve the treatment of the insane. To this end increased means and increased opportunity are offered. These imply increased work and enlarged responsibilities. Within the broader scope of the hospital there must be embraced means of study and investigation of everything which enters not only into the treatment of insanity, but its causes and prevention.

Here clinical and pathological studies may be pursued under the best advantages, and here may be obtained by those so inclined a knowledge of the clinical manifestations, and of the care and treatment of insanity, as in general hospitals general diseases are studied.

The state will then have the proud distinction of having added to the scientific and charitable institutions within her borders, one without a parallel in the character of its work and the nature of its endowment.

In the ninth annual report of the hospital the president of the board gives a succinct account of the whole contest over Mr. Pratt's will and reports that the value of the residuary estate after deducting all charges and expenses of litigation was $1,069,300.41.

During the summer of 1900 many improvements were made in the grounds, especially in the near vicinity of the buildings, under plans by a landscape gardener, and in the following year an attractive recreation building was erected upon a plateau opposite the hospital buildings overlooking terraced lawns and gardens.

In 1899 Dr. Stewart Paton was appointed director of the laboratory, which position he filled until June, 1904. He was succeeded by Dr. Clarence B. Farrar, who continued in service until July, 1912. Gradually the medical staff was enlarged, clinical assistants were appointed and a distinct effort made to take advantage of the resources of the hospital for clinical instruction and for the purpose of adding "something valuable to the knowledge of insanity." Clinical lectures have been since given to the senior class of The Johns Hopkins Medical School by Dr. Wm. R. Dunton, Jr., and to the senior class of the College of Physicians and Surgeons by Dr. Brush.

In May, 1904, a well-equipped hydrotherapeutic plant was put in operation and has been in continuous use since.

In 1907 a dining room and kitchen block was erected, connected to each building by a corridor. The dining rooms are separate for each sex, four being provided on each side, with small tables seating four patients at each, thus permitting the arrangement of patients into congenial groups or divisions at meals. These dining rooms are immediately in connection with a large serving room, which in turn opens directly into the large kitchen.

Diet kitchens were at the same time installed in each section of the hospital building. The second floor of the dining room block is used as a nurses' home. The kitchen is one story high, is well lighted from each side and by a large monitor sky-light, which also serves for ventilating purposes.

In accepting Mr. Pratt's bequest the trustees resolved to use the income only for the purposes of the institution.

In Mr. Pratt's will he says: "It is my wish and will that the income be used." Moses Sheppard did not bind his trustees by his will as to the conduct of his trust, but in a letter accompanying the will says, among other suggestions, "the income and not the principal shall be used." While such suggestion was of course not legally mandatory, the trustees have regarded it as a guiding principle and out of the income of the Sheppard trust the buildings and grounds were provided and the buildings furnished for the reception of patients.

No aid has ever been received from the state or any other public source. On the contrary, state, county and municipal taxes absorb about 15 per cent of the gross income. The trustees report, as required by their charter, annually to the Governor, under oaths, the condition of the trust and of the institution and are subject to the supervision of the Legislature and the courts.

The charitable work of the hospital has steadily grown until in the 24th year 19 per cent of the entire number of days' care was given to free cases and another 19 per cent to patients paying less than one-third the average per capita cost. These two groups, to whom 38 per cent of the entire days' care was given, brought the hospital an average income of but 38 cents per week. Adding to these other patients who paid less than the per captia cost, over 62 per cent paid but one-fourth the per capita cost. At the same time the care of those who could pay for treatment has not been neglected and within the last year special suites, with private baths in addition to those already in use, have been provided for those who may desire them.

The training of nurses, which was undertaken at the opening of the hospital, has been upon a well-established basis for ten years. The course comprises three years, one-half of which is spent by pupils in affiliated general hospitals.

The trustees of the hospital have consistently attempted to carry out the intention of the founder to "carry forward and improve" the treatment of mental disorders and to that end have generously sustained the medical superintendent in all of his plans and aspirations.

Up to the close of the 24th fiscal year November 30, 1915, 3070 cases have been admitted, 687 have been discharged recovered, 487 much improved, 249 have died and 178 were discharged not insane.

The trustees are self-perpetuating, filling by vote any vacancies which occur in their number, but the life of the corporation is insured by a provision in the charter that, should the number of trustees be permitted by neglect to fill vacancies to fall below four at any time, the Governor shall fill the vacancies.

The trustees who have served from the granting of the charter in May, 1853, to the present time are:

PRESIDENTS BOARD OF TRUSTEES.

Moses Sheppard 1853-1856
John Saurin Norris......1882-1887
William Riley, M. .D......1882-1887
George A. Pope..........1887-

TRUSTEES.

Moses Sheppard 1853-1857
David M. Perine.........1853-1878
Wm. Riley, M. D.........1853-1887
Archibald Stirling 1853-1856
Charles Howard 1853-1856
William M. Medcalf......1853-1856
Richard H. Townsend....1853-1879
John Saurin Norris......1856-1882
Gerard H. Reese.........1856-1879
Gerard T. Hopkins.......1856-1900
William H. Graham......1858-1885
E. Glenn Perine..........1878-1897
J. H. Worthington, M. D..1879-1884
George A. Pope..........1882-
Richard D. Fisher........1883-1887
William T. Dixon........1885-1890
J. Olney Norris..........1887-1912
Charles H. Riley, M. D....1887-
John S. Gilman..........1889-1889
Charles C. Homer........1890-1914
George M. Lamb.........1898-1900
Edward A. Robinson.....1898-1900
Henry B. Gilpin..........1900-
Robert K. Waring.......1901-1913
W. Champlin Robinson...1908-
William K. Bartlett......1912-
Wilton Snowden 1913-
Charles C. Homer, Jr.....1914-

The medical staff from the opening of the hospital has been:

PHYSICIAN-IN-CHIEF AND SUPERINTENDENT.

Edward N. Brush, M. D.

ASSISTANT PHYSICIANS OR CLINICAL ASSISTANTS.

L. Gibbon Smart, M. D.
Edwin R. Bishop, M. D.
William Rush Dunton, Jr., M. D.
Charles Mayer Franklin, M. D.
Clarence B. Farrar, M. D.
Glanville Y. Rusk, M. D.
Seymour D. Ludlum, M. D.
William Burgess Cornell, M. D.
George E. Chinn, M. D.
James H. Randolph, M. D.
Charles Ricksher, M. D.
John G. Fitzgerald, M. D.
Edward F. Malone, M. D.
Francis M. Barnes, Jr., M. D.
George F. Sargent, M. D.
Burt J. Asper, M. D.
George B. Wolff, M. D.
Frederick P. Weltner, M. D.
Stewart Paton, M. D. (director of laboratory).

THE HENRY PHIPPS PSYCHIATRIC CLINIC.[1]

The Henry Phipps Psychiatric Clinic, one of the divisions of The Johns Hopkins Hospital, was opened April 16, 1913.

Stewart Paton's untiring efforts to direct the interest of the leaders of The Johns Hopkins Medical School and Hospital towards the growth and needs of psychiatry had led Dr. William Osler to put a psychiatric clinic in the first position among the desiderata depicted by him in his farewell address before he went to Oxford. When Mr. Henry Phipps asked Dr. William H. Welch what he considered the greatest need of The Johns Hopkins Medical School, he answered: "a psychiatric clinic." And out of this in June, 1908, came a most generous gift: funds for the construction and equipment of a modern type of hospital with laboratories, and for expenses of an adequate staff and of the hospital for a period of ten years. The architect chosen by Mr. Phipps, Mr. Grosvenor Atterbury, and the head of the new department chosen by The Johns Hopkins authorities, Dr. Adolf Meyer, developed the plans of this new department. They were adopted in 1909 and the building was opened to receive patients May 1, 1913.

The organization is unique in this: It is the first university clinic, in this country at least, free to receive its patients according to the judgment of the staff, and without any compulsion or conditions or obligations imposed by any city or state authorities.

The Clinic comprehends an out-patient department; a public ward service with 66 beds, and provision for 18 private patients; a department of hydrotheraphy and a gymnasium; occupation and recreation departments and three laboratory units, one for the investigation of the problems of internal medicine, one for psychology and psychopathology, and one for investigations in neuropathology in its functional and histological aspects.

The building is so designed that all the quarters for patients are located to the south of the main corridors, and the administrative and laboratory quarters to the north. The wards occupy four superimposed floors. Each one of the three public wards for each sex has one large room for eight cases and from two to four single rooms and day room space, and the necessary rooms for the admin-

[1] By Dr. Adolf Meyer, director of the Clinic.

istration. The first floor is planned for bed cases and patients requiring special attention on account of excitement. It has two entrances, one from the corridor and one from the court, so as to make possible a division if quarantine is needed. Two tubs for continuous baths for public ward patients and a separate tub room for private patients and three single rooms comprise the accommodations of the portion of the ward which is thus shut off; they are all usually thrown together with the large room. The second floor, for semi-quiet patients, has, besides the ward for eight patients, two single rooms, a special occupation room, a day room, and an open porch and provisions for two continuous baths. The third floor has three single rooms, and the ward is subdivided by low partitions, giving the individual eight beds a certain privacy. The fourth floor has two suites of sitting room, bedroom, bath and closet; two rooms with bath and closet; and two sets of rooms using bath room and closets conjointly; moreover, an alcove and a day room and a dining room. The recreation room on the fifth floor, with stage and organ and piano, and billiard room, and two roof gardens, complete the equipment.

The basement is taken up by the out-patient department (waiting-room, social-service department, four examination rooms and a demonstration room), the department of hydrotherapy and gymnasium, a work-shop and orderlies' rooms.

An account of the opening exercises and a series of lectures given by guests from Europe and this country was published as a special number of the *American Journal of Insanity* (Vol. lxix, pp. 835-1086). The hospital was honored by addresses and papers from Sir William Osler, William McDougall, E. Bleuler, August Hoch, Frederick Lyman Wells, F. W. Mott, O. Rossi, Harvey Cushing, Stewart Paton, K. Heilbronner, Ernest Jones, George H. Kirby, Charles B. Dunlap and Albert Moore Barrett.

The Clinic aims to be able to furnish adequate provisions for any type of mental disorder, from the simplest psychopathological problems to the more difficult and disturbing cases. No cases are admitted without a full account of their development sufficient to decide whether there are any diagnostic or therapeutic problems to warrant admission. The admission is primarily for diagnostic purposes; the selected cases which present problems for further study and therapeutic openings can be kept as long as the psychiatrist-in-chief sees fit. The admissions are practically limited to cases which come voluntarily. No distinction is made between " non-insane " and " insane " patients; in exceptional cases only patients who object to treatment are retained under the commitment provisions of the State of Maryland (examination and certification by two physicians not connected with the Clinic, without any court action).

The staff of the Clinic consists of the psychiatrist-in-chief of The Johns Hopkins Hospital, who is also professor of psychiatry in the medical school of The Johns Hopkins University (Adolf Meyer); the associate psychiatrist of The Johns Hopkins Hospital and associate professor of psychiatry (C. Macfie Campbell); the resident physician (David K. Henderson, 1912-1915; Roscoe W. Hall, 1915-), two assistant resident physicians (Edward J. Kempf and Ralph P. Truitt, 1913-1914; Roscoe W. Hall, 1914-1915, and Augusta Scott, 1915- ; Charles B. Thompson, 1914- ; and five house officers. The laboratory for internal medicine was organized by S. R. Miller and is now in the hands of C. A. Neymann. The other laboratories are not provided for as yet.

The out-patient department has seen the following number of cases: 1913 (8 months), 479; 1914, 671; 1915, 840.

The number of admissions to the Clinic were: 1913 (8 months), 237; 1914, 432; 1915, 426.

The teaching comprehends courses for the second, third and fourth year classes of the medical school and students of the psychological department of the University; elective work in the clinical and laboratory departments and research work.

ROSEWOOD STATE TRAINING SCHOOL.

Owings Mills, Md.

The Maryland Asylum and Training School for Feeble-minded was incorporated by the General Assembly in 1888, and its name was changed by the General Assembly of 1912 to Rosewood State Training School. It is a permanent charitable institution, owned and entirely supported by the State of Maryland.

The movement to establish a training school for feeble-minded patients had its origin largely in the efforts of Dr. Richard Gundry, then superintendent of the Spring Grove State Hospital, who in several reports called the attention of the state to the great need of doing something for the care and training of feeble-minded children. In consequence of his initiative, much interest was developed in several public-spirited philanthropists, among whom were Dr. J. Pembroke Thom, Gen. Herman Stump and Milton G. Urner. A small appropriation was obtained to establish such a school in the former residence of Dr. Wood, of the Navy, near Owings Mills, known as Rosewood. The first superintendent was Miss Martha M. Gundry, a daughter of Dr. Gundry, who, with a single teacher, opened the school in a small way in 1888. Miss Gundry continued in responsible charge for several years, and resigned to establish a school in Virginia. She was succeeded by several medical gentlemen, who held the office for comparatively brief periods. Dr. Thom continued much interested, and two of the cottages, Pembroke and Thom, bear his name. Gen. Herman Stump and Milton G. Urner are still connected with the board. Later the full development of the institution resulted in the appointment of Dr. F. W. Keating, who has been responsible for its work for the past 16 years.

The object of the institution is to furnish a home and a practical education for the feeble-minded children of the state who are not provided for in the public schools. Many children are of such defective understanding as to render them incapable of receiving proper training in the public schools, where they are brought into competition with those of normal intellect and where they cannot receive the especial care and attention absolutely necessary to secure mental development. In most instances they require training specially adapted to their condition, or they will become a burden upon their friends or the community; but by receiving kind and painstaking care and tuition at the hands of competent, experienced persons many of them become partly self-supporting under proper supervision. To care for and train such children to accomplish the results indicated, is the purpose of this institution.

Rosewood is situated about one-half mile from Owings Mills, in Baltimore County, and is accessible by the Western Maryland Railroad and the Emory Grove electric cars. It is in the Green Spring Valley, and is beautifully and healthfully located upon a farm of 537 acres of land.

Children between the ages of 7 and 17 years who, by reason of mental defect, cannot be educated in ordinary schools, and who are not insane or greatly afflicted or deformed physically, are admitted into the institution free of charge for board and tuition, upon evidence being furnished of their inability to pay. Reasonable compensation is charged to those able to pay. It has a capacity of 700 children.

The group of buildings consists of a main or administration building and cottages which have been added from time to time, furnishing accommodation for 492 inmates, a school building and the necessary farm structures. In addition a custodial building for girls of low-grade type was completed in the spring of 1914, providing additional accommodations for 260 girls. This building is furnished with dormitories, day rooms, toilet and bath rooms, dining rooms and a scullery. On the first and second floors are large sleeping porches and in the basement is a large play room, which is used in inclement weather. The third floor is occupied by the nurses and attendants in the building, each having a separate bedroom, with a general sitting room for their comfort when not on duty with the children.

In the same year other improvements were made on the grounds. Two new stone barns and a large terra cotta silo were erected to replace old wooden structures, at a total cost of $10,584.41. An attractive stone gate lodge, with stone gateway, was also completed, at a cost of $3554, which adds greatly to the appearance of this entrance to the grounds.

The majority of the patients admitted are children under 15 years of age, at a time when they are susceptible of improvement by school instruction.

In the school department much attention is paid to manual training for the more advanced pupils and to kindergarten instruction for the younger ones. Each child is accorded the full advantages of class-room training when he or she is admitted to the institution within the limits of the school age. In the household department, sewing room, dining room, kitchen and laundry the work is entered into with much interest on the part of the patients. Their desire is great to do "something like work," and the improvement made in this branch of their training calls for still greater effort in the future, for such training saves them from a life of idleness and is one of the most important factors in developing the feeble-minded along lines of economic efficiency.

The farming and clearing of land have been of substantial benefit to the boys, and the good derived from this work cannot be too highly estimated. The produce raised on the farm has furnished the institution with a supply of fresh vegetables at all seasons. The entire supply of milk is obtained from the school's own herd, and a great deal of the fresh meat has been obtained from the live stock fattened and butchered on the farm. During the biennial period of 1913-14 the market value of the farm products aggregated $32,-923.63; also the value at local prices of work performed by farm teams in hauling and excavating would amount to $3977.10. The work on the farm furnishes one of the most effective means of developing, both mentally and physically, the boys committed to the institution. Some of those most useful on the farm were able to accomplish practically nothing in the school room, but the outdoor occupation seems to render them particularly docile and happy.

The per capita expense for maintenance during the period of 1913-14 was $4.58 weekly, an increase of 15 cents per patient over the preceding biennial period, which increase is due to the advance in the market price of many supplies and the general increase in the wages of employees.

SUPERINTENDENTS SINCE OPENING TO DATE.

Miss Mattie M. Gundry. February 19, 1889, to April 4, 1892.
Dr. B. D. Evans........April 4, 1892, to May 30, 1892.
Dr. B. A. Turner.......June 15, 1892, to May 7, 1895.
Dr. L. Gibbons Smart..June 5, 1895, to August 31, 1896.
Dr. Frank W. Keating..October 1, 1896, to date.

FIRST BOARD OF VISITORS.

J. Pembroke Thom, M. D., president.
Milton G. Urner, vice-president.
Levin F. Morris, secretary.
Henry S. King, treasurer.

Charles Ridgely Goodwin. J. Walter Carpenter.
John Morris, M. D. Richard H. Edelen.
Goldsborough S. Griffith. Herman Stump.
James A. L. McClure. Charles B. Roberts.
Thomas Hill. William T. P. Turpin.
J. Clarence Lane. John W. Dashiel, M. D.
Richard Gundry, M. D.

PRESENT BOARD OF VISITORS.

Herman Stump, president.
Charles G. Hill, M. D., vice-president.
Benjamin Bissell, treasurer.

Milton G. Urner.	John S. Biddison.
Henry S. King.	Julius H. Wyman.
Henry B. Whiteley.	William D. Corse, M. D.
Lemuel T. Appold.	William P. E. Wyse, M. D.
William H. H. Campbell, M. D.	John B. Hanna.
Thomas J. Ewell.	Robert Garrett.
C. Lyon Rogers.	W. Bladen Lowndes.

Frank W. Keating, M. D., secretary and superintendent.

OTHERS WHO HAVE SERVED ON THE BOARD.

Henry J. Hebb, M. D.	Louis F. Detrick.
Abraham R. Price, M. D.	William H. Rinehart.
James S. Woodside.	Milton G. Offutt.
Aubrey Pearre.	Edward E. Goslin.
Major N. H. Hutton.	Joshua W. Hering, M. D.

George May.

THE RELAY SANITARIUM.

RELAY, MD.

This institution is located at Relay, Baltimore County, Md., and was established in 1878, being founded by Dr. Conrad, and taken over and remodeled by the present management at a more recent date. The buildings are of frame and brick; they are lighted by electricity. The water supply is by the Baltimore County Water Company. There are 72 acres of land in connection with this institution. The number of patients is limited to 45. The detached buildings consist of a physicians' cottage, a farmer's cottage and servants' quarters. The patients are employed in the garden and on the grounds at farm work, etc. In the way of amusements there is croquet, tennis, golf, weekly dances and entertainments, pool, cards, library, etc. There are two medical officers, consisting of a superintendent and resident physician. Nurses are given practical training, but there is no training school. There are associate dining rooms. Cases of drug and alcoholic addiction are admitted as well as nervous and mental cases. The superintendent is Dr. Lewis H. Gundry.

MT. HERBERT.

CATONSVILLE, MD.

(FORMERLY FONT HILL, ELLICOTT CITY, MD.)

Mt. Herbert is a private home for the mentally deficient, established in 1886 in Howard County, near Ellicott City, Md., lately removed to the more modern and better equipped building in Catonsville. There are ample lawns and garden spaces; the house is well heated, ventilated and lighted, and situated far enough from Frederick Avenue to insure complete privacy and be within easy distance of the trolley between Baltimore and Catonsville. Both sexes are admitted and every effort is made to give a home environment without evident restraint.

Kindergarten training, wood-working, house and garden work are used for the employment of patients, with music, library facilities and family association as additional features of caretaking. The medical director is Dr. Samuel J. Fort.

THE RICHARD GUNDRY HOME.

CATONSVILLE, MD.

This institution was established in 1891 by Mrs. Mary M. Gundry and Dr. Richard F. Gundry, her son, being named in memory of Dr. Richard Gundry, Sr. Mrs. Gundry retired from the institution in 1898, since which time it has been conducted entirely by Dr. Richard F. Gundry. The buildings are frame and five in number, consisting of the main building and annex, men's bungalow, Harlem cottage and a small bungalow. They are heated by steam and lighted by electricity. The water supply is furnished by the Catonsville Water Works and the sewerage is taken care of by a septic tank and a sand and gravel filter. The grounds consist of 30 acres, which are well shaded. Fifteen acres are in lawns and the rest is under cultivation. The institution raises its own vegetables and a herd of Guernsey cows is kept. The capacity of the institution is 45 patients. The patients are employed in outdoor work, such as gardening, in the green house and on the lawn, and there is also a shop for the patients to work with tools. The outdoor amusements consist of tennis, golf, croquet, baseball and medicine ball. The medical officers consist of the medical director, assistant physician and interne. The average number of nurses is one to every four patients. Trained nurses are employed as required. There are both associate and private dining rooms. Cases of alcoholic and drug addiction, as well as nervous and mental cases, are received. All rational means of treatment are employed, such as electricity, hydrotherapy, occupation, amusement, etc.

THE LAUREL SANITARIUM.

LAUREL, MD.

The Laurel Sanitarium was established in 1905 by Jesse C. Coggins, for nine years assistant physician at the Maryland Hospital, and Dr. Cornelius DeWeese, formerly assistant physician and pathologist at the Maryland Hospital for the Insane, and for four years physician-in-charge of the clinical laboratory of the Government Hospital in Washington.

The sanitarium is a private hospital for the care and treatment of nervous and mental diseases, alcoholic and drug addiction. It is located about one mile from Laurel, Md., and comprises five buildings.

The female building is a three-story frame structure, containing 30 bedrooms and five bathrooms, music room, library, three sun-parlors and spacious porches. The female annex, a two-story fireproof brick building, is situated near the main female building and is connected therewith by a fireproof corridor. This building contains 14 bedrooms and two bathrooms, one equipped with a continuous bath; it also has a sun-parlor and large porch.

The main building for men is a two-story frame building containing 36 bedrooms and six bathrooms. The gymnasium in the basement contains bowling alleys, billiard table, shuffle-board, rowing machine, punching bag and other exercises. Adjoining this room is the hydrotherapeutic room containing hot air cabinets, shower baths and massage tables.

The bungalow, a one-story frame structure, has six rooms, one bathroom and a sun-parlor.

The central or administration building is a three-story fireproof structure containing the offices, drug-room, examination room, record-room, store-room, central kitchen, five dining rooms, and eight bedrooms.

All buildings are connected with the administration building by fireproof corridors, and are heated by a hot water system from the central heating plant in the fireproof basement of the administration building. The buildings and grounds are lighted by electricity; the water supply is from the City of Laurel; the drinking water is supplied from an artesian well 325 feet deep.

The nursing is done by experienced nurses. Nurses are quartered on the third floor of their respective buildings. A night nurse of each service and an outside watchman are on duty at all times during the night.

A teacher is employed to teach the women needle-work, raffia, basket making, etc. In the men's group patients are employed at gardening, road-making and painting. The indoor amusements consist of musicales, cards, bowling, billiards and other games. Outdoor amusements are tennis, croquet and ball-playing.

The farm surrounding the sanitarium comprises 163 acres, which is laid out in walks, lawns, garden and fields; and the table is supplied from the herd, poultry yards and garden belonging to the institution.

The physicians-in-charge are Dr. Jesse C. Coggins and Dr. Cornelius DeWeese, owners and resident medical officers.

PATAPSCO MANOR SANITARIUM.

Ellicott City, Md.

Patapsco Manor Sanitarium is a private home devoted to the care of drug, alcoholic, nervous and mild mental cases.

It is located at Ellicott City, Md., on one of the highest points of Howard County, overlooking the Patapsco Valley.

The buildings consist of a large main building of stone, containing spacious and airy rooms. Independent of and a short distance from the main building is a large modern cottage and also a modern bungalow, which have been erected for the purpose of maintaining a desirable classification of patients.

The buildings are situated in a private park of 55 acres and are equipped with every modern convenience.

The purest of artesian well water is of constant supply, and special attention is given to the diet of the individual patient. A large garden provides an abundance of fresh vegetables and fruit.

Amusements have been provided for by tennis courts, croquet lawns and a well-equipped billiard-room.

The superintendent is Dr. W. Rushmer White.

RIGGS COTTAGE SANITARIUM.

Ijamsville, Md.

Riggs Cottage Sanitarium, a private institution for the care and treatment of nervous and mental diseases, located on the main line of the Baltimore & Ohio Railroad at Ijamsville, Frederick County, Md., was established in 1896 and licensed by the Lunacy Commission in the same year for the reception of patients.

The property consists of 42 acres of land, on the southern end of which is the Baltimore & Ohio station and on the northern end is the sanitarium, consisting of three buildings, an annex, an engine house, barn, large ice house, corn house, poultry houses, tennis and croquet grounds.

The center building of the sanitarium consists of 14 rooms, large attic and cellar. This building has modern sanitary plumbing, baths and steam heat.

The west building is three stories high and consists of 10 rooms, with modern sanitary plumbing, baths and steam heat. It is occupied by men alone and is connected with the central building by a pavilion.

The east building is an eight-room cottage connected with the central building by an annex consisting of a large dining room and hall and bedrooms above.

The kitchen is in the rear of the central building. The water for the sanitarium is derived from an artesian well and forced to a large tank above the kitchen.

The sanitarium accommodates comfortably 25 patients. Both voluntary and committed patients are received, and many who are not mentally deranged and need rest come as boarders.

Aside from occupation there are a number of amusements and diversions. The patients enjoy fishing excursions, daily walks, lawn tennis, frequent games of baseball, croquet, pool, parlor games, music and dancing. During pleasant weather much of their time is spent out of doors.

Hydrotherapy is found indispensable, and continuous baths and packs are used.

Dr. George H. Riggs is the present resident physician.

THE CARE OF THE INSANE IN MASSACHUSETTS.

The earliest record of any legislation regarding the insane in Massachusetts was in 1676. In the records of the Massachusetts Bay Colony, Vol. V, page 80, there is the following law:

> WHEREAS, There are distracted persons in some tounes, that are unruly, whereby not only the families wherein they are, but others, suffer much damage by them, it is ordered by this Court and the authoritie thereof, that the selectmen in all tounes where such persons are are hereby impowred & injoyned to take care of all such persons, that they doe not damnify others; and also to take care & order the management of their estates in the times of their distemperature, so as may be for the good of themselves & families depending on them, and the charge to be paid out of the estates of all such persons where it may be had, otherwise at the publick charge of the toune such persons belong unto.

This delegates to the selectmen the care of the person and estate of the dependent insane.

In 1694, in an act entitled "An Act for the Relief of Idiots and Distracted Persons," the care of the insane is given to the selectmen and overseers of the poor, but the disposition of their estates and of their person is given to the justice of the peace. This is the only reference found in the law which might be construed as authorizing the letting out of the insane to families in the community who might perchance be the lowest bidders. This law provided that whenever a person should be "wanting of understanding, so as to be uncapable to provide for him or herself," or should become insane—

> and no relations appear that will undertake the care of providing for him, or that stand in so near a degree as that by law they may be compelled thereto: in every such case the selectmen or overseers of the poor of the town or peculiar where such person was born or is by law an inhabitant, be and hereby are empowered & enjoined to take effectual care & make necessary provision for the relief, support, and safety of such impotent or distracted persons at the charge of the place where he or she of right belongs. And the justices of the peace within the same county, at their county courts may order & dispose the estate of such impotent & distracted persons to the best of his or her support as also the person to any proper work or service he or she may be capable to be employed in at the discretion of the Selectmen & Overseers of the poor.

We find in 1736 the first reference to the methods of determining the insanity of the individual, in a law which puts it in the power of the judge of probate, on the request of friends or the overseers of the poor, to direct the selectmen to make inquisition, the final results seeming to depend upon the opinion of the selectmen or overseers of the poor and the judge.

The first indication of personal interest in the claims of the insane occurs in the will of Thomas Handcock, who died in 1764:

I give unto the Town of Boston the sum of six hundred pounds lawful money towards erecting and finishing a convenient House for the reception and more comfortable keeping of such unhappy persons as it shall please God, in His Providence, to deprive of their reason in any part of this Province; such as are inhabitants of Boston always to have the preference. This sum I order shall be paid into the hands of the Town Treasurer for the time being, viz: One-half thereof in three months after said House shall be begun, and the other half thereof when the same shall be finished and fit for said purpose. And in case said House shall not be built and finished in three years after my decease, I then declare this legacy to be void; or if I should in my lifetime erect it, this bequest then to be void. Dated March 5, 1763.

This legacy was declined by the selectmen of Boston for the reason that *there were not enough insane persons in the province to call for the erection of such house*.[1]

In 1784 a further law was passed in regard to guardianship of the insane, and in 1798 the law permitted the commitment of such lunatics as were "furiously mad so as to render it dangerous to the safety or the peace of the good people to be at large" to the House of Correction. This act, passed February 27, 1798, is entitled: "An Act in Addition to an Act entitled 'An Act for Suppressing Rogues, Vagabonds, Common Beggars and Other Idle, Disorderly and Lewd Persons,'" and was as follows:

---

[1] Seventy-five years after this generous proposal was declined, however, the need of such a house became urgent, owing to the overcrowded condition of the hospital at Worcester, opened but a few years before, which necessitated the return of a large number of patients to the almshouse and house of correction. This need was recognized in the spirit which has animated Boston in the care of her dependents, Mayor Elliott reporting that while the law required Boston to provide a receptacle for the insane of Suffolk County, humanity required her to provide a hospital for them. Thus it came about that in 1839 there was opened for the reception of patients the Boston Lunatic Hospital, the first municipal hospital for the insane in America.

SEC. 3. *Be it further enacted by the authority aforesaid,* That when it shall be made to appear to any two justices, *quorum unus,* that any person, being within their county, is lunatick and so furiously mad as to render it dangerous to the peace or the safety of the good people for such lunatick person to go at large; the said justices shall have full power, by warrant under their hands & seals, to commit such person to the house of correction, there to be detained till he or she be restored to his right mind, or otherwise delivered by due course of law. And every person so committed, shall be kept at his or her expense, if he or she have estate, otherwise, at the charge of the person or town upon whom his maintenance was regularly to be charged, if he or she had not been committed; and he or she shall, if able, be put to work during his or her confinement.

The next legislation was in 1811, when the Massachusetts General Hospital was incorporated and the McLean Hospital was established.

In 1816 the law directed the commitment of persons under indictment, who were acquitted because of insanity, to be committed to prisons and to be kept until it was safe for them to be discharged, or until some responsible person would go bond for their conduct.

In 1827 the law was changed in regard to the safekeeping of "lunatic persons furiously mad" so that they were committed to the hospital or lunatic asylum instead of to the jail.

An interesting light is thrown upon the early care of the insane in private establishments in the New England States by some remarks of Dr. Ray's, published in the *Journal of Insanity* in 1864. He says:

The history of the operations of these private establishments, the means and plans which they used, their discipline and methods of treatment were so different from ours that they would be highly interesting. Dr. Willard's establishment, which flourished in the early years of the century, was situated in a little town on the line between Massachusetts and Rhode Island. I am inclined to think it was the pioneer establishment in Massachusetts, which took the lead in New England in regard to such establishments. I happened to make the acquaintance of a couple of old physicians, who, when young men, had spent a week or two with Dr. Willard, and from them I learned many things in regard to the management of his institution. I never knew exactly where Dr. Willard got his knowledge about insanity or what induced him to open the establishment. My two friends were quite young at the time of their visit, and probably desired no information upon those points. They, however, took much interest in the management, and carefully watched the Doctor's proceedings. The main fundamental idea was to break the patient's will and make him learn that he had a master; to teach him that there was a mind and physical strength there all superior to his own. That was the principal object to be kept in view, and it was to be gained at any risk. If fair means would not do, other means should; if strong words or curses would not answer then resort was had to the knock-down arguments. This was thought to be the proper way; no secret was made of it, and the friends of patients understood it perfectly well. Among the methods of treatment was one which I am inclined to think was used in England, although I find no mention of it in any book. That was the process of submersion, and the idea was, probably, that if the patient was nearly drowned and then brought to life, he would take a fresh start, leaving his disease behind. The idea sprang, probably, from the well-known fact that occasionally a patient who attempted suicide by drowning and is barely resuscitated is thereby cured of insanity. However that may be, Dr. Willard had a tank prepared on the premises, into which the patient, enclosed in a coffin-like box pierced with holes, was lowered by means of a well-sweep. He was kept there under water until the bubbles of air ceased to rise, when he was taken out, rubbed and revived. What success followed this process I never knew. Of the fact itself I have no doubt, for I was told of it by those two gentlemen who had witnessed it themselves. I do not know how far that treatment prevailed in this country. I believe there is no doubt that it was practiced in one public institution, for the fact rests, I think, on the authority of Miss Dix, who witnessed the process. I presume that with that exception it was confined to private establishments.

About the same time Dr. Thomas Kittredge, and after his decease Dr. Joseph Kittredge, were in the habit of treating insane patients at Andover, Mass. The former had at times as many as 10 or 12 under his care, the latter somewhat fewer. They never received their patients in their own homes, but made arrangements for boarding them in two or three private families. These families were presided over by strong, fearless, capable and good-natured women, most of whom had husbands, and the patients were under little restraint, though subject to constant supervision. They do not appear to have belonged to the most violent class, as there do not seem to have been any strong rooms in which to confine them.

In this connection it is interesting to note the case of Colonel James Otis, the famous Massachusetts orator, who was injured in the riots preceding the attempt to enforce the Stamp Act in Boston. In consequence of this injury he suffered from mental disease for the remainder of his life and was eventually killed by a stroke of lightning in 1783, while living in the house of Mr. Osgood at Andover, Mass., where he was obviously under treatment for his mental condition.

In a series of reports relating to the State Lunatic Hospital at Worcester, published by order of the Senate of the commonwealth, it appears that on the 22d of February, 1829, Horace Mann, on behalf of the committee, reported orders for the appointment of a committee "to examine and ascertain the practicability and expediency of erecting or procuring, at the expense of the commonwealth, an asylum for the safekeeping of lunatics and persons furiously mad," which required the selectmen of the several towns to ascertain and make returns to the Secretary of the commonwealth of "the number, age, sex and color of all persons reputed to be lunatics and furiously mad belonging to their respective towns; whether at large or in confinement, and where and how long confined." These orders were subsequently adopted by the House.

In the following January (1830) the Secretary of the commonwealth communicated to the House of Representatives the bills which had been received as to the number of insane, and they were referred to the committee, of which Horace Mann was chairman. In February the committee reported that returns had been received from 114 towns, comprising less than one-half the population of Massachusetts, and that in 25 of these towns there were no insane persons; that in the remaining 89 towns there were 289 lunatics or persons "furiously mad"; and that 161 of that number were in confinement as follows: In poorhouses and houses of industry, 78; in private houses, 37; in jails and houses of correction, 19; in insane hospitals, 10; and other places of confinement, 17. In addition to these there were certainly at least 60 confined in the insane hospital at Charlestown. The length of confinement of 26 cases is not stated, but it appeared that 29 cases had been confined less than one year and were manifestly recent cases. Thirteen had been confined from one to two years, five for 10 years, two for 13 years, one for 15 years, four for 20 years, three for 25 years, four for 30 years, one for 35 years, two for 40 years, and one for 45 years.

The committee recommended that a building suitable for the accommodation of a superintendent, with right and left wings suitable for the reception of 120 patients, be erected at a cost of $30,000. A bill making this appropriation was passed at the same session and approved by the Governor in March, 1830, the institution being located in the Town of Worcester, where a plot of 12 acres of land was purchased at a cost of $2500. Three commissioners were appointed to superintend the erection of the hospital.

Subsequently an appropriation of $20,000 was made to cover the expense of furnishing the hospital. In the same year a bequest of $500 was received from Nathaniel MacCarty to defray the expense of planting trees and shrubbery and otherwise ornamenting the hospital grounds. In March, 1832, a Board of Trustees was appointed, which elected Dr. Samuel B. Woodward, of Wethersfield, Conn., superintendent. The trustees were empowered to make regulations for the government and discipline of the institution. This involved the consideration of two questions: 1. The class of patients to be committed to its charge; and the authority by which they were to be committed and by whom discharged, as well as the mode in which their expenses should be defrayed. 2. The regulations governing the treatment of the insane in the hospitals.

Their report divides all patients in the hospital into three classes, as follows:

The first class consisted of those whom the justices of the supreme judicial court or the justices of the peace had committed to jails or houses of correction by virtue of the statutes of 1797 (chapter 62) and of 1816 (chapter 28), because it was deemed incompatible with the security of the citizens generally to permit them to go at large.

The second class consisted of town pauper lunatics, who were mostly confined in poorhouses by order of the municipal authorities. In some towns it had been the practice to make private contracts with the keeper of the jail or houses of correction to take the insane poor at a low price and to imprison them in unoccupied cells, without assuming any responsibility for their proper treatment or any authority to examine into it. Other towns, it is said, had annually offered the keeping of their insane poor at auction and struck them off to the lowest bidder, by whom they were treated with various degrees of kindness or cruelty, according to the character of the individual, whose object in bidding for them was generally solely to make a profit by keeping them.

The third class consisted of all insane persons in the commonwealth not included in the other two classes. It included persons not "furiously mad" as well as those who had sufficient property for their own support or were supported by their guardians or relatives and did not, therefore, belong in the second class.

The language used by the committee, of which Horace Mann was chairman, in reference to the first class is of extreme interest in the light of what we now know as to the possibility of making such persons comfortable. The committee complained that the law which permitted the incarceration of persons " furiously mad " in jails and houses of correction really placed them beyond the reach of recovery, for the commissioners had never heard of more than three or four instances of restoration among all who had been subjected to the rigors of confinement in a jail or house of correction, whereas in well-regulated institutions for the reception and treatment of the insane, 50 per cent, 60 per cent or in some instances 90 per cent had recovered. To quote some of the striking passages of this report:

> To him whose mind is alienated, a prison is a tomb, and within its walls he must suffer as one who awakes to life in the solitude of the grave. Existence and the capacity for pain alone are left him. From every former source of pleasure or contentment he is violently sequestered. Every former habit is abruptly broken off. No medical skill seconds the efforts of nature for his recovery, or breaks the strength of pain when it seizes him with convulsive grasp. No friends relieve each other in solacing the weariness of protracted disease. No assiduous affection guards the avenues of approaching disquietude. He is alike removed from all the occupations of health, and from all the attentions everywhere but within his homeless abode bestowed upon sickness. The solitary cell, the noisome atmosphere, the unmitigated cold and the untempered heat, are of themselves sufficient soon to derange every vital function of the body, and this only aggravates the derangement of his mind. On every side is raised up an insurmountable barrier against his recovery. Cut off from all the charities of life, endued with quickened sensibilities to pain, and perpetually stung by annoyances which, though individually small, rise by constant accumulation to agonies almost beyond the power of mortal sufferance; if his exiled mind in its devious wanderings ever approach the light by which it was once cheered and directed, it sees everything unwelcoming, everything repulsive and hostile, and is driven away into returnless banishment.

This bears out the following statement contained in the second report of the " Prison Discipline Society," as regards the condition of the insane in prisons in Massachusetts:

> In Massachusetts the statement is made that about 30 lunatics have been found in prison; in one prison there were three, in another five, in

another six, and in a fourth ten. The sheriff and jailers complained that they were compelled to receive such patients and had no suitable accommodations for them.

Of these last mentioned, one was found in an apartment in which he has been nine years. He had a wreath of rags round his body, and another round his neck. This was all his clothing. He had no bed, chair or bench. Two or three rough planks were strewed around the room, a heap of filthy straw, like the nest of swine, was in the corner. He had built a bird's nest of mud in the iron grate of his den. Connected with his wretched apartment was a dark dungeon, having no orifice for the admission of light, heat or air, except the iron door, about two and a half feet square, opening into it from the prison.

The other lunatics in the same prison were scattered in separate cells which were almost dark dungeons. It was difficult, after the door was open, to see them distinctly. The ventilation was so incomplete that more than one person on entering them has found the air so fetid as to produce nauseousness and almost vomiting. The old straw on which they were laid and their filthy garments were such as to make their insanity more hopeless, and at one time it was not considered within the province of the physicians' department to examine particularly the condition of the lunatics. In these circumstances any improvement of their minds could hardly be expected. Instead of having three out of four restored to reason, as is the fact in some of the favored lunatic asylums, it is to be feared that in these circumstances some who might otherwise be restored would become incurable, and that others might lose their lives, to say nothing of present sufferings.

In the prison in which there were six lunatics their condition was less wretched. But they were sometimes an annoyance, and sometimes a sport to the convicts, and even the apartment in which the females were confined opened into the yard of the men; and there was an injurious interchange of obscenity and profaneness between them, which was not restrained by the presence of the keeper.

In the prison, or house of correction, so called, in which were ten lunatics, two were found about 70 years of age, a male and a female, in the same apartment of an upper story. The female was lying on a heap of straw under a broken window. The snow in a severe storm was beating through a window, and lay upon the straw around her withered body, which was partially covered with a few filthy and tattered garments. The man was lying in the corner of the room in a similar situation, except that he was less exposed to the storm. The former had been in this apartment six and the latter 21 years.

Another lunatic in the same prison was found in a plank apartment of the first story, where he had been eight years. During this time he had never left the room but twice. The door of this apartment had not been opened in 18 months. The food was furnished through a small orifice in the door. The room was warmed by no fire; and still the woman of the house said "he had never froze." As he was seen through the orifice in the door, the first question was, "Is that a human being?" The hair was gone from one side of his head and his eyes were like balls of fire.

In the cellar of the same prison were five lunatics. The windows of this cellar were no defence against the storm, and, as might be supposed, the woman of the house said, "we have a sight to do to keep them from freezing." There was no fire in this cellar which could be felt by four of the lunatics. One of the five had a little fire of turf in an apartment of the cellar by herself. She was, however, infuriated if any one came near her. This woman was committed to this cellar 17 years ago. The apartments are about six by eight feet. They are made of coarse plank, and have an orifice in the door for the admission of light and air, about six inches by six. The darkness was such in two of these apartments that nothing could be seen by looking through the orifice in the door. At the same time there was a poor lunatic in each. A man who has grown old was committed to one of them in 1810 and had lived in it 17 years. An emaciated female was found in a similar apartment in the dark without fire, almost without covering, where she had been nearly two years. A colored woman in another, in which she had been six years; and a miserable man in another, in which he had been four years.

In the light of these conditions the commissioners recommended that since the hospital at Worcester had been prepared for the reception of the insane, the statute of 1797 and of 1816 be so modified that such patients should be committed to the hospital at Worcester instead of to any jail or house of correction, and that any insane persons who were confined in any jail or house of correction under order or sentence or decree of any court or any judicial officers should be removed to the state hospital and that "the power of enlargement" be given to boards of visitors, to the justices of the supreme judicial court and to the court of common pleas, and should be exercised upon the written application of any person. It also recommended that keepers of jails or houses of correction be prohibited under penalty from making profit contracts for the custody and support of insane people within the county buildings without the consent and approval of the mayor, aldermen of the City of Boston, or of the county commissioners of the respective counties. It also recommended that patients should be kept at the actual expense incurred for their support.

When the institution was ready for the admission of patients a proclamation was made by Governor Lincoln that from and after the date of his proclamation the lunatic who by virtue of the statute of 1797 and of 1816 had been sent to jail or the house of correction in future was to be committed to the State Lunatic Hospital at Worcester.

On January 12, 1833, Governor Lincoln issued a proclamation declaring the State Lunatic Hospital at Worcester to be legally open for the reception of patients, and seven days afterwards the first patient was received.

In 1836 the pauper lunatics of the City of Boston were confined in the House of Industry and the House of Correction at South Boston. An act of the Legislature of that year made it imperative upon the several counties of the commonwealth to provide suitable accommodations for those paupers within their limits who, being idiotic or incurably insane, were too unsafe, either to themselves or others, to be allowed to go at large, and who, on account of their condition and the crowded state of that institution, could not be received at the Lunatic Hospital at Worcester.

This resulted in the establishment of the Boston Lunatic Hospital, which was opened for the reception of patients on December 11, 1839. This institution was under the control of the City of Boston until its transfer to the state December 1, 1908. It is now known as the Boston State Hospital.

An act of the Legislature approved May 24, 1851, authorized the erection of a second state hospital for the insane, which was subsequently located at Taunton. It was opened in 1853, under the name of the State Lunatic Hospital at Taunton, which was later changed to Taunton State Hospital.

As a result of the labors of a commission, of which Dr. Edward Jarvis was chairman, authorized by the Legislature of 1854, for the purpose of ascertaining what further accommodations, if any, were needed for the relief and care of the insane, the Legislature of 1855 appropriated $200,000 for an additional hospital to accommodate 250 patients. The new hospital was located at Northampton, and was opened in August, 1858. It is known as the Northampton State Hospital.

An act of the Legislature of May 20, 1852, authorized the building of three state almshouses to accommodate not less than 500 inmates each. The locations chosen were Tewksbury, Bridgewater and Monson.

In 1856 certain of the harmless and incurable insane were sent to the almshouse at Tewksbury, as they could be cared for there at a much less cost than at the lunatic hospitals. By an act of 1866 Tewksbury became an asylum for the harmless and incurable insane, the crippled, the epileptic, idiotic children, and for such other persons who, on account of their infirmities, were unable to support themselves. An appropriation made in 1874 enabled the insane to be cared for in a separate building.

In 1909 the name of the institution was changed to State Infirmary, Tewksbury, Mass., by which it is now known.

An act of the Legislature of 1866 added to the almshouse at Bridgewater the functions of a workhouse, to which could be committed so-called vicious paupers. By an act of 1886 provision was made for a building for the chronic insane at the State Workhouse at Bridgewater.

In 1887 the name of the institution was changed to State Farm, and in 1888 $60,000 was appropriated for the construction of a strong building for insane criminals. In 1895 the insane department of the State Farm was designated the State Asylum for Insane Criminals, which name was changed in 1909 to Bridgewater State Hospital. Since 1895 it has been devoted to the care of the criminal insane of the state.

Danvers State Hospital was established in 1873, but was not opened for the reception of patients until May 13, 1878.

An act of May 15, 1877, established a temporary asylum for the chronic insane to occupy the buildings which had belonged for 40 years to the Worcester Lunatic Hospital. The new institution was known as the Worcester Insane Asylum, and, although an individual institution, was under the management of the trustees of the Worcester Lunatic Hospital, but with a separate superintendent and staff. In 1909 the name of the institution was changed to Worcester State Asylum, and in 1915 to Grafton State Asylum, in accordance with the act of May 29, 1912, providing for the removal of the institution to its colony at North Grafton.

Westborough State Hospital was established by the Legislature of 1884 for the homeopathic treatment of the insane of the state. It was opened for the reception of patients on December 1, 1886.

The Massachusetts Hospital for Dipsomaniacs and Inebriates, later changed to Foxborough State Hospital, was established by the Legislature of 1889 and opened for the reception of patients in 1893. In 1905 its wards were opened for the reception of insane patients from other state institutions. In 1914 all the inebriates and drug cases under treatment at Foxborough were transferred to the newly created Norfolk State Hospital. The Foxborough State Hospital continues to receive transferred insane from other state institutions, but will shortly be made an admitting hospital for both sexes.

Medfield State Hospital was established in 1890 as an asylum for the chronic insane in Eastern Massachusetts and opened for the reception of patients on May 1, 1896.

In 1895 the Massachusetts Hospital for Epileptics was established for the care and treatment of 200 adult epileptics, and was endowed with the lands belonging to the State Primary School for Boys at Monson, originally one of the three almshouses established by the state in 1852.[1]

In 1910 the name of the institution was changed to Monson State Hospital and the provision that restricted admission to adults was removed.

Gardner State Colony, established for the care of the chronic insane by the Legislature of 1900, was opened on October 22, 1902.

Norfolk State Hospital, established in 1810, was opened on June 1, 1914, by the transfer of all inebriates and drug cases from Foxborough State Hospital, as has been already indicated. It is for the treatment of male inebriates and drug habitues and is under the supervision of the State Board of Charity.

In 1906 the State of Massachusetts established at Wrentham the Wrentham State School, for the care of feeble-minded children.

Since 1904 the state has provided for the care, control and treatment of all insane, feeble-minded and epileptics, also for persons addicted to the intemperate use of narcotics or stimulants, No county, city or town has a right to establish or maintain any institution or receptacle for the care and attention of insane people. The whole duty of caring for the insane is committed to the State Board of Insanity, consisting of three persons, one of whom at least must be an expert in insanity.[2]

[1] Tewksbury, Bridgewater and Monson.

[2] Prior to the passage of Chapter 762, Act of 1914, this board consisted of five persons, two of whom were required to be experts in insanity; they served without compensation, but were paid actual expenses in the discharge of their duties.

They are appointed by the Governor, by and with the consent of the Council, and any member may be removed for cause. One member is designated by the Governor as chairman, and one member is chosen by the board as secretary. All of the members are required to devote their entire time to the duties of the board. The chairman receives an annual salary of $5500, and the other members $5000. Of the members of the board just appointed under the act, one was appointed for a term of one year, one for two years and one for three years. Vacancies may be filled by the Governor with the consent of the Council.

The State Board of Insanity has charge of all insane, feeble-minded and epileptic persons and persons addicted to the intemperate use of narcotics or stimulants, the care of whom is vested in the commonwealth by law, and of all institutions or buildings now or hereafter owned or maintained by the commonwealth for the care of such persons. This does not include the Norfolk State Hospital or the Hospital Cottages for Children, which are under the control of the State Board of Charity.

The State Board of Insanity appoints its subordinate officers and fixes their compensation. It makes its own by-laws and reports annually to the Governor.

In these reports it is required to present properly qualified tabular statements of the receipts and expenses of the board of each of the state institutions under its supervision for the previous year, also estimates of expenses for the ensuing year and such suggestions and recommendations as may be considered essential to the best interests of all the persons under the control of the board. The board also is required to encourage scientific investigation and to publish from time to time a bulletin of the reports of scientific and clinical work.

It is also required to prescribe to the superintendents or managers of the several institutions in its supervision the forms of statistical returns and the periods of time to be covered by them.

The board has, in addition to general supervision, powers over all public and private institutions and receptacles for the insane, feeble-minded, epileptics, or inebriates. It may also, when so directed by the Governor, exercise the powers of the Board of Trustees in any way relating to the management of the institutions. The board has the same powers relating to state patients as the overseers of the poor in towns and counties for the relief of paupers.

The board also is required to inspect and approve all plans and specifications for new buildings which are to be used by the state as institutions coming under the supervision of the board. It further has the power to act as commissioners of insane, to investigate the institutions, and the condition of any person who is confined in an institution for the insane, public or private, at any place within the commonwealth, and if the board discovers that such person is not insane or can be cared for without danger to others, it is empowered to discharge such person. All questions about the supervision of inmates of penal, reformatory or other institutions of the commonwealth are to be referred to this board and determined by them.

The board must also prescribe the forms of applications, medical certificates or commitment required by law. It must keep a record of such commitment and admissions, and must secure compliance with the provisions of the law. If the board has reason to believe that an insane, epileptic or feeble-minded person, who ought to be in a state institution, is confined in the almshouse or other place of a public charge, or otherwise, it must cause application to be made to a judge to commit such person to the institution.

Each one of the state institutions is under the government of seven trustees, five of whom are men and two women, except in the case of the Foxborough State Hospital, where all the trustees are men. The period of service of the trustees of the State Hospital is seven years and their terms are so arranged that one person is appointed annually by the Governor. The trustees form a corporation and have general charge of the interests of the institution and are required to see that its affairs are conducted according to law, and that the by-laws and regulations for its government are established by them. They receive no compensation beyond the necessary expenses incurred in the performance of official duty. They are required to appoint a superintendent, with the approval of the board, and subordinate officers and as many medical officers as may be required. If the number of assistant physicians is more than two one of them shall be a woman. The superintendent and the assistant physician at the Westborough State Hospital are required to belong to the homeopathic school of medicine. The trustees are required to appoint two of their number to visit the institution monthly and the majority of them to visit the institution quarterly and the whole board semi-annually. They also are required to make an annual report to the Governor and Council, accompanied by an inventory of the list of salaried officers and all matters requiring attention of the Governor.

The State Board of Insanity may license a suitable person to establish or keep a hospital or private house for the care and treatment of the insane, epileptics and feeble-minded and persons addicted to the intemperate use of narcotics or stimulants.

The State Board of Insanity is required to divide the state into hospital districts, from which the insane, epileptics and feeble-minded may be assigned to the institution in the district.

The Governor has power to transfer any inmate of a state institution under the charge of the State Board of Insanity to another institution when in his judgment such removal is desirable. The State Board of Insanity may also similarly transfer patients from one institution to another. All commitment papers, together with abstracts of the hospital case record, are to be transmitted with him to the institution to which he is transferred. Private patients shall not be transferred except upon application of a legal or natural guardian of the person, and a voluntary inmate shall not be transferred except with a written request.

Any person in an institution, public or private, who is quiet and not dangerous, and who is not committed as a dipsomaniac or inebriate, may be placed to board in a suitable family or placed in the commonwealth or elsewhere at a weekly cost not to exceed $3.25 for each person and the bills shall be paid by the state. Such boarding-out patients shall be visited at least once in three months, and if upon visitation they are found to be abused, neglected or improperly treated they are to be returned to the institution or removed to a better boarding place. Permission is also given to the superintendent or manager of any hospital or receptacle to allow the inmates to leave the institution in charge of guardians, relatives or friends for a period not exceeding six months. If the patient does not do well the superintendent may terminate such leave of absence at any time and authorize the arrest and return of the patient. If the patient on parole is not returned at the end of six months he shall be discharged. No unrecovered patient who is known to have committed or attempted violence or who is likely to become dangerous to others can be discharged without such discharge being approved in writing by the State Board of Insanity.

On October 1, 1912, there were remaining in state insane institutions 795 private patients. Receipts for the fiscal year ending November 30, 1912, for the support of private patients at 13 state institutions, including the sane and insane departments of the Monson State Hospital, the inebriate and insane departments of the Foxborough State Hospital, the two schools for the feeble-minded, and also the insane state institutions, amounted to $247,735.08.

The Board of Insanity has a support department, which takes the history of each patient committed as a public charge, to determine if the patient has a claim upon Massachusetts for support, and whether any one liable under the law for support is able to pay. If the investigation shows that the patient cannot be made private, but is able to reimburse the state in part, the amount which can be paid is submitted to the board for its approval in accordance with Section 82, Chapter 504, of the Acts of 1909, which provides that the price of support of state charges shall be determined by the State Board of Insanity at a sum not exceeding $5 per week for each person. During the year 1912 the amount received at the 13 state institutions above referred to for reimbursements amounted to $126,756.34.

Classes Committed.—All insane persons except feeble-minded are entitled to admission to the state hospitals.

Legal Procedure in Commitment.—Commitment may not be made unless there has been filed with the proper judge or justice a certificate of the insanity of the person by two physicians nor without an order signed by the proper judge that he finds the person insane. The judge must see and examine the person if he deems it advisable and must certify to his residence. He may call in a third physician if he thinks it advisable.

A physician making a certificate of insanity must be a graduate of a legally chartered medical school, in actual practice for three years and for the three years last preceding, and be registered. His standing, character and professional knowledge of insanity must be satisfactory to the judge. He must have examined the person within five days. A copy of the certificate, attested by the judge, must be sent to the superintendent of the hospital, who in turn sends copies to the State Board of Insanity.

The judge may summon a jury of six men to hear and determine whether the alleged insane person is insane. The verdict of the jury is final.

The superintendent of any hospital may, without an order, receive and detain for not more than five days any person whose case is certified to be one of violent and dangerous insanity or of other emergency by two physicians qualified as provided by law.

If a person is found by two qualified physicians to be in such mental condition that his commitment is necessary for his proper care or observation, he may be committed to a state hospital for the insane or to the McLean Hospital, under such limitations as the judge may direct, pending the determination of his insanity.

Voluntary Patients.—The superintendent of any institution may receive any person as a voluntary patient who makes written application and is mentally competent to make it. A voluntary patient may not be detained for more than three days after having given notice in writing of his desire to leave.

Insane epileptics may be committed to the Monson State Hospital in the same manner as other insane persons are committed. Voluntary patients may also be received in this hospital if of such age and mental condition that they are competent to make application. No voluntary patient of the Monson State Hospital may be detained more than three days after notice in writing of his intention to leave.

Appeal from Commitment.—There is no provision for appeal from an order of commitment.

Cost of Commitment.—The expenses of committing and delivering an insane person are chargeable to the county.

McLEAN HOSPITAL.[1]

Waverley, Mass.

At the beginning of the nineteenth century Massachusetts had no hospital, either general or for the insane, although institutions had for some years been established in New York and Pennsylvania, while Virginia boasted the first, and, until 1808, when the insane of the New York Hospital were removed to a separate building, the only hospital solely for the insane, in her asylum at Williamsburg. There had been some agitation of the subject and one or two attempts had been made to found such an institution in Boston; the earliest in 1797, when William Phillipps devised $5000 towards the building of a hospital, afterwards increased to $20,000 by his heirs and paid to the trustees of the Massachusetts General Hospital Corporation. The circular letter, however, prepared in August, 1810, by Drs. James Jackson and John C. Warren was the first definite appeal to the public, and may be regarded as the beginning of the present Massachusetts General Hospital, of which McLean is a part. This circular sets forth at some length the need of a hospital for the sick and the insane, especially the sick and insane poor, for whom at that time there was no place except in the almshouse at Charlestown, where not more than eight persons could be cared for; the various town almshouses, or the jails, to which the "furious insane" were sent; the need of clinical instruction for medical students which such a hospital only could supply; and, finally, the obligation entailed upon the wealthy and influential to help their sick and suffering neighbors.

The response to this appeal was immediate, and in January following (1811) a charter was obtained from the Legislature. It incorporated James Bowdoin and 55 other citizens of the various towns of the commonwealth, under the name of the Massachusetts General Hospital, with power to hold real and personal estate yielding an annual income not exceeding $30,000, the same to be placed under the care of 12 trustees, four of whom were to be chosen by the Board of Visitors, which was composed of the Governor, Lieutenant-Governor, President of the

[1] By George T. Tuttle, M. D., superintendent.

Senate, Speaker of the House and the chaplains of both houses of the Legislature. A grant was made by the commonwealth of the "Province House Estate" (then valued at $20,000), upon the condition that within ten years an additional sum of $100,000 should be raised by private subscriptions. In return for the grant of this property by the state, the charter imposed upon the corporation the obligation of supporting a number "which shall at no time exceed 30" sick or insane persons chargeable to the commonwealth. This condition was afterwards modified to make the number of such patients depend upon the actual income derived from the Province House property, and finally, in 1816, was repealed because such provision tended to make of the hospital a pauper institution.

Province House had an interesting history. Built in 1679 by Peter Sargeant, nearly opposite the Old South Meeting-House on Washington (then Marlborough) Street, in Boston, it was purchased in 1716 by the Provincial Legislature for the residence of the royal Governors, and was used as such until the Revolution. After the separation of the colonies from England it became "Government House" and was held by the state until 1811, when it was presented to the Massachusetts General Hospital Corporation. In 1813 plans were made to remodel the house for a hospital and asylum, and a Mr. Hornby, of Newport, R. I., was selected to have charge of the proposed institution. This project was found to be impracticable, however, and in 1817 the estate was leased to David Greenough for a term of 99 years. He erected stores in front of the house and converted it to uses of trade. It later became a tavern, and figures in Hawthorne's "Twice-told Tales." In 1864 it was destroyed by fire.

The war of 1812 delayed the plans for building the hospital, but in 1816 the Board of Trustees instituted a house-to-house canvass and received such liberal responses that within a week $93,969 was subscribed, $43,997.47 of which was contributed specifically for the asylum. There were 1047 original subscribers.

Negotiations were at once opened for the purchase of a site suitable for an asylum for the insane, the need of which branch of the proposed hospital was considered to be more urgent than a general hospital. In December of 1816 the Joy, or Barrell, estate (known also as Poplar Grove and Cobble Hill) at Charlestown, was bought for $15,650.

This estate contained approximately 18⅓ acres. Here, on Cobble Hill, in 1775, General Putnam and Colonel Knox laid out a fort, which received the name of "Putnam's Impregnable Fortress." At the foot of the hill flowed a small stream, Miller's River, a tributary of the Charles, and for some years to come McLean Asylum did nearly all its transportation by water. Upon this hill, surrounded by trees and gardens, stood a colonial dwelling house built in 1792 by Joseph Barrell. Charles Bulfinch designed this mansion, which, enlarged and altered, was used as the administration house of the asylum for 77 years. In 1817 two three-story brick houses, known as the East Houses, accommodating 30 patients each, were built adjacent to this mansion, but on diverging lines from it. The Joy estate and the additional buildings and alterations prior to 1818 cost $89,821.16. The first patient was admitted October 6, 1818—a young man whose father thought him possessed with a devil which he had tried to exorcise with the rod. The trustees spent three hours discussing his case, but finally decided to receive him. It is recorded that he made a complete recovery, became a pedlar, and acquired a property of $10,000 or $12,000. At the end of the first year 13 patients had been admitted.

Until 1826 the Charlestown branch of the Massachusetts General Hospital was known simply as the "Asylum," to distinguish it from the "Hospital," which was opened for patients in 1821. It was officially named The McLean Asylum for the Insane on June 12, 1826, and as such was known until 1892, when it was re-christened McLean Hospital. The name of McLean was given to it in honor of John McLean, a Boston merchant, who in 1823 left the corporation $25,000 and naming it as his residuary legatee. Eventually the corporation received nearly $120,000 from the McLean estate. To further perpetuate his memory, the trustees commissioned Gilbert Stuart to paint his portrait, which was finished in 1825 and now hangs in the library at Waverley.

The first superintendent of the asylum was Dr. Rufus Wyman, elected March 23, 1818. During the 17 years of Dr. Wyman's superintendency several changes were made in the asylum. There was of necessity much pioneer work to be done and much remodelling of buildings to suit the peculiar needs of this asylum. Rooms for "the occasional seclusion of refractory boarders" were required, and accordingly, in 1822, five "strong rooms for raging female patients" were constructed, which were removed in 1836 when the new "cottage" for "female patients in seclusion" was erected. A similar addition to the men's department was built in 1826. This was the "lodge" or "retreat," a brick building of two stories, costing $22,700. During 1826-29 still further additions and improvements were made, to the amount of $91,822.33. These included the "lodge" referred to above; a new five-story building for men called the North Building, costing $65,000; a new roof for the mansion house, with an additional story in the middle and extensive repairs throughout; improvements in ventilation; the addition of a laundry and a new kitchen. No further additions appear to have been made until 1835, when $28,000 was voted to be used for a new building for women known as the Belknap House, named in honor of Miss Mary Belknap of Boston, who, in 1832, left the asylum a sum of nearly $90,000.

In the matter of the treatment of patients, from the first great stress was laid upon the "system of moral management" under which the asylum was conducted. The attendants were carefully chosen and were instructed to treat their patients with kindness and gentleness. In 1833 Dr. Wyman writes that "chains or strait jackets have never been used or provided in this asylum" and that "no attendant is allowed to put the smallest restraint upon a patient without the direction of the supervisor, who enters the fact in a book and reports it to the physician"; also that "no person is ever allowed to strike a patient, even in self-defence."

In the first report published by the hospital (1822), Dr. Wyman speaks of the advantage of occupation and diversion in the treatment of the insane, and says that the "amusements provided, as draughts, chess, backgammon, nine-pins, swinging, sawing wood, gardening, reading, writing, music, etc., divert the attention from the unpleasant subjects of thought and afford exercise both of body and mind." He further argues that regularity in meals, exercise, work and rest "have a powerful effect in tranquilizing the mind, breaking up wrong associations of ideas and inducing correct habits of thinking as well as acting." Outdoor exercise was insisted upon, and in 1828 the first carriage and pair of horses for the use of the patients were bought.

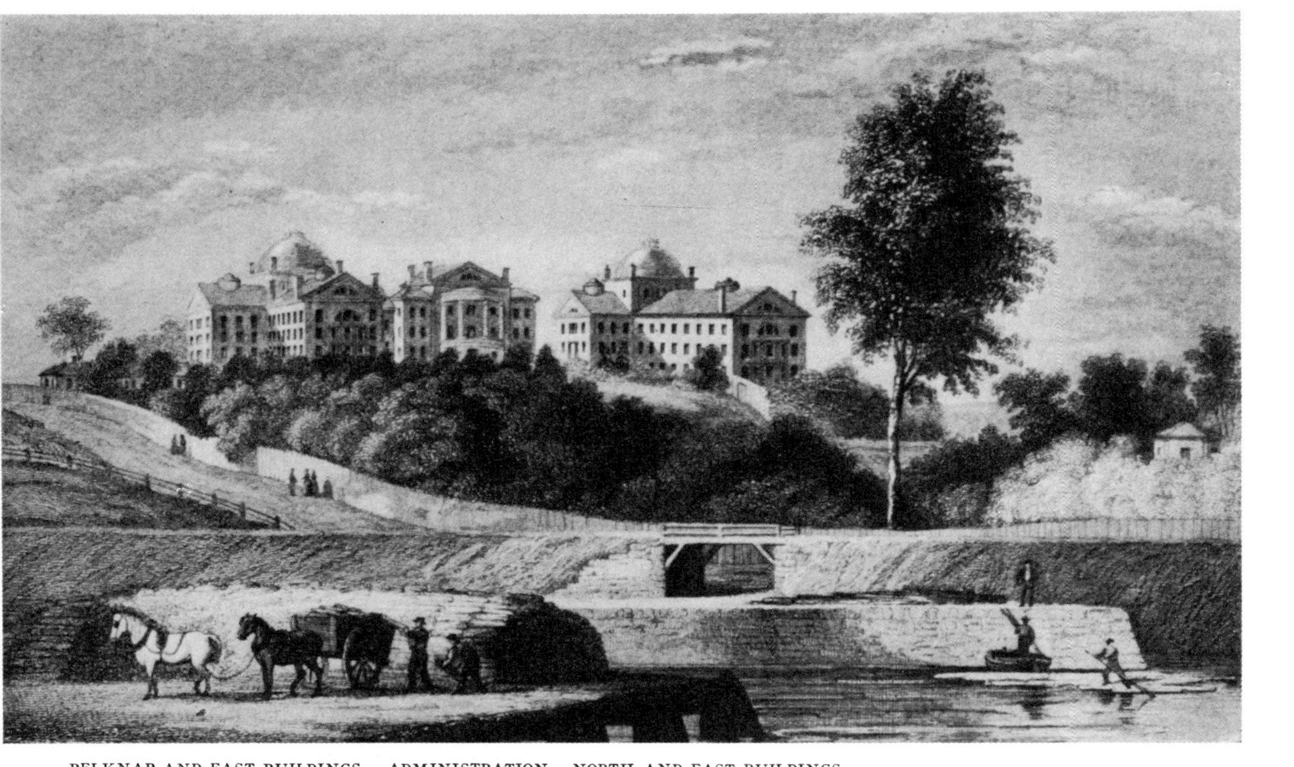

BELKNAP AND EAST BUILDINGS. ADMINISTRATION. NORTH AND EAST BUILDINGS.

McLEAN ASYLUM FOR THE INSANE, SOMERVILLE, 1844.

Dr. Wyman retired in 1835 and Dr. Thomas G. Lee, assistant physician, was promoted to the office of superintendent. Dr. Lee died in October, 1836, at the age of 28, while on a visit to his friend, Dr. Woodward, at the newly opened Worcester Asylum. He was a man of remarkable brilliancy and lovableness, and his one report is a unique document in its grasp of the needs of the asylum and in its moral force. So much impressed by it were the trustees that Dr. Lee's successor, Dr. Bell, was instructed by them to carry out the rules of government and suggestions of treatment therein outlined.

During the year 1835-36, under Dr. Lee's administration, the first piano and the first billiard table were purchased; the general library was started with 120 volumes; religious services were introduced; the "Belknap Sewing Society" for women patients was organized, and the carpenter shop for the use of the men patients was opened. One evening in each week those patients who were well enough were invited for dancing and conversation to the oval room at the administration house. The men patients worked on the farm and the women in the laundry and kitchen. Dr. Lee says in his report that "useful labor is the best employment," but his successor was obliged to abandon many of these industries, as the class of patients later received at McLean was not accustomed to such manual labor and refused to do it. Under Dr. Lee's administration six acres of land were purchased for $6000; the "strong rooms" before mentioned were removed, the "cottage" was built, and the "Belknap House" for 50 women begun.

The next superintendent of the asylum was Dr. Luther V. Bell,[1] one of the foremost psychiatrists of his day. During the 19 years of Dr. Bell's service the asylum grew in all directions. The Belknap House was finished in 1837, costing $43,000, with $2500 extra for furnishings; 12 new rooms were finished in the North Building in 1838 at a cost of $1490.79, and billiard rooms and attendants' rooms were converted into quarters for patients, making accommodations for 61 men patients in all; new rooms, at an expense of $1600, were built into the fourth story of the Belknap House in 1839, increasing the capacity of the whole asylum to 145 patients.

[1] See Biographies, Vol. IV.

By 1840, owing to the opening of the various state hospitals in New England, the social status of the patients in McLean Hospital had changed, making it necessary to provide more commodious and luxurious quarters for them in order that they might not miss their home surroundings. Therefore carpets, wall-paper, mirrors, mantels and better furniture were introduced, and in order that still further luxuries might be available, in 1850 William Appleton, president of the corporation, donated $20,000. To this gift was added the bequest of $20,000, received in 1839 from Joseph Lee, of which a separate investment had been made and which in 1851 exceeded $45,000. With these two gifts two houses for men and women, accommodating eight persons each and providing a suite of sitting room, bed room and bath for each patient, were begun in 1850 and finished in 1853. By the desire of the Lee family Mr. Appleton's name was given to these houses, and at their suggestion the North Building, for which the name of Lee had been proposed, was officially changed to Dix Ward, in honor of Miss Dorothea Dix.

The ventilating and heating plants were completely made over in 1848, hot water heating being introduced. According to Dr. Bell, McLean Asylum was the first institution for the insane in the country to try this method. Cochituate water from Boston was brought into the asylum under the railroad tracks in block tin pipes in 1851 and gas was introduced in 1854. New bowling alleys and billiard rooms for men and women were provided in 1855; also in the same year six rooms and a corridor below the dome in the North Building were removed and made into one large dormitory for 10 or 12 patients.

As may be gathered from the record of these alterations and additions, McLean Asylum had begun to outgrow its quarters. In 1844, for the first time in its history, patients were refused admission for want of room, and in 1852 more were turned away than were admitted. As early as 1839 Dr. Bell had foreseen this situation and had then proposed several schemes by which the number of patients could be limited. The one which was adopted was an increase in the rate of board.

The rates at first charged in the asylum ranged from $2.50 to $5 per week. These rates gradually increased. In 1827 the Visiting Committee reported that the rates should never be less than $3 nor more than $12, but later they were made sometimes as low as $2 and as high as $20 a week; at that time the expenses of the asylum were about $18,000 a year. In 1839, in the effort to relieve the overcrowded condition and limit the number of applications, a rate was made of not less than $4.50 for persons outside the state and $3 for those from Massachusetts. It was then estimated that one-third of the patients admitted to McLean came from other states.

In 1832 the opening of the State Asylum at Worcester, and in 1839 of the Boston Lunatic Asylum, freed McLean from a large number of her lower-rate patients, but the new asylums founded during this period in the other New England States drew away many of those who had paid higher rates. To meet expenses and not turn away desirable patients who could not afford to pay even the $3 rate, William Appleton gave $10,000 in 1843 and Samuel Appleton added another $10,000 to this fund in 1854. In 1844 there were reported 30 patients who paid only $1.50 a week; in 1846 $500 from the Belknap fund was placed at Dr. Bell's disposal for poor patients.

From its earliest days McLean Hospital has done much for charity. There has usually been a larger number of patients in the hospital who pay less than the actual cost than of those who pay more, and it has been, and is, the policy of the trustees to apply the excess of income from the latter to meet the expenses of the former. Should a surplus occur at the end of the year it is devoted to the other department of the corporation (the Massachusetts General Hospital) to help meet the expenses of its non-paying patients.

Of the 170 patients in the asylum at the end of the year 1847, 153 paid $5 a week or less; the expenses for that year are reported as being $32,500. In 1864 the cost per patient is computed at $9.77 and the rates were again raised. In 1875 the average cost was $21.07, with the expenses increased to $165,000. In 1912 the average cost per patient was reckoned as $25 and the expenses for the year amounted to $359,038.15.

The different railroads now merged into the Boston and Maine system began to encroach upon the asylum grounds in 1837. Various law suits resulted, and from 1837 until the removal of the hospital in 1895 to Waverley, when the entire property was sold to the Boston and Lowell Railroad, there were frequent struggles with the railroads. In 1871 the Boston and Lowell took a strip of land through the front of the asylum grounds across the main avenue. The final result was that the asylum was virtually situated in the midst of a large freight yard, being entirely surrounded by tracks. Moreover the neighborhood grew further undesirable because of adjacent factories, pork-packing establishments and cheap tenements.

After his first visit to Europe in 1840 Dr. Bell was more than ever interested in the new science of psychiatry. In 1843 he wrote an analytical summary of his experience during the preceding eight years from a medical point of view, in which his discussion of the causation, classification and treatment of insanity was well abreast of his time.

His ideas on restraint and non-restraint are set forth in this report and also in the earlier one of 1840 and the later one of 1855. Although not a believer in absolute non-restraint, he says in 1840 that very little restraint is used at McLean and that " for some years the average number of patients under the restraint of leather mittens has not exceeded one per cent, and often week after week elapses without a single instance."

For the first 16 years of McLean Asylum the superintendent was the only physician employed, though a medical student acted as apothecary with some duties on the wards. The first assistant physician, Dr. Thomas G. Lee, of Hartford, Conn., afterwards superintendent, was appointed in May, 1834, at a salary of $700. In April, 1854, it was decided that an additional physician was needed, and Dr. Ranney, of Butler Hospital, was engaged at a salary of $600. A third assistant was appointed in 1887, and junior assistant physicians have been employed since 1897. Medical students acted as apothecaries until 1880 and as internes with more important medical duties, but without money compensation, from 1880 to 1897.

In those early days the superintendents and assistant physicians devoted themselves to a greater extent to the entertainment of their patients than they do at present. They ate with them, drove with them, worked and played with them; they rarely absented themselves from the asylum. No vacations were given till 1873, when it was voted that each member of the staff should be allowed

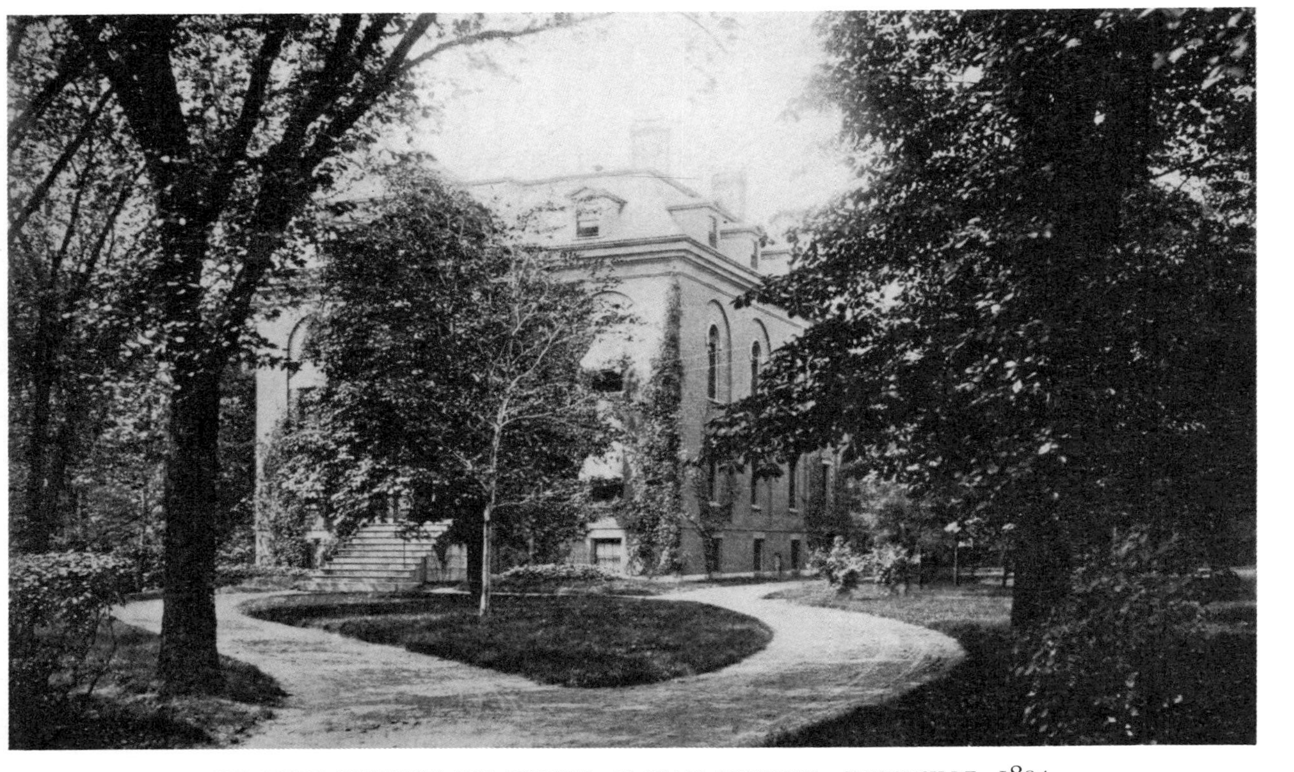

APPLETON BUILDING FOR WOMEN, McLEAN HOSPITAL, SOMERVILLE, 1894.

two weeks during the year. Previous to this, upon very rare occasions, leave of absence for a week or two was asked and granted. The Visiting Committee of the trustees also took a serious view of their duties and made it a point to see personally each patient in the asylum once a week, checking his name off a prepared list.

The nurses of that time were for the greater part school teachers. In 1843, with 150 patients, 25 nurses were considered "a very liberal number of attendants."

In his report for 1848 Dr. Bell mentions the fact, not generally recognized at that time but since become of national importance, that other countries were sending over their vagrants, paupers and insane and casting them upon our shores to rid themselves of their care.

By 1847 the asylum was full, with 173 patients, and only two-thirds of all who applied could be admitted. In his report for 1848 Dr. Bell states that there are 184 patients in the asylum and that "the architecture is hopelessly inadequate" to accommodate that number. Accordingly, in 1852 he began to advocate building another asylum and using one for men and the other for women. Meantime the number of patients increased, and in 1852, with comfortable accommodations for 160 patients, there were at times 210 crowded into attics, dormitories and the fifth stories. The external dimensions, with the exception of the two Appleton houses, just finished, were the same as in 1837, when there were one-half as many patients.

Dr. Bell resigned December 31, 1855, and Dr. Chauncey Booth,[1] who had filled the position of first assistant physician for 13 years, was appointed in March, 1856, to the office of superintendent. Dr. Booth had suffered for many years from tuberculosis; later on Bright's disease developed. Because of his serious condition, in November, 1857, Dr. Bell was recalled to take charge of the hospital, and upon Dr. Booth's death, January 12, 1858, was desired to remain until his successor should be appointed. He therefore continued to act as superintendent until March, 1858.

Dr. John E. Tyler[1] was the next superintendent, being appointed in 1858 and serving till 1871.

[1] See Biographies, Vol. IV.

Dr. Ray was temporary superintendent from July to October, 1871, before the appointment of Dr. Tyler's successor.

The 13 years of Dr. Tyler's administration were noted for the continued encroachments of the railroads, the enlargement of the asylum grounds, and the building of the new cottage and Bowditch House for excited patients.

In his second year of office Dr. Tyler asked for and received a regular appropriation of $300 for the general library, which appropriation continues to the present day. He devoted a great deal of attention to the amusement and diversion of patients in the way of weekly entertainments, sleigh rides, singing classes, an orchestra composed of men patients, drawing and French classes for the women and the like. Believing thoroughly in the idea that bodily infirmities influence the mind for ill, he engaged Dr. Dio Lewis as gymnastic teacher in 1860. Of an extremely religious temperament himself, he encouraged the wave of religious revival which swept over the institution in 1858, and in 1867 succeeded in getting a chaplain appointed—the Rev. David G. Haskins.

In 1860 five acres of land were bought adjoining the northeast boundary of the grounds and a release of some restrictions on the land originally acquired was secured. In 1862 the Joy and Woodworth estates were added (the former costing $15,000) and in 1867 the Barrell Farm, leased for many years, was bought for $20,000. In 1864, the Cochituate water supply being insufficient, the institution was connected with the Charlestown water works, then just completed.

Perhaps the greatest achievement of Dr. Tyler was the planning and erection of the new cottage for excited women, begun in 1860 and finished in 1862, and the Bowditch House for excited men, finished in 1865. For the building of the latter, $44,500 was raised by public subscription within four weeks. It was named for Nathaniel I. Bowditch, for many years secretary of the Board of Trustees.

In 1866 a large sum of money was expended for repairs and improvements; the grounds were graded and improved and the farm buildings removed from their former close proximity to the front entrance and repaired.

Upon Dr. Tyler's resignation in 1871 and the resignation at the same time of his first assistant, Dr. James H. Whittemore, Dr. George F. Jelly, second assistant physician, was appointed superintendent, which office he held for eight years.[1]

The eight years of Dr. Jelly's term of office as superintendent were years of retrenchment in all departments. The trustees had decided in 1871 that, owing to the continued encroachments of the railroads and the other objectionable features of its location, the asylum must be removed, and, therefore, for the next few years practically no repairs, alterations or improvements were made. In 1875 107 acres of land on Wellington Hill, Belmont (Waverley), were purchased for $75,000. In 1878 the trustees entered upon negotiations to sell the Somerville property, and in 1880 the Fitchburg Railroad bought 23 acres of their land for $70,000, which, with damages awarded from various law suits, created a fund of $122,076.30 for the new hospital buildings at Waverley.

In 1879 Dr. Edward Cowles was appointed superintendent to succeed Dr. Jelly, Dr. Frank W. Page acting as superintendent from July until December of that year.

Dr. Cowles came to McLean with the experience of 16 years in the army and as superintendent of a large city hospital behind him. He at once proceeded to make of the asylum a distinctly modern hospital. In 1880, his first year, the bars were taken off some of the windows and unobtrusive screens were put in. The following year he tried the experiment of unlocked doors between the wards of some of the buildings for convalescent patients; the women nurses on the men's side introduced by Dr. Jelly were increased to four; ward maids were employed, and visitors were admitted freely to the patients.

The same year (1881) was the first in which patients were admitted voluntarily to the hospitals, and McLean had one such. In 1882 there were 11 voluntary admissions and in 1883 33. Since January 1, 1883, when the admission of patients on the voluntary basis had become an established custom, 43.5 per cent of all admissions have been voluntary.

In 1882 the McLean Hospital training school for nurses was established, the first formally organized training school in a hospital for the insane in the world. The "attendants" were called

[1] See Biographies, Vol. IV.

"nurses" and put in uniform; a superintendent of nurses, Miss Mary F. Palmer, was appointed; a two-years' course of lectures and clinical work was laid out. The first class to graduate was that of 1886, when 15 women received their diplomas; the same year saw the formation of a class of men, and in 1888 20 women and four men were graduated. In the 30 years of the school (1882-1912) 708 nurses have been graduated—458 women and 250 men.

In 1884 Miss Palmer resigned as superintendent of nurses and Miss Lucia E. Woodward was appointed in her place, and held that position until her resignation in the fall of 1912. Miss Woodward came to the asylum as an attendant in 1864; was made supervisor in 1870 and superintendent of nurses in 1884, having previously spent some months in the training school for nurses at the Boston City Hospital. For 48 years Miss Woodward was identified with McLean Hospital, and the success of the training school owes much to her personality.

As the removal of the hospital from Somerville to Waverley was delayed from year to year, it became absolutely necessary to make alterations and repairs. In 1886 accommodations were made for 14 women nurses in a large dormitory under the dome of the Belknap House, and in 1888 changes were made in the cottage; there were minor repairs till 1892, when the buildings at Waverley were at last begun. In that year the trustees bought a house and barn at Waverley for $8000 and voted to erect on the land previously acquired there two buildings for patients—the Belknap and Appleton houses for women, and the stable, appropriating for these buildings $288,622. In 1893 the Upham Memorial Building, gift of George P. Upham, was begun.

On May 14, 1894, the Upham Memorial House was formally presented by its donor to the trustees, and on October 1, 1895, the new McLean Hospital, offering accommodations for 180 patients, was open for inspection. The entire plant to date (1912) cost $1,395,404.29 and includes the Pierce Building (administration house), the Upham Memorial, the Belknap, Proctor and Bowditch houses for men; the Belknap, East, Appleton and Wyman houses for women; the stable, laboratories and various service buildings. In the following year the two gymnasiums were finished and the Hope Cottage, built by Mrs. Sarah S. Matchett.

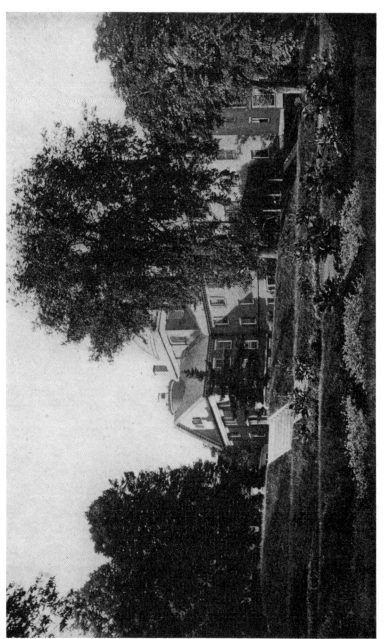

NORTH AND EAST BUILDINGS, McLEAN HOSPITAL, SOMERVILLE, 1894.

The new hospital is built on the cottage plan, with houses quite widely separated, but with corridor connection, and located as far as possible with reference to view and sunlight in the patients' rooms.

The first patients were transferred from Somerville to Waverley in April, 1895—two women to the Appleton and one man to the Upham House. Gradually others were brought over, a few at a time, until the final transfer November 15, 1895. On November 16 the grounds where the asylum had been started 77 years before were delivered to the Boston and Lowell Railroad.

Dr. William Noyes was appointed pathologist in 1888, and in 1889 the trustees appropriated $600 for the development of the pathological department. Dr. William W. Gannett, of Boston, had served as pathologist for several years, and aside from his other duties had given instruction to the medical staff. Dr. Noyes, besides acting as pathologist, began research work in connection with the patients and was the pioneer in the establishment of a clinical laboratory. He resigned in 1893 and Dr. August Hoch was appointed in his place. Under the latter's leadership Kraepelin's classification of mental disease was adopted, case-records were kept in a much more scientific manner, and cases were studied and compared and research work was carried on. Dr. Hoch resigned in 1905, when he was appointed assistant physician at Bloomingdale Hospital, White Plains, N. Y., and Dr. Frederick H. Packard, junior assistant physician, who had studied with Dr. Hoch, took his place. In December, 1909, he exchanged positions with Dr. E. Stanley Abbot, then first assistant physician.

The chemical laboratory was established in 1900 and Dr. Otto Folin was appointed chemist, in which capacity he served until 1908, when he was elected professor of biological chemistry in the Harvard Medical School. During this time extensive researches in physiological chemistry were carried on, new methods of analysis were devised, and many important investigations and valuable contributions to science were made by Dr. Folin, which gave him an international reputation. He was succeeded by Mr. Charles C. Erdman.

The psychological laboratory was opened in 1904, with Dr. Shepherd Ivory Franz at its head. Dr. Franz did much valuable work in physiological psychology during the two years he remained at McLean. Upon his resignation in 1906 Dr. F. Lyman Wells succeeded him. Dr. Wells has devoted his attention to experimental and abnormal psychology.

In 1899 hydrotherapeutic apparatus was installed at a cost of $10,000.

One of the pleasantest features of the institution is the collection of paintings in the art room, which was started in 1898 upon the suggestion of a former patient. While it began as a loan exhibition, many pictures have since been given to the hospital.

In 1903 the trustees of the hospital voted that the medical superintendent and the first and second assistant physicians "shall be retired upon reaching the age of 64 years, and if so retired after a service in the hospital of not less than 14 years they shall receive thereafter a retired salary equal to 60 per cent of the salary they received at the time of their retirement."

Accordingly, Dr. Cowles, having reached this age limit, was retired in December, 1903, carrying with him the loyal affection of all who had been associated with him in his work.

Upon Dr. Cowles' retirement Dr. George T. Tuttle, who had been associated with Dr. Cowles as second and then first assistant physician for 25 years, was appointed medical superintendent, taking office January 1, 1904.

At the same time a change was made in the administration of the corporation, whereby the Massachusetts General and the McLean hospitals were combined under one administrative head, responsible for the finances of both hospitals and holding the purchasing power. The various mechanical and industrial departments were merged so as to combine the greatest economy with the greatest efficiency. Dr. Herbert B. Howard, resident physician of the Massachusetts General Hospital, was appointed administrator and served until 1908, when he was succeeded by Dr. Frederick A. Washburn.

Since 1904 three new houses have been built—the Samuel Eliot Memorial Chapel, dedicated May 31, 1906; Codman House, named for Edward Codman, from whose bequest it was erected in 1906, and a single-story cottage for one patient, begun in 1912.

All the houses have been redecorated and partially refurnished; both gymnasium buildings have been thoroughly renovated and made more comfortable and attractive, and a recreation room for

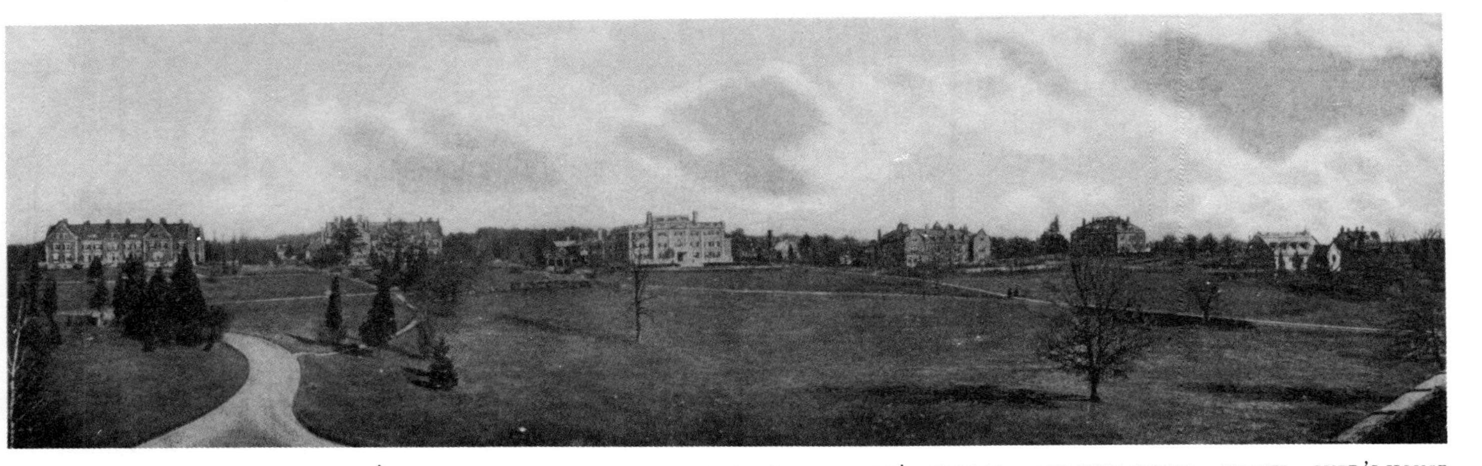

PROCTOR HOUSE. MEN'S BELKNAP. PIERCE BUILDING. WOMEN'S BELKNAP. APPLETON HOUSE. CHAPEL. SUPT.'S HOUSE.

McLEAN HOSPITAL, WAVERLEY, 1916.

Proctor House patients fitted up in the basement of the men's gymnasium. The original library room was refurnished in 1908, and in the following year the large front room known as the "Trustees' Parlor" was added.

The Wyman House for excited women was remodelled in 1908-09, the ventilation and lighting improved and a one-story wing added containing two rooms for continuous warm baths.

The Bowditch House for excited men was altered along similar lines but more extensively. Upon the addition of the Codman House, which added 36 to the number of women patients, the proportion of excited women admitted to the hospital was increased to a number greater than Wyman House could accommodate. Therefore the lower floor of the East House was reconstructed to adapt it to the care of this class of patients. Partitions were taken out, improving the ventilation and lighting, and an addition built containing service rooms, two rooms for patients and two rooms for continuous warm baths.

Much attention has always been paid in this hospital to physical exercise in the treatment of patients. To promote this, a static machine, a mechanical vibrator, and a set of Zander apparatus were installed in connection with the baths in the gymnasium building for women in 1904; a golf course of nine holes was laid out and is kept in good condition; three tennis courts have been built, and all forms of outdoor exercise encouraged.

The importance of various forms of diversion, and especially of manual occupation, has been recognized in this hospital from its very beginning. As early as 1822 Dr. Wyman writes of their value, and Dr. Bell, in 1839, says that "the experiment of mechanical labor was here first introduced, and the safety, expediency and immense utility of putting tools into the hands of the patients entirely and satisfactorily decided." Although later, owing to the class of patients received at McLean, mechanical and agricultural labor was abandoned for "some form of busy idleness," yet each superintendent has done his share in developing this method of treatment. For the men, as long ago as 1836 the carpenter's shop was opened for their use and of late years woodcarving and cabinet making have been taught; while the women have had lessons in drawing and painting and have done various forms of fancy work. In 1910 two rooms in the women's gymnasium were prepared for industrial occupations of a somewhat different type; a teacher of handicrafts was engaged, and instruction is now given daily in basketry, leather work, lace making, weaving and other forms of industry.

Another important factor in the healthful diversion of the patients is the library, which was placed upon a systematic basis in 1904. During the nine years following about 3000 volumes have been added, making a total of more than 7400, and the circulation has increased from approximately 5000 books a year to nearly 8800.

In November, 1909, the hospital first received an annual bequest from the estate of Miss Sarah C. M. Lovering. Under the terms of her will this money was to be used "to promote the comfort and happiness of the inmates," and with it many substantial benefits have been obtained for the patients which otherwise they could not have had.

Scientific research work has been carried on in various laboratories and the medical library has increased to more than 5200 volumes. At present 85 medical and scientific periodicals are taken in connection with this library.

In the training school the course of study has been lengthened and improved. The term is now two and one-half years, with the privilege, for the women, of entering the training school at the Massachusetts General Hospital, taking an 18 months' course of study and receiving a diploma from that hospital as well as from McLean. The number of ward maids has been increased in order that the nurses might be released from drudgery and allowed more time for the care of the patients. Ward maids are now employed on all the men's wards.

More land has been acquired during the last nine years. In 1907 one acre with house and barn was bought; in 1908 71,800 square feet of land on Mill Street was purchased, also the "Brown Farm" of a little more than 56 acres, containing a spring which supplies all the water for the hospital. In 1909 a lot of land containing seven and one-half acres and a house on Mill Street was bought to provide a third residence for married physicians.

McLean Hospital, at the beginning of the year 1913, occupies an estate of 317 acres on the southwestern extremity of the

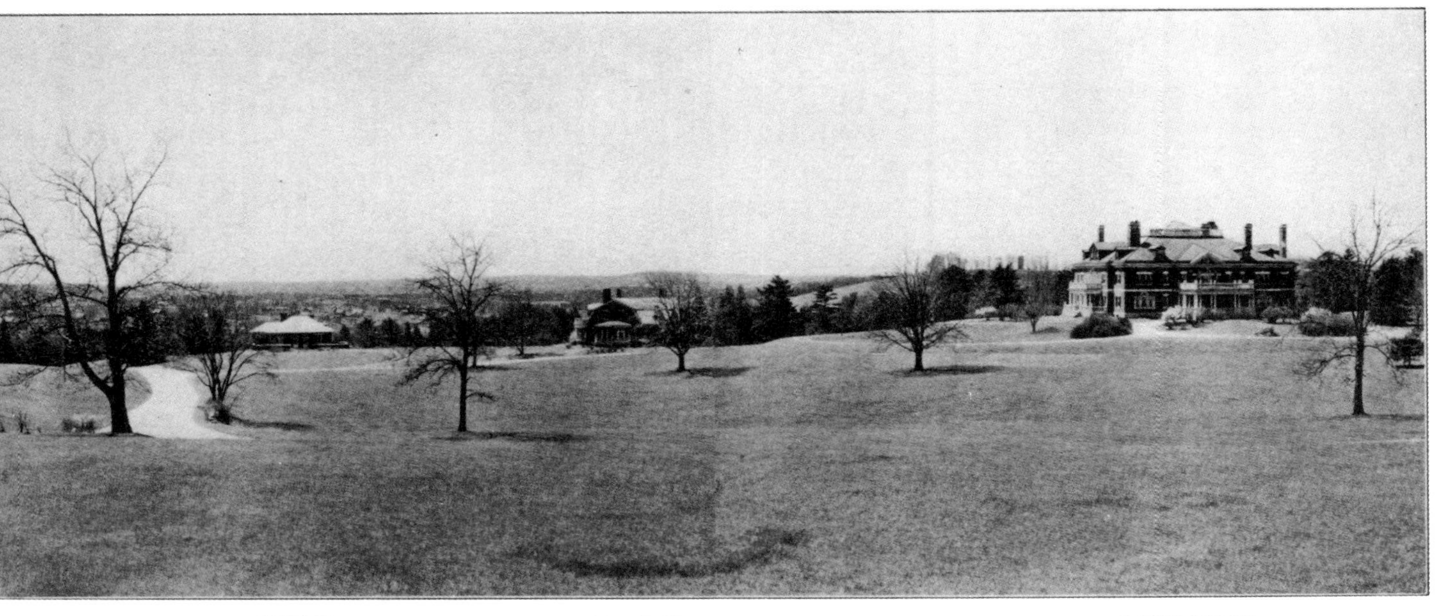

COTTAGE. HOPE COTTAGE. UPHAM HOUSE.

McLEAN HOSPITAL, WAVERLEY, 1916.

Arlington Heights range of hills overlooking the Charles River Valley. It accommodates 220 patients in eleven houses.

Patients are received according to the laws of Massachusetts, voluntarily or by commitment. The hospital is not large enough for reception wards, nor are they needed, for no one is admitted except by previous arrangement and after sufficient information has been obtained to make it reasonably certain that there is room in the house where the patient would properly belong. With opportunity for making many classes of men and women in houses quite widely separated, there is little difficulty in making a proper assignment of rooms at the time of admission. Each patient is given special nursing care during the first few hours, to lessen the shock of admission to a hospital for mental diseases and to obtain further information for the attending physician.

The hospital is administered by the Massachusetts General Hospital Corporation. The value of the entire plant, including service buildings, stable, farm, etc., is estimated at $1,914,157.52. The income from invested funds for 1912 amounted to $20,383.23. The cost of maintenance for the year 1912 was $359,038.15, and the income from the patients was $343,785.07. The average expense of each patient to the hospital is about $25 a week.

SUPERINTENDENTS.

Name	Years
Rufus Wyman	1818-1835
Thomas G. Lee	1835-1836
Luther V. Bell	1837-1856 1857-1858
Chauncey Booth	1856-1857
John E. Tyler	1858-1871
George F. Jelly	1871-1879
Edward Cowles	1879-1904
George T. Tuttle	1904-

FIRST ASSISTANT PHYSICIANS.

Name	Years
Thomas G. Lee	1834-1835
Edward Rowland	1835-1836
John R. Lee	1837-1839
John Fox	1839-1843
Chauncey Booth	1843-1856
Mark Ranney	1856-1865
James H. Whittemore	1865-1871 1873-1876
Orville E. Rogers	1871-1872
Charles F. Folsom	1872-1873
Charles E. Woodbury	1876-1877
James B. Ayer (temporary)	1876-1877
A. R. Moulton (temporary)	1877-
Frank W. Page	1878-1879
George T. Tuttle	1879-1904
E. Stanley Abbot	1904-1909
Frederic H. Packard	1909-

SECOND ASSISTANT PHYSICIANS.

Mark Ranney 1854-1856
Jerome C. Smith........ 1856-1861
J. Blackmere 1861-1862
James H. Whittemore... 1862-1865
Isaac H. Hazelton....... 1865-1867
James H. Denney....... 1867-1869
George F. Jelly.......... 1869-1871
Ferdinand A. Stillings... 1871-1873
Charles E. Woodbury.. 1874-1876
Wilbur F. Sanborn..... 1876-1879
Winfred B. Bancroft... 1879-1880
Frederick M. Turnbull.. 1880-1885
Henry C. Baldwin....... 1885-
James W. Babcock..... 1885-1891
Daniel H. Fuller........ 1891-1897
E. Stanley Abbot....... 1897-1898
Charles S. Little........ 1898-1902
Guy G. Fernald......... 1902-1908
Earl D. Bond........... 1908-1912
Theodore A. Hoch...... 1912-

THIRD ASSISTANT PHYSICIANS.

Horace M. Locke....... 1887-1889
E. Stanley Abbot....... 1893-1897
Charles G. Dewey...... 1894-1895
Frederick W. Pearl..... 1898-1913
Ray L. Whitney........ 1913-

PATHOLOGISTS.

William Noyes 1888-1893
August Hoch 1893-1905
Frederic H. Packard.... 1905-1909
E. Stanley Abbot........ 1909-
Emma W. Mooers (assistant) 1900-1903

CHEMISTS.

Otto Folin 1900-1908
Charles C. Erdman..... 1907-
Philip A. F. Schaffer (assistant) 1900-1903
Lucian A. Hill (assistant) 1903-1904
Christian Oestergren (assistant) 1904-1907

PSYCHOLOGISTS.

Shepherd Ivory Franz... 1904-1906
F Lyman Wells........ 1907-

JUNIOR ASSISTANT PHYSICIANS.

George E. Emery...... 1897-1898
Howard W. Beal........ 1897-1898
Edwin Leonard, Jr...... 1897-1898
George W. Blanchard... 1898-
Albert E. Loveland..... 1898-1899
Harry W. Miller....... 1898-1900
Charles B. Dunlap...... 1898-1899
William G. Ward........ 1899-1900
Guy G. Fernald........ 1899-1902
Martin J. Cooley........ 1900-1903
Frederic H. Packard..... 1902-1905
Albert E. Steele......... 1902-1903
William F. Roberts..... 1903-1905
Gilbert V. Hamilton..... 1905-1907
Ralph C. Kell........... 1906-1908
Frederic B. M. Cady.... 1907-1908
Earl D. Bond........... 1908-
Edmund M. Pease...... 1908-1912
Howard T. Child....... 1909-1910
Clarence M. Kelley...... 1910-1914
Henning V. Hendricks.. 1911-1912
Clifford G. Rounsefell.. 1913-
Carl F. Vernlund........ 1913-1914
Charles M. Flagg....... 1914-1914
Carl B. Hudson......... 1914-1914

MEDICAL STUDENTS.

Walter J. Norfolk	1872-1874	Lucius J. Curtis	1876-1877
Wilbur F. Sanborn	1874-1876	Charles F. Denny	1877-
Charles P. Bancroft	1875-1876		

INTERNES.

Royal Whitman	1880-1882	E. Stanley Abbot	1890-1891
Henry F. Adams	1881-1882	Edward M. Foote	1890-
George C. Shepherd	1882-	Charles D. Young	1890-
George E. Thompson	1882-1883	George W. Fitz	1890-
Asbury G. Smith	1882-1883	Gilman D. Frost	1890-1892
Israel P. Dana	1883-1884	Walter E. Sawyer	1891-1892
Joseph H. Potts	1883-1885	Follen Cabot, Jr.	1891-1893
Edward B. Lane	1884-	Charles B. Stevens	1892-1893
Alanson J. Abbe	1884-1885	George A. Harlow	1892-1893
James W. Babcock	1885-	Abel A. Davis	1892-
Horace M. Locke	1885-1886	Edward P. Starbird	1893-
Howard Lilienthal	1885-1886	Frederick W. Pearl	1893-1894
Edward M. Greene	1886-1887	Cleon M. Hibbard	1893-1895
Warren R. Gilman	1887-	Harry L. Houghton	1893-
Addison S. Thayer	1887-1888	Henry P. Lovewell	1894-1895
Albert C. Stannard	1888-	Joseph A. Capps	1894-1895
John H. Huddleton	1888-1889	Edward N. Libby	1894-1895
Joel E. Goldthwaite	1888-1889	John P. Torrey	1895-1896
Daniel H. Fuller	1889-1890	Fred. G. Burrows	1895-1897
Arthur C. Jelly	1889-1890	Arthur R. Perry	1895-1896
Frank B. Mallory	1889-1891	George E. Emery	1896-1897

THE LABORATORIES OF THE McLEAN HOSPITAL FOR RESEARCH IN PATHOLOGICAL PSYCHOLOGY AND BIOCHEMISTRY.[1]

Research in the pathology of mental disease has a history of peculiar interest; progress has been indirect and difficult in this branch of the medical sciences because of both favoring and conflicting influences. In modern psychiatry laboratory investigations were first employed to find in anatomical pathology explanations of mental disorders. Great progress has been made in the 70 years since Griesinger published his work on mental disease. During the first 20 years of that period he was the first to establish psychiatry upon the basis of scientific research and pathological principles. During the next 20 years several contributing movements, having their genesis in the advancement of general medicine, gained headway or had their inception; in America, a new interest arose in pathological investigations in institutions for the insane, and among them the plan was formed at the McLean Asylum (Hospital after 1892) to add to the pathological laboratory two other laboratories in order to combine researches in physiological and pathological psychology and biochemistry with the clinical work. In 1889, after ten years of preparatory observation, under the inspiration of general medicine and the "new psychology," these combined laboratories were fully organized and equipped for beginning researches by the methods then available.

In the laboratory movement of the time the new combination here described was the outcome of definite concurring influences, which, with their sources, should be recognized for their historical significance. The McLean Hospital laboratories reflected contemporary trends leading to the momentous changes which are now revolutionizing ideas that have long dominated psychiatry; it is important to note what these changes have contributed to a stage of progress that has been slow in awakening the attention of alienists. In the asylums, as they were constituted in the decade of 1880-90, the medical service was concerned with a number of quite distinct major problems in theory and practice; these related to the methods by which explanations of mental disorder were sought in the findings of the pathological laboratory; the generally

[1] By Dr. Edward Cowles.

accepted psychological conceptions and formulæ descriptive of mental physiology and of mental diseases for their classification; the physical conditions associated with mental diseases and their causes with respect to the principles of general physiology and of general medicine; the practical methods of treatment of the different forms of these diseases.

The General Position of Psychiatry in America in its Theory and Practice, 1880-90.

The attitude of the alienists toward their problems was one of newly stimulated interest. Some of the difficulties met with and the obstructive effects of certain misleading contradictions in the formulations of the problems should be noted; they will appear in the following account of the McLean laboratories as an example of the general efforts toward progress. The purpose, course pursued and results accomplished can be better understood by indicating here the observations concerning the nature of the major problems that prompted the laboratory investigations. The alienists were subject, by general consent, to the claims of pathological anatomy as the master science in general pathology; they looked to it for a basis of scientific psychiatry, but it was hope deferred, and they remained under the reproach of being unscientific. Although the new science of neurology, claiming psychiatry as a part of itself, was then bringing much aid, yet within 20 years thereafter it reached one of its authoritative conclusions that "pathological anatomy is of more academic than practical interest to the psychiatrist . . . . the burden of our work should be away from morphology and more in physiologic lines." This of course did not deny the essential value of pathological morphology in association with these fields of investigation.

Mental physiology, with true explaining principles in the physical mechanism, was the immediate need of the alienists for the investigation of abnormal behavior, and the first step in "tracing back symptoms to structural changes in accordance with the principles of general pathology." Lacking such explanations and limited to descriptive classifications of clinical symptoms, the alienists avoided the speculations of academic psychology which gave little aid. Thus, in common with all the world, they adopted the general empirical conception of the intellect, feelings and will; and in terms of these conceptions they framed their descriptions of the mental activities. Twenty years prior to the time under consideration Griesinger was making the bequest of his conceptions of mental pathology universally followed in modern psychiatry; his formulations of the symptom-complexes of melancholia and mania still dominate our descriptions of melancholia as "states of mental depression," and mania as "states of mental exaltation."

These phrases condense one of the most fundamental and general concepts of psychiatric theory into two words, "depression" and "exaltation," used as physical metaphors for the contrast of the feelings of pain and pleasure, which present a true "oppositeness" of *quality* of feeling or emotion—both normal and morbid. But while "depression" always fitted melancholy states, "exaltation" was found to be far from constant in maniacal states and not to fit the physical facts; and the make-shift word "excitement" came into use in its motor sense. To-day we frame our descriptions around "depression" and "excitement," making a false differential of emotion and activity, which always seems to imply a *quantitative* contrast of decrease and increase; whereas, on the contrary, in the states of real physical depression with constant mental pain there is always increase of its intensity and often motor agitation, while in the states of excitement—of shifting emotion and motor activity—there are further real decreases of integrity of both mental and physical functions and descent to "deeper levels of destruction." Such are some of the contradictions in this slough of despond for scientific psychiatric thinking and experiment. There is no way of escape but to abandon it. It is an inheritance from the most primitive experiences of an ever-widening range of such concepts of the feelings, as of pleasure and pain, joy and sadness, hope and fear, as expressed in such figures of speech as exaltation and depression, being uplifted or downcast, and innumerable analogues of highness and lowness in the moral sense; thus have been drawn into the complex conceptions of the feelings the physical meanings of such ambiguous words.

There can be no change in the common usage of such picturesque analogies and physical metaphors; but in the present instance they are destructive and unfit. The remedy must be by passing from facile description to the explanatory level; and to the advancement of laboratory investigations in psychology, psychiatry and physiology are due the definite signs of emergence in recent years. In 30 years, since the beginnings of Wundt's psychophysic experiments to Pawlow's and Cannon's latest discoveries in the physiologic relations of protective bodily changes to emotional reactions, there has been a revolution of ideas through the contributions of physiology to psychiatry.

The physical conditions associated with mental diseases were of constant interest to the alienists; systems of classification were attempted, based upon the etiology of mental disorders as sequences of general diseases. This tended to aid in prompting the purpose of the laboratories which grew out of the conditions observed in the preceding ten years, showing the need of physiological investigations to explain the psychological problems. Some of the fallacies of the conceptions of them have been noted in the foregoing statements to show the reasons for the attempt to apply new methods. The attitude of inquiry is indicated by the position taken in respect to Griesinger's description of contrasting mental states before quoted. Beginning in 1885, and since then carried forward in annual courses of lectures and in projecting these laboratories, the view has been presented as the belief of many alienists that melancholia and mania constitute one disease, with stages declining to dementia. It was proposed two years later, in an unpublished paper on classification, to amend Griesinger's formulations to read "states of depression of feeling" and "states of derangement of intellect," for the reasons that while the persistent mental pain characteristic of the first stage reflects truly the bodily malaise, the second stage is characterized by graver derangements of thinking and unstable emotional states, showing their disordered relations with the bodily ill-being and the losses of functional power and control. This was known to have been essentially the position taken by Griesinger, but it can be better appreciated in the light of later understanding by newly studying his writings, which reveal his vigorous but unheeded protest against the immediate misinterpretation by his contemporaries of his psychological meanings. Limiting the present view of the situation to what it was in the decade prior to 1889, it can now be seen that he used the words "depression" and "exaltation" in their figurative sense, as did the contemporary alienists, psychologists and all the world besides, following the ancient and fixed usage. But he meant simply "mental pain" and the emotional contrast; he did not mean an oppositeness of "mental torpor" and "mental irritation"—an "increase" or "decrease" of something. Yet the psychiatric world still clings to the ancient, unscientific conception of a physical *something, up or down,* although the physiological investigations of the laboratories have been proving for 30 years that Griesinger was right.

The following narration of events will show the course of progress, and what was done with the ancient conceptions when the new psychology brought psycho-physic experiment into psychiatry.

The most significant indication of the attitude of the alienists of 30 years ago toward general medicine was their position with respect to the practical methods of treatment. They had been the leaders in the adoption of the " supporting treatment " for many years in advance of general medicine—a logical, though empirical, expression of their comprehension of the physiological principles of the energy concept. Here was the basis of the vogue of the neurasthenic concept developed in the science of neurology. This was the crux of the matter from which came the inspiration to research in the chemistry of nutrition. The " fatigue question " and the " nutrition question " were " believed to be of primary importance in psychiatry." Hence as an outcome the laboratory of biochemistry. The psychological laboratory was added by direct importation from the laboratory of Ludwig at Leipsic, through Dr. Stanley Hall and the department of psychology at The Johns Hopkins University. These preliminary comments have a certain historical interest; they are also needed not only to show the origins of this laboratory movement, but to state the problems with which it had to contend, and which essentially form the basis of the conclusions that emerge from the broader review of the whole matter.

The Organization of the Laboratories.

The new laboratories at the McLean Hospital were early attempts to combine the methods of physiological, biochemical and psychological experiment, under the principles of general medicine, in the clinical work in such institutions. The general progress made was noted in the annual reports; of special interest are those from 1888 to 1892, describing the establishment of the three laboratories, and a review of the work of the hospital in the reports for 1901 and 1902. Biological chemistry and physiological psychology were held to have an essential dependence upon each other. The conception of the chemical laboratory as a clinical aid in psychiatry had a longer incubation and was the direct expression of the neurasthenic concept, or, better, the energy concept. Here, as before noted, there was a direct sequence of events. From the time of the "supporting treatment" Griesinger's recognition of the principle of reduction of energy in the relation between melancholia and mania, the energy concept had been gaining its place of fundamental importance in general medicine, and has held it in the practice of psychiatry, though much obscured and mostly lost to sight in theory.

The aims of the combination of the laboratories were comprehensively stated in a report on the psychological laboratories in America, contributed to the *Année Psychologique* in 1894 by Dr. Delabarre, in which the McLean Hospital psychological laboratory and its equipment were described as follows:

> The purpose of establishing and developing the laboratory has been carried on under much difficulty, naturally due to the newness of the attempt to combine with psychiatry the other departments of scientific medical research. The pathology of the terminal stages of insanity must be studied as heretofore, and it is necessary to add that of the initial conditions which lead to mental disorder. Such studies must therefore be combined with physiological psychology in the attempt to determine the exact nature and causes of departures from normal mental function. Also in the dependence of these changes upon general physiological processes, and in order to take into account all the elements of vital activity involved, it is supremely necessary to study both physiological and pathological chemistry in their direct and indirect relations to mental changes. It will be seen by the foregoing report that the fatigue question, and its relation to auto-intoxication, is believed to be of primary importance in psychiatry. It is inevitable that progress must be slow in developing these several concurrent lines of inquiry; but the researches already begun are most interesting and promising, and encourage the hope that the work which is contemplated will so effectively combine them all as to yield worthy results.[1]

The laboratory, with its two purposes, was described by Dr. Delabarre as "the only one in America which united psychiatry and physiological psychology. In Germany there exists only one like it—that of Professor Kraepelin at Heidelberg. It attempts to combine the studies of the clinic and of neurology with those of chemistry on the one hand, and with those of psychology on the other."

[1] "Les Laboratoires de Psychologie en Amerique," by E. B. Delabarre, L'Année Psychologique, 1895; also "Laboratory of McLean Hospital," by G. Stanley Hall, Amer. Jour. Insanity, 1895.

In a lecture on "Neurasthenia" in 1891, and in other papers,[1] there is an extended discussion of the energy concept as it is involved in the successive reductions of functional capacity in neurasthenia, melancholia and mania, considered as stages of one disease—meaning that a *neurasthenic condition* underlies all of these phases.

The laboratories were under the direction of Dr. Noyes, appointed in 1888 and continuing till 1893, including that of pathological anatomy; and a seminary was organized by the medical staff for study in psychology and psychiatry. The equipment for psychological experiment was guided by that of Dr. Hall at Johns Hopkins University and at Harvard Medical School, aided by the counsel of Dr. Bowditch and Prof. James; the chemical work had the valuable advice of Dr. Wood and Dr. Chittenden. The direction of the three laboratories was continued by Dr. Hoch for nearly ten years, beginning in 1894, after six months' studies in Europe with Mosso, Wundt, Nissl and Kraepelin. The provision of ample rooms and equipment for research in the new McLean Hospital, opened in 1895, was justified by the early experience. The claim of the chemical laboratory to a place in clinical psychiatry was established by the investigations of Dr. Folin, who took charge of it in 1900, when he applied the methods of pure chemistry and gave it a recognized distinction. The development of the work as a whole was aided directly by the conceptions of the English physiologists. It was noted at the outset that the clinical questions were characteristically associated with causes producing neurasthenic conditions, and with recoveries through restoration of the general health and strength. As stated later by Dr. Folin, "the problem to be dealt with in such cases is very largely that of nutrition, and the nutrition question is fundamentally a chemical one; also that it is disorders of metabolism that have a large part in the derangements of nutrition and dependent functions of the nervous system; and it is to such derangements that disorders of the mental function may be due in many cases." The purpose from the first was to approach such problems from the side of general medicine and

[1] "Neurasthenia and its Mental Symptoms," Shattuck Lecture, E. Cowles, Amer. Jour. Insanity, 1891; "The Mental Symptoms of Fatigue," Trans. N. Y. State Med. Assn., 1893; also "The Problem of Psychiatry in the Functional Psychoses," Amer. Jour. Insanity, 1905. See also "The Mechanism of Insanity," *Ibid.*, 1889-91.

to determine "what conclusions can be reached concerning the important question whether any tangible relation between faulty nutrition or other faulty metabolism and different forms of mental disease can be established." This implies the study of the influence of functionally disordered bodily conditions and organic sensations causing alteration of the "sense of well-being" and "personality," and of the "sense of adequacy," producing obstructive interferences with the processes of feeling, thinking and doing. The reactions of the emotions were recognized, when first undertaking the joint investigations, as essential factors of the utmost importance, in "the changes in nervous reactions in health and disease, the relation of the mental element as to its interferences with these reactions, and the counter influence of bodily conditions upon mental states." The conclusion was drawn that "in acute neurasthenia and in true melancholia and mania there is always nutritional and toxic functional weakness, fundamentally, in the organism; it is from this that the influences arise which affect the conscious feeling and thinking, making these higher mental states the sensitive indices of the lower physical changes." [1]

[1] Op. cit. Neurasthenia and its Mental Symptoms, 1891. The quotation continues: "When all goes well with the organism and it is in a condition of unfelt equilibrium, the processes of thinking and feeling are adjusted, more or less logically, to the varying environment upon a basis of a sense of well-being and normal love of life. On the other hand, a morbid process may be started in these higher activities, in a previously healthy and strong organism; but until the organism itself suffers a change to the specified nutritional and functional weakness there can be no such mental symptoms as are being studied here. Normal mental activities cannot produce 'mental symptoms' except by first causing the characteristic 'weakness' somewhere in the physical basis of all of them."

It is of great historical interest in this connection that one who newly reads Griesinger's conceptions of more than 70 years ago may trace the substantial evidence throughout of their underlying continuance and growing force to the present time. The words he wrote in 1861 have lost none of their significance: "I would therefore beg the readers wherever doctrines, pages, and even chapters, occur similar, or nearly similar, to what they may shortly before have read in books or journals, simply to compare them with the first edition of this work which appeared in 1845." Describing the states of melancholia as most frequently appearing to be the direct continuation of some painful emotion dependent upon some external influences, he notes the cases without apparent moral causes in which it "does not originate as their direct continuation, but only shows itself after these affections have wrought considerable disturbance in the func-

In this view it was believed that all the operations, physical and chemical, of the nervous and mental mechanism, should be studied as being conditioned by the contributing and concurring activities in both fields, and as having a primary and necessary relation to the supporting energy. The conscious attitude of the moment, having its inseparable emotional factors, affecting both the mental response and the physical reactions, these in turn must condition, and may determine, a persistent affective tone, especially when of pathological intensity. "The phenomena of nervous life are the outcome of a contest between what we may call inhibitory and exciting or augmenting forces" (Foster, Physiology). Voluntary action is at all times the resultant of the compounding of our impulsions with our inhibitions (James).

The point of present interest is that these laboratories and their combination were simply outcomes of principles then generally recognized, but awaiting effective acceptance in psychiatry. The significant exception to this was that the energy concept which, having given psychiatry the leadership as its long-used practical guide for treatment, had gained only a slow and limited appreciation of its special physiological and biochemical import for mental diseases. The result followed that psychiatry has engaged itself in working out other trends of inquiry and has neglected the study of its most pregnant problem, leaving it to the physiologists and the chemists to be solved for us.

The Chemical Laboratory.

The chemical laboratory was the one first conceived to be a clinical need. Psychiatry was not yet ready for biochemistry 25 years ago, nor for explanations in disordered metabolism of morbid mental moods and activities; neither was organic chemistry yet able to offer practical aid to the mental clinic. But the principle being established and the way opened for its methods, the later

---

tions and nutrition of the nervous system, or have undermined the entire constitution." We have learned to distinguish neurasthenic conditions from the "hypochondria" of those days; Griesinger observed that the states of painful emotion may "proceed from a strong *feeling of bodily illness.*" Going further, he regarded the "states of mania as engendered by melancholia" and as a "still deeper destruction"; he never lost sight of the principle which is fundamental in all progress in the modern treatment of insanity.

history of these laboratories shows the somewhat indirect and obstructed path by which psychiatry is now coming to know its need. In the last 20 years there has been wrought a great transformation, culminating in the new conception of the psychopathic hospital. Dr. Folin gave new character to the expert application of pure chemistry to the problems of nutrition in psychiatry; his research work continued from 1900 to 1909, when, having an appointment in the department of biological chemistry in Harvard Medical School, he was succeeded by Mr. Erdmann; in connection with clinical pathology there was a steady advancement in the recognition and formulation of new and definite problems for chemical investigation. Established since 1900, there are now at least 14 other psycho-pathological laboratories in connection with institutions for the insane and defective in this country; in a few of them research in biochemistry is also included in their investigations, notably at Vineland by Dr. Goddard. It could not be learned at the time of the founding of its own chemical laboratory at the McLean Hospital that there was any other one of the kind in existence, in like institutions, aiming at a permanent association with the clinical work. The exception should be noted of the chemical laboratory of the new asylum at Claybury (1896), where the idea of Mott and Halliburton appears to have been to find what chemical changes took place in definite diseased tissues. Individual researches in such subjects were published prior to 1900, and under the influence of the later widely extended interest in pathological chemistry; but comparatively recent have been the efforts to discover metabolic abnormalities in the insane as a special problem by organized methods for prolonged investigation. It should be mentioned that in 1910 a laboratory of this kind was opened at the Munich Psychiatric Clinic, where the tendency of research is toward the study of changes in definite forms of organic disease. It can be said at least that the chemical laboratory at the McLean Hospital was an early attempt to carry out the "hospital idea."

The Psychological Laboratory.

The psychological laboratory, under the conditions which grew up around it, as we are now prepared to see, pursued a productive course with well-known results. We are brought here to a point of critical interest in the great change in psychiatry in America—

a movement still increasing in volume, though discarding much that is found wanting. The McLean Hospital laboratory typically illustrates some important factors in the general change. The psychological department, while pursuing its own special line of work in applying physiological experiment in abnormal psychology, had its course and development peculiarly subjected to collateral influences. To prove this one needs only to look through the brief summaries of work done, in the hospital reports, especially that of 1901 and the following years. The first of these concurrent and more or less controlling influences was in the clinical field, through bringing to this hospital the teachings of the Heidelberg school in 1897 as then developed, when Doctor Hoch was sent there for that purpose on his second mission. We know how these teachings spread and dominated psychiatric thinking in America. The greatest significance belongs to the fact that, on the one hand, the methods of physiological experiment had been brought years before through Stanley Hall direct from Leipsic, and his extended course of study in the laboratory of Ludwig, and moreover had been established here, coupled with concepts of biological chemistry; and that, on the other hand, certain methods of experimental psychology designed for the study of motor and intellectual function by measurement of time factors applied to psychiatry, came here later, also from Leipsic, by way of Heidelberg, but making no use of biochemical and little of physiological explanation. A great contribution to descriptive psychiatry was made by the doctrines of the Heidelberg school in arousing interest in descriptions of mental states. But they perpetuated with some changes of terms the long-accepted formulæ ascribed to Griesinger, except that Kraepelin passed wholly from the emotional criterion of Griesinger to that of activity by " increase or decrease " and " oppositeness," represented by " retardation " and " excitement." This appears to have led largely to the limiting of experimentation to reaction-time and motor effects, and to the insistence upon the analysis and classification of behavior thus differentiated into set clinical pictures and disease forms.

For the good of psychiatry, there should be noted in this connection the extraordinary fact that the extremes of divergence from the real teachings of Griesinger have grown out of the immediate misconception of them when they were first published, and against which he made formal protest; but this was disregarded to the effect of making him responsible for an interpretation of his conceptions that he never meant, but that has ever since dominated psychiatry.[1] Believing that these states of melancholia and mania represented simply successive degrees of disorder of the mental and cerebral processes to the " deeper destruction " of their functional integrity, he used the term " depression " clearly in the qualitative sense of mental pain, not confusing it with the notion of something less than normal in contrast with something in " exaltation " more than normal in a quantitative sense. To the soundness of his real conceptions, contemporary with the beginning of the last half-century, is due their vitality and lasting influence.[2] These should not be forgotten when we recognize the fact that the greatest of the factors of progress formulated in the energy concept,

[1] Griesinger, Mental Diseases, second edition, 1861: "In employing the term 'states of mental depression,' we do not wish to be understood as implying that the nature of these states or conditions consists in inaction and weakness, or in the *suppression* of the mental or cerebral phenomena which accompany them. We have much more cause to assume that very violent *states of irritation* of the brain and excitation in the mental processes are here very often the cause; but *the general result* of these (mental and cerebral) processes is *depression* or a *painful state of mind.* It is sufficient to recall the analogy to physical pain; and to those who imagine that they make things better by substituting '*cerebral torpor*' and '*cerebral irritation*' for 'depression' and 'exaltation' it may fairly enough be objected that in melancholia there is also a state of irritation."

[2] Richard Mead, Medical Precepts and Cautions, 1755: "Medical writers distinguish two kinds of madness . . . . but with this difference, that the one is attended with audaciousness and fury, the other with sadness and fear; and that they call mania, this melancholy. But they generally differ in degree . . . . sometimes take each other's place and undergo various degrees of combination." Among the leaders in modern British psychiatry Clouston wrote 30 years ago of the "Descent to Dementia" through melancholia and mania. Twenty years ago Bevan Lewis wrote of melancholia and mania: "Yet, fundamentally different as these mental states would appear to be, we have little doubt that the process of reduction is the same for both, but in maniacal states the dissolution is to a *greater depth*—the difference is one of *degree.*" . . . . "In mania we must recognize that the excitement of lower levels is one of disorderly, ungoverned license, indicative of the removal of the influence of higher controlling planes." Here are applied in psychiatry the physiological conceptions of Hughlings-Jackson; they are in harmony with Wundt's theory of functional capacity, and the teachings of Sherrington, which are having a notable influence upon modern thought.

with a steadily moving force toward culminating results, has been determining the long-impending revolution now going on in psychiatry. Its tendency to this in recent years has been simply a pervasive coordinating movement toward the principles established in general medicine, to which Barker refers with respect to the value of a functional conception of pathology; medicine becoming more scientific, classifications of "clinical types" are replaced by those of "a developmental or genetic character."[1] True to the genetic method are the new investigations and discoveries in experimental physiology and biological chemistry, proving the remarkable influences of the interdependence of mental and emotional states and physiological adaptations. The new knowledge of such normal reactions is of the utmost importance for psychology and psychiatry; interferences with normal mental reactions in the functional pathology of behavior demand the tracing back to the most fundamental of all the forces that act; there can be no action, however complex the "contest of forces," that is not conditioned by the degree of integrity of the potential energy. The new psychiatry must be founded upon such explaining elementary principles. Anatomical pathology gives us end results.

Proof of the foregoing statements appears in the operation of the concurrent influences that qualified the work of the laboratories here described. The second of these major influences in relation to the course of development of the psychological department was its immediate association with the biochemical research. This is a part of what is shown by the briefest outline of the later stage of progress and by the titles of papers published. The psychological laboratory was newly organized upon a special fund in 1904; under the direction of Dr. Franz, then appointed; it demonstrated the value of such research in pathological psychology through his qualifications as a trained psychologist and his experience in the teaching of nervous physiology. Continuing till 1908, he was then appointed to establish a like service at the Government Hospital

[1] Barker, L. F.: Methods in Medicine, Boston Med. & Surg. Jour., June, 1905: "As medicine has become more scientific, the mind has ceased to be satisfied with such descriptive classifications as the clinical symptoms and syndromes represent and with 'clinical types' set up, and is ever on the alert to replace them by classifications of a developmental or genetic character."

in Washington. His successor in the former service, Dr. Wells, has maintained its continuity and carried forward its development by his well-known original investigations. The record of the work done in the three laboratories indicates their stimulating influence as intimate adjuncts of the clinical service. Certain subjects of research show not only the local trend, but the general movement in psychiatry toward the conceptions of general medicine.

While psychiatry has been seeing the remarkable extension of interest from a rigid morphologic neurology on one side, to the extremes of speculative psycho-analysis on the other, it keeps to its course on the middle ground of the graver insanities where psychology and psycho-pathology are held to the stern facts of associated physical disorders. The laboratory movement, for the bringing together of the long-disjoined paths of progress of psychology and psychiatry, has a significant example in the present work of the combined clinic and three laboratories at the McLean Hospital, an environment in which academic psychology has had some years of continuous collaboration.

Some particulars of this combined service should be cited here to explain the conclusion to which this review is leading. "A constant attempt has been made to find and apply such psychological and other scientific methods as can be made practical." "A stage of transition in the general laboratory policy was reached when the former conventional methods of experimental psychology proved to be of limited usefulness; the earlier methods of the experimental study of motor and intellectual function by measurement of time factors tended to be outgrown." "In accord with the tendency of the time, a wider use of physico-chemical methods in biological research" was adopted; "attention was given to serological investigations," studies of "psycho-galvanic phenomena in relation to emotional reactions" were published. "The principles involved in the biological point of view in psychiatry" were applied; "new means were sought for experimental observation," the laboratories were extended and refitted to meet the new problems. In the later chemical work a method for the determination of the "surface tension of liquids for biological purposes" was published, and a "research on alkylamines" was concluded. "Experimental studies in association opened new fields of research, one of these being concerned with the use of a method of this nature in different forms and stages of the psychoses, and the other with "the traits of personality which it reflects among individuals in general." "In the development of a method for the systematic observation of the personality, susceptible to quantitative treatment, emphasis was laid upon the actual mental difficulties to which the individual is subjected and their proper means of adjustment." "Recognizing the most hopeful tendency in psycho-pathology and normal psychology as founded on the conception of the mind as an adaptive mechanism, an experimental method is needed for the estimation of the adaptive reactions."

The process of applying the methods of normal psychology to the problems of abnormal conditions, and of testing the validity of current contributions to psychology, has had a free and liberal field and competent direction. "The clinical ideal of the study of the whole life and personality of each patient as an individual special problem has become also the psychological ideal." This implied "the need of studies in dynamic psychology, and the investigation of the relation of mental states to the disorders of digestion and nutrition." Time was spent at the Carnegie Nutrition Laboratory in Boston. The immediately available expert aid of "physico-chemical methods in biological research" had its influence and "determined their wider use here in accordance with the now recognized tendency of the time." (From annual reports of the McLean Hospital.)

The productive results of the combined operation of these laboratories are traceable directly to the projects of the decade 1880-90; they justify the forecast of the essential value of the dynamic concept in psychiatry, although the recognition of it has needed the labor of many years to make its wider use the tendency of the time.

The outcome here is typical of the great interest that has arisen in a considerable number of the institutions throughout the country and of their increasing productiveness within a few years. The laboratories of the McLean Hospital and the U. S. Government Hospital have tended to specialize for the longer time in psychological studies, the former giving more attention than any others to biochemical investigations. A special significance also attaches to the events at the McLean Hospital because of the introduction there of the variations in the formulation of psychiatric doctrine brought from the Heidelberg school, and because of the results of the contact there of the still prevailing system of essentially descriptive psychiatry, with the movement for broader biological explanations. The tendency of the former has been to perpetuate the fallacies of metaphorical descriptions of behavior, and to continue to seek to differentiate new "disease forms" under new names while now becoming constrained to place its failures in a growing group of "unclassified forms"; the tendency of the latter is to the practical conclusion that a functional conception of mental diseases leads to treatment through the study of the whole personality of each individual case. "Psychiatry belongs to general medicine, and mental disease, like bodily disease, is not an entity nor an agency, but the result of normal forces acting under abnormal conditions; the problem requires the investigation of the developmental and genetic character of functional modifications." [1] Osler asserts: that "the battle ground of medicine in the near future will lie in the fields of clinical chemistry and metabolism."

Conclusion.

The foregoing recital in outline of events in the progress of psychiatry has needed some detail to show their historical import. While the account in part relates largely to one line of advancement and to one institution, for the sake of its continuity and coherence, it is still only typical of the great movements and progress of the time. It is shown that in the march of development certain forces, alike in general medicine and psychiatry, and not less in psychology, have held their course, though with unequal steps. The historical meaning, revealed by a brief tracing of these trends to their recent leadings, betokens the momentous change now going on in the conceptions of mental diseases.

The problem of overcoming the barrier between mental physiology and mental pathology is one of the greatest importance to psychiatry. That medical training in psychology is desirable needs no saying. It is needed to consider whatever there may be in the methods of normal psychology that does not fit with the problems of pathological psychology.[1] What is there in the mental attitude of the psychologist which differs from that of the research worker in the physiological or physico-chemical laboratory, who has to deal with the physical facts of the mechanism of life?

The history of the laboratories here described reveals such a difference of attitude, and shows that both the psychologist and psychiatrist have been halting between the two leadings—the latter having to compound this disharmony in his practical work. In the course of these two trends of progress in modern psychiatry, there

[1] Op. cit. "The Problem of Psychiatry in the Functional Psychoses," 1905.

[1] F. L. Wells, "The Advancement of Psychological Medicine," the Pop. Sci. Monthly, Feb., 1913. The discourse of the medical man is one of problems, of the psychologist, one of methods; which under present conditions could scarcely be otherwise. The difficulty is that the methods of normal psychology and the problems of pathological psychology do not fit.

were conflicts and mergings, and the tendency to the emergence of clearer conceptions of scientific psychiatry. In the contemporary movements on the normal plane, beginning about 75 years ago, Johannes Müller, the founder of modern physiology, and his followers developed the methods of experimental research contributing to the rapid advancement in general medicine. Wundt, who had been with Helmholtz at Heidelberg, went to Leipsic in 1872, where Ludwig's laboratory became a center of interest for American physiologists. Academic psychology was seeking in the physical field explanations to support its views of psychic activity. Wundt established his laboratory in 1879 for applying the new mode of the exact methods of physical science to psychology.

The point of present interest in this movement is in the psychology of the emotions and the accepted fixed conceptions of their associated physical contrasts. Wundt's theory of the "three dimensions of feeling" expressed in pairs of "opposites"—"excitement-repose," "strain-retardation," "agreeableness-disagreeableness"—became a large problem of psycho-physical research. This great experiment and the vast literature written around it in 30 years in volumes of description and discussion, to fit with conscious experiences a like oppositeness of normal organic reactions, has been most productive in broadening the fields of research, although a negative conclusion has emerged concerning the "three-dimension theory." The psychologists have done their part along their lines of approach to the recognition of the problem of the mind as an adaptive mechanism. But to the same end, and proceeding from the rapid advancement in physiological and physico-chemical experiment, a revolution of ideas has been wrought, of which an example is the final dislodgment of the ancient conception of an oppositeness of physical reactions of "integration and disintegration," through the later discoveries proving the protective relations between normal emotional and physiological reactions. In the normal field this strengthens the foundations for cooperation in the merging of the problems and methods of psychology and medical research.

In the abnormal field the special place of these laboratories may now be pointed out by briefly recapitulating the meaning of some of the main events here narrated. In conclusion it remains also, with respect to the notable influence of the Heidelberg school, to specify more particularly what its doctrines were with reference to the results of their contact with the purposes of the combined laboratories; the manner of their introduction has been described. The beginnings of modern psychiatry are ascribed to Griesinger, who, in the awakening of his time, recognized the deeper physiological truth which he failed to impart. In the order of nature and universal experience the contrasts of mental pleasure and pain have been associated with many of the implications of exaltation and depression. The alienists, resting upon Griesinger's verbal formulations, have served the purpose of describing "clinical types set up," and even tended to antagonize the seeking for explanation through physiological principles with which, in fact, they do not fit.

The psychiatric movement has been substantially governed by the practical principles of the "supporting treatment"—the energy concept, under the influences of general medicine, which prompted the founding of the McLean laboratories, in their combination, and the change proposed in 1887 of the Griesinger formulæ to fit both the mental and physical facts. The inspiration to psycho-physical research then brought by Stanley Hall from the laboratories of Ludwig and Wundt, chiefly the former, did not change the physiological attitude; it was sought to escape from the domination of the ancient descriptive conceptions lacking explanations of the obvious changes of physical functions. When later the teachings of the Heidelberg school were brought in, they proved to revive the doubted formulæ; with some words of elaboration upon the model of the "three-dimension theory" the "triad of opposites" was framed and came into general use: "exaltation-depression," "excitement-relaxation," "flight of ideas-difficulty of thinking," with differentials of "increase and decrease" and determinations of disease-forms by reaction-time experiments.

This position was essentially descriptive and exactly contrary to that of Griesinger and the original purpose of the laboratories. It had no leaning toward the proposed physiological and physico-chemical explanations; the four missions of inquiry to psychiatric centers in Europe, 1888-1901, found no prolonged measures established for such combined research, but rather a lack of hopeful views of it. The clinical field of the McLean laboratories became the scene of an attempt to harmonize the perpetuated descriptive attitude and the explanatory attitude. In the first years the former flourished more, but the latter persisted. In the later period of nearly 15 years of expert work in "pure chemistry" and "pure psychology" conjoined in the clinic there emerged another change of scene indicated by the quoted description of some of the work done. The earlier conventional methods of measurements by time factors were proved to be of limited usefulness. There was increasing recourse to physico-chemical investigations of nutrition and other problems, and to new collaboration in methods for "studying the problems of the whole man" immediately presented by the physical facts of the clinic.

In the greater experiment formed by the years of work of these laboratories the primary problem was held in the proposition that all the activities represented by behavior, whether normal or abnormal, are always conditioned by the state of the energy potential, whether adequate or inadequate, modified or inhibited by interferences. The field of mental disorders is nature's laboratory, where the psychologist's methods of analysis must fit both the mental and physical problems of the psychiatrist. The energy concept being held as implying the storage of energy in living substance, and the law of physiological use as implying growth in functional power, these physical facts are extended by the new advances in the physiology of protective and defensive reactions. This new proof sustains for psychiatry the conception of the effects of overuse, waste in excess of repair, irritable weakness with lowering of thresholds, failing inhibition with increasing activity tending to losses through exhaustion by degrees of sensori-motor function to states of lethargy, and death. In the growing recognition of the constant presence of such elementary principles conceptions of a developmental or genetic character emerge for dealing with the complexes of abnormal mental and physical conditions. Thus there is revealed the broader field of explanation for the new psychiatry.

The dynamic principle long recognized in practice has prevailed in the work of these laboratories, although usage still clings to the old formulæ, which do not fit the physical facts. Psychiatry, by laying broader foundations, is becoming more completely free to frame its creed with a new ritual upon the coming revelations of physiology.

WORCESTER STATE HOSPITAL.[1]

WORCESTER, MASS.

On the 23d of February, 1829, Horace Mann, of Dedham, in behalf of a committee of the House of Representatives, appointed to consider the subject of the presence of considerable numbers of insane persons in the community who were either cared for in their own homes or in jails and almshouses, reported orders for the appointment of a committee "to examine and ascertain the practicability and expediency of erecting or procuring, at the expense of the commonwealth, an asylum for the safekeeping of lunatics and persons furiously mad," and requiring the selectmen of the several towns to ascertain and make returns to the Secretary of the commonwealth of the "number, age, sex and color of all persons reputed to be lunatics and furiously mad belonging to their respective towns, and whether at large or in confinement, and where and how long confined"—which orders were subsequently adopted by the House, and Messrs. Mann, Loud, of Dorchester, and Denny, of Leicester, were appointed to constitute said committee.

On the 7th of January, 1830, the Secretary communicated to the House of Representatives the returns which had been received in his office, in pursuance of the order above stated, which returns were referred to Messrs. Mann, of Dedham, Loud, of Dorchester, Strong, of Pittsfield, Oliver, of Boston, and Frothingham, of Newburyport. This committee reported, through Mr. Mann, a recommendation for the erection of a lunatic hospital, suitable for the accommodation of a superintendent, with wings sufficient for the reception of 120 inmates. For the accomplishment of this work the sum of $30,000 was asked. In accordance with this report the Legislature passed a resolve on February 7, 1832, authorizing the Governor to purchase a lot of land within the commonwealth suitable for a lunatic hospital, and to appoint a board of three commissioners for the erection on this site of a hospital for the accommodation of a superintendent and 120 insane

[1] By E. V. Scribner, M. D., superintendent.

persons. This resolve having passed the Legislature, received the approval of the Governor on the 10th of March, 1830. Under the power therein conferred the town of Worcester, "after diligent inquiry, and a faithful comparison of various proposed situations, was selected by the Governor and Council for the location of the hospital, and a plot of 12 acres of land purchased at the cost to that town of $2500." "Horace Mann, Bezaleel Taft, Jr., and William B. Calhoun were appointed commissioners to superintend the erection of the hospital thereon." On the 5th of July, 1832, the Governor and Council appointed Horace Mann, Bezaleel Taft, Jr., William B. Calhoun, Francis C. Gray and Alfred D. Foster as a Board of Trustees for the management of the institution, with power to appoint all other necessary officers. On January 12, 1833, Governor Levi Lincoln issued a proclamation declaring the State Lunatic Hospital at Worcester to be legally open for the reception of patients. The first patient was received into the hospital on the 19th day of January, 1833.

Meanwhile, in pursuance of the authority given, the trustees appointed as first superintendent of the new institution Samuel B. Woodward, M. D., of Wethersfield, Conn. Dr. Samuel Bayard Woodward was the son of a physician and a native of Connecticut, born on June 10, 1787, and licensed to practice medicine at the age of 21. His attention was called to this special department of the profession by the occurrence of several cases of insanity in his own practice and in that of his professional brethren whose adviser he was. The difficulty of managing these cases in their private practice led Dr. Woodward and his particular friend, Dr. Eli Todd, to take the first step towards the establishment of the Retreat for the Insane at Hartford, and he took credit to himself in having secured for it its present delightful location. He was appointed superintendent of the State Lunatic Hospital at Worcester, Mass., in September, 1832; went to Worcester in December following, and moved into the hospital as soon as rooms could be finished and furnished for the reception of his family. He retired on June 30, 1846, on account of failing health, and moved to Northampton, Mass., where he died quite suddenly on the evening of January 3, 1850.

That the hospital filled a public need was shown by the rapid influx of patients. In their report of December 31, 1833, the trustees stated that the hospital was then in a very crowded condition and that many applications for admission had been necessarily rejected because of lack of accommodations. Immediate measures were taken to increase the capacity of the institution and on April 7, 1835, the sum of $25,000 was appropriated for the enlargement of the hospital. Later in the session an appropriation of $3000 was made for the erection of a chapel and $7000 for the purchase of additional land for the use of the hospital. This increase in capacity was soon followed by others and at the time of the retirement of Dr. Woodward the patients in the hospital numbered 360—three times the amount of the accommodation furnished at the erection of the original building.

In their choice of Dr. Samuel B. Woodward as their first superintendent the trustees were singularly fortunate. Under his wise and humane administration the treatment of the insane in this hospital, one of the early state institutions in this country, was placed at once upon a high level.

Following the resignation of Dr. Woodward, Dr. George Chandler was appointed superintendent of the State Lunatic Hospital on July 1, 1846. Dr. Chandler began practice in Worcester in 1831 and a few years later was appointed assistant physician at the State Lunatic Hospital at Worcester. From 1842 to 1845 he was superintendent of the insane hospital at Concord, N. H. With this experience Dr. Chandler came well equipped for his work. His administration of affairs was successful. He was a good manager and in many ways improved the institution's equipment. He lighted the hospital with gas, introduced steam heating and greatly improved the ventilation. He did considerable in the way of educational instruction of the patients. He increased the capacity of the institution to keep pace with the ever-increasing numbers of the insane. As early as 1847 Dr. Chandler called attention in his reports to the increasing numbers of foreign born among the insane, showing the influence of immigration in the filling of our hospitals.

When the institution was first established its location was considered sufficiently removed from the residence center of the town to be unobjectionable. With the growth of the community the town steadily encroached upon the hospital and there began to be a feeling in the minds of many that another site should be found, to which the institution should be later transferred. Dr. Chandler suggested that it would be wise to consider a relocation at a more remote point.

Dr. Chandler resigned his superintendency April 1, 1856. After his retirement to private life he spent his time in travel and in biographical work. He died May 17, 1893, at the age of 97 years.

Succeeding Dr. Chandler, Dr. Merrick Bemis was promoted from the office of assistant physician, which he had acceptably filled, to that of superintendent. Under Dr. Bemis the good traditions of the hospital were preserved. He proved an efficient and capable man. He, like his predecessors, constantly enlarged the institution in response to the public need. He placed great stress on occupation in the treatment of mental disease and lessened restraint and seclusion. He employed the first female physician. The removal of the institution from its original location was again actively agitated, and in 1869 Dr. Bemis, under the direction of the trustees, bonded land in the outskirts of the town, on a site overlooking Lake Quinsigamond. The Legislature approving, the land was purchased the next year. The plan of the new institution, as formulated by Dr. Bemis, was ambitious and ideal. He advocated a central hospital plant for the actively disturbed, giving accommodation to perhaps one-third of the cases. The remaining two-thirds, the quiet and the convalescent, he proposed to care for in groups of 15 to 20, located in separate cottages. This would provide a family care approaching the more natural life in the community.

After a service of 24 years as assistant physician and afterwards as superintendent, Dr. Bemis resigned from the public service and established a small private hospital in Worcester. He also conducted a private practice in the community. He lived to a ripe old age, dying October 3, 1904.

The trustees elected as superintendent to succeed Dr. Bemis, Dr. Bernard D. Eastman, first assistant physician at the National Hospital, Washington, and formerly assistant physician at Concord, N. H. Upon Dr. Eastman, with the assistance of the architect, Mr. Rand, devolved the task of the preparation of plans for the erection of the proposed new hospital in the suburbs.

These plans struck " a happy medium between the older fashioned system of aggregation and the theoretical system of segregation."

In 1873, the plans for the new hospital buildings having been approved by the Governor and Council, the Legislature authorized the erection of the new institution, limiting the number of inmates for whom accommodation was to be provided to 400. As the number then in the parent institution was nearly 500, the pressure for a still further increase was very great. In view of this fact the plans were modified to provide accommodation for 500 and the work of construction entered upon. Building operations were actively prosecuted. The new hospital buildings received their first patients on October 8, 1877, but it was not until the 23d of the same month that the transfer was completed, 430 persons being removed. The old buildings were devoted to the purposes of the newly created Asylum for the Chronic Insane.

On February 6, 1879, Dr. Eastman resigned from the superintendency of the hospital. He later went to Kansas and was long identified with the insane hospital at Topeka.

Dr. John G. Park, formerly assistant physician at the hospital and later superintendent of the Asylum for the Chronic Insane, assumed the superintendency of the hospital on March 1, 1879. His administration perfected the organization of the service in the new hospital buildings and did much in the improvement of the grounds. He took a deep interest in the physical activities of his patients and recognized occupation as one of the best and most important of remedial measures. He introduced various industrial activities, as spinning, knitting, the use of the hand weaving loom and other forms of employment. He early advocated the establishment of a separate institution for the male criminal insane. The continued increase in numbers of patients necessitated the still further enlargement of the institution. Dr. Park erected the two circular observation wards, which have proven so well adapted for their purpose. During his administration the Hillside Farm, of 130 acres, in the town of Shrewsbury, was purchased to provide pasturage for the increasing herds.

In September, 1890, Dr. Park resigned his position as superintendent. After his retirement from this institution he served as chairman of the commission which erected the buildings of the Medfield State Asylum. Later, with the occupancy of the buildings, he was appointed to the Board of Trustees of that asylum, which office he held at the time of his death on August 9, 1905.

Dr. Hosea M. Quinby assumed the superintendency of the hospital on November 25, 1890. Dr. Quinby was previously assistant physician at the hospital and superintendent of the Worcester Asylum from 1879 to 1890. During his administration a farm building was erected for the accommodation of working patients, two nurses' homes built, infirmary buildings and a bath house completed, the domestic departments added to and the capacity of the institution generally increased, the number of patients rising from 785 to 1401.

One of the chief contributions of Dr. Quinby to the improvement of the care of the insane and the study of insanity was the employment of a special pathologist and clinician, who reorganized the record-taking and the general methods of examination and study of insanity. A training school for assistant physicians was organized, which was highly successful and attracted many capable men to the service of the institution. A laboratory building was erected to provide special facilities for scientific research in connection with the care and treatment of the insane. Dr. Quinby was also greatly interested in the development and beautifying of the grounds and conducted this work with much ability. April 1, 1912, he retired from the service to the enjoyment of private life.

April 1, 1912, Dr. Ernest V. Scribner, formerly assistant physician at the hospital, and more lately for some years superintendent of the Worcester State Asylum, succeeded Dr. Quinby as superintendent of the hospital and is now in office.

During the life of the institution 113 different persons figured as assistant physicians in its service. Some of these men have achieved renown in their chosen specialty. To enter in any way into their individual histories would exceed the proper limits of this brief account. Suffice it to say that nearly a score have risen to the management of institutions.

SUPERINTENDENTS.

Dr. Samuel B. Woodward 1833-1846
Dr. George Chandler.... 1846-1856
Dr. Merrick Bemis...... 1856-1871
Dr. Barnard D. Eastman. 1871-1879
Dr. John G. Park....... 1879-1890
Dr. Hosea M. Quinby... 1890-1912
Dr. Ernest V. Scribner.. 1912-

The following is a list of the assistant physicians who have been connected with the institution since its opening in 1833:

George Chandler.
John R. Lee.
Rufus Woodward.
Thomas E. Hatch.
Merrick Bemis.
Edward A. Smith.
Frank H. Rice.
Thomas H. Gage.
Harry C. Prentiss.
Joseph Draper.
Alfred E. Walker.
Mary H. Stinson.
H. O. Palmer.
Daniel H. Lovejoy.
John G. Park.
H. M. Quinby.
F. H. Gifford.
W. H. Raymenton.
A. R. Moulton.
Samuel M. Garlick.
Enoch Q. Marston.
Walter P. Bowers.
Charles A. Peabody.
W. E. Sylvester.
Omer P. Porter.
Ernest V. Scribner.
Everett Flood.
John A. Houston.
Frederick H. Daniels.
Bessie Earle.
Alfred I. Noble.
Harstein W. Page.
Laura Hulme.
Elmer E. Brown.
J. Frank Edgerly.
Maurice W. Pearson.
Clarence Pelton.
Lyman A. Jones.
Appleton H. Pierce.
Adolf Meyer.
Edwin D. Boynton.
Margaret A. Fleming.
George A. Tripp.
A. Ross Diefendorf.
Revere R. Gurley.
Edwin Leonard, Jr.
Walter J. Webb.
Emma W. Mooers.
Henry W. Miller.
Walter D. Berry.
Albert E. Loveland.
Albert M. Barrett.
Thomas Van Urk.
Otto P. Geier.
David R. Talbot.
Frank T. Budd.
Albert C. Thomas.
George H. Kirby.
Downey L. Harris.
Ross C. Whitman.
Isador H. Coriat.
William W. Newcomb.
Charles B. Dunlap.
Henry A. Cotton.
Cornelia B. J. Schorer.
Theodore A. Hoch.
George M. Kline.
Peter Bassoe.
Henry S. Chaffee.
Charles T. Fisher.
William E. Kornegay.
H. Walton Wood.
George H. Lynch.
Melvin J. Rowe.

James H. Turner.
G. Franklin Sargent.
E. Moore Fisher.
William E. Eaton.
Edward Mellus.
Walter C. Haviland.
Freeman A. Tower.
George B. Landers.
Harry W. Hammond.
Robert O. LeBaron.
Ray L. Whitney.
Mason W. H. Pitman.
James A. Mackintosh.
George F. Sullivan.
Florence H. Abbot.
Howard A. Knox.
Fred G. Campbell.
Percy L. Dodge.
William M. Dobson.
John R. Ross.
Frank L. S. Reynolds.
George A. McIver.
Nelson G. Trueman.
Samuel T. Orton.
Frank H. Matthews.
John G. Streigel.
Harry G. Hagerty.
James H. Cook.
Harry A. Clark.
Paul K. Sellew.
Walter H. Crandall.
Floyd A. Weed.
Henning V. Hendricks.
Francis A. Taylor.
Frank E. Lewis.
S. Carleton Gwynne.
J. Abel Thibodeau.
Mary E. Morse.
Wallace L. Orcutt.
Harold C. Arey.
Roy C. Jackson.
B. Henry Mason.
Sidney M. Bunker.
Benjamin F. Andrews.
William H. MacKay.
George E. Mott.
Jennie G. McIntosh.
R. Grant Barry.

BOSTON STATE HOSPITAL.[1]

DORCHESTER CENTRE, MASS.

No more fitting introduction to the history of the Boston Lunatic Hospital could be penned than the following, from the first annual report of the institution by its superintendent, Dr. John S. Butler:

In the first annual report of this institution there appears a propriety in briefly alluding to the circumstances which led to its establishment, and to the means which it presents for the successful accomplishment of its objects. By an act of the Legislature, passed in the year 1836, it was made imperative upon the several counties of the commonwealth to provide suitable accommodations for those paupers within their limits who, being idiotic or incurably insane, were too unsafe, either to themselves or others, to be allowed to go at large, and who, on account of their condition and the crowded state of that institution, could not be received at the Lunatic Hospital at Worcester. The pauper lunatics of the City of Boston were at this time confined in the House of Industry and the House of Correction at South Boston. They were numerous, and many of them, especially those in the House of Industry, were, under the circumstances of restraint in which they were unavoidably placed, violent and dangerous. No special accommodations or attendance were allowed for them by the city government, and, though all which the circumstances of their situation allowed had been done for them, much remained to be done. In discharge therefore of the duties imposed upon it by the law of the commonwealth and by the law of humanity, the government of the city with great unanimity voted to erect a hospital for the insane. The building, calculated to accommodate 100 patients, was commenced in 1837, and was ready for its intended inmates in the autumn of 1839. It was erected principally by the inmates of the House of Correction at an expense of $32,000; is plainly but substantially built, is convenient and comfortable, and well answers its intended purposes. It consists of a main building, 40 feet square, five stories high, including the basement, and two wings, each 40 feet by 60, which are three stories high, with a large and commodious room in the attic. The basement story of the building is occupied by the kitchen, washing room and laundry; the second, by the superintendent's office and dining rooms; the third, by the public and private parlors and the family dining room; the fourth, by the chambers of the families of the superintendent and steward, and the sewing room; the fifth, which is still unfurnished, is intended for the chapel, and above, the attic, containing the store room, chambers, etc. Each story in

---

[1] By Henry P. Frost, M. D., superintendent.

the wings contains 12 rooms, which, with the attic, will conveniently accommodate 50 patients in each wing. By forcing pumps in the cellar, water is thrown into large tanks in the attic, from which the water closets, sink and bath rooms in each story are supplied with an abundance of excellent water. Two large cisterns in the yard, supplied from the roof of the building, afford our family a good supply of soft water.

The location of the hospital is delightful; situated half way between the House of Industry and Correction, it commands on the front a view of the extensive gardens and highly cultivated grounds of the adjacent institutions, and in the rear the panorama of the harbor and City of Boston.

The Boston Lunatic Hospital originated from the necessity of constructing some suitable place or receptacle for the safekeeping of the idiotic and incurable insane. But whatever may have been the original design, it is now evident that the exigencies of the community require that it assume the same general character as those public state institutions which are in progress around us, and that amid the accumulation of old and incurable patients its wards should be open to the reception of those more recent cases whose recovery may after all be the best measure of its benefits.

The hospital was opened December 11, 1839, and had received up to July 1 of the following year, the date of this report, 104 patients, of whom 44 came from the House of Industry and 21 from the House of Correction. An experience of the first year was the introduction of smallpox, of which there were 12 cases, with one death.

In this and in his two subsequent reports Dr. Butler gave much attention to the subject of treatment, emphasizing the importance of occupation, diversion, outdoor exercise and hydrotherapy, mentioning with respect to the latter the satisfactory employment of the common garden watering pot in default of more elaborate apparatus.

The hospital was fortunate indeed in securing as its first superintendent a man of Dr. Butler's culture, enlightened sympathy and scientific attainments. Hampered as he was by meager equipment, insufficient funds, and lack of appreciative support in his relations with the business head of the institution, which led to his retirement at the end of three years' service, he established the care of the insane in the City of Boston on a high moral plane and implanted as its fundamental quality his own spirit of kind, considerate and helpful treatment.

An interesting incident in the history of the Boston Lunatic Hospital during Dr. Butler's superintendency was a visit from

Charles Dickens in 1842, who in "American Notes" recorded his agreeable impressions of the institution and its superintendent:

At South Boston, as it is called, in a situation excellently adapted for the purpose, several charitable institutions are clustered together. One of these is the hospital for the insane; admirably conducted on those enlightened principles of conciliation and kindness which 20 years ago would have been worse than heretical, and which have been acted upon with so much success in our own pauper asylum at Hanwell.

Each ward in this institution is shaped like a long gallery or hall, with the dormitories of the patients opening from it on either hand. Here they work, read, play skittles and other games; and, when the weather does not admit of their taking exercise out of doors, pass the day together. In one of these rooms, seated calmly, and quite as a matter of course, amid a throng of mad-women, black and white, were the physician's wife and another lady, with a couple of children. These ladies were graceful and handsome; and it was not difficult to perceive at a glance that even their presence there had a highly beneficial influence.

Every patient in this asylum sits down to dinner every day with a knife and fork; and in the midst of them sits the gentleman whose manner of dealing with his charges I have just described. At every meal, moral influence alone restrains the more violent among them from cutting the throats of the rest; but the effect of that influence is reduced to an absolute certainty, and is found, even as a measure of restraint, to say nothing of it as a means of cure, a hundred times more efficacious than all the straight waistcoats, fetters, and handcuffs that ignorance, prejudice and cruelty have manufactured since the creation of the world.

In the labor department every patient is as freely trusted with the tools of his trade as if he were a sane man. In the garden and on the farm they work with spades, rakes and hoes. For amusement they walk, run, fish, paint, read, and ride out to take the air in carriages provided for the purpose. They have among themselves a sewing society to make clothes for the poor, which holds meetings, passes resolutions, never comes to fisticuffs or bowie-knives as sane assemblies have been known to do elsewhere; and conducts all its proceedings with the greatest decorum. The irritability which would otherwise be expended on their own flesh, clothes and furniture is dissipated in these pursuits. They are cheerful, tranquil and healthy.

It is obvious that one great feature of this system is the inculcation and encouragement, even among such unhappy persons, of a decent self-respect. Something of the same spirit pervades all the institutions at South Boston.

Dr. Butler was succeeded as superintendent by Dr. Charles H. Stedman, whose service extended from 1842 to 1851, a period of nine years. Like his predecessor, he was charged with the medical care of the inmates.

The third superintendent was Dr. Clement A. Walker, appointed July 1, 1851. He had previously been in the service of the city as physician to the House of Industry, after taking his medical degree at Harvard. Dr. Walker, as superintendent, conducted the affairs of the institution for 30 years, retiring December 31, 1881, on account of ill health, which caused his death April 26, 1883. During this long period the troubles due to overcrowding in the building and lack of ground for exercise and occupation were often very serious. With proper accommodations for less than 200, the population ran as high as 275.

Dr. Walker repeatedly urged upon the city government the purchase of land in a suburban location and the building thereon of a new hospital with ample grounds, and in default of that he advocated enlargement on the existing site by building on the grounds of the House of Industry after removal of that institution to Deer Island. This property, however, was sold by the city and a shipbuilding and boilermaking business established on it right under the windows of the hospital. From time to time some steps were taken towards removal into the country and plans were even drawn and a site selected in 1866, but nothing came of it till many years later.

At intervals, when physically impossible to care for any more patients, the reception of new cases was discontinued, but as a rule the policy adopted in the first year of the hospital's operation, to treat recent and acute cases, and not simply to house chronic patients, was adhered to in spite of the great difficulties encountered in carrying it out.

The gradual transition from what we would now call primitive conditions to comparatively modern methods is interestingly shown by a brief record of the principal events and changes noted in the reports of these 30 years: 1853—Solar lamps were introduced in all the wards, with great rejoicing. Male attendants discontinued for female wing. 1855—Gas introduced. 1859—Undergraduate interne as assistant. 1863—Assistant physician appointed for the first time. 1875—Second assistant physician provided.

Dr. Walker was succeeded by Dr. Theodore W. Fisher, who had previously served the hospital as an assistant and had spent several months abroad studying hospitals for the insane. He had also had experience as examiner for the city in lunacy cases. Dr. Fisher assumed charge of the institution with the understanding that it was to be renovated and provided with the essentials for proper care and treatment of the patients. He succeeded in getting these plans put into execution without delay and his administration throughout was marked by efficient and progressive measures. His description of the hospital and of the conditions under which its work had been carried on up to that time forms an instructive chapter in its history:

The ideas which prevailed half a century ago concerning the treatment of insanity may easily be discerned in the construction of this hospital. A central administration building, with short wings, containing 84 rooms, was built in 1839. It accommodated 66 patients, distributed in three wards for each sex. The hospital faced the south, and the rooms for patients were located in front and rear of the wings, with corridors 12 feet wide between, lighted only at the ends. Each room was 12 feet long by eight feet wide, and about nine feet high. The doors were thick and solid, the windows heavily barred, and in one corner of each room was a triangular plank seat built into the brick walls. In some of these seats were staples, to which a violent lunatic in restraint could be fastened in a sitting posture. An attempt at ventilation was made by means of a system of horizontal and perpendicular flues in the outer walls, between each tier of windows, opening into each other at their intersections, and at the eaves into short, chimney-like airshafts without heat. A six-inch opening in each room over the window afforded an excellent hiding place for rags, paper and rubbish, but could never have been of any service as a ventilator. A small transom, six inches by 18, completed this absurd system of ventilation. No provision was made for heating any room independently. Those on the south side were sunny and warm in pleasant weather, but those on the north side were always sunless, and very cold in winter. Sick and excited patients could only receive such heat as might find its way through the transom. The corridors were also dark and sunless, and are so still, with no possibility of a change, except at the loss of sleeping accommodation. All the living rooms and half the sleeping rooms of the hospital were without the sun. It seems incredible that such a position and construction should have been adopted. The dark and narrow corridor was at first the only day room. It was heated originally by a stove, and afterwards by a furnace in the basement. The register openings were protected by strong iron fenders, which were very useful, but had a cage-like appearance. The walls were whitewashed, and the furniture strong, scanty and plain. The corridors were not lighted in the evening until 1851, when hanging solar lamps were introduced into the two upper wards, with cheering effect. Gas was first used in 1855.

The provision for feeding the patients was equally primitive, and in fact remained so for many years. A dining room in the center building adjoining each wing, which also served as the passageway into the wards, seating about 25, was the only accommodation for eating in a hospital at one time containing 271 patients. All but 50 patients have been obliged to eat in the day room or sleeping rooms of their wards. The food and waste have for 45 years been carried up and down stairs by hand. The dining rooms were furnished with unpainted pine tables and wooden benches without backs. The rooms in the lower wards had in each door a trap or observation hole, through which food could be passed to an excited patient. Wells and privy vaults, found in digging for foundations, attest the fact that Cochituate water had not been introduced. The location of the hospital suggests the manner in which insane persons were disposed of before the era of asylum accommodation. It was plainly built of brick and situated between two massive stone structures in one enclosure, the House of Correction being on the left and the almshouse on the right. It was a necessary complement to both these institutions then, receiving, at its opening, patients from both, as well as the overflow of city cases from the State Hospital at Worcester.

In 1846 an addition was made to each wing, containing dormitories for about 100 patients, but no single rooms. The attics had long been used for quiet patients at night, the first instance in the United States of the use of associated dormitories for the insane. This use suggested further accommodations of the same kind in the extension. The old corridors were continued into the new part and expanded into large parlors or day rooms, which required an additional furnace in the basement. These day rooms were somewhat lighter than the corridors, but still almost sunless, and had for their outlook the prison on the female side, and the almshouse, now Harrison Loring's Iron Works, on the male side. Probably at the time, or soon after the construction of the main building in 1839, a small one-story structure, known as the cottage, was erected in the rear, containing a block of cells, like those of a police station, for 10 violent patients. Here they remained, summer and winter, without constant attendance either day or night. This kind of building was at that time regarded as necessary for every hospital. It was enlarged in 1849; but by Dr. Walker's humane efforts was gradually disused, and finally abandoned in 1858, being then remodeled into the present kitchen and laundry.

The physical improvements made at this time were: Building dining room extensions, general repair, renovation and refurnishing of the wards, replacing dilapidated outbuildings, and improvement and extension of the grounds. The medical administration was improved by the adoption of a better system of case records. In 1881 a pathologist was appointed and the clinical instruction of medical students at the hospital was begun. In 1884 graduate internes were added to the staff, women attendants were put in uniform, and systematic instruction by lectures was given to the attendants. In 1887 dental students were admitted to care for the patients' teeth. Eighty-four chronic cases were transferred to the Retreat for the Insane at Austin Farm, in Dorchester, formerly used by the city as an almshouse. In 1889 the Retreat was made part of the Boston Lunatic Hospital and 200 patients of both sexes were accommodated there under the charge of Dr. Edward B. Lane, first assistant physician.

Dr. Fisher having, as he said, "gotten one foot into the country," pressed vigorously the proposal to erect other buildings there and desert the old institution. He had the satisfaction of seeing his policy carried out, though failure of health did not permit him to continue in charge after its consummation. New buildings were occupied at Austin Farm in 1893 and 1894, and at Pierce Farm, adjoining, in 1895, at which time the South Boston building was given up, to be demolished a few years later.

No one can read the reports of these 56 years during which patients were cared for in the South Boston institution without being profoundly impressed by the genuine interest displayed in their welfare by the four big-hearted men who have been named as successively in charge, and by the evidence throughout that in spite of many handicaps a great deal was done for their happiness and benefit. The ruling spirit was kindness from the very beginning. There was a family or household atmosphere pervading the establishment, such as we know not in these days of larger growth. Intimate acquaintance with the patients, and even affectionate regard for them, is manifest in many passages, and the record is full of wise and helpful accomplishment and of earnest desire to add to it. The policy was always enlightened and reflected the best thought of the period. How very modern the chapters on avoidance of restraint and sedative drugs, on the value of comparative freedom and healthful activity, on the importance of proper classification, of individual study and treatment, of high-grade medical and nursing care!

Every point was strained to admit patients at an early stage of their disorder and with as little delay and formality as the law allowed. Emergency and voluntary commitments were early and freely used. Visitors were admitted daily and practically at all hours. In these and many related ways was shown a sincere desire to fulfill to the uttermost the beneficent purpose for which the hospital stood.

Dr. Fisher resigned November 1, 1895, and Austin and Pierce farms, though known collectively as Boston Insane Hospital, were organized as separate institutions, with Dr. Edward B. Lane, superintendent of the former, and Dr. William Noyes of the latter. In 1897 the hospital was placed in the charge of a Board of Trustees, succeeding the Commissioner of Institutions, and the two units were consolidated under one management, Dr. Lane being made superintendent and Dr. Noyes associate superintendent. Austin Farm then became the department for women and Pierce Farm the department for men.

The new institution was of the cottage type, consisting of groups of detached buildings, some with and some without corridor connections. They were constructed of wood, with cement stucco outside, and were attractive in appearance, being pleasingly designed with ornamentation in the "half-timbered" style. To the women's group three substantial brick buildings were added in 1904, providing excellent wards for the treatment of acute cases.

Dr. Lane resigned from the superintendency in 1905 to engage in private practice and was succeeded by Dr. Noyes, the position of associate superintendent being at the same time abolished.

The next important step in the further development of the hospital which should enable it adequately to care for the insane of Boston was its transfer to the state December 1, 1908, its reorganization as the Boston State Hospital and the immediate preparation of plans for its enlargement and equipment. By acquiring 79 acres of adjoining land the institution has a site of 232 acres, containing high ground suitable for buildings and a rich meadow for cultivation. The tract being divided unequally by Morton Street, the smaller area to the east of this highway is to become a reception and treatment center for both sexes, while on the larger portion, where the farm land lies, is to be a custodial and infirmary group, flanked by groups of smaller cottages for patients capable of employment.

Building operations under this plan have been quite active, beginning in 1910. One infirmary and one building for violent patients have been built, both of which it is proposed to duplicate later; also three of the industrial cottages and a reception pavilion for male patients, increasing the capacity to 1500 (1914). A central heating and power plant, a building for stores and a new laundry have been erected. The completed institution will accommodate 2000 to 3000 patients, according to the size of the cottage groups. Looking forward to a large future growth and hoping to avoid an ancient evil of large institutions—enforced idleness for the majority of patients—the present management is interested in extending occupational training, paying special attention to the employment of the demented class. Industrial activity, non-restraint and a large measure of personal liberty enjoyed by the patients are the chief features of the administrative policy, while on the medical side systematic staff meetings, the equipment of operating rooms, the establishment of a pathological and bacteriological laboratory and the extensive employment of hydrotherapy are in line with modern methods.

The present superintendent is Dr. Henry P. Frost, who was appointed April 15, 1910, after a service of some years as first assistant at the Buffalo State Hospital in New York, succeeding Dr. Noyes, or, rather, Dr. Owen Copp, who, while executive officer of the State Board, had consented to take charge of the hospital after its transfer to the state, and who gave to the trustees the benefit of his extensive experience in planning its further development.

Psychopathic Hospital.

Under the same Board of Trustees, and organized as a department of the Boston State Hospital, the psychopathic hospital, located on Fenwood Road, in Boston, was opened in June, 1912. This department was established by an act of the Legislature in 1909, which appropriated the sum of $600,000 for land, buildings and equipment for the purpose of "establishing in the City of Boston a hospital for the first care and observation of mental patients and the treatment of acute and curable mental diseases and for an out-patient department, treatment rooms and laboratories for scientific research as to the nature, causes and results of insanity."

Its capacity is 100 beds, with provision for future extension if required. The location enables it to serve especially Boston and vicinity, whose mental patients aggregate about one-half the insane of the state, but it holds an important relation to the other state hospitals in the study and treatment of exceptional patients, as a center of clinical and scientific investigation of special problems and of co-operative effort in other directions. The director of the psychopathic department since its opening is Dr. Elmer E. Southard, Bullard professor of neuropathology in Harvard Medical School and pathologist to the State Board of Insanity. The hospital has a very active service, the admissions having been at a rate of over 1500 a year. Patients are received on the voluntary basis, or under the several provisions of law which authorize temporary care and observation to determine the necessity for commitment. These two classes of patients as a rule occupy about two-thirds the capacity, while the remainder is taken up with patients who have been committed after observation and are later transferred to the main hospital in Dorchester.

Dr. Southard and his assistants, including a technical and out-patient staff, have been occupied with a variety of laboratory, clinical and social problems and with clinical teaching, which is one of the important functions of the institution.

The building, which is four stories high, of brick and terra cotta, occupies a spacious corner lot, commands a pleasing outlook across the parkway and has unrestricted air and sunlight. The arrangement is such that all excited and noisy patients can be cared for in a pavilion extending to the rear, well removed from neighboring residences; and a special system of forced ventilation permits closed windows in this section, these being double glazed to prevent the transmission of noise. The entrance for patients is from an ambulance court in the rear, giving access to the admitting office and reception wards on the first floor of the pavilion, where provision is made for seven patients of each sex in a dormitory and two single rooms, with toilet, bath, fumigating chamber and other utilities. On the second and third floors of the pavilion are wards for men and women, respectively, each accommodating 24 patients, seven of these in single rooms at the extreme end of the section, the remainder in small wards of four and six beds each. Each of these wards has six tubs for prolonged baths, an examination and treatment room, and a clinical laboratory. There are in this part of the building no day rooms or dining rooms, the design being to treat the patients in bed, but there is a solarium and roof garden on the fourth floor, which is reached by elevator.

In the front portion of the building are reception rooms, offices, living quarters for officers and nurses, an extensive laboratory suite, and an out-patient or social-service department. These features occupy the first, second and third floors; the fourth contains two wards for 20 patients of each sex, which will be devoted to cases requiring special study and treatment, while the reception wards will take care of a more rapidly changing population.

The resident officers since the founding of the institution have been:

John S. Butler	1839-1842	William Noyes	1896-1909
Charles H. Stedman	1842-1851	Samuel W. Crittenden	1900-
Clement A. Walker	1851-1881	Augustus T. Marshall	1902-1904
Theodore W. Fisher, superintendent	1881-1895	Mary E. Gill (Gill-Noble)	1904-
Theodore W. Fisher, assistant supt.	1863-1868	George H. Maxfield	1905-1910
		Francis X. Corr	1905-1909
George H. M. Rowe	1868-1880	George E. Emerson	1904-1904
John T. Carter	1874-1878	Ermy C. Noble	1909-
Elisha S. Boland	1878-1885	Stephen E. Vosburgh	1910-1912
Manuel Schwab	1880-1883	Henry P. Frost	1910-
Simeon M. Metcalf	1883-1884	William M. Dobson	1912-
Edward B. Lane	1885-1905	Cyril G. Richards	1912-1914
Robert Swift	1885-1889	Joseph H. Toomey	1912-1912
Charles G. Dewey	1888-1893	John P. H. Murphy	1912-1912
Charles J. Bolton	1889-1896	Harry M. Nicholson	1910-1911
Linnaeus A. Roberts	1892-1902	John E. Overlander	1911-1911
Arthur C. Jelly	1892-1895	Guy D. Tibbets	1912-1913
Fred B. Colby	1896-1904	John I. Wiseman	1911-
Henry A. Roberts	1896-1900		

PATHOLOGIST.

Myrtelle M. Canavan.... 1910-

PSYCHOPATHIC DEPARTMENT.

Dr. Elmer E. Southard	1912-	Dr. George E. Eversole	1912-
Dr. Herman M. Adler	1912-	Dr. Charles O. Maisch	1913-1914
Dr. Victor V. Anderson	1912-1913	Dr. Thomas H. Haines	1913-
Dr. William P. Lucas	1912-1913	Dr. Frankwood E. Williams	1913-
Dr. Abraham Myerson	1912-1913	Dr. Harriet M. Gervais	1914-
Dr. A. Warren Stearns	1912-		

NON-RESIDENT PATHOLOGISTS.

Dr. W. W. Gannett	1881-1891	Dr. John J. Thomas	1898-1903
Dr. William T. Councilman	1893-1894	Dr. Elmer E. Southard	1904-1908

The trustees appointed by the Governor to take charge of the Boston State Hospital December 1, 1908, were: Chairman, Walter Channing, M. D., Brookline; Secretary, Henry Lefavour, Ph. D., LL. D., President of Simmons College, Boston; Mrs. Henrietta S. Lowell, Brookline; Joseph Koshland, Mrs. Katherine G. Devine, Mr. George H. Leonard, and Michael J. Jordan, Boston. Mr. Leonard died a very short time after the organization of the board and was succeeded by William Taggard Piper, of Cambridge. Dr. Channing's long connection and intimate acquaintance with the care of the insane, President Lefavour's skill as an organizer and administrator, Mr. Jordan's familiarity with the affairs of the institution as chairman of the City Board of Trustees, and Mr. Piper's experience as chairman of the board of a large general hospital were special qualifications which, in happy combination with the business ability of Mr. Koshland and the philanthropic interests of the two ladies, constituted an organization well fitted for its task. The board sustained a loss in the resignation of Mr. Koshland, October, 1910, and another in the death of Mr. Piper, July, 1911. Lehman Pickert, of Boston, and Melvin S. Nash, of Hanover, were appointed in their places; with these exceptions the original members continue to give their service to the hospital and effectively to forward its development.

TAUNTON STATE HOSPITAL.[1]

TAUNTON, MASS.

The Taunton State Hospital was the second state hospital to be built in Massachusetts, the first being the Worcester State Hospital. An act of the Legislature, approved May 24, 1851, authorized the erection of a second hospital for the insane, which at first bore the name of the State Lunatic Hospital at Taunton.

The same act empowered the Governor, with the advice and consent of the Council, "to appoint a board of three commissioners to purchase an eligible site in such a section of the commonwealth as they should deem expedient and cause to be erected thereon a suitable hospital for the cure and care of the insane—the accommodations of such hospital to be sufficient for 250 patients.

This commission, after due inquiry and consideration, decided to locate the hospital in the town of Taunton.

In July, 1853, the Board of Trustees was appointed and in October of that year the first superintendent, Dr. George C. S. Choate, of Salem, Mass., was selected. The superintendent and members of the Board of Trustees were enlightened and progressive men, with advanced views as to the treatment of the insane, as was shown from the first by their administration.

In their first report the Board of Trustees writes as follows:

> In one respect the trustees have deemed it advisable to make a material change. As originally constructed, there were 42 rooms designed for the reception of violent and filthy patients, called *strong rooms*. These rooms were built of stone, brick and iron, and were finished throughout with a view chiefly of strength. The walls were of brick, 16 inches thick, and were whitewashed on the brick. They were placed along the center of the wing which was devoted to them, having a narrow passageway before and behind, and consequently having no windows opening to the outer air, and few of them any view but of the gloomy white prison walls.
>
> A small opening in the rear of each cell, guarded by strong iron bars, answered for a window; the doors were narrow, and made of the same material, each provided with two formidable locks. By the side of the door was a small aperture, just large enough to pass in food. The floors

[1] By Arthur V. Goss, M. D., superintendent.

in the two upper stories were of wood. In the lower story, which was designed probably for filthy patients and such as should refuse to wear clothes, floors were of stone, made sloping, and terminating in front of the cells in a stone gutter, for the convenience of washing them out. The stones were also heated, to afford warmth to the naked inmates who were expected to rest upon them.

The trustees are aware that it has been considered necessary to have rooms of this description or strong rooms, for the use of patients difficult to control or to keep properly clothed; but, apart from considerations of humanity, they are now satisfied that it can never be necessary thus to confine even the most furious, and they are happy to be able to say that it has never been found necessary in this institution to resort to such extreme modes of restraint in a single instance. The length of the time during which the system of dispensing with the use of such rooms has been tried, the fact that many patients previously so confined have manifested a decided change for the better, and the general good order and quiet which reigns throughout the hospital under its operation, convince the trustees that the safety of such a course is no longer a matter of experiment; and it is a matter of great gratification to them that, so early in the history of the hospital, so important a point in the treatment of the furiously insane has been satisfactorily established. For these reasons, and because the space occupied by the strong rooms was needed for other purposes, the trustees have caused them to be demolished and other and more suitable apartments to be constructed in their places.

These *strong rooms* were consequently never occupied.

Dr. Choate in his first report also advocates the disuse of all mechanical restraint in most cases and states that only two forms of mechanical restraint were used, the belt and wristers for men and the camisole for women, and these only in a very limited number of cases.

He also advocated in the strongest manner the employment of patients as a means of treatment, and although he considered farm work the best for men, in view of the long winters during which there was practically no farm work, he recommended the erection of workshops for both sexes. The money for workshops was not forthcoming and Dr. Choate had to seek elsewhere for means of employment; fortunately they were at hand. In the various domestic departments there were ample means of employment for women, while the farm and grounds afforded plenty of the best employment for men.

The hospital buildings were situated upon a low, barren, sandy hill, surrounded by an exhausted farm of 140 acres, with con-

TAUNTON STATE HOSPITAL, 1854.

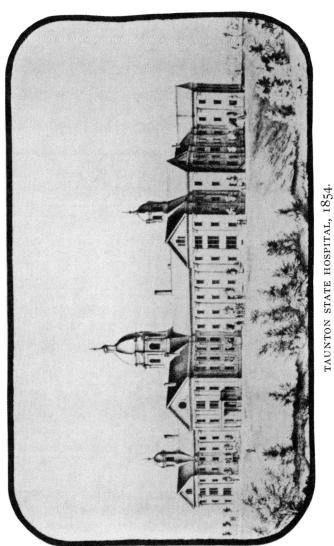

siderable swamp and brush land, the whole plentifully sprinkled with boulders. Dr. Choate employed his patients in removing the stones, with which a substantial wall was built surrounding the entire property, draining the swampy portions, and gradually restoring the exhausted soil. The results of Dr. Choate's policy are still felt and the works of his patients remain lasting memorials to the wisdom that directed them.

The hospital was built for 250 patients, but it was soon overcrowded and in 1860 had between 300 and 400 patients. Dr. Choate, however, did not believe it practicable to enlarge the hospital and that work was left for his successors.

After a long and successful administration Dr. Choate resigned in December, 1869, feeling "the necessity of change and relief from the trying and harassing cares of my position here and the growing importance of removing my family from the influences inseparable from a large public institution." Dr. Choate removed to New York, where he had a long and successful career conducting a private hospital for mental cases.

He was succeeded by Dr. William W. Godding, of Winchendon, Mass., who at the time of his appointment was first assistant physician at St. Elizabeth, the national hospital at Washington, D. C. When Dr. Godding assumed charge of the hospital it was much overcrowded and in 1872 the population of the hospital had reached the number of 400. In his annual report for the year 1872 Dr. Godding asked for an appropriation to build two new wings to increase the normal capacity of the hospital to 500, which number at that time he considered the best unit for a hospital. The money was appropriated and the extreme east and west wings were built to accommodate 150 patients. Dr. Godding's term of service was a busy one, not only in construction and reconstruction, but in meeting the problems that a rapidly changing population presented. He resigned in 1877 to accept the superintendency of St. Elizabeth, the government hospital at Washington, D. C., which position he held until his death, May 6, 1899.

Dr. Godding was succeeded in 1878 by Dr. John P. Brown, of Concord, N. H., who at the time of his appointment was first assistant physician of the New Hampshire State Hospital. During the whole of his long service he was actively engaged in extending the institution and making additions to increase its efficiency.

Dr. Brown, until the last years of his administration, when failing health rendered it necessary for him to husband his strength, kept in his own hands the administration of all departments and had a personal oversight over the entire institution. His first act was to protect the main plant by fire walls extending from basement to roof. Twenty-five years later these walls doubtless saved the institution from total destruction when a devastating fire broke out in the extreme east wing.

In 1892 and 1893 two infirmary buildings to accommodate about 75 patients each were completed and occupied. The east infirmary (for women) was named the "Howland Infirmary," in memory of George Howland, of New Bedford, trustee of the hospital for 37 years; and the west infirmary, the "Brown Infirmary," in honor of Dr. Brown. These buildings marked a distinct advance in the treatment of the insane in Massachusetts.

In 1894 a training school for nurses of both sexes was established, which has been in successful operation ever since.

In 1895 a pathological laboratory was constructed and a pathologist was appointed in 1897.

In 1899 a farm colony was established by the purchase of a 150-acre farm in the adjoining town of Raynham, which in 1905, by the erection of suitable buildings, was able to care for 72 patients. The benefit that these patients receive from healthy out-of-door life and greater freedom has been more and more evident each succeeding year.

Dr. Brown was a firm believer in useful employment as a remedial agent in the treatment of mental diseases and during his administration he labored to render the system established by his predecessors more effective. An industrial building was constructed in 1895, which afforded much-needed workshops.

In addition to the training school, Dr. Brown did much to render the life of the nurses employed more pleasant and their work more efficient. In 1902 a "home for women nurses" was completed and a corresponding "home for men nurses" in 1904. In this last building were 12 large rooms for the accommodation

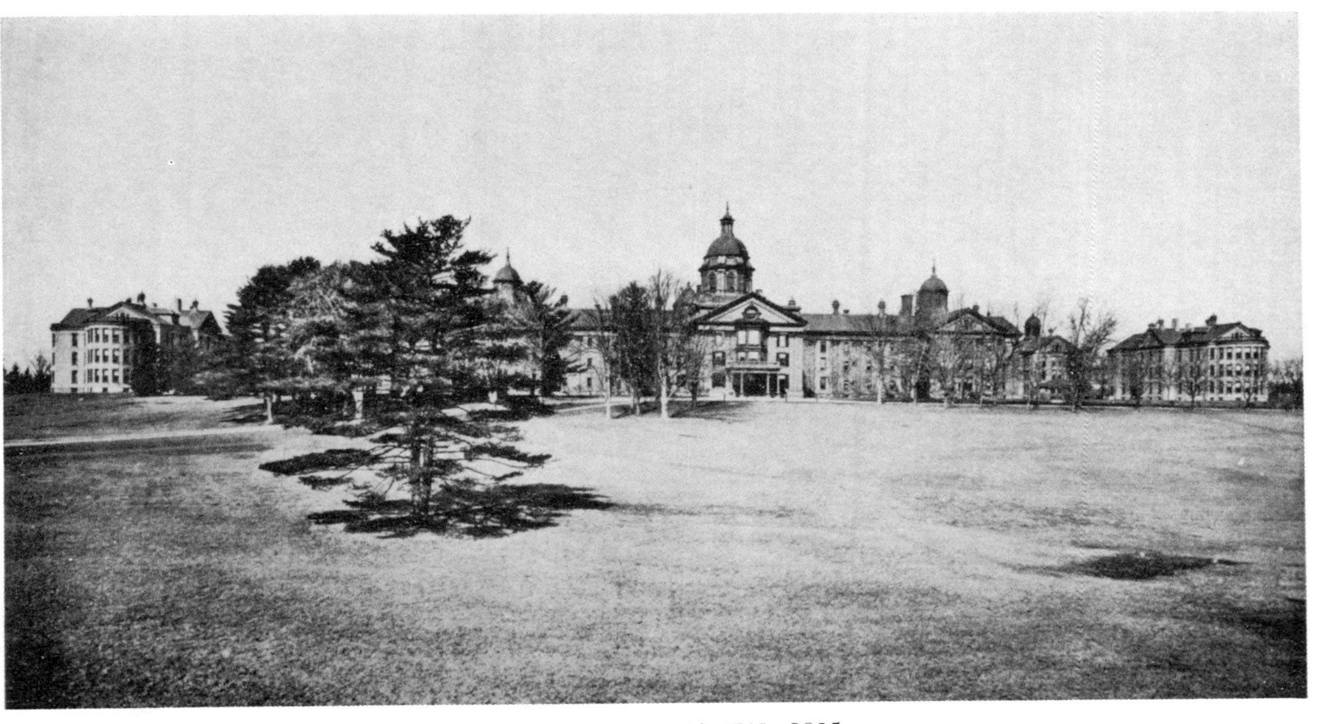

TAUNTON STATE HOSPITAL, 1915.

of married couples, a provision that experience has proved to be most wise. Among the last of Dr. Brown's official acts was one limiting the hours of duty of nurses to 70 hours per week, with one day of rest.

When Dr. Brown was appointed the hospital contained 633 patients and his official staff consisted of two assistant physicians and a treasurer and clerk united in the same person. When advancing years and failing health compelled him to resign in 1906 the hospital contained 905 patients and his official staff had increased to six assistant physicians, a pathologist, a treasurer, a steward, a clerk and three stenographers, while the number of employees in each department had correspondingly increased. With it all the hospital was practically a new institution, having been reconstructed throughout and greatly developed in all departments. It is impossible to review adequately the successful administration of Dr. Brown within the limits of the present article. On November 15, 1906, he retired to private life and died at the home of his daughter September 19, 1908.

He was succeeded by the present superintendent, Dr. Arthur V. Goss, who had been an assistant physician since 1892. During the past seven years the employment of patients as a remedial agent has been developed chiefly along utilitarian and co-operative lines and the number employed has steadily increased, until in 1912 75 per cent of the whole number under treatment were employed to a greater or less extent. Diversional forms of employment have not been neglected, but are secondary to utilitarian forms. Industrial instruction has also been made part of the training school course. The treatment of acute patients has been much advanced by the construction of extensions to the east and west wings, affording treatment wards for acute cases, equipped with continuous baths, a hydrotherapeutic room and spacious verandas for out-of-door treatment. Since the occupancy of these wards in November, 1912, the use of mechanical restraint, which had been gradually decreasing, has been practically abolished, while seclusion has been greatly reduced. These same extensions provide two large dining rooms, equipped with the necessary appliances for serving food and also two wards for tuberculosis patients, in which by monitor roofs the atmosphere is kept practically in out-of-door condition.

The colony method of caring for patients is also in process of development, by which 25 patients will be added to the colony farm and a colony for women of 100 patients created.

The training school for nurses has been reorganized and for the past three years attendance upon it has been obligatory for both sexes.

At the beginning of the hospital year, 1913, the number of patients under treatment was 1103.

TRUSTEES.

Name	Years
Marcus Norton	1853-1854
William Sutton	1853-1856
Charles Edward Cook	1853-1857
George R. Russell	1853-1858
George A. Crocker	1853-1861
Charles R. Vickery	1854-1855
George Howland, Jr.	1855-1892
Menzies R. Randall	1856-1862
James W. Seaver	1857-1858
Charles Edward Cook	1858-1873
John M. Kinney	1858-1864
Charles R. Atwood	1861-1877
Oliver Ames	1862-1877
LeBaron Russell	1864-1889
Simeon Borden	1873-1896
William C. Lovering	1877-1910
Samuel L. Crocker	1878-1883
Oakes A. Ames	1883-1899
Mrs. Ruth S. Murray	1884-1901
Mrs. Grace S. Bartlett	1884-1891
John J. Russell	1889-1896
Mrs. Susan B. Learoyd	1891-1912
Henry R. Stedman, M. D. (in office)	1892-
Gerard C. Tobey	1896-1902
Milton Reed	1896-1901
Oliver Ames	1899-1901
Nathaniel B. Borden	1901-1908
Mrs. Elizabeth C. M. Gifford (in office)	1901-
Loyed E. Chamberlain (in office)	1902-
James P. Francis (in office)	1903-
Simeon Borden, Jr. (in office)	1909-
Edward Lovering (in office)	1910-
Mrs. Margaret Smith (in office)	1912-

SUPERINTENDENTS.

Dr. George C. S. Choate, Oct. 4, 1855, to May 1, 1870.
Dr. William W. Godding, May 1, 1870, to Sept. 20, 1877.
Dr. John P. Brown, March 1, 1878, to Nov. 15, 1906.
Dr. Arthur V. Goss, Nov. 15, 1906-in office.

PATHOLOGISTS.

Dr. Frederick S. Ward. Dr. Henry W. Miller.
Dr. Charles P. McGaffin.

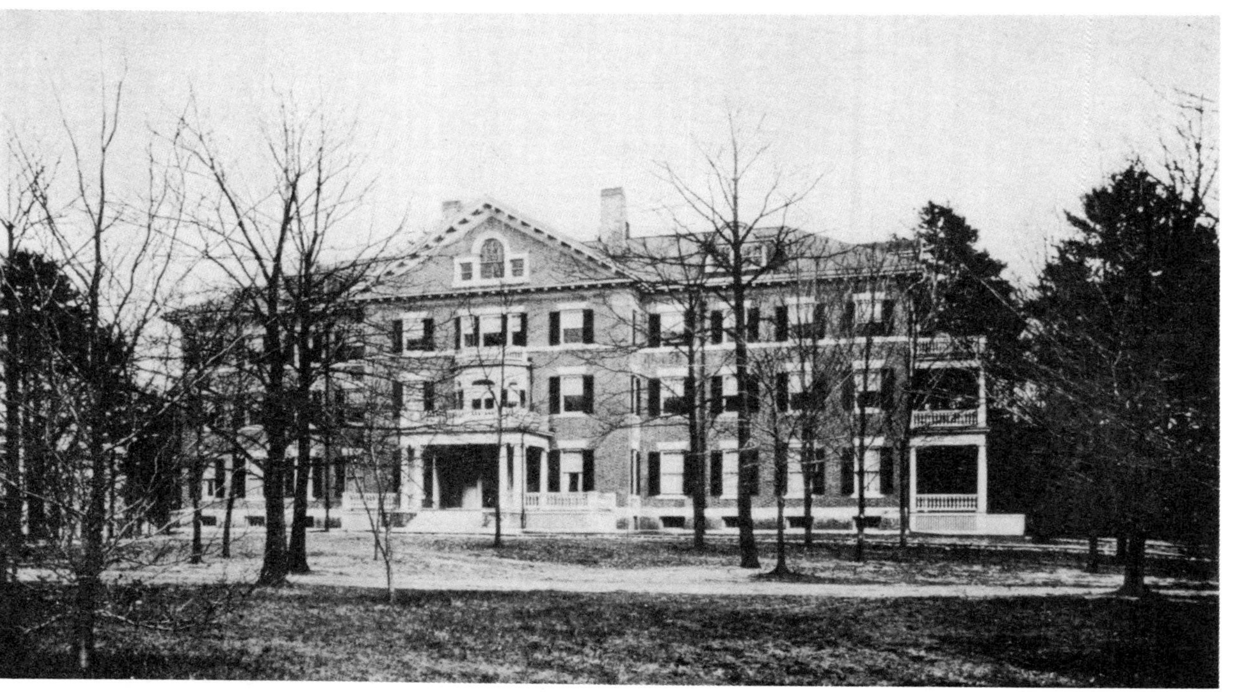

NURSES' HOME, TAUNTON STATE HOSPITAL.

ASSISTANT PHYSICIANS.

Dr. S. A. Holman.
Dr. Normus Page.
Dr. Norton Folsom.
Dr. William H. Gage.
Dr. George L. Ellis.
Dr. Marcello Hutchinson.
Dr. Alice Rogers.
Dr. Charles A. Drew.
Dr. Owen Copp.
Dr. Charles G. Dewey.
Dr. Whitefield N. Thompson.
Dr. George A. Bancroft.
Dr. Chauncey Adams.
Dr. Ida M. Shimer.
Dr. Frank S. Hamlet.
Dr. Arthur V. Goss.
Dr. Ernest H. Wheeler.
Dr. Ida L. Brimmer.
Dr. Charles E. Adams.
Dr. George B. Coon.
Dr. Mary Jameson Gates.
Dr. Frederick S. Ward.
Dr. Frederick B. Jewett.
Dr. John E. Fish.
Dr. Tertia G. Wilton.
Dr. Benjamin W. Baker.
Dr. R. V. Baketel.
Dr. W. H. Lane.
Dr. Henry T. Marshall.
Dr. Harry M. Lowd.
Dr. Frederick R. Sims.
Dr. George K. Butterfield.
Dr. H. Walton Wood.
Dr. Florence H. Abbot.
Dr. William T. Hanson.
Dr. Horace G. Ripley.
Dr. Dora W. Faxon.
Dr. Raoul G. Provost.
Dr. John J. Thompson.
Dr. Charles G. McGaffin.
Dr. Fred H. Freeman.
Dr. G. B. McMurray.
Dr. J. P. H. Murphy.
Dr. John H. Travis.
Dr John F. O'Brien.
Dr. Lester F. Norris.
Dr. Francis H. Slack.

NORTHAMPTON STATE HOSPITAL.[1]

NORTHAMPTON, MASS.

No provision for the public care of the insane was made in Massachusetts till the opening of the McLean Asylum, now McLean Hospital, in 1818.

McLean Asylum, only partially under state control, proved quite inadequate to care for all the insane of the commonwealth. Accordingly a state hospital was opened at Worcester in 1833, and another at Taunton in 1854.

The demand for further accommodations for the insane becoming so insistent the Legislature of 1854 authorized the Governor to appoint a commission to examine into the condition of the insane in the commonwealth; to ascertain their numbers; the number who were confined in institutions; to distinguish between the insane and idiotic, between the harmless and the furious, the curable and the incurable, the native and foreign; and to see what further accommodations, if any, were needed for the relief and care of the insane.

There were at that time throughout the United States 37 hospitals for the care of the insane, state and private or incorporated. In Massachusetts there were the three already mentioned and the Municipal Hospital at South Boston.

Probably the most exhaustive survey of the subject ever made in our country was made by the commission thus authorized, of whom Dr. Edward Jarvis was chairman.

It was found that all the institutions of the state were crowded and that more than 600 proper subjects for hospital treatment were at their own homes, 205 of whom were curable and others were troublesome or dangerous. Influenced by this report, the Legislature of 1855 made an appropriation of $200,000 to buy the land and erect buildings to accommodate 250 patients. The commissioners appointed to carry on the work were Luther V. Bell, Henry W. Benchley and S. S. Standley.

The plans prepared by Jonathan Preston, a Boston architect, were largely designed by Dr. Bell, one of the ablest and most

[1] By Dr. John A. Houston, superintendent.

experienced of the superintendents of asylums in the country at that time.

Northampton was selected as the site for the new hospital. The argument in favor of this location was that the people of the western part of the state were insufficiently provided for as to the care of their insane, being too remote from the two existing state hospitals.

After the hospital was begun a sentiment adverse to its construction became so effective that in a subsequent Legislature the purpose would have been abandoned if its friends had not used every effort to prevent that result. To many it seemed a mistake to locate it so far from the center of population. The prediction was freely made that it would never be filled with patients from the western part of the state. As it happened, this prediction proved true for many years, the hospital being filled with patients transferred from the hospitals in the eastern part of the state.

The hospital was opened for the reception of patients in August, 1858, and within six weeks had received within 32 of the number which it was planned to care for, but of these only 16 came from the four western counties, the district it serves; 212 were sent from the hospitals at Worcester and South Boston. Parenthetically, it may be added that 43 of these remained at the hospital till released by death.

Before the expiration of two years, the number maintained exceeded its capacity by 65; a like condition has persisted to the present day.

The first purchase of land comprised 175 acres which have been added to from time to time till at present there are 513 acres.

The plan of the institution comprises an administrative building, four stories high, with an extension in the rear for store rooms, kitchen and bakery, "chapel," dormitories for employees and the like and a range of wings on each side, three stories high, for patients. It follows closely the plans for similar institutions in vogue at the time of its erection, and has but one detached building for the accommodation of patients.

To the rear of the main building are the shops, boiler and engine rooms, laundry, paint shop and farm buildings.

The administration building, with its wings on either side, is on an elevation about 100 feet above the Connecticut River, about a mile west of the City of Northampton, and commands a beautiful prospect of meadows and the two ranges of mountains, Holyoke and Mount Tom, with the Connecticut River finding its outlet between them.

Beginning in 1892 extensive changes and additions have been made, of which only brief mention is made.

A new building to accommodate the heating plant, machine shop, and carpenter shop, made room for enlarged kitchens, sewing and mending room, and above them a beautiful assembly hall for religious services and for amusements. The old so-called "chapel" in turn provided a small laboratory, an operating room and library on the second floor, and above, a large room for a gymnasium, now used also as an industrial room.

As originally built, the windows that lighted the bays and corridors were narrow. All these windows have been enlarged and others have been added, so that the wards are now flooded with light. Some of the wards have been further improved by the addition of bay windows and piazzas.

Following these changes, new heating, ventilating and lighting systems were installed.

In 1898-99 a large addition to the main building was erected, providing increased office room and living accommodations for the officers.

In 1900 a cold storage plant was installed wherein can be stored 30,000 dozen eggs, several tons of butter, many sides of beef, 2000 barrels of apples, and several thousand bushels of potatoes.

In 1900 a new stable for the carriage horses was built.

In 1903 a new cow barn was built, accommodating 70 cows, 14 oxen and other stock.

In 1904 a reception building and infirmary for women patients was built, and one similar to it for the men in 1905 .

In 1911 a new laundry was built, and in 1914 a fire pump house and a stable for farm horses, made necessary by a fire in the old stable in the winter of 1913-14.

Two additions worthy of note are buildings erected for the entertainment and recreation of patients—both gifts to the hospital. Both are situated in the grove in front of the main building. One is a large enclosed pavilion for the women, presented by the grateful sister of a former patient. The other is a club house

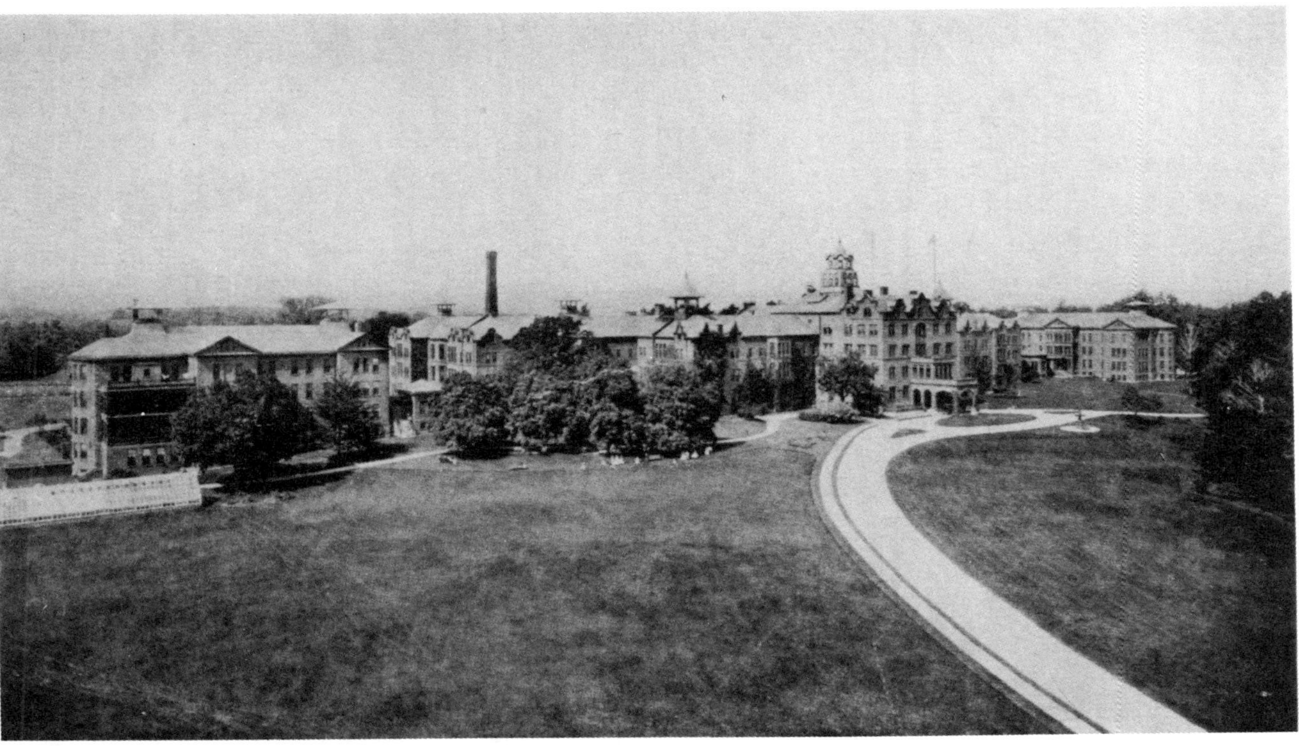

NORTHAMPTON STATE HOSPITAL, NORTHAMPTON, MASS.

for men, containing bowling alleys, a billiard room, and a reading and smoking room, presented as a memorial of a trustee whose services to the hospital had covered a period of 24 years.

A review of the early annual hospital reports reveals much of historical interest as well as much that is instructive to the present generation

From these reports we can measure whatever progress has been attained at the present day in the care and treatment of the insane, in most of which progress the earlier superintendents blazed the way. The same problems puzzled them that still perplex us and usually the same solutions were proposed that are approved at the present time. Indeed, in most particulars and in essentials the early reports read as if they might have been written but yesterday.

Some of the subjects written about are introduced into this history to show that 50 years ago the best thought on such matters was abreast of what obtains at present. Running through all the earlier reports of the hospital are comments, suggestions, recommendations, on all the things that are still alive; economy of administration and yet absence of parsimony; the nursing question; the influence of occupation and recreation; medical and moral treatment; restraint and non-restraint; classifications of patients and of institutions; recoveries and the curability of insanity, and like matters.

The powerful influence for good or ill of nurses, who are in constant contact and in unrestricted intercourse with their patients, on the importance of which so much emphasis is placed to-day, was recognized in the first annual report of the superintendent in these words:

> The success of a hospital as a curative institution is to a considerable extent dependent on their fidelity and natural adaptation to the performance of the duties of the office. There must be an active sympathizing interest felt in their unfortunate charge, a desire to promote the cure of the patients committed to their care, by constant watchfulness over their conduct, their amusements and daily habits, and a determination to make their comfort and well-being the object of paramount importance.

The second superintendent, more than 50 years ago, commented thus: "The nurses, on whose fidelity so much of comfort and happiness depends," and again, quoting Dr. Kirkbride, "Tact in exciting the interest of patients in their occupation and amusements should always be regarded as among the qualifications to be possessed by those who are to be in the immediate care of the insane."

The early reports had frequent reference to treatment which was classified as "medical" and "moral." Some of these references are of sufficient historical interest to warrant their mention here.

Of medicines used this was said: "This brief epitome comprehends the whole of the therapeutics of insanity," namely, tonics, stimulants, "alteratives," and cathartics.

In 1865 the "hypodermic" method of administering morphine was mentioned as having been used in several cases and the method was recommended as a resource of great value in hospitals where many of the patients refuse to swallow any medicines.

In 1866 the "new cure" for epilepsy, bromide of potassium, was reported as having been freely used in a considerable number of cases, without other favorable results than a mitigation of the severity of the disease in a few of them; but it was admitted that the cases were all chronic when admitted to the hospital. The remedy might be more efficient in the earlier stages of the disease.

In 1870 the "new remedy, the hydrate of choral, was used to a considerable extent during the year, but our experience with it is still insufficient for the basis of a fair judgment of its merits."

As to treatment, it was recognized that "there is no drug specific for disordered minds"; that the most potent remedial agents were those measures that constitute the so-called moral treatment. "By this term is included all agencies the direct and immediate operation of which is upon either the intellect, the passions, the propensities or the moral and religious sentiments. All the details of what is called discipline are included under this head"; such agencies as "manual labor, religious worship, intellectual employment, and recreation and amusement in their diversified forms."

The importance of both employment and amusement or recreation as curative agencies, recently rediscovered by enthusiasts not long in the service, was dwelt upon at length in nearly every report of the hospital.

Fifty years ago it was noted that three-fourths of all the work done in the institution was done by patients.

Daily records of the number of patients at work were kept thus early.

Employment as a means of treatment was not restricted to purely utilitarian pursuits. In the first annual report this is said: "One patient who has passed several years of her life in the very closest confinement, with scarcely the vestige of humanity remaining, is now daily employed in this way (knitting) with much benefit, although she has not recovered the power of speech nor the upright position since her release from close confinement some years since." And the report of 1862 says: "In the hospital let us have labor, hygienic, but not necessarily profitable. Let it cure if it may; but in the name of humanity do not oblige it to be profitable. Let it soothe and heal and amuse if it can, but let us look elsewhere for its profits."

As was noted in 1863, "this subject" (the importance of efforts to introduce a more varied system of labor and to instruct those on the lower strata of weakened intellect in some of the useful departments of labor) "is now attracting the attention of scientific, learned, skillful and long-experienced superintendents of lunatic hospitals, and of medical gentlemen of the highest rank in their profession, both in this country and in Europe."

It may be of interest in these days of diversional occupation, of industrial departments and industrial instructors; of basketry, rug making, weaving and the like, to read that at Northampton 1000 baskets were made in 1862, and that "the manufacture of mats" (of husks) "has well answered its purposes of pleasant diversion and the supply of a constantly recurring want of the house."

The manufacture of palm leaf hats was also attempted in that year.

The inestimable curative value of recreation was written about annually, often at great length; of the value of books, pictures, music and flowers, of bowling, billiards and other indoor games, of dancing, of out-of-door exercises, of ball games, of picnics, and the like.

A singing class was organized in the first winter after the opening of the hospital. Within three years billiards were introduced, a bowling alley was built, a boat was put in commission on the river, a reading room was established with writing table and stand for daily and weekly papers.

A new amusement was introduced in 1866: in the words of the report, "and not to be forgotten, lest we might be thought unfashionable, croquet (or, as one of the *diletantte* patients writes it, *krow-keigh)*." Football was played that year and within a year or two what has since become our national game, baseball.

From the time the hospital went into operation religious exercises have been held every Lord's day. The by-laws of the hospital also required that there be some service or exercise in the chapel on the week day evenings. At first these exercises were conducted by the superintendent and were semi-religious, in that a part of the exercise consisted in the singing of a hymn or two and the reading of a chapter in the Bible. Later this was restricted to Saturday evenings and other exercises were held on the other evenings of the week.

In one year the superintendent notes that assemblies of patients were held on every day of that year except 16, these being days of official visits of trustees, of the Governor and Council, and of the legislative committees. Dr. Earle notes in one place that "as an indication of 'time changes' it may be mentioned that the first sermon ever addressed in America to an audience in an institution like this was preached on the 31st of August, 1819, by the Rev. John Sanford at the New York Hospital."

In 1867 Dr. Earle delivered a course of six lectures to the patients upon diseases of the brain which are accompanied by mental disorder, the "first time that an audience of insane persons ever listened to a course of lectures upon their own malady."

The subject of classification of patients and of institutions for them, always present, ever new, was a frequent one for discussion. It may be added that time has brought about a realization of most of the recommendations made so many years ago.

In 1862 a judicious system of colonization was suggested for the separate support of the incurable pauper insane. As early as 1872 Dr. Earle advocated a separate hospital for insane convicts and the homicidal insane. In 1874 he called attention to defects in the laws bearing upon the subject of inebriation and urged the establishment of a state institution for inebriates. In this year he also emphasized what he had written of before: the desirability of founding a hospital for epileptics alone. He further outlined a scheme for the future by which small hospitals, for 250 patients, might be disseminated throughout the commonwealth according to the massing of its population in the different sections. These should be essentially curative, organized for curables, even if receiving all classes. He deprecated the large institution and the maintaining of institutions solely for chronic cases.

Non-restraint was as live a subject for discussion 60 years ago as it has been in recent years. In the first annual report Dr. Prince writes:

> We have been enabled thus far to dispense with the use of all means of personal restraint, no apparatus of any kind having as yet been used upon any patient. One patient who, from want of proper accommodations in her former place of confinement, had for some time before her admission been chained by the waist, has now the range of one of our halls and by the change wrought in her temper and habits shows that she appreciates the greater liberty allowed her.

It seems to have been the policy of those in charge to use sparingly both restraint and seclusion. During the past 18 years not only has there been a policy of absolute non-restraint in the hospital, but no patients have been allowed to be secluded, and, furthermore, no drugs have been allowed to take the place of either restraint or seclusion. No hypnotics or sedatives are allowed to be used. Their ill effects more than counterbalance any good results from their use.

During the past 15 years extensive use has been made of hydrotherapy.

A training school for nurses was established in 1897.

Since January, 1885, there has always been a woman on the staff of assistant physicians. This hospital was one of the first two in this country to employ more than one woman physician on its staff. Since 1903 the women patients have been entirely cared for by women physicians. At present there are four women assistant physicians in the service of the hospital, including the physician to the out-patient and after-care service.

In order to extend its sphere of usefulness as widely as possible the hospital has encouraged persons mentally ill, or their relatives, to come for free consultation and advice. To increase this work still further, and in a more systematic way, a medical officer was added to the staff in 1911, whose duties are to procure boarding places and to supervise patients placed in family care; to care for the out-patient and social service; to visit patients away from the hospital on probation; to visit patients who are mentally disordered; to advise whether commitment or home treatment is desirable in cases whose commitment is being considered; to investigate home conditions of patients whose release is being considered, and other duties of a similar nature.

In 1914 a series of weekly clinics was established in the principal cities of the hospital district to which anyone in need of advice may come for free consultation. To these clinics come also patients who are out on probation, to report; and relatives to ask about patients at the hospital; and to them are referred doubtful cases by the courts and by societies established to help the unfortunates, as the Society for the Prevention of Cruelty to Children and allied charitable associations. These clinics are attended by the superintendent or by one of the assistant physicians.

The hospital was first called "The Northampton Lunatic Hospital." Thirty years ago Dr. Earle requested of the Legislature that the title "Northampton Hospital for Insane" be substituted, thus eliminating the objectionable word lunatic, but this request was not heeded. However, the name was changed in 1899 to the "Northampton Insane Hospital," and at the request of the present superintendent it was again changed in 1906 by a special act of the Legislature to its present title, "The Northampton State Hospital."

During the 58 years of its operation there have been but four superintendents. Dr. William H. Prince was its first superintendent, serving from 1858 to 1864. Though inexperienced in the care of the insane prior to assuming the position, the trustees bear testimony to his high ideals, to his capacity, and to an adaptation to his duties of a high order. He was succeeded by Dr. Pliny Earle, a gentleman of classical education, with large experience in the care of the insane and management of institutions, both in this and in foreign countries, extending over many years. His ability as a writer and his reputation in this country and abroad are too well known to require more than a brief mention in this history. A voluminous writer, his best known contributions to the literature of the specialty are his articles on the "Curability of Insanity," which appeared in the reports of 1876 and several following years, in which he so thoroughly demonstrated the fallacies that were then held by many of the leaders in the specialty that the methods of estimating recoveries and of recording the statistics of the insane were revolutionized. He served 21 years, retiring in 1885, but he continued to reside at the hospital till his death in 1892.

He was succeeded by Dr. Edward B. Nims, who had been his assistant physician for nearly 17 years. He came to the hospital in 1869, after a service of three years as assistant physician at the Brattleboro (Vt.) Hospital for the Insane. Previous to that he had had medical and surgical service for 15 months in the Civil War as assistant surgeon in the First Regiment of Vermont Cavalry. He served 12 years as superintendent, retiring in 1897, after the longest medical service in the history of the hospital, 29 years as assistant and superintendent.

His successor, John A. Houston, the present superintendent, came to this hospital as assistant physician in 1889, after a service of one year in the Maine General Hospital and seven years in the Worcester Lunatic (now State) Hospital.

The following medical officers have served as assistant physicians:

Austin W. Thompson, M. D.	1858-1859
C. K. Bartlett, M. D.	1859-1869
Edward B. Nims, M. D. (later supt.)	1869-1885
Edw. R. Spalding, M. D.	1870-1874
Alonzo S. Wallace, M. D.	1874-1874
Samuel M. Garlick, M. D.	1874-1876
Wm. G. Kimball, M. D.	1876-1877
Daniel Pickard, M. D.	1877-1887
David G. Hall, M. D.	1882-1888
Emily F Wells, M. D.	1885-1892
Charles G. Dewey, M. D.	1886-1887
Edward B. Lane, M. D.	1888-1889
Chas. M. Holmes, M. D.	1889-1898
John A. Houston, M. D. (later supt.)	1889-1897
Jane R. Raker, M. D.	1892-1897
Payn B. Parsons, M. D.	1897-1900
William H. Coon, M. D.	1897-1898
Emma W. Mooers, M. D.	1898-1899
Justus G. Hanson, M. D.	1898-1903
E. Stanley Abbot, M. D.	1898-1899
Charles H. Dean, M. D.	1900-1913
Harriet M. Wiley, M. D.	1900-
Arthur B. Moulton, M. D.	1901-1904
Helen T. Cleaves, M. D.	1901-1901
Grace E. B. Rice, M. D.	1903-1909
Edw. W. Whitney, M. D.	1905-1911
Chas. S. Raymond, M. D.	1906-1912
Mabel C. Cruttenden, M. D.	1909-1911
B. Angela Bober, M. D.	1911-
Eliza P. Brison, M. D.	1911-1912
Charles E. Perry, M. D.	1912-1914
Anne Humphreys, M. D.	1912-1913
Mary C. Couch, M. D.	1912-1913
Arthur N. Ball, M. D.	1912-
Geraldine Oakley, M. D.	1913-
Jean MacLean, M. D.	1914-
Edward C. Greene, M. D.	1914-

STATE INFIRMARY.[1]

TEWKSBURY, MASS.

An act of the Legislature of Massachusetts, May 20, 1852, Chapter 275, authorized the building of three state almshouses to accommodate not less than 500 inmates each. An appropriation of $100,000 being granted for the construction of the three, locations were selected and wooden buildings erected in the towns of Tewksbury, Bridgewater and Monson. The State Almshouse, Tewksbury, Mass., was opened for inmates on May 1, 1854, under proclamation of Governor Emory Washburn. The government of the almshouse was vested in a board of three inspectors, E. Huntington, George Foster and J. G. Peabody, and the executive department in a superintendent, physician and chaplain, as follows: Isaac H. Meserve, superintendent; Jonathan Brown, physician; Joseph M. Burtt, chaplain.

At the end of the first week 668 inmates had been admitted, and by May 20, 800. "For the first year 2193 pauper inmates were admitted, comprising men, women, boys, girls, infants; sane and insane."

By an act of 1855, children between 5 and 15 years of age were sent to Monson.

In 1856 certain of the harmless and incurable insane were sent to Tewksbury, as they could be cared for there at a much less cost than at the lunatic hospitals.

In the annual report of 1857 occurs the following:

"Within the last year arrangements have been made for the accommodation and safekeeping of the insane, of which class we always have more or less. A cheap building has been put up within the enclosure of the yard, where these unfortunates can be properly guarded and kindly cared for." This building was fitted up for the care of the insane women, but for the insane men there was no distinct department, and it was recommended that they be quartered in the "old school room."

[1] By John H. Nichols, M. D., superintendent and resident physician.

In 1858 Isaac Meserve was succeeded as superintendent by Thomas J. Marsh.[1]

In 1861 there was a weekly average of 900 inmates, and the want of suitable quarters for the insane was urgent, as large numbers of insane had been transferred to Tewksbury from the lunatic hospitals.

In 1864 the Board of Charities transferred to Tewksbury 58 harmless and incurable insane patients from the hospitals at Worcester and Taunton. A few were also voluntarily sent from the various towns. The Legislature accordingly appropriated $10,000 to erect a suitable building for this class, and $15,000 more was appropriated to provide for the criminal insane, but this latter class was never transferred to Tewksbury. The action of the board appears to have been induced by the following reasons:

First. The necessity of relieving overcrowded insane hospitals, and thus making room for new applicants.

Second. The belief that the recovery of curable cases was retarded, if not prevented, by the presence of so many pitiable objects, who were themselves gaining nothing by a longer residence.

Third. The hope that their condition might be bettered by assigning all able to do a trifling amount of work to some suitable department of labor.

Fourth. The opportunity thus afforded for a better classification within the hospitals.

Fifth. The obvious economy of the change.

In 1865 a fence was built around the institution. The men and boys and the insane men all had different recreation yards; and the women and girls and the insane women also had separate recreation yards.

By the act of 1866 creating a State Primary School at Monson and a State Workhouse at Bridgewater, Tewksbury was relieved of the care of children mentally and physically well, and of the

[1] It is of interest to know that the change of superintendents was made by the Governor simply to find a job for Thomas J. Marsh, as a purely political favor for some acknowledged obligation. Entirely unexpectedly Mr. Marsh appeared before Supt. Meserve at the office with his commission from the Governor in his hands, and said, "I wish to be your guest for to-night and to-morrow I wish you to be my guest."

adult, vicious paupers, and became an asylum for the harmless and incurable insane, the crippled, the epileptic, idiotic children, and for such other persons, who, on account of their infirmities, were unable to support themselves.

The Tewksbury institution, besides being a place for harmless and chronic insane, became a state asylum for those who, through misfortune and poverty, had become dependent on state care.

In 1866 an asylum for the insane was completed at a cost of $33,910.98 to accommodate 120 harmless insane paupers. This building was four stories in height, 125 feet long by 45 feet wide, and constitutes to-day one-half of the old brick building which is used for insane women. It was opened on October 21, 1866, and a special register for the insane was ordered, which has been kept separate ever since. There were 145 inmates placed upon the register, consisting of the insane, the idiotic and the feeble-minded.

On July 1, 1866, there were 126 insane in the almshouse. There are no data by which the number of insane can be ascertained prior to that date, as there were no separate records of the insane prior to 1864.

On October 1, 1866, 145 persons were transferred by order of the Board of State Charities to the asylum for harmless insane—74 males and 71 females. Eighty-three resided in the new building—38 males and 45 females. Forty-nine were detailed for labor and were domiciled among the inmates of the almshouse. Two men and three women were put in the hospital for the sick.

Jonathan Brown, M. D., the first physician, appointed in 1854, resigned January, 1866, and Dr. Horace P. Wakefield was appointed to succeed him.

In the report of Dr. Horace P. Wakefield for 1867 occurs the following:

The attention of the medical world is being directed to the condition of the harmless and incurable insane. The American Medical Association, at its annual meeting held in Cincinnati in May last, after discussion on this subject, passed the following resolution:

Resolved, That the example of Massachusetts in establishing asylums for the accommodation and humane treatment of the chronic insane is worthy of all praise and commendation, and in the opinion of this association such institutions, if rightly inaugurated and judiciously carried on, will be a benefit to the state in an economical point of view, will raise the character of the state hospitals, and will greatly subserve the interests of the insane generally.

The establishment of such a department connected with one of our state almshouses has given rise to much controversy in this state, and has elicited much discussion among the members of the medical profession and philanthropists particularly interested in the insane throughout the United States. It has cost some effort to initiate this experiment. The thorns have been thicker than the roses. Massachusetts, which has been the pioneer in many noble works, struck out boldly, and, while others have hesitated, after having provided liberally for her recent insane, has concluded to do something for her chronic insane, her idiots, epileptics and imbeciles.

In 1868 Dr. Wakefield resigned to accept the superintendency of the State Primary School, Monson. Dr. Joseph D. Nichols was appointed his successor after eight years' experience in a similar institution at Monson. The whole number of insane in the institution was 267, and a large amount of the work was being performed by these patients. This year the sum of $6000 was appropriated for reservoirs, cisterns, steam pump and hydrants for fire protection.

In 1870 the number of insane reached 294—201 women and 93 men. An appropriation made for a new hospital led, in 1874, to a better classification of the inmates, namely:

1. Insane cared for in separate building (asylum).
2. Sick cared for in separate building (hospital).
3. Poor cared for in separate building (almshouse).

In 1871 the Legislature appropriated $25,000 to provide accommodations for 150 more insane. This enlargement caused the erection of the second part of the brick building used for insane women.

In 1871 the management of Tewksbury was vested in: First, a board of three male inspectors; second, an advisory board of three women; third, a superintendent; and, fourth, a resident physician.

In 1874, as a matter of reorganization, Dr. J. M. Whitaker was appointed physician, and assigned to the exclusive charge of the insane, and Dr. Nichols and "Miss Marsh, M. D.," were placed in charge of the sick. At the same time six nurses were added to the number on duty in the hospital. Here water closets had been established in place of the earth closets, and improvements made in the ventilation.

According to the report of 1874, the institution could hardly be longer called a poorhouse in the ordinary sense of the term, but rather a combination of an asylum for the demented, an infirmary for the sick, and a nursery for foundlings. Forty per cent of the inmates were patients deemed by experts to be hopelessly insane; 15 per cent were hospital patients, 12 per cent foundlings, or children under four years of age, making the classes of defectives or dependents 67 per cent of the entire population, while all of the remaining 33 per cent were incapacitated by age or some infirmity of mind or body.

Dr. Joseph Nichols resigned during the year after 15 years' service at Tewksbury and Monson.

In 1876 the number of physicians and nurses was increased. Dr. William H. Lothrop was appointed as physician-in-charge, and Dr. E. Putney and Dr. E. Q. Marston appointed as first and second assistants to Dr. Lothrop. In his report for the year the thanks of the superintendent are expressed to W. W. Godding, of Taunton, for counsel and assistance to the insane.

In 1877 new water sections were established throughout the asylum building. Mention is made of the fact that many insane have been sent to Tewksbury from the different towns who should have been properly committed to regular insane hospitals. There were seven cases requiring restraint, and one, seclusion. One hundred and fifty-seven inmates in the asylum were able to do no work whatever.

In 1878 Dr. Charles Foster succeeded Dr. Marston, who went to the asylum at Worcester, and Dr. Putney made a series of stethoscopic examinations of the insane for thoracic diseases, finding 16 cases of phthisis and 17 of organic heart disease.

In 1883 there were 293 insane inmates, only 18 of whom were men. In this year the number of attendants in the insane wards was increased, and "the husbands of the female attendants who formerly assisted their wives in the care of the insane women" were either assigned positions elsewhere or were discharged.

In the 30th annual report of the almshouse, as written by the Board of Lunacy and Charity, acting as trustees, the trustees having been suspended by Governor Butler, April 23, the following change is announced:

" By authority of the Legislature the whole establishment, which has long been a hospital in fact, though almshouse in name, was put under the direction of a competent medical officer, the present superintendent and resident physician." This change was long since recommended by the State Board, which, in January, 1876, said in its yearly report: " None but a physician could properly regulate the daily discipline of a hospital, and any competent physician in full charge might, in a short time, remove most of the objections which have been made to this great State Almshouse as a place for treatment of disease and insanity."

The resident physician declined re-election. The former superintendent, Thomas J. Marsh, declined to present a new bond, and therefore ceased to hold office, continuing certain duties until July 1, when he closed his long period of service at the State Almshouse. The union of the office of resident physician and superintendent in one person which was made this year much promoted the comfort of the sick and the insane.

Dr. C. Irving Fisher, formerly port physician of Boston, was placed in charge as superintendent and resident physician.

On July 1, 1884, Tewksbury entered upon a new organization. The government was vested in a Board of seven Trustees, composed of five men and two women, as follows: J. White Belcher, chairman; Weaver Osborn, Sarah D. Fiske, Catharine Lothrop, E. W. Hoyt and Dr. Thomas Dwight. The executive power was vested in a medical superintendent.

Dr. Anna M. Wilkin resigned to accept the position of resident physician in the Women's Reformatory, and Dr. M. Emily Pagelson was appointed in her place. Dr. Herbert B. Howard was appointed to the position left vacant by Dr. Cole.

The insane asylum contained 297 women. The few insane men did not require separation. The number of the insane had been recently increased by large transfers from Worcester, Taunton and Danvers. Besides the whole work of their own department, the insane aided in sewing for other departments. Music was furnished and the patients were encouraged to dance and sing, and daily walks were made with attendants through the woods and country roads. Iron fire escapes were established on asylum buildings.

Colonel W. D. Tripp, who was placed in charge when the Board of Lunacy and Charity assumed control, and who remained as acting assistant superintendent, was recalled August 1 by the State Board of Lunacy and Charity.

In 1885 there were 250 women in the asylum, and mention is made of their usual recreations, walks, dancing, etc., and sleigh rides. For the first time "the insane in the asylum receive daily visits from physicians."

Dr. Herbert B. Howard resigned to enter private practice, and Dr. M. Emily Pagelson resigned to become resident physician of New England Hospital for Women.

In 1886 there were 375 insane, only 11 of whom were men; 2140 had been admitted since the beginning of the register in 1866.

In November, 1886, 43 insane men were transferred to the almshouse without previous notice being given, and accommodations for them were arranged in the "old chapel building," 51 beds in all.

Dr. E. C. Norton and Dr. Ella M. Patton were assistant physicians during this year.

In 1888 Tewksbury had become a large hospital divided into:

1. Three separate hospitals for male and female patients.

2. Two separate asylums for male and female insane.

3. Pauper department, occupying several wards in different parts of the institution. In consequence of which the trustees in 1888 suggested to the Legislature that the institution be called "State Hospital."

Dr. H. B. Howard, mentioned in previous reports, was appointed first assistant physician on December 15, 1888, and Dr. Myra D. Allen assistant physician on January 15.

There were 90 admissions to the insane asylums. These patients made their own clothing as well as that for the whole institution. Sixty-three patients were boarded out. Reference is made to the work of the insane in gathering fruits, etc.

The report of 1888 records the resignation of Dr. Patton and Dr. Norton, to go into private practice.

A system of electric lighting was introduced throughout the whole institution. Rearrangement of heating appliances in the insane asylum connected with boilers of the new hospital made it possible to remove the men from the basement of the women's asylum, where it was necessary for them to attend to the fires. This year a fine piano was provided by the trustees.

In 1889 a Board of Consulting Physicians was established, as follows: John Homans, M. D.; Maurice H. Richardson, M. D.; B. Joy Jeffries, M. D.; J. C. Irish, M. D.; Cyrus M. Chamberlain, M. D.; J. J. Putnam, M. D.; Gustav Liebman, M. D.

In 1891 an idea of the general conditions and standards of the almshouse at the end of Dr. Fisher's administration is expressed in the trustees' report, as follows:

> The State Almshouse differs in character and requirements from the other institutions supported in whole or in part by the commonwealth. It not only contains a pauper department, for which a portion of the present building was originally intended, but a male and female hospital, recently erected, and a male and female insane asylum; and while there are thus five different and separate departments, they are in reality five different institutions combined under one management.

At the end of this year Dr. C. Irving Fisher tendered his resignation in order to accept the superintendency of the Presbyterian Hospital, New York City, after eight years' service as superintendent.

Dr. John H. Nichols, of the Harvard Medical School, was appointed interne on July 1.

In the department for the insane there were 364 present—68 males and 296 females. Mention is made that a large amount of work is done by the insane, including all of the milking and gathering and preparing for cooking of a large amount of products of the farm. Ten to 20 men are employed on the farm.

In his final report Dr. Fisher modestly says, referring to his eight years of service: "I have been enabled to institute and bring to completion many improvements."

Dr. Herbert B. Howard was appointed to succeed Dr. Fisher in November, 1891. He was, at the time, first assistant physician and acting assistant superintendent. Dr. Howard first came in relation to the institution in 1883 when a student in the Harvard Medical School.

In 1892 Dr. John M. Gile was appointed first assistant physician and assistant superintendent. The immediate care of the insane was placed in the hands of Dr. Fred. B. Jewett.

The tables of "uniform statistics," 19 in number, relative to the department for the insane, appear for the first time in this report for 1892. The individual history of every insane patient in the institution is the basis of this work. Spacious summer houses with concrete floors had been built in the yard for insane women. The ward of the women's hospital, second floor, had been fitted up with window guards, etc., and was used as an infirmary for the insane women.

In 1893 $34,000 was appropriated for new kitchen, boiler house, bakery and dining room near the center of the yard, giving a large dining room in the basement for the insane women. The insane men were provided for at separate tables in the main dining room for men on the first floor of this building.

Dr. Harvey P. Towle, first assistant physician, resigned to become assistant superintendent of the Boston City Hospital. He was succeeded by Dr. John H. Nichols.

The men's asylum was occupied on the 1st of October, 1892. It has proved a most admirable building for the class of cases for which it was designed. The ventilation has been good, notwithstanding that 40 more patients have been housed in it than the original design contemplated.

The old building vacated by the men was moved across the yard, in accordance with the suggestion of the Board of Lunacy and Charity, and was occupied by 60 insane women.

The lectures of the training school continued from October 1 to June 1. The asylums for the insane were brought under the same superintendent of nurses, and the training school work was extended to the asylum department.

In 1895 $50,000 was appropriated for a building for insane women.

In 1896 Dr. John M. Gile, assistant superintendent for five years, resigned to become professor of theory and practice in the Dartmouth Medical School. Dr. J. F. Edgerly was called to the Pennsylvania Hospital for the Insane as one of its assistants. Dr. Elizabeth Newcomb accepted a call as lecturer of physiology and director of girls' gymnasium at Oberlin College. Dr. Nichols was granted three months' leave of absence in which to visit institutions for the poor, the sick and the insane in England and Scotland.

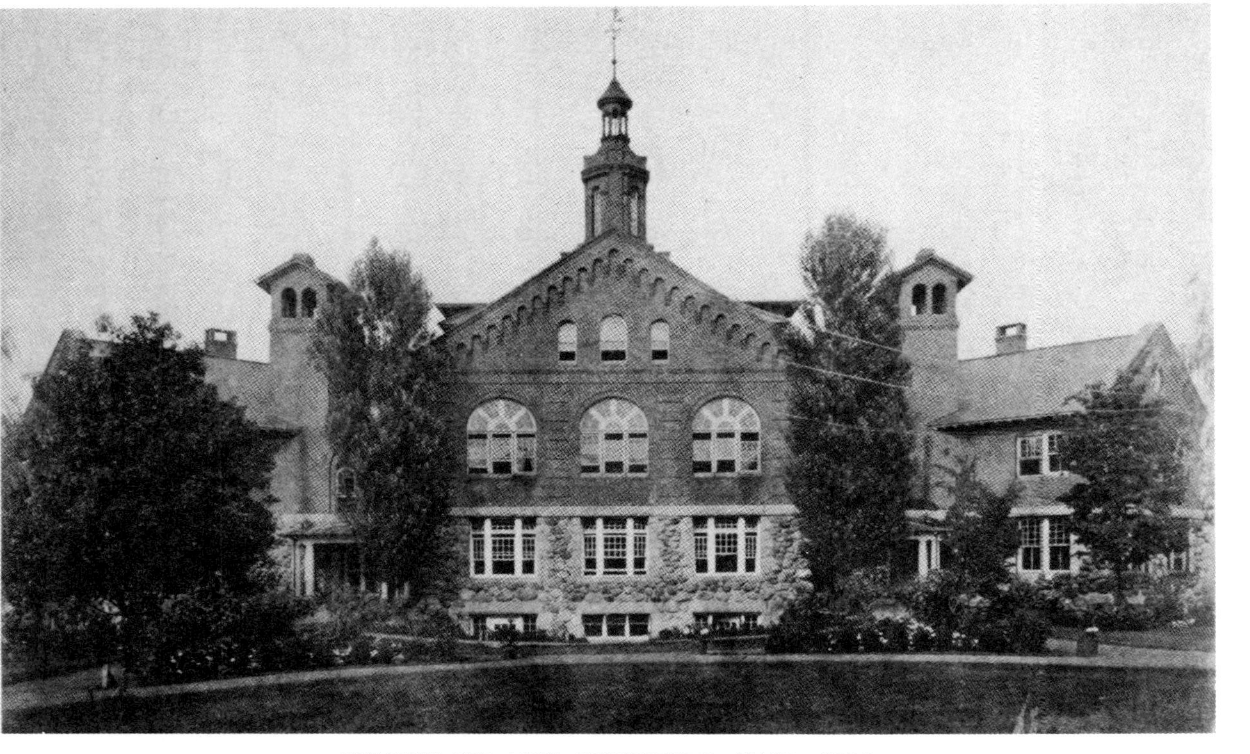

BUILDING FOR MEN, TEWKSBURY, MASS., 1902.

This year the first diplomas were granted from the training school, four nurses receiving diplomas. The men's hospital was brought under the charge of the superintendent of nurses and the training school work extended to reach this department.

Dr. John H. Nichols was appointed to succeed Dr. Gile as assistant superintendent. Dr. Emily Pagelson Howard was appointed assistant physician in charge of the department for the insane.

In 1897 "the faithful and efficient administration of Dr. Herbert B. Howard came to an end." He resigned June 1 to become superintendent of the Massachusetts General Hospital. Dr. John H. Nichols was made acting superintendent for four months, at the end of which time he was made superintendent.

The new asylum for women was opened on May 1 and proved a great help toward better care and classification of the insane. The violent cases were transferred to this ward and further classification of patients in the old asylum effected, much to the benefit and comfort of the milder cases.

The resignation of Dr. Emily Pagelson Howard, assistant physician-in-charge of the department for the insane, took effect soon after that of Dr. H. B. Howard on July 1, but not until after a careful classification of the patients in this department, made possible by the new building for women, had been carried into effect.

In 1898 85 patients were received in the asylum during the year. The daily average was 461; 29 patients were transferred to the hospital for epileptics at Palmer. The good effects of the classification of the patients of the previous year and the improvement in their general deportment were manifest during the year, as well as the general efficiency of the nurses in charge. Three thousand three hundred dollars was expended in repairing and improving the old asylum buildings for women. Improvements in sanitary sections, remodelling, and addition of special comforts in sitting rooms, and improvements in heating and ventilating in both sitting rooms and dormitories, and the bringing of this building up to the modern requirements, were effected at this time.

An improved daily report for the asylum department was established; also a table to show the amount of days' work done by patients. Of the whole number present, 56 per cent were employed daily. This improved report provided for a detailed account of everything going on in the wards not only during the day, but also through the night, requiring a record of every incident in connection with the patients. These reports were reviewed and signed by the physicians every morning. All of the patients requiring restraint or seclusion had been removed the previous year to the new asylum for women, and in order to reduce the matter of mechanical restraint to the minimum possibility, such restraint was removed from all of the patients for a period of two weeks, after which it was found necessary to apply a mild form of restraint to a few of the patients, because of the small number of nurses available in the department and because of the destructiveness to the building, the fixtures and their own clothing on the part of some of the patients.

The work of the training school for nurses was extended to a three-years' course, to include the asylum as well as the hospital; especially to improve the general care of the patients in the asylum wards, and also to give advantage to the pupil nurses of a broader field in experience and usefulness.

The number of insane patients remaining at the end of the year 1899 was 494; in the asylum 118 patients were admitted during the year. Besides the reconstruction of the old asylum for women, considerable work was accomplished in refurnishing these wards with furniture especially adapted to the requirements of the insane, and made in the asylum shops.

During the year 1903 infirmary records of the insane department were established and appear in additional tables at the end of the report for the insane, so this year for the first time the physical diseases were not included in the regular hospital statistics, but appeared in the additional tables of the asylum department.

In 1901 Dr. A. J. Ranney, assistant superintendent, specially assigned to the care of the department for the insane, resigned to become superintendent of the Long Island Hospital, Boston Harbor. He was succeeded by Dr. Joseph B. Howland, first assistant physician.

In 1902 $60,000 was appropriated for an additional asylum for 100 insane women. In this year Dr. Joseph B. Howland resigned to become superintendent of the Gardner State Colony for the Insane, then under construction.

A new asylum for men was completed with three separate sections, two of which contained 30 patients each, and the middle section 40. This building is two stories in height and has a habitable basement for kitchen, dining rooms, industrial rooms, etc., and six rooms on the third floor for nurses. Dr. Harold C. Goodwin from this department resigned to take a position of greater responsibilities at the State Hospital for Insane, Concord, N. H. Dr. Charles E. Thompson was assigned to duties in the laboratory and department for the insane.

In 1904 a new asylum for men was opened and furnished with furniture of asylum design and construction; this brought the department for men up to the most recent standards.

This year Dr. Arthur K. Drake, assistant superintendent, resigned to become superintendent of the Lowell General Hospital, and Charles E. Thompson, pathologist, resigned to accept a position at the State Colony for Insane, Gardner. Dr. George L. Baker, of the interne service, was appointed assistant in bacteriology at the Harvard Medical School.

In 1906 the death of J. White Belcher, chairman of the Board of Trustees since its organization in 1884, is recorded. "The whole rebuilding of the institution until 1906 took place under Mr. Belcher's chairmanship, until it was recognized as one of the best of its kind, and will ever be a great monument to his labors. Although holding many high positions it did not prevent him from answering every call at the State Hospital." The last new building constructed under his administration (building for insane women) is designated by the name "Belcher."

The occupation of the new building for insane women made it possible to effect much better classification, added much to the general comfort of the patients and greatly diminished the excitement and confusion on the wards which necessarily exists in an institution of this kind. One-half of this new building was devoted to acute and infirmary cases, the other half to excited patients.

In this year a hospital for consumptive women was erected, one-half mile distant from the other buildings, and also a building for male nurses and attendants. A new wire fence with stone columns and iron posts was erected around the yards for the insane, which greatly enlarged the enclosed area of this department, replacing old wooden fences. This is one of the most satisfactory improvements of recent years, especially in the yard for insane women, which now comprises about five acres of land without sub-divisions. The patients are able to see all that is going on near the institution, their distant view is not restricted, the circulation of air is not prevented during the sultry days of summer, the visitors to the grounds of the institution and those passing by are able to observe the patients within at all times; thus, there is practically a constant inspection of all that is going on within the yard, contentment is promoted among the patients and greater care and pride in their personal appearance and behavior are manifested in a large number of the cases. Additional attractiveness or pleasure is afforded by very extensive gardens of perennial and bedding-out plants well cared for, presenting a mass of continuous change of form and color throughout the season.

In 1907 Dr. George A. Pierce, first assistant physician for nine years, and during the last two years in charge of the department for insane, resigned to take the position of assistant superintendent of the State Colony for Insane, Gardner. Dr. Burt F. Howard, of the Eastern Maine Hospital, Bangor, succeeded Dr. Pierce.

Dr. Ernest B. Emerson, assistant superintendent and in charge of the department for the insane, resigned in 1908 to organize and build the new consumptive hospital at North Reading. Dr. Howard F. Holmes succeeded him in charge of the insane.

From this hospital had gone out within a decade eight men who are now hospital superintendents.

Dr. Carl J. Hedin, assistant in the department for insane, resigned in April to accept a position at the hospital for insane in Augusta. Dr. Samuel R. Haythorn, pathologist, resigned, to take a position in the pathological department of the Boston City Hospital, and is now professor in the Alleghany Medical School in Pittsburgh.

By the Acts and Resolves of 1909, Chapter 504, the name of the State Hospital was changed to "State Infirmary." This was because the same act eliminated the word "insane" from the titles of the numerous institutions for the insane, naming them state hospitals, and designating them by the town in which they

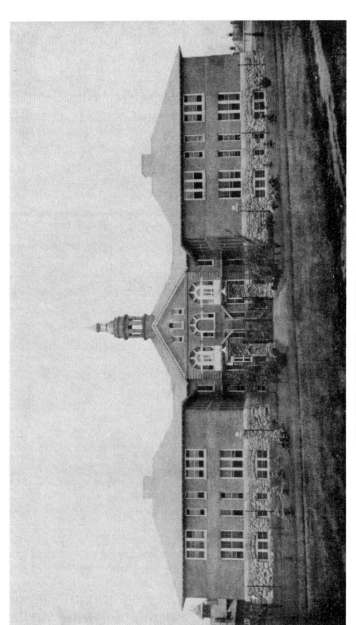

BELCHER BUILDING, TEWKSBURY, MASS.

were located, which would have left this institution without a special distinctive name, and would have been misleading as to the general hospital character.

In the insane department there were admitted 226 patients, 78 of which were committed from the hospital wards. There remained at the end of the year 704—508 women and 196 men.

The work of extending and improving the dining room and kitchen building gave a new, attractive dining room for the insane men. The insane women, who had previously occupied the dining room in the basement, were allowed to occupy a large dining room on the first floor.

In 1910 the average number of insane was 738. Dr. T. F. Richards resigned this year to become assistant in pathology at the Harvard Medical School.

In 1911 Dr. John C. Lindsay resigned to take a position in the State Hospital for the Insane, Augusta, Me.

Although frequent mention is made of the work and industries of the insane throughout the entire history of the institution, a more systematic development of the industries was attempted during this year. Industrial rooms were established in the basement of several of the buildings and larger numbers were employed. A greatly increased industrial output was accomplished as well as a marked improvement in the interest and deportment of the insane patients. Remaking and repairing of old articles and remaking of old junk and attempts at recovering the valuable by-products became a special matter of interest this year.

In the department for the insane 129 patients were admitted in 1912. A dentist was added to the staff, especially benefiting the children and those in the department for the insane.

A new building, an observation ward for women, for cases of probable insanity or feeble-mindedness, was built. The chapel was enlarged, increasing the seating capacity from 500 to 900. Besides the religious services on Sunday, a large stage enabled the hospital to present effective dramatic and other entertainments. Social and other gatherings are held in this chapel. The circulating library was removed and shelves placed in the alcoves and along the outer aisles; reading tables were established and everything planned to enable this building to serve as a neighborhood house during the times when it is not used for religious services.

During the 12 months beginning October 1, 1913, and ending September 30, 1914, there were admitted to the insane department 138 cases—65 by transfer, 55 by commitment from the general hospital department, 15 nominally and 3 from visit and escape. The daily average number of patients was 722. The number remaining September 30, 1914, was 741—538 women and 203 men. There were 56 deaths—27 men and 29 women. There were discharged 17 cases improved, 10 not improved, 7 on visit, 9 transferred to other institutions and 8 escaped.

Dr. Harry R. Coburn was placed in charge of the department of the insane, assisted by Dr. John C. Lindsay, Dr. Earl C. Willoughby and Dr. Hattie E. Chalmers.

The new laboratory building was completed, with ample opportunities for post-mortem examinations, with seats for instruction of nurses and students, with museum section, consulting room, office, one large laboratory for general pathology, one smaller section for biological chemistry and one for bacteriology, with three smaller rooms for the heads of these different departments.

By the Acts of 1904 authority was given for commitment of patients judged to be insane, received in the general hospital wards, into the department for the insane. It is by this process that the hospital receives the new acute forms of mental disease, although they are not committed to the asylum from the courts outside.

At present the insane are housed in buildings separated by a large yard from the building of the general hospital department, surrounding a large rectangular piece of ground, in the southernmost part of the main group. They occupy separate grounds and separate dining rooms, and a large part of them assist in the regular work or activities of the institution. They are cared for by four physicians who give almost their entire time, and three others who give partial time to their care. Besides the general work in which they have assisted from the beginning, they have also accomplished, during the last four or five years, a vast amount of work in a great variety of lines under the direction of industrial teachers.

At occasional intervals since 1900, when the general care of the insane was taken from the Board of Charity and the State Board of Insanity was established, the State Board of Charity has urged that the insane should be removed from the State Infirmary. Opposition has been maintained by the Board of Trustees for the reason that this department greatly aids in the general up-keep and work of the rest of the institution.

The patients enjoy a great deal of freedom, and, by being in relation with a large, well-equipped general hospital, are able to command many medical and surgical advantages and considerations which are not provided in institutions entirely for the insane.

Although all of the patients are now legally committed cases, the fact of their being here does not necessarily establish the stigma of insanity upon them, they being in an institution of which they form one-third of the population, and which is generally known as a large hospital for general diseases, with large separate departments for children and for tuberculosis as well.

One special matter of good fortune and comfort in regard to the housing of the insane at the infirmary is that with all the overcrowding it has never been necessary to encroach upon the very ample and attractive sitting rooms, which they occupy during the day.

Among the physicians who have assisted or who have been trained in this department and have gained distinction in matters relating to the problems of the insane are: Dr. Herbert B. Howard, former superintendent at Tewksbury, subsequently one of the original members appointed to the State Board of Insanity in 1900, chairman of the Board of Trustees for State Colony for the Insane, Gardner, during the building and organizing of that institution, later member of the Board of Insanity and chairman of the board from 1908 to 1913. Dr. John M. Gile, formerly one of the Commissioners of Insanity for the State of New Hampshire, professor of theory and practice of medicine, later professor of surgery and dean of the Dartmouth Medical School. Dr. Joseph B. Howland, for five years superintendent of the State Colony for the Insane, Gardner, during the construction and organization of that institution. Dr. Jane R. Baker, superintendent of the County Hospital for the Insane, Embreeville, Pennsylvania, from 1902 to 1912. Dr. Fred. B. Jewett, recently superintendent of the department for the insane, Howard, R. I. Dr. Charles E. Thompson, superintendent of the State Colony for the Insane, Gardner, from 1909 to 1911, executive officer of the Massachusetts State

Board of Insanity from 1911 to 1914. Dr. Charles S. Little, superintendent of the School for Feeble-minded, Laconia, N. H., now superintendent School for Feeble-minded, Letchworth Village, Rockland County, Thiells, N. Y. Dr. Ernest B. Emerson, medical director at the State Hospital for the Insane, Bridgewater, Mass. Dr. Carl J. Hedin, superintendent of the School for Feeble-minded, West Pownal, Me., 1911-. Dr. Frederick M. Hollister, superintendent of the County Hospital for the Insane, Embreeville, Pennsylvania, from 1912, and Dr. Forrest C. Tyson, superintendent of the State Hospital for the Insane, Augusta, Me., 1914.

To-day the State Infirmary is situated on a tract of land comprising 750 acres; carries on three distinct farms, one of these operated wholly by the insane men; maintains its own waterworks, a system of driven wells; has seven acres of filter beds for the disposal of sewage; central heat, lighting and power department; cold storage and mechanical department. It consists of about 50 buildings of brick or fire-resisting construction, and 25 or more wooden out-lying buildings; has four separate buildings for nurses' home and employees' department; a separate building for children; two large hospitals for tuberculosis (men and women); five isolation wards for infectious diseases; an observation ward for mental cases (women); a surgical building; a laboratory building; a separate building for administration offices and officers' quarters; a house for the superintendent; detached buildings for laundry and store or freight-house, with a separate siding for coal and freight; two large pavilion buildings (men and women) for the crippled and infirm, and also for convalescent patients; five general hospitals in separate buildings; a maternity hospital; a centralized domestic building; five separate buildings for the insane—two for men and three for women. With the exception of five main buildings, which are distantly located, these main departments are included in an enclosed area of about 26 acres, with very attractive grounds, courts and gardens, with large airing spaces between each of the separate departments.

The register for the insane indicates that 5467 patients have been admitted and cared for in the institution since 1866. The number of insane in the wards is 741—540 women and 201 men. The total census of the institution to-day (1914) is 2800 (largest in the history of the institution). The total admissions to the infirmary since it has been established are 183,278.

Throughout the history of the institution mention has been constantly made and great appreciation expressed of the value of the insane to the institution, and although there has been phenomenal growth in all the other departments for which the institution is specially intended and designed, still the thought for the care, comfort and the happiness of this portion of the institution has been continuously in evidence, as manifested by the new buildings and the many matters of interest and improvements effected especially for them; and the constant genuine attempt to keep this department at least up to the standards of institutions especially designated for the insane.

In closing this history it seems pertinent, owing to the fact that agitation is still active for removing this department from the State Infirmary, to say that the opposition of the management to this proposition is maintained for reasons as follows:

"The buildings in which the insane patients are housed form practically a distinct group, occupying the southernmost portions of the grounds. The organization and the administration of this department are distinct from the others, so that it is nearly like an independent establishment. The patients who are able, however, as has always been the case, contribute very largely to the operation and economy of the whole institution by doing such work as it is suitable for them to perform in general housekeeping, laundry, kitchen and work on the farm, stable and grounds. The patients not only do that which they would necessarily do in relation to the running of their own department, but are able to do a large amount of the same sort of work for the other departments, at the various points where large amounts of work can be centralized, in the institution, of which numerically they make up but one-third of the population; the other two-thirds occupying the general hospital, tuberculosis, house and convalescent departments, are mostly physically able to render but little aid in the necessary daily activities of the large institution. Briefly spoken, the insane patients, without prejudicing their own well-being, can and do render much service for the welfare of others, which is also an essential to the real treatment and to the general happiness of themselves."

Throughout this review of the insane there has been continued mention and record of statistics, conditions and improvements relative to the other departments for reason that the unusual character of the State Infirmary, and the important bearing of the relation of all of the different departments and interests with the others are essential. The welfare of any one or more departments also affects the others, and it would be like recording the history of a large family and omitting to take account of a number of its members if mention should be omitted of the nature and progress of the other work while recording that of the department of the insane at the State Infirmary.

The resident officers since the founding of the institution have been:

Name	Years
Isaac H. Meserve	1854-1858
Dr. Jonathan Brown	1854-1856
Thomas Marsh	1858-1883
Dr. ——— Wood	1862-
Dr. ——— Brigham	1862-
Dr. W. C. Tracy	1866-
Dr. George W. Marsters	1866-
Dr. Horace Wakefield	1867-1868
Dr. Joseph D. Nichols	1868-1875
Dr. Helen M. Marsh	1872-1876
Dr. James M. Whitaker	1874-1875
Dr. William Lothrop	1875-1883
Dr. George E. Putney	1876-1878
Dr. Enoch Q. Marston	1876-1878
Dr. Charles Foster	1877-1880
Dr. Edwin F. Cummings	1878-1879
Dr. Wendall P. Kenney	1880-1881
Dr. Julia P. Pease	1880-1881
Dr. Stephen W. Abbott	1881-1882
Dr. Julia P. Abbott	1881-1882
Dr. Edward J. Cutter	1882-1883
Dr. Anna W. Wilkin	1882-1884
Dr. C. Irving Fisher	1883-1892
Dr. David Dana	1883-
Dr. William D. Otterson	1883-
Dr. R. M. Cole	1883-1884
Dr. F. W. Kennedy	1883-
Dr. Herbert B. Howard	1884-1885 1888-1897
Dr. Emily Pagelson	1884-1885
Dr. Anna M. Dorr	1884-
Dr. Eben C. Norton	1885-1887
Dr. Ella M. Patton	1885-1887
Dr. George E. Livermore	1886-1888
Dr. Eliza B. Lawrence	1887-1888
Dr. Myra D. Allen	1888-1889
Dr. Eliza D. Comly	1889-1890
Dr. Ida M. Porter	1890-1892
Dr. John M. Gile	1892-1896
Dr. F. B. Jewett	1892-
Dr. J. H. Ford	1892-
Dr. Elizabeth Newcomb	1892-1898 1913-
Dr. H. P. Towle	1892-1893
Dr. John H. Nichols	1891-1892 1893-
Dr. Emily Pagelson *Howard*	1896-1897
Dr. Archibald J. Ranney	1896-1901
Dr. J. F. Edgerly	1896-
Dr. C. S. Little	1897-
Dr. Arthur T. Mann	1897-1899
Dr. F. G. Mansom	1897-1898
Dr. Jane R. Baker	1898-1900
Dr. Edmund F. Curry	1898-1899
Dr. Arthur K. Drake	1898-1903
Dr. Robert H. Purple	1898-
Dr. Ernest B. Emerson	1899-1908
Dr. Joseph B. Howland	1900-1902
Dr. Arthur J. Dresser	1900-

Dr. George A. Pierce...	1900-1906 1908-
Dr. Harold C. Goodwin..	1901-1903
Dr. Hannah Lowell.....	1901-1903
Dr. Howard F. Holmes.	1903-1915
Dr. Charles E. Thompson	1903-1904
Dr. Hannah Lowell *Emerson*	1904-1908
Dr. Julius M. Dutton....	1904-1905
Dr. Carl J. Hedin......	1905-1908
Dr. Walter C. Kenney...	1905-1910
Dr. Freeman D. Bosworth, Jr.	1906-1907
Dr. Samuel R. Hathorn	1906-1908
Dr. Alfred J. Roach....	1907-
Dr. Burt F. Howard....	1907-1909
Dr. Carl C. MacCorison.	1908-1909
Dr. Carleton R. Metcalf	1908-1909
Dr. Howard K. Tuttle..	1908-1910 1911-1915
Dr. Carroll D. Partridge	1908-1910
Dr. J. Lee Robinson.....	1908-
Dr. Anna E. Barker.....	1908-1912
Dr. E. T. F. Richards....	1909-1910
Dr. Charles O. Day......	1909-1909
Dr. Harry R. Coburn....	1909-
Dr. Walter H. Crosby...	1909-1912

Dr. George P. Laton....	1910-1911
Dr. Sherman Perry......	1910-
Dr. Hanford Carvell....	1910-1912
Dr. Thomas V. Uniac...	1910-1913
Dr. Fred M. Hollister...	1910-1911
Dr. Dennis L. Black....	1911-1912
Dr. Edward E. Linderman	1911-
Dr. Charles L. Trickey..	1911-1912 1915-
Dr. George McWaldie..	1912-
Dr. Charles O. Maisch..	1912-1913
Dr. Earle C. Willoughby	1912-
Dr. Eleanor M. Slater...	1912-1913
Dr. John C. Lindsay.....	1912-
Dr. Frederick E. Twitchell, D. M. D.	1912-
Dr. Charles E. Dunbar..	1913-
Dr. Hattie E. Chalmers.	1913-
Dr. Charles W. DeWolf.	1913-
Dr. Thomas H. Odeneal.	1914-
Dr. C. Stanley Raymond	1914-
Dr. Mabel C. Raymond..	1914-
Dr. Marie Strom Lindsay	1914-
Dr. Adolph Kohn.......	1915-
Dr. William T. Hanson.	1915-

BRIDGEWATER STATE HOSPITAL.[1]

BRIDGEWATER, MASS.

About the middle of the last century, as the result of an increasing foreign population, the State of Massachusetts was forced to provide for a class of helpless dependents without residence or claim on the municipalities.

In 1852 the commonwealth met this situation by appropriating $100,000 for the construction of three state almshouses, each to accommodate not less than 500 inmates.

The sites chosen were Bridgewater, Tewksbury and Monson, and the amount of the appropriation necessitated wooden structures.

By proclamation of Governor Emory Washburn, the institution at Bridgewater was opened May 1, 1854, under the management of Abraham T. Lowe, Bradford L. Wales and Nahum Stetson, inspectors, and Levi L. Goodspeed, superintendent.

The government of the institution remained under a Board of three Inspectors until 1879, when it was placed under a Board of five Trustees until 1884, since which time there have been seven trustees, two of whom have been women.

At first dependents were received with little regard for classification. Young and old, sick and infirm, feeble-minded and insane were brought together under one roof. Later children were placed in the institution at Monson, the infirm and truly unfortunate were sent to Tewksbury, while the more needlessly dependent were segregated at Bridgewater. At a later date the insane were removed to other institutions.

An act of the Legislature of 1866 added to the almshouse the function of a workhouse, to which could be committed so-called vicious paupers. Later legislation designated it as a place to which misdemeanants could be sent. In 1872 the name of almshouse was omitted and the institution became known as the State Workhouse, although paupers were and still are received.

In 1887 the name was changed to State Farm. Levi L. Goodspeed, the first superintendent, retired in 1870, after a service of

[1] By Ernest B. Emerson, M. D., medical director.

15 years. He was succeeded by Captain Nahun Leonard, who held the office 13 years. The third and present superintendent, Hollis M. Blackstone, assumed control July 5, 1883. Thirty-six hours after his arrival the entire institution, with the exception of a few out-buildings, was destroyed by fire, fortunately without loss of life. By prompt action the paupers were transferred to Tewksbury and the prisoners to the Reform School at Westborough, where the workhouse was temporarily established in unused buildings.

The destruction of the original building marks the beginning of the present institution, now consisting of three distinct departments, covering approximately 40 acres of land; a prison for the custody of misdemeanants; an almshouse located one-halt mile from the main group; and a hospital for the insane, a part of the main group, but entirely separated from the prison department. The capacity of the three departments is respectively 1700, 400 and 1000.

The real estate valuation of 1911 was: Land, $69,470; buildings, $1,105,800; all other property, $439,892.14; total, $1,615,162.14. The approximate value of the hospital department, including buildings and equipment, is $450,000.

There are 1200 acres of land, the greater part of which has been reclaimed from forest and waste land.

The entire institution is of brick and concrete construction, of simple architectural design, all practically fireproof.

Farm work for the prison population has been developed to a high state of efficiency, the indeterminate sentence and the moral influence of the institution being the two great restraining factors.

Provision for the custody of the criminal insane of Massachusetts was provided for by statute in 1815. Under this statute persons held for crimes and offenses, if found to be dangerously insane, might be committed to prison by the proper legal authorities. This law remained in forçe until 1832, when the Legislature, recognizing that the insane, regardless of social or moral status, were entitled to the care and treatment afforded by the hospital, passed an act authorizing the commitment of persons designated in the act of 1816 to the State Lunatic Hospital at Worcester. This was soon followed by an act authorizing the commitment of all penal cases becoming insane to the State Lunatic Hospital.

The difficulties of restraining as well as the injustice of treating and housing the criminal and non-criminal insane in the same institution became apparent, and in 1864 an effort was made to establish wards for the criminal class at the State Almshouse, Tewksbury, but nothing was accomplished, however, towards the separation of the two classes until the matter was taken up in 1886 by H. M. Blackstone and the trustees of the then State Workhouse at Bridgewater.

At this time the institution was composed of two departments: a workhouse for the custody of drunkards, vagrants and other misdemeanants serving short sentences and an almshouse. The population of the two departments varied with the seasons, there being overcrowding in the winter and a corresponding diminution of inmates during the summer.

The State Insane Hospitals being overcrowded with the chronic and harmless insane, a plan was suggested whereby these cases might be transferred to the State Farm, thus relieving the hospitals and furnishing the State Farm with a more permanent population, which should be used advantageously during the summer season when inmate labor was needed. The scheme was approved by the Legislature and under Chap. 219, Acts of 1886, entitled "An Act to Provide a Building for the Chronic Insane at the State Workhouse at Bridgewater," $50,000 was appropriated for the construction of a building to accommodate 125 chronic insane persons. Before its completion 50 cases were transferred from the hospitals and housed in temporary quarters.

Upon the opening of this building it was soon discovered that, in addition to the chronic and harmless insane, many criminal cases were being transferred, and that the wards planned originally for the demented and inoffensive were inadequate to hold the more dangerous and troublesome patients who were arriving.

To meet the difficulty under Chap. 89, Acts and Resolves of 1888, $60,000 was appropriated for the construction of a strong building for the care of insane criminals and for an addition for the care of the sick insane. The following year $10,000 was appropriated for furnishing and equipment. The building was opened for patients October, 1890, and filled by transfers from the several state hospitals.

All available space was soon filled and in 1893 the Legislature appropriated $35,000 for the construction of a building with rooms to accommodate 75 patients. Seven thousand dollars was appropriated for an attendants' dormitory, and the following year $8400 was appropriated for furnishing and equipment.

Under Chap. 66, Resolves of 1899, $56,000 was appropriated for alterations and additions to provide not less than 140 strong rooms. The following year a new wing was added with 134 single rooms and a total capacity of 150 patients.

On recommendation of the superintendent $20,000 was appropriated in 1899 for the construction of a high wall inclosing some 17 acres on the west side of the institution. The wall was constructed from stone taken from the farm and built largely by the labor of inmates. Within this enclosure many patients find employment who would otherwise be more closely confined on account of their runaway habits.

Under Chap. 414, Acts of 1903, $100,000 was appropriated for an additional building, which was ready for occupancy the following year. Its upper floor, provided with two open wards, single rooms, a small surgery and diet kitchen, is used as an infirmary and is in charge of a woman nurse.

Under Chap. 500, Acts of 1906, $20,000 was appropriated for a building designed for industrial purposes. This is a plain concrete structure forming the north boundary of a large courtyard connecting the two buildings which form the east and west boundaries.

Under Chap. 522, Resolves of 1909, $90,000 was appropriated for further additions to the insane department, consisting of two reinforced concrete structures, forming practically a separate unit with kitchen and dining room accommodations. These buildings are in separate yards with subway connection to the main group.

One of these buildings is made especially secure to care for the more troublesome and ingenious; the other is designed for an admitting ward and infirmary.

The growth and development of that part of the State Farm known as the Bridgewater State Hospital represents the state's effort to care for its troublesome, though unfortunate, citizens. Since its inception the policy has been to introduce and carry out hospital ideas so far as the same were consistent with the safekeeping of its inmates.

In 1894 the superintendent and trustees, recognizing that the original purpose of the asylum department had been defeated and finding themselves burdened with the care of all the male insane criminals, in place of the harmless and chronic cases which were anticipated, recommended that this department be placed under medical control as an independent institution with a separate board of trustees. The legislative committees, however, thought differently. A compromise was finally effected and a bill known as Chap. 390, Acts of 1895, prepared by representatives of the legislative committees of the state hospitals, of the State Farm and others, became a law June 17, 1895.

Under this act so much of the State Farm as was established for the care and maintenance of insane men was designated the State Asylum for Insane Criminals. The appointment of a medical director, who should have the care and custody of the inmates and govern the same in accordance with the regulations approved by the trustees, was authorized.

The bill also authorized the removal of insane convicts directly to the asylum instead of to the hospital, and further provided that the court cases, persons under indictment by reason of insanity, indicted persons found insane at the time of trial, and persons acquitted of murder or manslaughter, should be committed directly to this asylum according as the court determined, whether or not the individual was criminal or vicious. Under Chap. 504, Acts of 1909, the name State Asylum for Insane Criminals was changed to Bridgewater State Hospital.

The State Farm and Bridgewater State Hospital represent the product of inmate labor as developed under the guidance and wise supervision of the present superintendent, Hollis M. Blackstone, for nearly 30 years the chief executive officer.

J. White Belcher was appointed inspector February 10, 1874, and served as such until he was designated a member of the Board of Trustees in 1879. He was made chairman in 1884 and so continued until his death, February 9, 1906. He was a man of integrity, sound judgment and skilled in the business committed to his trust.

Following the passage of the act which gave the asylum department identity, Dr. Arthur H. Harrington, of the Danvers Hospital staff, became medical director, and served until 1898, when he resigned to accept the superintendency of the Danvers Hospital.

Dr. Charles A. Drew, first assistant at the Medfield State Hospital, succeeded Dr. Harrington in 1898 and served until he resigned in 1909 to accept the superintendency of the Worcester City Hospital. He was succeeded by Dr. Alfred E. Elliott, a former assistant, who served until 1911.

The present incumbent, Dr. Ernest B. Emerson, assumed control October 1, 1911.

INSPECTORS.

Abraham T. Lowe.
Bradford L. Wales.
Nahum Stetson.
J. F. Murdock.
Marshall Lincoln.
William B. May.
James Ford.
James H. Mitchell.
Irah Chase.
Charles Shute.
Joseph Thaxter.
Asa Millet.
John B. Hathaway.
Joshua E. Crane.
J. White Belcher.
Seabury W. Bowen.

TRUSTEES (SUCCEEDING BOARD OF INSPECTORS).

Joshua E. Crane.
J. White Belcher.
Weaver Osborn.
Catherine P. Lothrop.
Mary E. Crafts.
Lyman A. Belknap.
Thomas Dwight, M. D.
Sarah D. Fiske.
Eli W. Hoyt.
Anna F. Prescott.
Oliver R. Clark.
William F. Corolin, M. D.
Jacob H. Hecht.
Clarence P. Lovell.
Warren E. Rice.
Leonard Huntress, M. D.
Cecil F. P. Bancroft.
Joseph A. Smart.
John B. Tivnan.
Emery M. Low.
Helen R. Smith.
Annie Fields.
Galen Stone.
Mrs. Nellie E. Talbot.
John W. Coughlin, M. D.
Rev. Payson W. Lyman.
Francis W. Anthony, M. D.
Walter F. Dearborn.
Dennis D. Sullivan.
Mrs. Mary E. Cogan.

RESIDENT PHYSICIANS.

Dr. George H. Oliver... 1855-
Dr. Charles A. Ruggles. 1856-1857
Dr. C. B. Cogswell...... 1857-1858
Dr. Henry C. Shaw..... 1859-1860
Dr. S. H. Carney........ 1861-
Dr. Morril Robinson.... 1862-1863
Dr. Samuel L. Young.... 1864-1865
Dr. Edward Sawyer..... 1866-1891
Dr. F. E. Corey......... 1884-
Dr. Charles A. Blake.... 1888-1895
Dr. J. Frank Blair...... 1897-1900
Dr. Reuben J. Marvel... 1904-1907

CONSULTING PHYSICIANS.

Dr. S. A. Orr...........	1862-1863	Dr. Gustav Liebman....	1895-
Dr. Asa Millet.........	1864-	Dr. Samuel J. Mixter...	1895-
Dr. J. E. Harlow.......	1865-1871	Dr. Maurice H. Richardson	1895-1912
Dr. Morril M. Robinson	1871-		
Dr. Calvin Pratt........	1874-		

ASSISTANT PHYSICIANS.

Dr. Henry A. Roberts.	Dr. A. J. Nugent.
Dr. H. Walter Mitchell.	Dr. Harry O. Johnson.
Dr. Butler Metzger.	Dr. Alfred A. Elliott.
Dr. Frank E. Farmer.	Dr. Cyril G. Richards.
Dr. Allen Troxell.	Dr. Clarence B. Kenney.
Dr. Frederick M. Hollister.	Benjamin Kasson, M. D.
Dr. H. Louis Stick.	Minot W. Gale, M. D.

The following Board of Consulting Physicians was established by the trustees in 1895 and has given continuous service since then with the exception of Dr. George F. Jelly, who resigned in 1898: Dr. George F. Jelly, Dr. Walter Channing, Dr. Philip Coombs Knapp, Dr. Henry R. Stedman, Dr. Edward W. Taylor, consulting pathologist.

PRESENT MEDICAL STAFF (1014).

Dr. Ernest B. Emerson..................Medical director.
Dr. Leonard A. Baker...................Assistant physician.
Dr. John H. Weller.....................Assistant physician.
Dr. Lonnie O. Farrar....................Assistant physician.
Dr. Wilmot Y. Seymour.................Assistant physician.

DANVERS STATE HOSPITAL.[1]

HATHORNE, MASS.

In 1873, Act 239 of the General Court, appointing commissioners to establish a hospital for the insane in the northeastern part of the state, was passed in response to a general demand for the increased accommodation of the insane and a special petition from the City of Boston, which desired to be relieved from the burden of supporting its insane in a local institution and at the same time paying a large portion of the expense of supporting the insane of other cities and towns in the state institutions.

The building commissioners, who were appointed on April 29, 1873, and entered upon their duties May 17 following, were Samuel C. Cobb, C. S. Esty and Edwin Walden.

They advertised for a suitable site for a hospital and out of more than 40 places offered finally selected on October 6 the Dodge Farm, in the western part of the town of Danvers, containing 197¼ acres.

The first estimate of the cost of the new institution had been $600,000. The commissioners, however, before contracts were signed, asked and received $900,000, and when the work was under way the revised plans called for $600,000 more, which the Legislature of 1876 granted.

The building commissioners in October, 1877, delivered the property into the hands of the first Board of Trustees, who found much work to be done before the building could be made ready for patients.

The hospital was first opened to patients on the 13th day of May, 1878. The trustees issued the by-laws in the same year. Worth noting among these is Chapter 1, Section 12:

> The number of cases of chronic insanity admitted to the hospital shall not consist of a larger proportion than one-third of the total number of patients, so far as can be accomplished under the laws of the commonwealth.

The Dodge farm included a hill 180 feet above the level of the railroad, and on the top of this hill the hospital, a long line of turreted buildings of Gothic type, was established. The

[1] By Dr. George M. Kline, superintendent.

main group was composed of 10 buildings, connected by fireproof passages, each building falling back about 64 feet behind the one central to it.

The two extreme buildings, called A and J, lying obliquely, were intended for and have been used for the reception of the more excited patients. It was planned to accommodate 270 patients in single rooms, a total of 468.

The rear center building contained kitchen, pantry, laundry, linen room, bake room, dining and sitting rooms.

At the same time a reservoir was constructed through a mutual agreement between state and town, by which the town was to furnish water and the hospital to build a reservoir, keep it in repair, and pay $1000 a year for 20 years to the town. On December 31, 1886, the contract as to yearly payments expired, and the town asked a yearly payment of $5000. After six years of costly negotiation, in which no satisfactory conclusion was obtained, an act of 1905, authorizing the hospital trustees to provide an independent supply, was passed.

The value of the whole plant November 30, 1911, was estimated at $1,842,143.

The main building stands at present almost exactly as built with the addition of large projecting out-of-door porches and dormitories with connecting bed-rooms for buildings A and J.

In 1905 the largest single addition was made in the establishment of a colony for women, located just beyond the line separating Danvers from Middleton. One hundred and seventy-eight women occupied these buildings in 1905, and this number has been increased to about 250 at the present time. All patients' quarters are located on the ground floor. Each ward has a large platform or veranda along its front, upon which the patients spend the greater part of the day. Windows are wholly unbarred. Under such conditions only able-bodied and quiet patients can be maintained there, although constant supervision day and night is provided.

In 1907 two one-story buildings were completed for male and female tubercular patients. These accommodate 18 patients each.

A building equipped for surgical purposes was attached to building A in 1903.

A home for women nurses was completed in 1898.

Grove Hall, a building at the foot of the hill and standing by itself, has proven to be an attractive home for those of the patients who are able workers and need little supervision. It was completed in 1902 and accommodates about 50.

Dayton Hall, a much smaller building, attached to the filter beds, has for the last 14 years accommodated about 11 patients and one attendant, whose business it is to see to the proper working of the filters.

At present 125 acres are under cultivation, the produce amounting to about $7000 a year. From 30 to 40 patients are usually engaged in the farm work. One hundred and three men and 106 women find employment on the wards only. A few inadequate rooms over the boiler house are used as workshops, but poor facilities have not prevented the hospital making its mattresses as needed, its brooms, harness and shoe repairing, caning chairs, upholstering and renewing much of its furniture. Sewing rooms for women have been established both at the main hospital and at Middleton Colony. Seven hundred gallons of tomatoes and also 500 quarts of berries, picked by patients, have been canned and 30 barrels of pickles prepared. Many patients are employed in the laundry.

In all 308 women and 355 men are usefully employed, 38 per cent and 56 per cent respectively, a total of 45 per cent for the total population.

In 1889, with the daily average of 744 patients, the total expenses for maintenance were $148,461.92, an average cost per patient per week of $3.89. In 1911, with 1452 patients as a daily average, the total maintenance expenses had risen to $365,-242.77, an average cost per patient per week of $4.857.

A new purchasing system was inaugurated at the beginning of the fiscal year 1910-11. All requisitions for supplies to be purchased are presented Monday mornings by the heads of departments to the superintendent for approval. Requests for quotations are then sent out. This method has produced very gratifying results. Before this system of sending out bids was inaugurated it was necessary for the steward to spend two days a week in Boston; now one day is sufficient. It was found that nearly everything could be purchased by sample.

The triplicate order form has been put to a year's test. It has resulted in the careful receipt of all stores; count, weight, or measurement being taken before any bill was approved. The freight charges have been entered on the orders and these charges have been deducted from the invoices. Attention has been given to the return of empty receptacles for which the hospital has received credit. This has been in a great part due to the use of this order form.

The unbusinesslike method of issuing storeroom supplies merely by exchanging worn-out articles at the store for new articles has been discontinued. All stores have been issued on signed requisitions. A perpetual stock book is now being kept which shows always the balance on hand. This book also shows the departments to which supplies are issued, affording a means to correct excessive issues.

Patients are received by a physician and supervisor and are assigned to ward A-1 or I-1 for observation. A cleansing bath is given at once, immediate records are made of patient's general condition, scars, bruises, temperature, pulse, and the patient is put to bed. A sample of urine is collected for examination, a 24-hour amount when possible.

In the meantime the friends of the patient who have accompanied him are detained for a history. When no one appears to give a history within the first two or three days an attempt is made to reach those interested in the patient by letter, and since October 12, 1912, it has been possible for a field worker to look up matters in the patient's home.

The physician's certificate follows the history in the typewritten records and this is in turn followed by the routine physical examination, under the headings general appearance, chest, circulatory system, digestive system, abdomen, genito-urinary system, including the laboratory report on the urine. This is in turn followed by a special neurological examination under the headings neuromuscular condition, cranial nerves, reflexes, sensations and subjective sensations.

An orientation blank containing questions on consciousness and orientation, school knowledge, arithmetical problems and a specimen of handwriting serves as a basis for the mental examination, which is intended to be a summary of the physician's observations from the first few weeks in the hospital. This is given under the formal headings of general appearance and attitude, conversation, handwriting, school knowledge, intelligence, consciousness and orientation, apprehension, attention, memory, associations, hallucinations, disturbance of judgment, emotions and will.

Considered of more importance than this formal summary are the running notes which follow the schedule—day of admission, three days after, one week after, every two weeks for two months, and then every month for six months, all these records being headed by a short summary. In the case of accident, escape, discharge, transfer from ward to ward, sudden change of condition, notes are made at once.

Among the running notes are the field worker's reports upon patients' home surroundings, occupation and condition of those out on a visit.

In the running notes are found the results of the Wassermann examinations, which, since July 1, 1912, have been made upon the blood of every patient admitted and on the spinal fluid of every case where there can be a suspicion of metasyphilitic disease.

In the preparation of these extensive notes two dictaphones have proven to be of great value.

In 1899 the daily clinic was begun at the hospital and accurate records were kept after 1902. All admissions and all discharges come before the physicians and the superintendent. Of late special invitations have been sent to the patients' local physicians, who have been able at the same time to observe closely the methods of the hospital to which they send their patients and to supply much-needed information as to the patient's history. A stenographer is present and a verbatim report of questions and answers is recorded under the running notes. Just before case reading an abstract is prepared, which precedes the history. At this time a list of symptoms is prepared for the symptom-index—an index which runs back to the beginning of the hospital in 1878.

The ordinary principle of keeping separate the different classes of patients has been followed with the acute cases, the infirm and the tubercular. No special provision has been made for the epileptic or alcoholic.

An entirely new dietary is made out every two weeks and care is taken not to place on it the same food for the same day of each week. A report of the waste of each meal is made to the steward and that report enables him either to find some sufficient reason for an unusual amount of waste or to cut out of the dietary those articles constantly refused by the patients.

Women nurses were employed on the male wards in 1897 and were soon removed, but in September, 1912, were again restored to the men's ward which contained the greatest number of bed patients.

Up to 1905 attendants were on duty 16 hours a day, with four hours off a week. From 1905 to 1910 one full day off was given, and in 1912 the hours on duty were reduced to 12, with one full day of free time. The minimum monthly wage for men attendants was raised to $25 in 1910.

In 1889 a two-years' course of training was established and a principal of the school appointed. In 1890 there were seven graduates, which is about the present average. No male attendant has as yet received a diploma.

An improvement which was first suggested in 1882 and finally carried into effect in 1897 was the establishment of a congregate dining room. At the first meal it accommodated 522 patients and 64 employees. The dining room is on the second floor behind the central building and is reached by covered galleries from the second floors of both wings. A floor area of 120 by 80 feet has air and light on three sides. Patients are in the room a full hour for dinner and a half-hour for breakfast and supper.

No food is placed upon the table until all patients have entered and are seated. As the kitchen is directly below the dining room, there is no difficulty in serving warm food to all. In practice it is found that the walk to and from the dining room, with two hours a day spent in changed surroundings, is an agreeable break to the ordinary routine of institution life. The two factors which led to its being retained, described by a later superintendent as a therapeutic measure, seemed to be that nothing is done in haste and that the music, if good, is eagerly listened to. A large expense in food transportation is, of course, done away with.

A scheme which this hospital shares with many other institutions of the state is efficiency in buying, attained by a voluntary association of the purchasing agents of the insane hospitals. Wherever possible it has been found that buying in large quantities in combination has resulted in a decided saving. Bids are given a much wider publicity than it is possible for one hospital to secure alone.

An incinerator in the basement of the rear center on the same level that all waste and rubbish of the buildings are deposited has proven a good sanitary measure and an economy.

In the first year of its history this hospital established open wards. Fifteen per cent of the patients were allowed to go home on a visit, to be terminated if things did not go well. While this custom has been followed ever since, it is only in 1912 that patients on visit have been followed up and definite information procured about them before they are discharged. In 1885 Dr. Goldsmith expressed himself strongly opposed to mechanical restraint, and suggested a system of boarding out as a means of relief from overcrowding.

A pathological laboratory was established in 1895 by Dr. Page and has been in continuous service ever since. In 1897 Dr. Page completed the uprooting of mechanical restraint in the hospital by formally prohibiting it.

In 1899, as before mentioned, the daily clinics for admissions and discharges were begun.

The year 1911 marked the establishment of two important innovations: the regular visits of a dentist and the beginning of eugenic work by a field worker under Dr. Davenport's direction. This field worker has been retained for the present year to make closer the contact between the patient's home and the hospital, by looking up patients on visits, patients whose friends have not come to see them and observing the home, occupation and family surroundings of the patient.

The year 1912 marked also the establishment of a routine Wassermann test on every admission, free access by patients to the halls at night and invitations to the local physicians of the patients to attend the case readings.

The hospital history has been marked by three alarming fires, which did no personal damage; one started from the drying room of the old laundry in 1899, one originated from defective electrical wiring in one of the towers connecting two of the buildings occupied by patients, in February, 1912.

The hospital has suffered epidemics of dysentery in 1908, and diphtheria in 1880, 1905 and 1910.

The Board of Commissioners appointed to establish the Danvers State Hospital were: Samuel C. Cobb, C. S. Esty, Edwin Walden, James F. Ellis, superintending architect; Nathaniel J. Bradlee, consulting architect; Charles A. Hammond, engineer.

TRUSTEES.

James Sturgis 1878-1882
Daniel S. Richardson... 1878-1890
Charles P. Preston..... 1878-1888
Samuel W. Hopkinson.. 1878-1910
Gardner A. Churchill.... 1878-1881
Charles F. Folsom, M. D. 1881-1883
Harriet R. Lee.......... 1882-1898
Solon Bancroft 1883-1909
Orville F. Rogers, M. D. 1884-1910
Florence Lyman 1884-1901
Augustus Mudge 1888-1889
Edward Hutchinson 1889-1892
John S. Colby.......... 1890-1894
William B. Sullivan.... 1892-1905
Zina E. Stone.......... 1894-1899
Grace C. Oliver......... 1898-1899
Mary Ward Nichols.... 1899-
Horace H. Atherton.... 1900-
Ada T. Brewster........ 1901-1909
Michael F. D'Arcy...... 1905-1906
George R. Jewett........ 1906-1910
Annie M. Kilham....... 1909-
S. Herbert Wilkins...... 1909-
Ernest B. Dane......... 1910-
Samuel Cole............ 1910-
Seward W. Jones....... 1910-

MEDICAL SUPERINTENDENTS.

Dr. Calvin S. May...... 1878-1880
Dr. William B. Goldsmith 1881-1886
Dr. William A. Gorton. 1886-1888
Dr. Charles W. Page.... 1888-1898
Dr. Arthur H. Harrington 1898-1903
Dr. Charles W. Page.... 1903-1910
Dr. Henry W. Mitchell.. 1910-1912
Dr. George M. Kline.... 1912-

ASSISTANT MEDICAL SUPERINTENDENTS.

Dr. Walter Channing... 1878-1879
Dr. Henry R. Stedman.. 1879-1884
Dr. William A. Gorton.. 1884-1886
Dr. Edward P. Elliott... 1886-1897
Dr. George P. Sprague.. 1897-1899
Dr. Henry W. Mitchell.. 1899-1907
Dr. Henry M. Swift.... 1908-1912
Dr. Ray D. Whitney.... 1912-1912
Dr. John B. MacDonald. 1912-

ASSISTANT PHYSICIANS.

Dr. Winfred B. Bancroft 1878-1879
Dr. Edward M. Harding 1879-1881
Dr. Julia K. Cary....... 1879-1897
Dr. Sanger Brown...... 1881-1882
Dr. William A. Gorton.. 1882-1884
Dr. F. W. Walsh........ 1882-1884
Dr. M. A. Jewett........ 1883-1892
Dr. Arthur H. Harrington 1885-1894
Dr. Joseph W. Jackson.. 1892-1893

Dr. Frederick L. Hills.. 1893-1896
Dr. George P. Sprague.. 1894-1897
Dr. Harry H. Colburn.. 1896-1899
Dr. Frank A. Ross...... 1898-1900
Dr. Mary Paulsell...... 1898-1907
Dr. James D. Madison.. 1899-1902
Dr. Harry L. Barnes.... 1900-1903
Dr. Phillip C. Bartlett.. 1901-1902
Dr. Henry M. Swift.... 1902-1905
Dr. Earl E. Bessey...... 1902-1907
Dr. Henry A. Cotton.... 1903-1907
Dr. Louis Hoag......... 1903-1906
Dr. F. Robertson Sims.. 1904-1906
Dr. Charles B. Sullivan. 1905-1909
Dr. Henry M. Swift.... 1906-1907
Dr. Anna H. Peabody... 1906-1913
Dr. John J. Walker..... 1907-1908
Dr. Gordon T. Brown... 1907-1908
Dr. Charles Ricksher.... 1907-1910
Dr. Edwin W. Katzenellenbogen 1908-1910
Dr. Leslie C. Bishop.... 1908-1910
Dr. Isaiah M. Halladjian 1908-1910
Dr. Harlan L. Paine.... 1909-
Dr. William B. Cornell.. 1910-1912
Dr. Nelson G. Trueman. 1910-
Dr. George Parcher..... 1910-1911
Dr. A. Warren Stearns.. 1910-1911
Dr. Allan D. Finlayson.. 1911-1912
Dr. Burton D. Thorpe... 1911-1913
Dr. F. D. Streeter...... 1912-1913
Dr. Rose Bebb.......... 1913-
Dr. Alice A. Steffian.... 1913-
Dr. Frederick P. Moore. 1913-1913
Dr. John H. Travis..... 1913-
Dr. David T. Brewster.. 1913-

PATHOLOGISTS.

Dr. James J. Putnam.... 1879-1880
Dr. William L. Worcester 1895-1901
Dr. Albert M. Barrett.. 1902-1905
Dr. Elmer E. Southard.. 1906-1909
Dr. James J. Ayer, assistant 1907-1908
Dr. Herman M. Adler... 1909-1912
Dr. Myrtelle M. Canavan 1908-1912
Dr. Earl D. Bond........ 1912-1913

GRAFTON STATE HOSPITAL.[1]

WORCESTER, MASS.

On May 15, 1877, an act was passed by the Legislature of Massachusetts establishing a temporary asylum for the chronic insane to occupy the buildings which had belonged for 40 years to the Worcester Lunatic Hospital.

Under this act the trustees of the Worcester Lunatic Hospital were invested with authority over the management and government of said asylum, the care of the inmates thereof, the custody of its funds and the collection and disbursement of moneys for and on account of it, and were authorized to sell any land heretofore used by said hospital not necessary for the purpose of the new asylum. Under this authority thus conferred upon the trustees of the hospital, who were then R. W. Hooper, William S. Lincoln, Thomas H. Gage, John D. Washburn and James B. Thayer, it was determined October 25, 1877, that the permanent officers of the asylum should be a superintendent, one assistant physician, a steward, a matron, a treasurer, a clerk, and an engineer, who should be elected by the trustees and whose salaries should be fixed by them. Dr. John G. Park was accordingly elected superintendent; Dr. Enoch A. Marston, assistant physician; Dr. Albert Wood, treasurer; C. R. Macomber, clerk; and William Sherman, engineer. At a subsequent meeting a matron and a steward were chosen and although the employment of a second assistant physician had not been mentioned previously, the trustees authorized the employment of Dr. William H. Raymenton in that capacity.

On the 13th of October, 1877, the trustees were directed by the State Board of Charities to transfer 200 state and town patients from the Taunton Lunatic Hospital, 100 from the Worcester Lunatic Hospital and 25 from the Northampton Lunatic Hospital to the asylum, the work of removal to begin at once and to be completed by the 18th of November.

On the day so designated every patient belonging to the hospital was domiciled in the new building except 100 chronic patients, who were proper subjects for the asylum and were left undisturbed.

[1] By Dr. H. Louis Stick, superintendent.

On the 23d of October 100 and on the 26th a second 100 patients were received from the Taunton Hospital, and on the 30th 25 more were received from Northampton, so that at the end of seven days 325 patients had become inmates of the asylum without any accident or escape. The largest number of patients within the year was 407.

The land occupied by the Worcester Lunatic Hospital, bounded by Summer Street, west, East Central Street, north, Mulberry Street, east, and Asylum Street, south, with the buildings thereon, was voted by the trustees on October 25, 1877, to be necessary for the institution; the temporary use of about four acres additional was also allowed.

The advisability of separating chronic from acute patients had been thoroughly discussed and opposed by most superintendents, but it was advocated by the State Board of Charities for reasons of economy. The question as to who were the chronic insane was decided by the dates of the commitment papers.

As the asylum buildings had been allowed to get much out of repair, it became necessary to make extensive improvements; the sum of $8767.86 was expended for this purpose. The old laundry formerly in the basement of the chapel wing was replaced by a new two-story brick building on the north side of the engine house.

Dr. John G. Park became the first superintendent of the asylum October 25, 1877. At the time of his transfer from the asylum to the hospital in 1879 the population was 375; the total number under treatment was 422. The weekly per capita cost was $2.79. Much attention was given to providing employment for the patients as a sanitary measure and every endeavor was made to have the patients do something useful.[1]

A water color painting of Lake Quinsigamond, executed by himself, was presented by Mr. Henry Woodward, a son of the first superintendent of the Worcester Lunatic Hospital, and one of its former treasurers.

Dr. Hosea M. Quinby, who received his first appointment as an assistant in the Worcester Lunatic Hospital in 1873, and had

[1] During this period Dorothea L. Dix frequently visited the asylum and presented it a number of copies of "Sacred Hymns and Tunes" for the chapel.

been transferred to the Lake institution, remained there as assistant until February, 1879, when he was appointed superintendent of the temporary asylum for the chronic insane, to succeed Dr. John G. Park, who had been appointed superintendent of the Worcester Lunatic Hospital.

He remained as superintendent of the asylum until November, 1890, when he was transferred to the Worcester Lunatic Hospital to succeed Dr. John G. Park, once more who resigned to resume private life at Groton, Mass. During his administration at the asylum the number of patients remained about 400.

Not much work, other than studying the patients and creating occupation for them, was done by Dr. Quinby during the early part of the first year. He found that he had one attendant to every 13 patients. During the latter part of the year the fences about the grounds were repaired and renovation of the wards was begun. Large air shafts were built in all the wards, running from the basement to the attic. In 1880 more improvements were made and wards were still further improved. A bay window was attached to the east end of the wings, enlarged air shafts running to the attic for ventilation were placed in every room, all water closets and bathrooms were remodeled and enlarged. A hot water system was installed. More than 4312 articles of clothing were made on the female wards during the year.

During his 11 years of active service many improvements by new additions to the old wards were made, materially enlarging them, and the grounds were improved as well. Summer Street was widened, which necessitated a heavy retaining wall at a large expense. As the asylum building had been erected more than 40 years before much necessarily had to be done in renovating and improving the ventilation, the heating and the plumbing. This work was done with the money saved from the income derived from the patients' board, which by an act of Legislature could not exceed $4.20 per week per patient, but the towns from which the patients came paid in addition any extra expense caused by their destructiveness to clothing or furniture. More than $10,000 was expended the first year of his administration in these improvements.

Patients' labor was utilized to a more or less extent and the amount of restraint and seclusion was materially lessened. During the last three months of the year 1886 no restraint or seclusion was necessary, and during the entire year 1889 there was a daily average of but three females and one male in restraint and but one or two of both sexes in seclusion. A great effort was made to keep the patients out of doors and occupied, especially during the warmer months of the year.

On the evening of February 8, 1890, a fire broke out in the attic of the north or female side, which spread rapidly. The patients were all quietly but forcibly taken from the north to the south or male wards by the attendants and nurses. Many former employees who lived in the city on seeing the fire came to the rescue. It was fought by the City Fire Department with difficulty. Most of the roof and attic floors of the Johonnots were destroyed. The wards were deluged with water, and, because of this condition, the State Board of Lunacy transferred 90 or more patients to the Worcester, Westborough and Taunton lunatic hospitals. The work of repairing was immediately begun, the money being appropriated by the Legislature and the Worcester Lunatic Hospital.

Dr. Ernest V. Scribner succeeded Dr. H. M. Quinby as superintendent in November, 1890.

During the first 10 years of his administration the number of patients in the asylum remained about the same. In October, 1890, there were 299 patients and but 464 individual cases were treated; on October 1, 1900, the number of patients was 482. Many repairs and improvements were made. The bays of the administration center were added, the basement of the south wing was made into a congregate dining room for patients, and later the north wing basement was made into a dining room. The ventilating system was improved. The chapel wing was rebuilt from a wooden interior to a fireproof construction; the draughts of the large chimney were relocated; the south dining room was enlarged, it occupying the entire basement space of the wing; the kitchen was changed and new cooking utensils were added; a new bakery with modern ovens was added; and the plumbing of all the wards of the north and south sides was changed. The nurses who roomed in single rooms on the different wards were removed to the upper north center by transferring the patients from this to other wards. A year later a similar change was made for the male nurses by vacating the middle south wing. This helped to make the home life more pleasant and agreeable for the nurses. The training school for nurses was started in 1890, but no graduation exercises for nurses took place until June, 1906, when there were six graduates.

Dr. Scribner remained as superintendent for a little more than 20 years and during this time over $100,000 were expended in repairs and improvements at the asylum alone.

When he resigned in March, 1912, the population of patients had increased to more than 1100. The names of more than 300 employees were also on the pay-roll.

In 1900 the State Board of Insanity asked the superintendent of this institution through its trustees to establish a colony for the asylum and he spent the greater part of a year in seeking a suitable site. In 1901 the Legislature granted for the purchase of such land as was necessary the sum of $25,000. Five hundred acres were purchased at first, comprising a number of small farms in the towns of Grafton, Shrewsbury and Westborough, on the water shed of Quinsigamond and Asabet rivers. More land has been added from time to time, so that now the colony contains about 882 acres, with more than 35 different buildings, accommodating more than 600 patients.

Up to April 1, 1912, more than $743,000 was expended in the erection of suitable buildings for patients, nurses and domestics and in the improvement of the land, which consisted of several abandoned farms. Twelve of the buildings are used for heat, light, power, storage, dining purposes and industrial work of the most necessary kind.

This colony has five different centers, four being for patients, while the fifth is the administration group. These centers naturally were developed about the old farm houses. New buildings are occupied by the excitable and turbulent class, while the Oaks and the Willows care for the purely colony type of patient.

Dr. Scribner encouraged open-air and out-of-doors work for both sexes and many patients who had been cared for on closed wards seemed glad to be out of doors, where fresh air, plenty of work and a different environment helped to change many of them from turbulent to quiet and industrious patients. More than 200 of them are now employed on the grounds and about the farm.

In 1909, after a careful study of all institutions by a commission of the State Board of Insanity designated by Governor

Draper, the names of the different institutions were changed and the Worcester Insane Asylum became the Worcester State Asylum, making the third change in the name of this asylum.

On March 5, 1912, Dr. Ernest V. Scribner resigned as superintendent of the asylum, to be appointed superintendent of the Worcester State Hospital to fill the vacancy caused by the resignation of Dr. Hosea M. Quinby.

Dr. H. Louis Stick was appointed his successor as superintendent of the Worcester State Asylum and assumed that office April 1, 1912, having been an assistant in the asylum since February 2, 1903.

GRAFTON COLONY.

Many changes were made during the year 1911 on account of a bill pending in the Legislature for the removal of the asylum to its colony at North Grafton, which was passed in both the House and Senate and signed by Governor Eugene N. Foss on May 29, 1912.

By this act the trustees of the Worcester State Asylum at Worcester were authorized to expend a sum not exceeding $400,000 in the construction, upon land owned by the commonwealth and situated at the Grafton Colony, of suitable buildings to accommodate 400 patients cared for at Worcester State Asylum.

The buildings were to be completed and ready for occupation not later than January 1, 1915, and upon their completion and equipment the trustees were to transfer from the Worcester State Asylum to the buildings at Grafton Colony 400 patients.

This law necessarily caused marked changes in the asylum and colony plans, which were developing slowly, by making it mandatory that the trustees should prepare buildings to be occupied by January 1, 1915. Plans were made and approved by the State Board of Insanity, then perfected, approved and accepted by the Governor on February 5, 1913. These plans are made so that expansion of the colony may be made at any time, and provide for the care of at least 1600 patients. The population of the asylum and its colony in 1912 was 1270, 650 of this number being at the colony.

It was found that the money appropriated for the removal scheme, namely, $400,000, was insufficient to care for the 400 patients as stated in the act and therefore it became necessary to ask for a larger special appropriation. This naturally necessitated the erection of new buildings, many of which are under process of construction.

The colony is divided into two distinct groups, so arranged that there are two centers for the male cases, one for the custodial type, while the second group contains the purely colony type. The buildings of this latter group are of a one-story wooden construction with cobble-stone basement. This same plan is followed out in the female groups.

During the past ten years the water supply has been developed and a new sewerage system installed, roads constructed, and a central electric plant and heating centers built. At first the old wood stove sufficed, but soon the turbulent class of patients made necessary a stronger type of building, thus necessitating new heating centers corresponding to the different groups. On account of the dangers of fire it was deemed wise to erect fireproof buildings. This was done until sufficient room to care for the excitable and turbulent cases had been provided. The purely colony groups have a simple type of construction, where a dormitory corresponds to the first story, and the basement is used for the day space, kitchen, dining room, sitting room, smoking room and industrial work of some kind. The patients living in them no longer feel that they are being kept in by locked doors, but that they can come and go about the grounds at their will and pleasure. The per capita cost per week for the year 1912 was $4.39.

The Legislature of 1913 made a special appropriation for the asylum, now hospital, amounting to $208,000, to provide for the construction of a male nurses' home, a female nurses' home and a new kitchen and dining room in the Willows group; also for repairs and renovation of the old farm house belonging to this group, an enlargement of the filter beds, the construction of a new reservoir of 2,000,000 gallons capacity, an additional boiler at the power house; and further a motor generation and new service building at Colony No. 4, or the Elms group. All the foregoing buildings and improvements have been completed, with the exception of the old farm house now under construction and the dining room and service building at the Elms group.

It proved impossible to erect the latter dining room and service building within the appropriation of $50,000 and the Board of Lunacy wisely decided to consent to a modification of the original plans. The Legislature, however, owing to the adverse report of the Economy and Efficiency Commission, in turn declined to appropriate additional funds for the same. As a result of these differences the removal of the whole institution from Worcester has now been deferred until January 1, 1917. Meantime there is serious doubt whether, if the service and dining room is completed in time, it will be practical to abandon the whole plant at Worcester because of the rapid increase in patients during the past two years. If such an increase continues at its present rate it is probable that by January, 1917, the number of patients at Worcester will exceed the capacity at Grafton by nearly 300 patients.

At least $750,000 will be necessary to increase the capacity of the colony to 2000 patients. To enlarge each of the four colonies to a capacity of 500 patients it will be necessary to erect an addition to the Pines service building, for which an appropriation was asked but was not granted by the Legislature of 1915.

The colony now has more than 901 acres of land, upwards of 400 of which are under cultivation and in gardens and lawns for the different buildings. Over 800 patients are cared for at present.

During the session of the Legislature of 1915 a bill was introduced by the State Board of Insanity to make the Worcester State Asylum a hospital for the insane, and to change its name to the Grafton State Hospital, which became a law May 18, 1915. The present is the fourth change in name since 1877. The asylum, which was an institution for the care of the acutely insane for more than 45 years, has come back to its own.

SUPERINTENDENTS.

Dr. John G. Park, from November, 1877, to February, 1879.
Dr. Hosea M. Quinby, from February, 1879, to November, 1890.
Dr. Ernest V. Scribner, from November, 1890, to April, 1912.
Dr. H. Louis Stick, from April, 1912, to present time.

RESIDENT OFFICERS.

Dr. Enoch A. Marston..	1877-1879	Dr. Ernest V. Scribner..	1884-1890
Dr. William H. Raymenton	1877-1881	Dr. Hartstein W. Page..	1891-1899
Dr. Charles A. Peabody..	1880-1881	Dr. Thomas Howell.....	1899-1902
Dr. E. Meade Perkins..	1881-1884	Dr. P. Challis Bartlett..	1902-1906
		Dr. H. Louis Stick......	1903-1912

Dr. Winfred O. Brown..	1905-1905	Dr. William T. Bailey...	1909-1910
Dr. Arthur E. Pattrell..	1905-	Dr. Jonathan H. Ranney	1910-1911
Dr. William T. Hanson.	1906-1908	Dr. Ransom A. Greene..	1910-1912
Dr. W. J. Churchill.....	1907-1907	Dr. Effie A. Stevenson..	1911-
Dr. Charles H. Wheeler.	1907-1908	Dr. Donald R. Gilfillan..	1912-
Dr. Ralph C. Kell.......	1908-1909	Dr. John B. Macdonald.	1912-1912
Dr. B. H. Mason.......	1908-	Dr. Hiram L. Horsman..	1912-

WESTBOROUGH STATE HOSPITAL.[1]

Westborough, Mass.

The Westborough State Hospital was established to provide homeopathic treatment for the insane of Massachusetts. For several years efforts had been made to obtain the use, in a limited way, of the existing hospitals; first, by having one assistant physician in each hospital who should care for homeopathic patients; and, second, to allow an outside homeopathic physician to care for certain patients within a state hospital, in similar manner to the practice in general hospitals. But these efforts were unsuccessful. It became necessary, therefore, to secure a new and separate hospital for homeopathic patients.

The first favorable opportunity came when the state authorities decided to make some change in the State Reform School at Westborough. In the end the school bought a new location a mile or two away in Westborough and became known as the Lyman School for Boys. The old buildings, together with the lands that had belonged to the school, were granted to the petitioners by act of the Legislature, June 3, 1884, and the Westborough Insane Hospital was established. It was the second in the world under homeopathic management. Especial credit for this success is due to Drs. I. T. Talbot and Samuel Worcester, who first suggested such a hospital in a paper before the Massachusetts Homeopathic Medical Society. Subsequently, in 1909, the name was changed to Westborough State Hospital.

The first Board of Trustees consisted of Charles R. Codman, Henry S. Russell, Lucius G. Pratt, Francis A. Dewson, Archi-

[1] Prepared by H. O. Spalding, M. D., with the assistance of Drs. Paine, of West Newton, and Klopp, of Allentown, Pa.

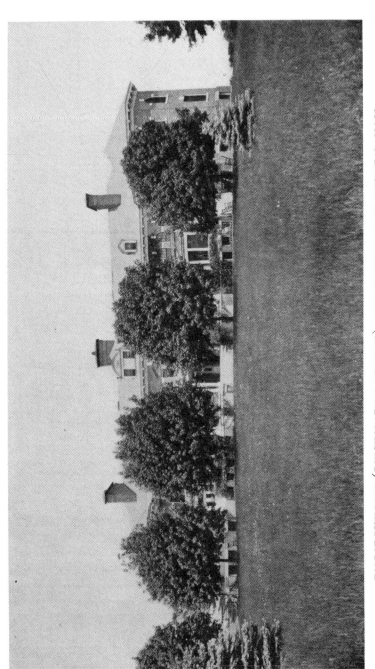

TALBOT BUILDING (PSYCHOPATHIC DIVISION), WESTBOROUGH STATE HOSPITAL, MASS.

bald H. Grimke, Phoebe J. Leonard and Emily Talbot. To them were granted the original school property, consisting of one large brick building, one small brick building and several cottages, outbuildings and barns, and about 275 acres of land, and also $150,000 for such alterations as would provide accommodations for 325 patients and necessary officers and employees. Their problem was to convert the old buildings of a prison into buildings suitable for hospital purposes.

About the 1st of May, 1885, plans had been prepared and the work of reconstruction was to begin, when the trustees appointed Dr. N. Emmons Paine as superintendent, in order to have the benefit of his experience and advice. The next year and a half were required for altering, furnishing and equipping the new hospital (for which an additional appropriation of $180,000 had been made in May, 1886, and for increasing the accommodations to 405 patients); and on December 1, 1886, it was declared open and ready for the reception of patients by proclamation of the Governor, George D. Robinson.

As patients came by transfer from other overcrowded hospitals and as new admissions were received, additional physicians were added, and in July, 1887, the medical staff was composed of the following: Dr. N. Emmons Paine, superintendent; Dr. George S. Adams, first assistant physician; Dr. Amos J. Givens, Dr. Edward H. Wiswall, Dr. George O. Welch, and Dr. Alice Nivison, assistant physicians.

The medical practice had been fixed by law "upon the principles of medicine known as homeopathic," which have been the dominating and guiding principles since its establishment, although other forms of treatment have been followed.

From the opening of the hospital rest treatment, with the new cases, has been a feature. All patients are placed in bed at the time of their admission and remain there for a varied length of time, dependent upon their mental state. With this comes forced feeding and massage. Although the hospital began with one group or block of old buildings, its development has been away from that type and into the cottage or isolated group plan. In 1898 the first building in the Massachusetts state hospitals for the exclusive care of the acute insane was erected as the beginning of the psychopathic department. This building, with accommodations for 60 patients and equipped with rooms for electrical treatment, proved most satisfactory.

This department was found to be so successful that in 1905 a second building, known as the Codman building, was opened as a part of this group, accommodating 50 patients. It was used for the reception of acute female patients and was divided into two wards. In 1911 the third building of the psychopathic group, Childs building, was opened, and was also used for the accommodation and reception of female patients suffering from acute disease. Codman building, formerly used by them, was devoted to the reception of male patients suitable for the psychopathic group. These last two buildings are both equipped with large porches for outdoor treatment, where patients spend their time day and night at all seasons of the year. They are also equipped for prolonged baths and electro- and hydrotheraphy.

Westborough was the first hospital to act upon the suggestion of the State Board of Insanity to establish a colony group in connection with its main plant, and in 1902 the Warren farm colony, accommodating 100 patients, situated about a mile from the hospital, was opened for men. In 1903 the second colony, Richmond, about half a mile from the hospital, was opened for women patients of the quiet chronic type. In connection with this there was provided a tuberculosis sanitarium, with a southern exposure and open to the air all day, especially adapted for these patients. The buildings were of one-story wooden construction and cost approximately $500 per bed, and were equipped throughout with heat, light, power and sewerage system complete. This colony group provided accommodations for 100 patients in units of 25 and a tuberculosis sanitarium with beds for 30 patients. In 1907 an adjoining farm, with a good set of farm buildings, was purchased and used as a farm colony for men, accommodating eight or nine patients. This has open doors, and under the charge of a man and his wife, the patients enjoy a life as nearly approximating normal farm life as possible. In 1911 the fourth colony group was added. This accommodated 100 women patients in units of 25, and provided tuberculosis wards, accommodating 40 patients. The women who had been at the Richmond colony were now moved to this new group and their former buildings given over to men patients. At this colony there is a laundry where all the work for that group is done, and also some from the men's colony.

When a patient is received at the hospital the admitting physician assigns him to the receiving ward of the psychopathic service if, after superficial examination, it appears that he is of the curable type. If, however, the patient is plainly of the chronic or organic demented type, he is admitted to the receiving ward of the chronic group; thus from the very beginning the psychopathic and the chronic departments are kept separate.

The open-ward policy has been pursued and developed as rapidly as circumstances would permit and at the present time 11 of the 49 wards are conducted as open wards.

For many years daily staff meetings have been held for the consideration of new cases and the discharge of old ones.

Occupational therapy and re-education of patients along industrial lines have been encouraged as well as the ordinary development of outdoor work and general work in the institution. At the present time, in addition to ordinary household and farm occupations, with the laundry and sewing rooms, there is an industrial room at the Warren farm colony for making and renovating mattresses, cane-seating chairs, repairing, renovating and making men's clothes. At the Richmond colony is located a shoe repair shop. At the main group there are employed two women industrial supervisors and teachers who devote their time exclusively to this work, carrying on rug making, basketry, stamped leather and other forms of arts and crafts work. There is also an industrial room in charge of a man who devotes his entire time to it, where male patients are employed, weaving rugs and towelling, and in broom and mat making. Patients' gardens, especially for the women, have been developed, and this year (1915) there are five gardens upon plots which have been set aside for five different classes or groups of patients.

The pathological department was established in July, 1887, and Dr. George O. Welch was appointed pathologist, this hospital being among the first in the state to take this step. For the past 17 years Dr. Solomon C. Fuller has occupied this position. His work has been noteworthy and a number of valuable contributions published in this country and abroad have come from this laboratory. The work has been largely upon clinical pathological lines; in 1914 the laboratory of the hospital was one of the two laboratories which did all of the Wassermann work for the Massachusetts state hospitals.

The training school for nurses was established in October, 1889, Westborough being one of the earliest of similar institutions to take this step. It included both men and women students; the course endeavors to approximate the courses in general hospitals, but is of two years' duration only. There has been affiliation with general hospitals and arrangements for freer and more extensive affiliation are under way at the present time. All of the women nurses are obliged to take the training, but for the men it is optional. The latter, however, if they do not attend the training school are required to take an attendants' course of 12 lectures given by one of the physicians. This course is continuous throughout the year and the attendant enters the course as soon as he enters the employ of the hospital, it being so arranged that each lecture is a unit in itself and he enters upon his studies at once without waiting several weeks or months for a new course to start. This was established about two years ago and is believed to have materially increased the efficiency of the male attendants.

A consulting board of physicians and surgeons was appointed in January, 1895, by the trustees, composed of 10 physicians, mostly specialists; and they have always responded to the call of the superintendent for assistance in eye, ear, nose and throat, heart, lungs, nervous and surgical diseases. Fees have never been paid for their valuable and generous services, except small honoraria for abdominal and surgical operations. The benefits to the hospital have been incalculable during the 20 years of skilled assistance of this consulting board.

For some years a dentist has been employed to attend to the wants of the patients, making regular weekly visits; at present he visits the hospital two mornings each week.

The problem of the care of the inebriates and habitual drunkards has passed through several stages in Massachusetts. They were formerly committed to the state hospitals, if " such person is not of bad repute or of bad character apart from such habits of intemperance." Later, in 1889, the Foxborough State Hospital was established especially for this class; but in 1905 commitments to Foxborough were limited to men, and women could be sent

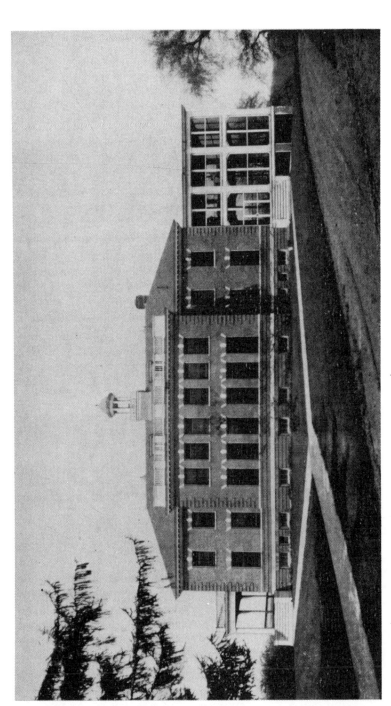

CODMAN BUILDING (PSYCHOPATHIC DIVISION) FOR MEN, WESTBOROUGH STATE HOSPITAL, MASS.

again to any of the state hospitals. In 1914 all female alcoholics and narcotic habitues in the state insane hospitals committed under the inebriate law were transferred by the State Board of Insanity to the Westborough State Hospital, where separate wards for their care and maintenance had been established.

A social worker was appointed in 1913 and spends her time visiting the homes of patients after their reception at the hospital, obtains additional information about patients, their families and the home conditions, and amplifies and perfects the case record with her observations and recommendations. This knowledge has been of advantage in the treatment of the invalid in the hospital and has been of great importance when the question of his discharge is considered. She also deals with the problems of after care.

The State Board of Insanity planned in 1914 for the several state hospitals to become responsible, in certain respects, for the insane persons in their districts. Their plan of grouping the boarded-out patients in the vicinity of the state hospitals under the surveillance of the local hospital is a practical and wise step, accomplishing what was recommended 26 years before in the Westborough Hospital report of 1888. Further, in harmony with the plans of the State Board of Insanity, Westborough, as the one homeopathic hospital of the whole state, attempts to reach as many as possible of the inhabitants who desire advice and treatment, by the following provisions: "Out-patient clinics will be held at the Westborough State Hospital each Wednesday from 2 to 3 o'clock and at the out-patient department of the Massachusetts Homeopathic Hospital, No. 31 East Newton Street, Boston, Mass., each Tuesday from 2 to 3 o'clock (holidays excepted)."

An idea of the present hospital may be obtained from these statistics: Land, 768 acres; buildings, 60; estimated value, $1,000,000; patients, September 30, 1914, 1213; total admissions within the year, 557; total admissions from opening of hospital, 11,492; total number of employees, 364.

SUPERINTENDENTS.

N. Emmons Paine, May 1, 1885, to February 1, 1892.
George S. Adams, February 1, 1892, to May 21, 1912.
Harry O. Spalding, May 21, 1912, in office.

ASSISTANT PHYSICIANS.

Name	Years
Amos J. Givens	1886-1889
George S. Adams	1886-1892
Edward H. Wiswall	1887-1889
George O. Welch	1887-1892
Alice Nivison	1887-1889
Ellen L. Keith	1889-1896
James F. Bothfield	1889-1890
W. O. Mann	1892-1895
A. Don Hines	1893-1894
Emilie Young O'Brien	1893-1894
D. Ette Brownell	1894-1902
Henry I. Klopp	1895-1912
George F. Adams	1895-1896
Mary F. Cushman	1896-1897
Solomon C. Fuller (in office)	1897-
John L. Bacon	1898-1901
Eva T. Swenney	1901-1902
Clifford J. Huyck	1901-1905
Ida J. Brooks	1902-1906
Wm. L. Soule	1902-1902
Frederick A. Webster	1903-1904
Alberta S. B. Guibord	1904-1905
William W. Coles	1904-1912
Michael M. Jordan (in office)	1905-
Ruth B. Coles	1905-1912
Mary Johnson	1906-1907
Esther S. B. Woodward	1908-1912
Clarence C. Burlingame	1908-1912
Walter A. Jillson (in office)	1910-
Alice S. Cutler (in office)	1911-
Emma H. Fay (in office)	1912-
Ruel A. Pierce	1912-1914
Everett W. Coates	1912-1914
Harriet Horner (in office)	1912-
Mark Mizener	1913-1915
M. Joseph Shealey (in office)	1914-
Willis W. Gleason	1914-1915

FOXBOROUGH STATE HOSPITAL.[1]

FOXBOBOUGH, MASS.

The law which authorized the establishment of the Massachusetts Hospital for Dipsomaniacs and Inebriates was enacted in 1889. It was approved on the 5th of June and took effect upon its passage. On the 10th of July the trustees were commissioned by the Governor and entered upon their duties.

A site, comprising 103 acres of land, was secured 25 miles from Boston. Dr. Marcello Hutchinson, formerly assistant physician at the State Hospital at Taunton, Mass., was appointed superintendent. The general outline of the buildings was indicated by the superintendent and a contract was made for five buildings to cost $91,000, as follows: Three cottages, a building containing a dining room and kitchen, an engine house and laundry. The hospital was opened for the reception of patients on February 10, 1893. The additions to the plant since the erection of these buildings have been as follows: Gymnasium, power

[1] By Irwin H. Neff, M. D.

house, laundry, insane ward, industrial shop and refrigerating plant. Including repairs and betterments, the total cost has amounted to $177,700. The present valuation of the plant is $349,280.88.

The State Board of Insanity was authorized to transfer insane patients from other institutions to the Foxborough State Hospital in 1905 (Chapter 400, Acts of 1905), and a special ward accommodating 128 patients was erected for that purpose. Since that time a daily average of 200 inebriate patients and 214 insane have been cared for at the hospital.

In 1907 Governor Curtis Guild effected a reorganization of the hospital by appointing a new Board of Trustees as follows: Robert A. Woods, chairman; William H. Prescott, M. D., secretary; Edwin Mulready, Philip R. Allen, Frank L. Locke, Timothy J. Foley, M. D., and W. Rodman Peabody. Dr. Irwin H. Neff was appointed superintendent, and entered upon his duties on April 1, 1908.

Recommendations were made to the Legislature that a special inquiry covering the classification, disposition of types of drunkenness, proper equipment for their treatment, after-care of discharged patients, co-operation of private citizens, etc., be formally authorized by the Legislature. By legislative enactment (Chapter 3, Acts 1909) a special report was made by the Board of Trustees on "Drunkenness in Massachusetts, Conditions and Remedies," House Document No. 1390.

By legislative action all the inebriates and drug cases under treatment at the Foxborough State Hospital were transferred to the Norfolk State Hospital on June 1, 1914. The Board of Trustees and the superintendent were also transferred to the Norfolk State Hospital, and a new Board of Trustees and a new superintendent appointed to replace them.

The Foxborough State Hospital continues under the State Board of Insanity, and will continue temporarily to receive transferred insane from other state institutions. A bill has been introduced which will make it an admitting hospital for both sexes.

SUPERINTENDENTS.

Marcello Hutchinson, M. D. 1893-1899
Charles E. Woodbury, M. D. 1899-1908
Irwin H. Neff, M. D.... 1908-1914
Albert C. Thomas, M. D. (in office) 1914-

RESIDENT PHYSICIANS.

Name	Years
William Noyes, M. D.	1893-1896
E. K. P. Fourtain, M. D.	1896-1899
Edgar T. Newsome, M. D.	1890-1900
Lewis M. Walker, M. D.	1900-1903
Edward Mellus, M. D.	1901-1904
Clarence J. Bell, M. D.	1903-1908
Leslie E. Coffin, M. D.	1903-1908
Frank H. Carlisle, M. D. (in office)	1908-
Fred. Porter Moore, M. D. (in office)	1910-
B. F. Lawley, M. D.	1912-1913
S. H. Rubin, M. D.	1913-1913
George E. McPherson, M. D. (in office)	1914-
John M. Thompson, M. D. (in office)	1914-

TRUSTEES.

Name	Years
Francis A. Walker	1893-1895
Samuel Carr	1893-1895
A. Lawrence Lowell	1893-1896
James J. Minot, M. D.	1893-1896
Anna Phillips Williams	1893-1907
Heman M. Burr	1895-1896
J. G. Pinkham, M. D.	1895-1902
Edward Cowles, M. D.	1896-1900
Benjamin H. Hartwell, M. D.	1896-1904
Robert H. Richards	1896-1898
Alfred E. Burton	1898-1899
S. Homer Woodbridge	1899-1903
John T. G. Nichols	1900-1907
Henry E. Cobb	1902-1904
Elwyn G. Preston	1902-1905
Samuel G. Webber	1902-1907
Leroy S. Brown	1903-1907
Frederick Fosdick	1904-1907
George L. Clemence	1905-1907
Leonard Wheeler	1905-1907
James H. Perkins	1907-1908
Robert A. Woods	1907-1914
Wm. H. Prescott, M. D.	1907-1914
Edwin Mulready	1907-1914
Timothy J. Foley, M. D.	1907-1914
Frank L. Locke	1907-1914
W. Rodman Peabody	1907-1914
Philip R. Allen	1908-1914
Henry T. Schafer (in office)	1914-
Isaac Heller (in office)	1914-
Dr. S. E. Coppinger (in office)	1914-
Geo. C. Shields (in office)	1914-
Dr. T. J. Scanlan (in office)	1914-
Mary A. Mahan (in office)	1914-
Joseph H. Guillet (in office)	1914-

MEDFIELD STATE HOSPITAL.[1]

HARDING, MASS.

In 1888 the condition of the insane in the State of Massachusetts was such that their friends and others interested in their care and treatment began to exert pressure for enlarged accommodation or some other means which would result in the improvement of the conditions in which they lived.

Dr. A. R. Moulton, inspector for the State Board of Lunacy and Charity at that time, stated as follows:

> The increase in the insane has been such that, although a new hospital had been opened in Worcester in 1877, one in Danvers in 1878 and the Homeopathic Hospital in Westborough only a few years previous, these three establishments alone housing about 1900 patients, there was a great crowding in all these institutions. Every hospital in the commonwealth was crowded much beyond its normal capacity, and in most of them many patients were obliged to sleep in cots placed on the corridor floors at night.
>
> The wards for the insane at the State Almshouse had been enlarged; provision for about 150 chronic insane of the criminal and vicious class had been made at the state farm and about 100 quiet chronic patients were boarding in families under the direction of the State Board.
>
> The natural increase in the number of insane was fully 200 a year. The only relief of the overcrowded state hospitals and asylums was that afforded by the boarding-out system, which provided for only a limited number by the removal of quiet and harmless patients from the state institutions to the local almshouse. Fully 1100 insane were under the care of the local overseers of the poor. In many the sexes were not properly separated. There was much filth and vermin and a condition of things in general existed that emphasized the fact that almshouse treatment was extremely bad and should be discouraged.

Finally, the State Board of Lunacy and Charity in their report for 1889 recommended the creation of a new asylum for the chronic insane, within a reasonable distance of Boston, which would provide for 1000 patients. The Willard plan was favorably commented on by this board.

In 1890 the Legislature passed an act to provide for the building of an asylum for the chronic insane in Eastern Massachusetts. The Governor was empowered to appoint three persons as a

[1] By Edward French, M. D., superintendent.

Board of Commissioners with full power to purchase or bond, subject to the approval of the Governor, suitable real estate in the eastern part of the state for a site for an asylum for the chronic insane to accommodate 1000 patients. They were also authorized to procure plans, specifications and estimates for the erection of suitable buildings, the first buildings to be constructed for 500 patients.

The sum of $25,000 was appropriated for the real estate and $5000 to carry out the provisions of the act.

The Governor appointed George L. Burt, Herbert Federhen and Dr. Albert R. Moulton as commissioners. They proceeded to advertise and to examine sites and finally a location was selected in Medfield and Dover of about 400 acres. This was bought at a cost of $25,250.

Dr. Moulton states that in the meetings of this commission with the Legislature a good deal of discussion was had as to the plan to be selected for the proposed asylum. Their opinion was strong that it should be on the cottage or detached plan, as affording better light, ventilation and classification. This commission visited many institutions and these visits further confirmed them in their idea of an institution on the cottage plan.

An act approved June 16, 1892, by the Legislature provided for a Board of Trustees consisting of seven persons, two of whom were to be women, and who should have authority to appoint a building committee of three members from their board to have entire charge of the Medfield Insane Asylum. This building committee was to receive compensation, the amount to be determined by the Governor and Council. The sum of $500,000 in addition to the amount necessary for compensation and the expenses of the trustees was appropriated; $250,000 of it in the year 1892; $200,000 in 1893 and $150,000 in the year 1894.

The price of the board of patients was also fixed by this act at $2.80 a week.

The original Board of Trustees consisted of Miss Elizabeth Thurber, Miss Mary H. Denny, Dr. John G. Park (late superintendent of the Worcester State Hospital), N. Hathaway, Jeremiah Murphy, H. M. Federhen and Frederick S. Risteen.

They held their first meeting on Thursday, July 21, 1892. It was voted that Messrs. Federhen, Hathaway and Murphy should be the building committee.

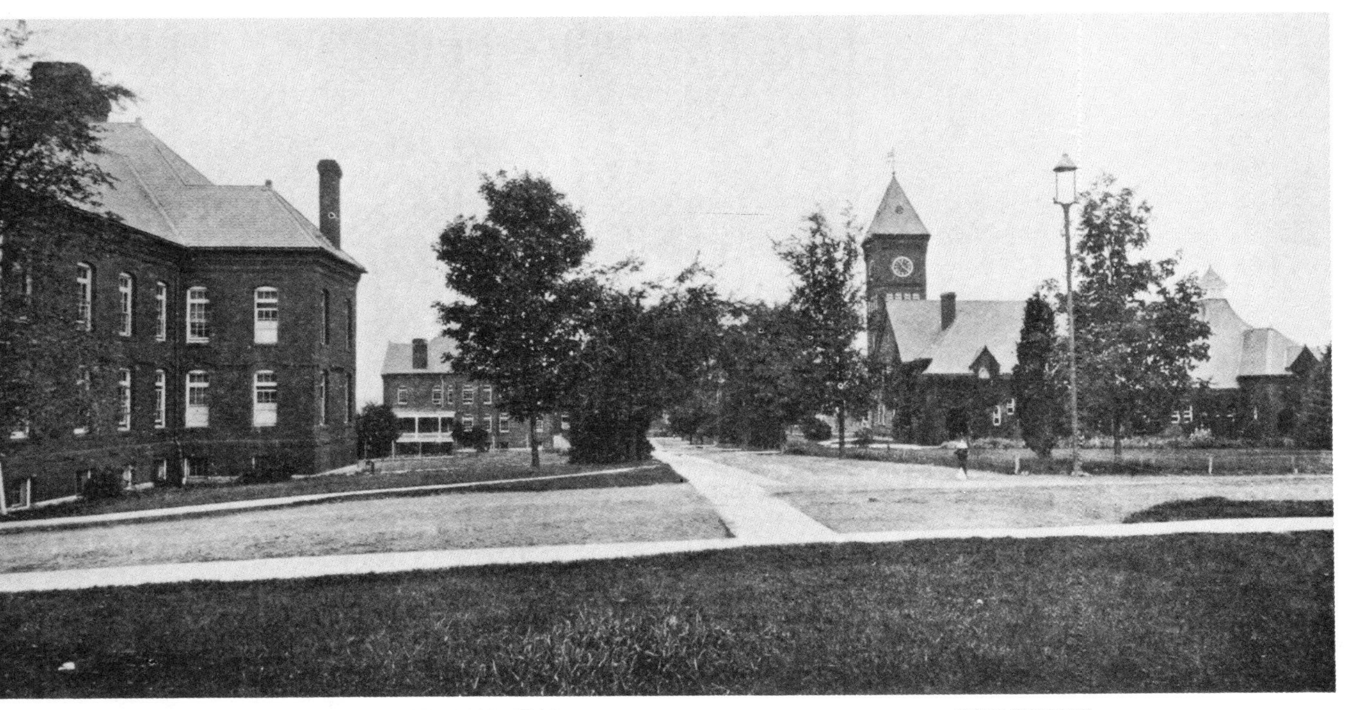

MEDFIELD STATE HOSPITAL. THE CHAPEL.

On January 2, 1894, a new building committee was appointed, as the members of the first building committee were no longer members of the Board of Trustees. The new committee consisted of Dr. Park, Mr. Hersey and William O. Blaney. The building of the institution had been going on during the previous year and it was practically completed under this building committee.

In 1896 a kitchen and two general dining rooms, a power plant, a laundry, an administration building and twelve buildings for patients being completed, the Governor was notified that the institution was ready to receive patients. On the first day of May, 1896, a transfer of 120 patients, 60 men and 60 women, was received from the Taunton State Hospital. In the previous February Dr. Edward French, of the New Hampshire State Hospital, had been appointed superintendent.

The original plans made by Dr. Moulton and the commissioners were but slightly modified. A building designed as a nurses' home was omitted. The location of the stand pipe was changed on the grounds and some minor changes in the partitions and construction of the ward buildings were brought about by the last building committee. On September 30, 1896, the end of the hospital year in Massachusetts and five months from the time of the reception of the first patients, there were 563 patients in the asylum.

A chapel, a stable and six more buildings for patients were completed this same year and the stock barn for farm operations was begun. The description of the institution at that time is as follows:

The completed plan shows 27 buildings facing along the sides and ends of a rectangle. The situation is upon the summit of a hill of about 250 feet elevation above the sea. The state owns 426 acres of land, part of it being situated in the town of Dover, all of it bordering upon the Charles River except upon the east side.

The top of the hill is graded on a gentle slope to the west. The prospect from all the buildings is beautiful and extensive. The woodland north of the institution borders on the river and offers an excellent opportunity for a park, and is already covered with well-grown trees. The ward buildings are situated upon the sides and ends and enclose the rectangle, all of them facing toward the center, in which are the chapel, laundry, general dining rooms, kitchen and power house. The buildings are separated from each other, the spaces between varying from four to eight rods, allowing air and sun upon the four sides of each building. Eighteen of these buildings are designed for patients, the second floor being used for sleeping purposes and the first story for sitting and work rooms. No patients are quartered above the second story. Most of the cottages accommodate about 50 patients, while two large ones are capable of accommodating 150 each. Some of these buildings are provided with dining rooms, but it is expected that the patients who are able will walk to the general dining rooms for their meals. Each dining room provides for 500 patients. The buildings are admirably lighted, with no dark corners, and are substantially and thoroughly built. Heat is forced into all the rooms by fans in each basement, from plenum chambers, which take fresh air direct from outside for heating purposes. Electric motors are used to drive these fans and also fans in the attic of all the buildings to exhaust the foul air.

At the end of the second hospital year there were 961 patients at the asylum. During the succeeding years additions and alterations have been made and the capacity has been increased from the nominal 1000 to 1800.

An industrial building, containing a machine shop, carpenter's shop and paint room on the first floor with two large shops on the second floor for the employment of patients, was commenced in 1898 and completed the following year. One room is used to manufacture all clothing for female patients; in the other room male patients cane chairs, make mattresses, repair iron beds, do upholstering and make trousers, shirts and coats.

In 1901 a farm house, arranged to provide living quarters for the head farmer and his family and to take care of 40 employees and patients, was completed. This was built near the stock barn.

In 1902 a nurses' home for 75 female attendants was completed.

In 1903 a large building for excited female patients was built outside of the rectangle and on the north end. This made additional room for 150.

In 1905 a nurses' dining room was erected to provide accommodation for all of the female employees and nurses at the asylum. Before this they had eaten in a portion screened off from the general dining room occupied by the female patients. During this same year two wooden cottages of simple construction for tuberculosis patients were erected, one for men and one for women. A new power house was also finished. This is located on the west side of the institution at a lower level in order to get a spur track from the railroad to the boiler house, thus avoiding the necessity of hauling coal with teams. This year also saw the completion of a home for male nurses with quarters for a medical assistant and his family, the male supervisor, a matron and 62 male attendants.

In 1906 a large building for excited male patients was completed, it being outside of the rectangle upon the west side. This increased the accommodation by 180 more. A large refrigerating plant was also installed. Three employees' cottages were built upon the grounds, providing in the same building tenements for married male attendants and accommodations for female attendants.

In 1907 the old power house, which was originally built in the center of the rectangle, was altered into a building for the cold storage of supplies and a new and modern bakery. This building was connected with the general kitchen and dining rooms by a tunnel. A cottage for the superintendent was built upon the grounds and occupied during this year.

In 1909 the name of the institution was changed from Medfield Insane Asylum to Medfield State Asylum.

The cottage plan for the care of the insane in Massachusetts had at Medfield its inception, and the results are all that could be expected.

Every building for patients has one or more verandas, some of them screened and some of them open. Some of these verandas are quite deep and have been utilized for open air hospitals, providing all the advantages of tents with greater conveniences and more security.

The buildings have from two to four day rooms, allowing, by this arrangement, intelligent patients to select their companionship, which would not be possible in one large day room.

The plan of having the patients live upon the first floor and sleep upon the second floor is more natural and home-like, and is appreciated by the intelligent patients.

With the location of the general dining rooms at a reasonable distance from these buildings the patients are obliged to take three walks a day in the open air to meals. This cannot be but of advantage. The absence of connecting corridors between the buildings and to the dining rooms has been found to be of no great disadvantage. Apart from the lessened expense of construction and necessary repairs to keep them in order, they have not been found necessary even in the rigorous climate of Eastern Massachusetts. The male patients have been able to reach the dining room for every meal in the history of the asylum. The women patients have been to every meal, with two exceptions, when there was a deep fall of snow with a high wind.

While the claim for economy in construction has been made for the cottage plan, experience has shown it to be untrue. It costs about one-sixteenth more to maintain a large institution on the cottage plan than it does one upon the block plan.

The increased advantages of sun, air, ventilation and exercise for the patients more than offset this increased expense.

In April, 1914, the State Board of Insanity, in joint action with the Board of Trustees of the Medfield State Asylum, introduced a bill in the current session of the Legislature to change the Medfield State Asylum from an asylum that receives chronic cases only, to a hospital. This change will allow the institution to receive acute cases from an appointed district. The name of the institution was changed to the Medfield State Hospital on the passage of the bill, which was signed by the Governor, April 28, 1914.

The following list of medical officers shows their time of service at the Medfield State Asylum from the time of its establishment to the year 1914:

SUPERINTENDENT.

Edward French (in office) 1896-

ASSISTANT PHYSICIANS.

Charles A. Drew........ 1896-1897
Thomas Howell 1896-1897
Lawrence F. Patton..... 1897-
Edward A. Andrews... 1897-1902
Harriet M. Doane...... 1897-
Fred C. Shultis......... 1898-1902
George B. Lockwood... 1898-1902
Florence H. Abbot...... 1898-1902
George C. Browne...... 1902-
Lewis M. Walker (in office) 1903-
Ralph S. Wilder........ 1903-1908
Helen T. Cleaves....... 1903-1910
G. Allen Troxell (in office) 1904-
Walter Burrier (in office) 1908-
Edmund C. Burrell...... 1909-
Jane B. Smith.......... 1910-1912
E. Mabel Thomson..... 1913-1914
Christina M. Leonard (in office) 1913-

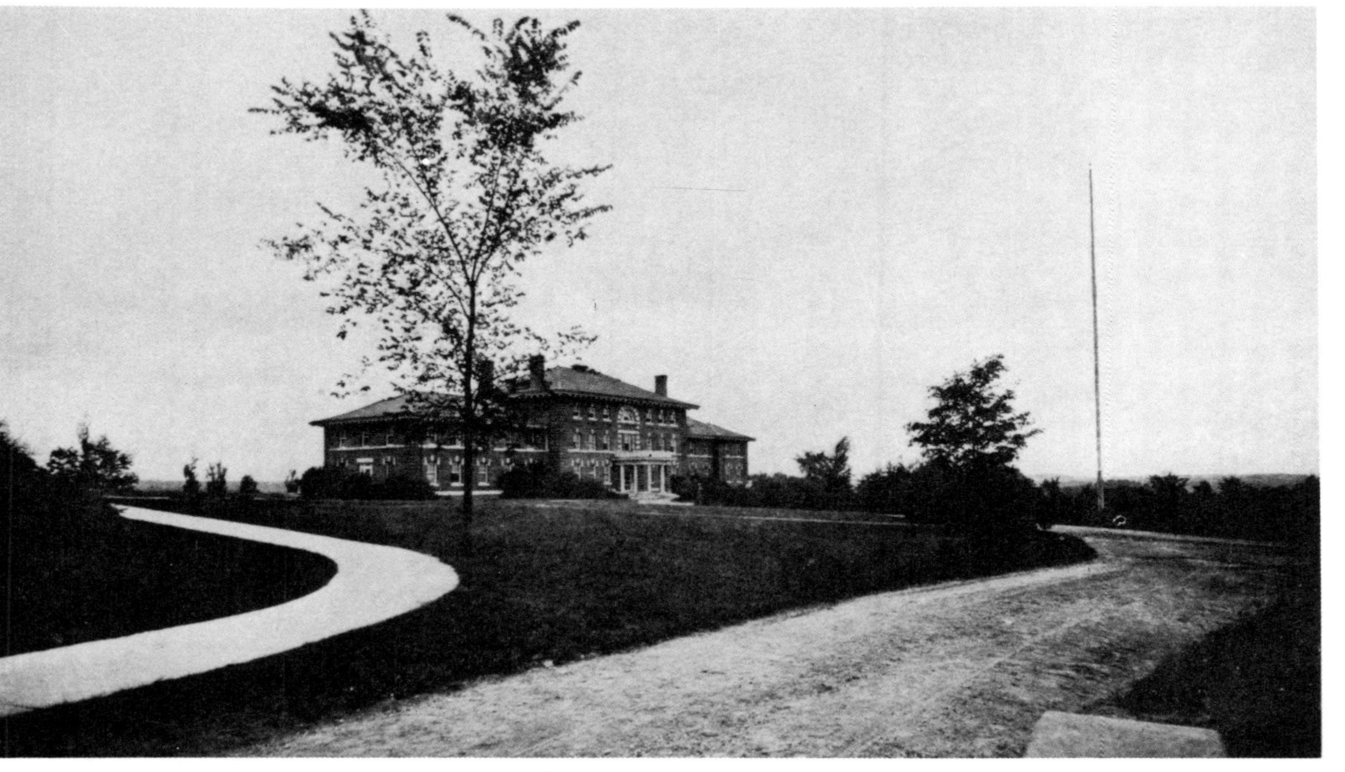

FEMALE NURSES' HOME, MEDFIELD STATE HOSPITAL.

MONSON STATE HOSPITAL.[1]

NEAR PALMER, MASS.

In 1852 Massachusetts established at Monson, near Palmer, on the Boston and Albany Railroad, one of three almshouses designed under the peculiar settlement law of the state for the care of state paupers. Later, when state paupers were transferred to the almshouses at Tewksbury and Bridgewater, the unoccupied buildings were placed at the disposal of the State Primary School for Boys. Subsequently the children of this school were placed in families and the school was discontinued.

In 1895 the Massachusetts Hospital for Epileptics was established for the care and treatment of 200 adult epileptics[2] and was endowed with the personal property, buildings and lands formerly belonging to the above-named institutions. The establishment of the Massachusetts Hospital for Epileptics had been the outcome of an agitation initiated by Drs. W. N. Bullard and H. R. Stedman, of Boston, who had labored for several years to awaken an interest in the medical profession and among the members of the Legislature as to the need of separate provision for epileptics. In 1895, through the active co-operation of an influential member of the Legislature and the support of the Governor, the desired legislation was secured and the second institution in the United States for the separate care of epileptics was established.

The trustees appointed Dr. Owen Copp superintendent and committed to him the supervision of the erection of the buildings and the development of the property. The original construction, which was of wood and not suited to the purposes of a hospital, was replaced by substantial brick buildings, arranged in detached groups for men and women, respectively, so situated as to give a proper separation of the sexes. The hospital was opened May 2, 1898.

At the present time there are several cottages for women, varying in capacity from 25 to 40 persons each, and a number of four-ward buildings, each ward accommodating 25 persons, all situated

[1] By Everett Flood, M. D.

[2] Chapter 483, Acts of 1895.

on the north slope of the hill; and on the opposite hillside, more than a half mile away, are similar cottages and four-ward buildings for men.[1]

In 1910 the name was changed from the Massachusetts Hospital for Epileptics to the Monson State Hospital and the provision which restricted admission to adults was removed.

Since the removal of the age limit a group of buildings for the accommodation of children, with suitable schools, has been constructed in still another direction upon a portion of the estate widely removed from the other divisions.

It is now the policy to develop the Monson Hospital in three separate and distinct departments, as above indicated.

The buildings are heated by central plants wherever they are situated in groups, but some of the cottages have a separate heating apparatus and the purpose is to continue the practice of establishing such separate heating in buildings which are not conveniently near to other buildings, but to bear in mind in all plans the desirability of uniting them with new groups when the vacant spaces become filled in.

The farm buildings are considerably removed from the three groups named, and their development will be carried on as means are provided. Already the institution has 120 cows and a sufficient force of employees and agricultural apparatus to take care of a large farm. Of the 700 acres of land owned by the institution the largest portion is in woodland and pasture. The amount of first-class land for tillage is small, but new areas are being cleared, the rocks taken from the land being crushed for road building.

Work shops and industries of various kinds are provided for the men and appropriate rooms for the women. It requires considerable oversight to keep epileptics busy and the pecuniary return is small, the actual advantage being mainly in the benefit which comes to each individual patient from his occupation. At present all mattresses and pillows are made and repaired when needed; also overalls and jumpers, mittens, shoes, door-mats and a large variety of women's clothing are manufactured. The women are employed in the laundry, kitchens, sewing rooms, etc.

[1] Two of the buildings have been named the W. S. Hyde Building and the Charles A. Clough Building, respectively, in honor of two deceased members of the Board of Trustees.

The value of the institution is estimated as follows: The aggregate of real estate is inventoried at $700,000 and of personal property at $129,000, making a total valuation of property used for the care of patients of about $829,000. The cost of maintenance has been about $4.50 per week for each patient, which charge during the past year has been increased owing to the establishment of the colony for children and the increased cost of supplies.

Three classes of cases are received:

1. Voluntary cases, whereby a patient either applies in person, or, if a child, application is made by a parent or guardian.

2. Patients who are considered to be "dangerous epileptics" and, although sane, need institutional care.

3. Cases who are positively insane.

The number of patients is now over 900 and buildings are in course of construction for about 200 more. It is expected that the institution will ultimately be required to take care of all epileptic persons who are at present in state institutions, to which end it will be necessary to expand its capacity to 1200 persons or more. The large number of buildings renders it possible to classify patients and divide them into many groups, which is undoubtedly better, although probably more expensive, than the congregate system.

When a patient is received he is examined, photographed and vaccinated and a method of treatment and work is prescribed for him. The administration of medicine is not encouraged until other methods have been used, such as the electric light cabinet bath and other forms of electric treatment, massage, appropriate work, diet, suitable hygienic measures and sleep, which are considered more helpful than the administration of drugs. Nevertheless recourse must occasionally be had to these latter in the treatment of intercurrent conditions. It is believed preferable, however, to persuade the patient to accept as more advantageous to himself the prevailing method of treatment without drugs. Incidentally he is more willing to regulate his diet and to do the moderate amount of work required.

Diet and routine are probably the most valuable curative methods and it should be added that suitable nourishment must not be stinted.

Laboratory work has been carried on and special investigations as to the cause of epilepsy have been made. The Brown-Sequard theory of inheritance has been practically disproved by experiment. It is not believed that acquired epilepsy is ever inherited.

Pathological studies are also in progress and a large amount of material partly worked up is already available. Field workers have been profitably employed to investigate the pedigrees of many patients. These are also social workers so far as time allows, and the records are made more vauable by the intimate acquaintance with the homes of the patients which is thereby gained.

Moreover, these inquiries are valuable not only to the hospital staff in dealing with individual cases, but as an educational and familiarizing influence in the public interest. They tend to bring the hospital and its patrons into a closer and more sympathetic union, and to make the friends and families of patients co-workers in the cause. It seems hardly too much to believe that they must in time increase our knowledge of epilepsy, the conditions of its origin and the means of its prevention. As the epileptic manifestation is nearly related to other forms of ancestral or collateral weakness, the scope of these investigations is seen to be far-reaching; and as their benefits mature, society must recognize their usefulness, and give the work its needed encouragement and support.

Since 1912 additional buildings have been added as follows: A cow barn, an employees' cottage, two ice houses, one greenhouse, three isolation shacks, one bungalow, one farm shed and a fireproof building for 130 patients.

TRUSTEES.

Wm. N. Bullard, M. D...	1895-	Henry P. Jaques........	1900-
Albert C. Gatchel, M. D..	1895-1900	Walter W. Scofield, M. D.	1901-1911
Burnhem B. Benner, M. D.	1895-1901	Winford H. Caldwell....	1902-1909
Adelaide A. Calkins....	1895-1904	Mary B. Townley.......	1904-
Charles A. Clough......	1895-1908	John B. Blake, M. D.....	1908-
William S. Hyde........	1895-1899	Edward P. Bagg........	1909-1912
Mabel M. Stedman.....	1895-	Michael L. Shea, M. D...	1911-
H. M. Phillips..........	1899-1902	George A. Moore, M. D.	1912-

SUPERINTENDENTS.

Owen Copp, M. D.......	1895-1898	Everett Flood, M. D. (in office)	1899-

PHYSICIANS.

Name	Years	Name	Years
Edgar J. Spratling......	1898-1899	Annie E. Taft..........	1909-1910
Arthur O. Morton......	1899-1905	Frederick W. Guild.....	1909-1912
Morgan B. Hodskins...	1899-	Edward A. Douglass....	1910-1912
Edmund R. Fourtain....	1899-	Charles A. Glancey......	1912-1912
Ransom A. Greene......	1902-1905 1912-	Helen Taft Cleaves.....	1912-
		Fred. S. Swain.........	1912-1912
Edward A. Kennedy....	1905-1910	Douglas A. Thom.......	1912-
Thomas A. Shaughnessy	1905-1905	George E. King........	1912-
Alden V. Cooper.......	1905-1912	Charles D. Leach.......	1912-1915
Charles A. Davis........	1905-1906	Donald J. McLean......	1912-
Melvin E. Cowan........	1907-1909	Erwin S. Bundy........	1913-

GARDNER STATE COLONY.[1]

GARDNER, MASS.

In the annual report of the Massachusetts State Board of Insanity for 1899, under the heading of "The Chronic Insane," the following statements are found:

Chronic cases of insanity constitute a large proportion of all the insane. Many of them are quiet, able-bodied persons. There are also some excitable patients, who would improve and become efficient workers under appropriate conditions. These classes, we believe, are suitable for colonization.

A colony for the chronic insane may be outlined thus:

It should start with a farm of not less than 2000 acres, near good railroad facilities. The land may be rough, hilly and stony, but should ultimately become fertile, when brought under cultivation by the labor of patients. There should be plenty of growing timber and wood, clay beds for brick-making, a quarry for stone cutting, water power, and other natural advantages for the formation of a village community.

From this stage the work should proceed under the general supervision of a Board of Trustees and in immediate charge of a superintendent, who, in addition to being a good medical man, should have practical business qualities. He should live at the colony and give his entire energies to its service. Starting with a good farmer, he should gradually gather a competent corps of assistants, namely, carpenters, masons and other mechanics, who, with the aid of patients, should continue the structural and industrial development. There should prevail a spirit of self-help and reluctance to call in outside assistance to do anything which could be accomplished through internal resources.

The construction of the buildings should be plain, simple and durable. The standard of workmanship should not be allowed to rise higher than the attainment of common mechanics and patients. At the start, only necessary and ordinary comforts should be expected. These should be supplemented later by every pleasure and improvement which a surplus of labor and the increasing skill of patients might be able to provide.

Such a tract of land would probably be an aggregation of several farms, with buildings already upon them. These should be utilized so far as possible. Gradually, here and there, in suitable locations groups of buildings of varying size and arrangement should be erected, sufficiently scattered to afford the necessary classifications as to sex, occupation and social and mental condition.

A small number of patients should be received as soon as possible to assist in the farming, excavating, road building and other work incident to

---

[1] By Senator John G. Faxon, Fitchburg, Mass.

construction. Thus should gradually grow up the first farmstead group. Others should follow as required to bring the patients near the fields which they are to till.

In time on the water-power site should be established carpenter, machine, blacksmith and paint shops, laundry, sawmill, and gristmill, and nearby homes for patients. Other industrial centers should form, one by one, for making necessary articles for use in the colony.

As soon as practicable, women should be provided for, at a considerable distance from the men. They would naturally fall in groups for sewing and mending, tailoring and hand laundering. They should make the butter, conduct the dairy, pick the fruits and engage in similar occupations.

Ultimately a stage should be reached when more would be produced than could be used in the colony. Then the surplus of labor should be sufficient to undertake many improvements which before had waited for more urgent necessities.

In accordance with the foregoing well-conceived plan, the State Board of Insanity recommended for immediate action "that a colony for the chronic insane should be established according to the general plan outlined in this report."

Accordingly the Legislature passed an act[1] to provide for the care of the insane by the State Board of Insanity and to establish the State Colony for the Insane. This act authorized the State Board of Insanity, with the approval of the Governor and Council, to take by purchase or otherwise a tract of farming or other land, suitable in its judgment for the establishment of a receptacle for the care, custody and control of the insane. "Said tract to consist of not less than 1500 nor more than 2500 acres, and may include buildings and other chattels thereon."

Section 4 provided for the appointment by the Governor of a board of seven trustees, which should have the government and management of the colony.

The trustees were to be removable only for cause, and their term of office was to be for five years; but of those first appointed one member was to hold office for five years, two for four years, one for three years, two for two years and one for one year. The trustees, upon their appointment, were to proceed to obtain plans and to construct the buildings required for the establishment of a farming colony for the insane, as well as to appoint a superintendent and such other officers and assistants as might be required.

[1] Acts of 1900, Chapter 451.

To meet the expenses to be incurred under the provisions of this act the State Board of Insanity was to expend a sum not exceeding $25,000 in acquiring the land, buildings and chattels provided for in Section 3 of the act; and a sum not exceeding $50,000, under the direction of the trustees, for repairs of such buildings as might be acquired, and for the construction of new buildings and for the care and maintenance of the colony.

Section 8 of the act provided that as soon as the colony was ready for the reception of patients the trustees were to give notice to the Governor, who should make proclamation that, upon a given day, the colony was to be opened for the reception of patients; and thereafter the State Board of Insanity was, at its discretion, to transfer from the state insane hospitals and asylums and from the state hospitals to the colony such of the chronic insane as were, in its judgment, the most suitable to be transferred. It was further provided that after the first day of January, 1904, the board was to transfer and remove to such state hospitals, state asylums, State Hospital, the Hospital for Epileptics, or the Colony for the Insane, as it would deem proper, all of the insane in any almshouse or other receptacle not maintained or controlled by the commonwealth; and the State Board of Insanity was to have power, in its discretion, to transfer insane patients to and from the State Colony for the Insane and the other hospitals, or asylums, or receptacles for the insane maintained or controlled by the commonwealth.

This act was approved July 11, 1900.

In obedience to the above legislative enactment the search for a proper location was undertaken and in due course some 1500 acres of land were purchased in the towns of Gardner, Westminster and Ashburnham, at and adjoining the common junction of these towns, of Northern Worcester County, and on the trunk line of the Fitchburg Railroad. These towns are some 1000 to 1200 feet above the sea level. There was arable land of sufficiently excellent quality to furnish acreage for farming. There was lumber enough to reduce the cost of materials for the buildings which soon began to take their places on these neglected acres. Stone abounded, of excellent quality for roads and walls and foundations, and in some cases for entire construction of certain buildings. There was water in abundance, and good drainage opportunities. The first appropriations in 1903-1904 amounted to $33,151, on which beginnings were made; one year later $150,000 was appropriated.

On December 18, 1901, Governor Winthrop Murray Crane appointed the first Board of Trustees, as folows:

Herbert B. Howard, M. D., chairman; Charles V. Dasey, Edmund A. Whitman, William H. Baker, M. D., Mrs. Alice Miller Spring, Mrs. Maie H. Coes, secretary, and George H. Harwood. Since that date other members have been: Dr. John G. Blake, appointed 1906, vice Mr. Dasey; Wilbur F. Whitney, appointed 1907, vice Dr. Howard. The present Board of Trustees is: Edmund A. Whitman, chairman; Mrs. Maie H. Coes, secretary; George H. Harwood, Wilbur F. Whitney, Mrs. Alice M. Spring, William H. Baker, M. D., and John G. Blake, M. D.

The chairman of the first board, Dr. Howard, had been a member of the State Board of Insanity since its organization in 1889, and resigned from that board that he might accept appointment on this new board. He was to a large extent the originator of the new plan for the care of the insane the state was undertaking. He had been superintendent of the State Hospital at Tewksbury, resigning to become superintendent of the Massachusetts General Hospital in Boston, later resigning to become superintendent of the new Peter Bent Brigham Hospital, Boston. After four years of service on the Board of Trustees of the colony, he resigned to become again a member and subsequently chairman of the State Board of Insanity.

Mr. George H. Harwood, of Barre, another member appointed to the first Board of Trustees, had previously been selected by the State Board of Insanity to conduct a search for a site for the colony.

The Board of Trustees was fortunate in securing Dr. Joseph B. Howland as its first superintendent. He was appointed April 1, 1902. To Dr. Howland great credit is due, for it was he who did the real "pioneer" work of the colony. Dr. Howland had been assistant superintendent at the Massachusetts General Hospital, Boston, whence he resigned to become assistant superintendent of the State Hospital at Tewksbury, resigning the latter position to become superintendent of the Gardner State Colony. He remained at Gardner as superintendent until April, 1907, when he resigned, having been appointed assistant administrator of the Massachusetts General Hospital, Boston.

The present superintendent, Dr. Charles E. Thompson, has been twice at the head of the colony. He came from the State Hospital at Tewksbury, where he had been assistant physician, in October, 1904, as assistant superintendent, and followed Dr. Howland as superintendent in 1907. Dr. Thompson resigned in September, 1911, having been appointed executive officer of the State Board of Insanity. He was succeeded by Dr. Charles T. LaMoure, assistant physician of the State Hospital at Rochester, N. Y., where he had done excellent work in the training of demented cases. Dr. LaMoure resigned in the spring of 1914 to accept the superintendency of the School for Imbeciles at Lakeville, and was replaced by Dr. Thompson. During Dr. LaMoure's administration the plant was not materially increased in size; when he resigned the registration was 438 males and 243 females.

Of the original buildings on the property, but one was deemed at all available for immediate occupancy. During the summer of 1902 enough repairing and renovating of this building was done to accommodate ten patients, and on October 22, 1902, Governor Crane declared the new institution to be open for the reception of patients, and in that same month five were transferred from the Taunton Insane Hospital and in December five more from Westborough.

These patients worked in the woods during the winter, cutting and drawing 46,000 feet of lumber. The following summer they worked on the farm and in excavating for the water supply. In the meantime the men's receiving ward, domestic building, power house, administration building and women's ward were nearing completion; in 1904 there were received 111 patients and in 1905 the number was 274.

At present the plant comprises 45 buildings. Their capacity is 740 patients and the number registered is 730. The buildings are: An administration building; ten buildings for male and six for female patients; one building each for heating plant, power house, greenhouse, isolation buildings for contagious cases; paint shop, three buildings for domestic service uses, four dwellings for employees, physicians and attendants, two for farmers and mechanics and two industrial buildings, one each for men and women.

The entire plant is electrically lighted and has a pressure water supply from a reservoir tank of 295,000 gallons capacity, and the drainage is in units for the different groups of buildings, largely on the filtration system.

The entire plot of 1500 acres is crossed and recrossed by macadam roads built by the patients, and the colony might not improperly be taken as a model spotless town in many ways.

The industrial buildings are amply equipped with tools and simple machinery needful for their purposes.

Instruction has been supplied in every branch where needed, and the gains made and benefits accrued have justified the pains-taking work and such expense as it has entailed.

It is especially noteworthy that the grounds of the colony are not in any way policed. To be sure an occasional "elopement" does occur, but the escaping patient is almost invariably apprehended and his return to the colony is effected without much trouble, and at present without notoriety, though the management had to contend for the first few years with the offensive publicity of certain newspapers which overrated the news value of an "escape."

In his report to the Board of Trustees for 1910 Dr. Thompson made the following statements which the conditions of this year amply confirm:

Special mention should be made of the fact that during the last year we have produced more than we have required for our own use of all clothing for both men and women: boots, shoes, and all slippers for men; handkerchiefs, neckties, mittens and hats; work, fancy and farm baskets; fiber and braided mats, and toweling for patients' use.

The report for 1911 said:

The two industrial buildings under construction at the time of my last report were completed early in the year and have proved very satisfactory. A large number can now be employed under systematic supervision, and a greater variety of articles made. At the present time 61 patients are regularly employed in these buildings, while of our total number of patients 85 per cent are daily employed in some useful and helpful occupation.

We are now making all clothing for both men and women except knitted underwear, all boots, shoes, slippers, gloves, mittens, hats, caps, stockings, while a large amount of mending, fancy work and basketry is done by the women patients.

Furniture purchased not being adapted to our use, we have opened a furniture department, under direction of a skilled instructor, and will hereafter make all of our own furniture of every description.

For several months we have knitted on hand machines all stockings worn by our men, and are now making all stockings required for our women patients.

Broom, brush and mattress making has been recently introduced. We have to deal with patients of reduced mentality, and our efforts are directed to the prevention of further loss of mind and the stimulation and training of that mind which still remains.

The gross weekly per capita cost, three years' average, 1909-1911, at the Gardner Colony was $3.651. The total average for the same time of all the state hospitals and asylums was $4.307. It is not improper to trace a portion of this lesser cost to the productivity of the labor of the patients as variously secured. The Gardner Colony cost is lowest of any institution for the insane in the commonwealth.

Since 1908 the farm has supplied all vegetables, while all milk and practically all eggs used have been produced by the colony.

In 1908 it was estimated that not less than 80 per cent of the patients were working. In 1911 90 per cent of the patients were occupied three or more hours per day.

The plant is inventoried in the last report at over $648,000, exclusive of the land.

At the railroad station is a storehouse and freight depot, where purchased supplies are received in bulk for distribution. A short walk brings one to the dignified administration building, which faces to the south, while opposite it across the lawns is the large domestic building. The other sides of the square are occupied by the men's and the women's receiving wards. Near by and toward the station is the power plant that heats the buildings of this central group and furnishes electric light and power as required about the colony. A greenhouse and stable are hard by, while adjoining the administration building, but not near enough to impair the architectural harmony of the plan, are the newer cottages for nurses, married couples and variously employed attendants, supervisors and others. On a high hill and giving adequate fire and domestic service pressure is a steel tank of nearly 300,000 gallons capacity, supplied from ample sources by high-pressure pumps.

The barns and necessary outbuildings are harmonious. In charge of each cottage group are such supervisors or house attendants as are needed. Attached to each cottage is its own farm, where are raised enough supplies from the ground to meet its needs or supply a surplus for other groups where the ground is called upon for other produce. A careful table of production is maintained, and through this and through the exchange and the exhibiting of the best specimens competition is stimulated.

Great care and wisdom in selection of attendants and supervisors have been shown and to this scrutiny may be traced no small measure of the results attained. Pleasant surroundings within, good color tones on the walls, light and air in unlimited quantities, wholesome food, recreation, every creature comfort, reading matter, games—all these things are at hand for every patient.

SUPERINTENDENTS.

Dr. Joseph B. Howland.	1902-1907	Dr. Charles E. Thompson	1907-1911; 1914-
Dr. Charles T. LaMoure	1911-1914		

ASSISTANT SUPERINTENDENTS.

Dr. Charles E. Thompson	1904-1907	Dr. Harlan L. Paine (in office)	1914-
Dr. George A. Pierce....	1907-1908		
Dr. Thomas Littlewood..	1908-1914		

ASSISTANT PHYSICIANS.

Dr. William F. Farmer..	1906-1907	Dr. Marion E. Kenworthy (in office)....	1913-
Dr. Harris C. Burrows..	1908-1910	Dr. Thomas W. Maloney	1913-1914
Dr. Paul R. Felt........	1910-1911	Dr. Chester A. Van Corr (in office)	1914-
Dr. Gardner N. Cobb....	1911-1912		
Dr. Harold H. Fox......	1912-1913		

NORFOLK STATE HOSPITAL.

PONDVILLE, MASS.

Acting upon the recommendation made in the special report by the Board of Trustees of Foxborough State Hospital on "Drunkenness in Massachusetts, Condition and Remedies," the Legislature of 1910 appropriated $50,000 for the purchase of land upon which a new and comprehensive institution for the care of inebriates by the state might be established. Following an extensive examination of sites the trustees purchased a tract of land comprising 1004 acres situated in the townships of Norfolk and Walpole, four miles from the Foxborough State Hospital, and 26 miles from Boston. The requisites for the colonies were as follows:

1. A colony for incipient or hopeful inebriate cases; for men who offer a considerable prospect of recovery, and who are willing to co-operate in all measures put forward for their betterment.

2. Colonies for the more advanced male cases; patients who are supposedly incurable and who are in need of custodial care.

3. A colony for refractory male cases; men who do not lend themselves to ordinary measures of treatment.

4. A colony for inebriate women; this colony at first to care only for women of the hospital type, namely, cases which are likely to be benefited by hospital treatment.

In order to permit of segregation and to allow for individualization in treatment, these colonies will be suitably situated and distributed over the large tract of land. The colonies, with the possible exception of the colony for refractory male cases, will consist of cottages containing a minimum number of 15 or a maximum number of 20 persons. These cottages will be under adequate supervision, but will be cared for largely by the patient occupants. Each cottage or habitation will be a unit.

Following the original appropriation for land (Chapter 635, Acts of 1910), appropriations of $115,000 (Chapter 124, Acts of 1912) and $89,000 (Chapter 133, Acts of 1913) were allowed for suitable buildings. Upon the recommendations of the board six cottages, two reception hospital pavilions, and administration building, power house, laundry and service building have been erected and the inebriates and drug habitues cared for at the Foxborough State Hospital were moved to the new hospital on June 1, 1914.

The Board of Trustees and the superintendent of the Foxborough State Hospital were transferred in office to the Norfolk State Hospital.

At that time the available beds at the Foxborough State Hospital, 200 in number, were utilized for the care of the insane under the continued care of the State Board of Insanity.

The Norfolk State Hospital has therefore been in existence since June 1, 1914, and is a state hospital for the treatment of male inebriates and drug habitues, and is under the supervision of the State Board of Charity.

BOARD OF TRUSTEES.

MEDICAL STAFF.

Dr. Irwin H. Neff.....................Superintendent.
Dr. Frank H. Carlisle...............Assistant.
Dr. Frederick P. Moore.............. Assistant physician.
Dr. Solomon H. Rubin...............Acting physician to out-patient dept.

WRENTHAM STATE SCHOOL.[1]

Wrentham, Mass.

The Wrentham State School, Wrentham, Mass., was established in 1906, and is situated on a tract of about 500 acres of land one mile from the village of Wrentham. The institution consists of two groups of buildings, built in the midst of pine groves, which afford play grounds for the children in summer.

The main group includes an administration building, five dormitories, a school building, laundry, service building and power house and six homes for employees. In addition to these there are now under construction a hospital and three new dormitories; two of the latter are of the same type of building as those already occupied, while the third is especially constructed to care for the defective delinquent type of boy.

The farm group is situated about a quarter of a mile from the main buildings and includes the original farm house remodeled and enlarged and two dormitories, together with the farm buildings, cow barn, horse stable, carriage house, etc.

The institution dormitories are two-story brick buildings, of fireproof construction, built with extra large windows, so as to admit the maximum amount of fresh air and sunlight. In each of the dormitories, besides the regular wards, day rooms, etc., is an industrial room, where is held the sewing classes, basketry, lace and weaving classes, etc., and the boys' industrial classes, including brush making, etc.

The school building contains several class rooms on the second floor, while the first floor is divided into music rooms, gymnasium and assembly hall, the latter being used for entertainments, school exhibitions, etc.

The service building contains the kitchen, bakery and storeroom, the dining rooms and a few sleeping rooms. The laundry is a separate building, as is the paint shop. In the power house are contained the boiler room, engine room, carpenter and repair shop.

[1] By George L. Wallace, M. D., superintendent.

The school is organized on an educational basis, the inmates attending either the regular school classes, industrial classes, or both. The work consists of graded school and kindergarten work and the various training methods that have been used in the schools for feeble-minded for many years. The children are also instructed in both instrumental and vocal music, gymnastics, sloyd and domestic science, sewing, fancy work, basketry, weaving of towelling, etc.

All of the outside work is done by the boys and includes the care of the farm, grounds, gardens, the barns and stock, etc., and is under the direction of competent trainers. The farm is considered the most valuable adjunct of the educational system, as it improves the boys physically as well as making them self-respecting and reliant.

The capacity of the institution is 448 beds.

The school is under the charge of a Board of Trustees, a medical superintendent and three assistant physicians.

TRUSTEES.

Albert L. Harwood, chairman ....1906-in office
Ellerton James, secretary ....1906-in office
Herbert Parsons 1906-1909
John J. Connor 1906-1909
Walter Channing 1906-1908
Mary Stewart Scott ....1906-in office
Susanna W. Berry ....1906-in office
George W. Gay, M. D. ....1908-in office
Patrick J. Lynch ....1909-in office
Harry T. Hayward 1909-1913
Herbert Parsons ....1913-in office

SUPERINTENDENT.

George L. Wallace, M. D. ....1907-in office

ASSISTANT PHYSICIANS.

Franklin H. Perkins, 1st assistant ....1910-in office
Eudora W. Faxon, 2d assistant ....1913-in office
Arthur R. Pillsbury, 3d assistant ....1914-in office

CHANNING SANITARIUM.[1]

BROOKLINE, MASS.

When this institution was opened in 1879 very few mentally-ill or nervous persons in this country were cared for by physicians in private houses. Patients who were not provided for in public hospitals or in their own homes were sent to such large endowed institutions as the Pennsylvania Hospital for the Insane in Philadelphia, the McLean at Somerville, Bloomingdale in New York, and the Butler Hospital in Providence. Some beginnings had, however, been made in Massachusetts, there being at the date mentioned two physicians at least who received several patients in their houses.

Dr. Edward Jarvis, a well-known authority on mental diseases, who, as one of a Commission on Lunacy, had prepared a valuable "report" for the state in 1855 "On Insanity and Idiocy in Massachusetts," and had himself for some years received patients in his house in Dorchester, Mass., gave encouraging advice, and finally it was decided to try the experiment in spite of rather a cold attitude on the part of some of the physicians connected with the large hospitals, who were of the opinion that risks would be considerable and the benefit to the patient less than in the then existing type of institution.

No name was given to the institution, it being called simply a private hospital for mental diseases. A few years ago, when it seemed desirable to adopt a specific title, the present one was chosen. When first opened a license was obtained, as was then necessary, from the Governor, on recommendation of the State Board of Lunacy and Charity. From the beginning the sanitarium has been under the jurisdiction of the former board, which supervises its management, exercising the same control as over the large hospitals, except in financial affairs. Patients are admitted by commitment or voluntary agreement.

The sanitarium being avowedly for mentally diseased persons, there has been a preponderance of such cases, but as time has gone on the number of mild cases has increased, and it is hoped

[1] By Walter Channing, M. D., superintendent.

to further limit the scope of the work to these and border-line cases, in order that its efforts may be largely concentrated on prevention. The fact that the small institutions have multiplied rapidly in this state during the last 20 years, there being more than 20 at the present time, proves that there is a field for them, though they receive a very small percentage of the total number of cases admitted to the hospitals.

The sanitarium is situated on high land, about 200 feet above sea level, in one of the most beautiful parts of Brookline. The grounds, comprising about 10 acres, were formerly part of an old farm and contain many fine shrubs and trees, some of the latter being 150 years old.

The first building occupied, now called the "Hayden," an old mansion house, was opened in 1879. Only a small number of patients was received into the family of the superintendent, the idea being, as already said, to preserve as far as possible the character of the surroundings from which they had come. After the lapse of a few years this house proved inadequate, not only for the accommodation of those seeking admission, but for proper facilities for treatment. It was therefore decided in 1888 to erect another building. This was called the "Mott" and provided for 10 patients, and was at a distance of about 100 feet from the Hayden building, the two being connected by a broad enclosed arcade which could serve both as a protected means of communication and a place to exercise in when the weather was bad.

In 1892 a third building, called the "Hayden Annex," was added. In the annex a ward was arranged for the care of five male patients and for some time was made use of for that purpose. After a while, however, it was decided that it would be desirable to treat only one sex and since that time the institution has been largely given over to women, though exceptions are sometimes made.

In 1895 an entirely separate estate, with a good house several hundred feet away from the main building, was acquired. This was called the "Fuller House," and arranged for a limited number of patients who might require some degree of isolation. At the present time it is chiefly used for nurses.

For the past 20 years a house at the sea-shore has been rented and during the summer months several patients have been sent there from time to time. They have been practically free from the necessary restrictions in the home institution at Brookline and are benefited by the change of air and scene.

The four buildings described, with the superintendent's house, the laundry and a small work shop, constitute the entire institution, furnishing accommodations for 25 patients. The number of buildings makes it possible to fairly diversify classification. In the Mott building there is a small hall with gymnastic apparatus, which hall is also used for parties and other entertainments, and the offices and dispensary are in this building. The rooms are arranged both in suites and singly. In 1909 the entire institution was renovated. Electric lights were installed throughout all the buildings and many bathrooms added.

The necessary staff to carry on the institution is composed of two physicians, at least 30 nurses, a head nurse, a bath masseuse nurse and a clerk. The latter typewrites the records, which are similar to those of large institutions, and attends to many business details. With 25 patients thorough individual treatment is possible, yet on the other hand the number is large enough, especially if the general type of cases is essentially the same, to bring several together for amusements, occupations and classes. The effort has always been made to maintain a home environment with the advantages of hospital treatment.

This institution was among the earlier ones to make use of so-called physical training in the treatment of patients and perhaps the first to thoroughly equip a gymnasium with apparatus for the purpose.

In 1900 a hydrotherapy plant was installed, being arranged after the plans of Dr. Simon Baruch, of New York.

The following physicians have been associated with the superintendent in the management of the institution either as resident physicians or as assistants:

Dr. Eben Norton........	1885-1885
Dr. Wallace M. Knowlton	1888-
Dr. J. Frank Edgerly....	1890-1892
Dr. Martin Barr........	1892-1892
Dr. Frank W. Pierce....	1894-1895
Dr. L. Vernon Briggs....	1900-1901
Dr. E. E. Bessey........	1901-1903
Dr. George A. Yeaton..	1902-1903
Dr. C. H. Downing......	1903-1904
Dr. W. Ferrin..........	1904-1905
Dr. Alva Mills..........	1905-1906
Dr. Carroll Still........	1906-1907
Dr. W. Ducy...........	1907-1908
Dr. Mabel D. Ordway..	1908-1909
Dr. J. E. Overlander....	1909-1911

THE NEWTON NERVINE.

WEST NEWTON, MASS.

The Newton Nervine, a private hospital for mental and nervous patients, is situated in West Newton, Mass., nine miles west of Boston.

It was established February 1, 1892, by N. Emmons Paine, M. D., immediately after his resignation from the superintendency of the Westborough Insane Hospital. Originally there were 12 acres of grounds and one building, the "Main House." As the number of patients increased, however, other buildings were added, beginning with the "Cottage," 1733 Commonwealth Avenue, which was added in October, 1892, and accommodates four patients. "The Colonial," 1760 Washington Street, was built to care for 10 patients, and was opened in July, 1896. Another cottage, 1640 Washington Street, was built for one special patient and her nurse as her home, and was occupied in December, 1906. These four buildings have ample accommodations for 21 patients.

On the first of January, 1910, Dr. Paine found it necessary to retire from active medical work, and Dr. Edward Mellus then rented three of the buildings, and has since carried on the Newton Nervine as his private hospital for mental and nervous diseases.

THE NEWTON SANATORIUM.

WEST NEWTON, MASS.

The Newton Sanatorium is a private hospital for nervous invalids and is situated in West Newton, Mass.

After Dr. N. Emmons Paine had been carrying on the Newton Nervine for about two years, and realizing the demand by certain nervous patients for treatment apart from mental cases, even of the mildest forms, he made provision for these nervous persons in private homes in the neighborhood of West Newton, and designated them collectively as the Newton Sanatorium. The number of these houses varied from one to eight, according to the needs from time to time. Each house had one or more competent nurses in charge of the medical and nursing requirements, under direction. Later, the time and labor in visiting these scattered houses became too great and Dr. Paine erected for them a new building, " The Brick House," 1660 Washington Street, next to his own residence, with accommodations for 12 patients, and it was opened in October, 1902. To it was given the name of The Newton Sanatorium, and the private residences were gradually discontinued.

RING SANATORIUM AND ARLINGTON HEIGHTS HEALTH RESORT.

Arlington Heights, Mass.

This institution consists of two distinct and separate plants. The Ring Sanatorium was opened in 1879. No mental cases are received in this institution. The Arlington Heights Health Resort is located a block away and consists of spacious grounds on which are three buildings for mild mental diseases. Two of these houses are for women and one for men. A hydropathic room is provided and the kitchens are modern and arranged to carry out special dietary. Occupational treatment is used, there being a special teacher who devotes her time to this work. Basket making, clay modeling, weaving, etc., are utilized. There is also a training school for nurses with a three-years' course, the last year being given in a general hospital.

The physicians in charge are Arthur H. Ring, M. D., Barbara T. Ring, M. D., and Wallace M. Knowlton, M. D.

There were 35 patients in the institution June 1, 1913.

THE CARE OF THE INSANE IN MICHIGAN.

In the year 1790 Michigan was known as the Northwest Territory and comprised all the country now embraced in the State of Michigan and parts of Wisconsin, Illinois, Indiana and Ohio. In the same year an act was passed respecting the division of the counties into townships and for the appointment of constables, overseers of the poor and clerks of the townships. It provided:

> That the justices in session in their respective counties shall annually appoint one or more overseers of the poor in each and every township of the county to serve for the term of one whole year, and it shall be the duty of each such overseer to make report to any justice of the peace in and for the county of all vagrant persons likely to become chargeable to the township for which he is appointed overseer, and also to take notice of all the poor and distressed families and persons residing in his proper township and inquire into the means by which they are supported and maintained. And whenever he shall discover any person or family really suffering through poverty, sickness, accident or any misfortune or inability which may render him, or her, or them, a wretched and proper object, or objects, of public charity, it shall be his duty, and he is hereby strictly enjoined, to give immediate information thereof to a justice of the peace, acting in and for the same county, that legal means may then be taken by such justice to afford the person or persons so suffering proper and seasonable relief.

In the above act the word inability refers to persons who were suffering from mental trouble.

In 1796 Wayne County was organized and embraced within its limits all the State of Michigan and parts of Illinois, Ohio, Indiana and Wisconsin.

The first reference to the care of the insane in Michigan is to be found in an act creating the Board of Superintendents of the Poor in Wayne County approved March 7, 1834. This board is therefore not only the oldest board in Wayne County, but is also the oldest in Michigan and the oldest in the vast Northwest Territory.

The act is entitled "An Act in Addition to the Several Acts for the Relief and Maintenance of the Poor." Section 1 reads:

Be it enacted by the Legislative Council of the Territory of Michigan, That it shall hereafter be lawful for the directors of the poor of the several townships of this territory and for the mayor, recorder and aldermen of the city of Detroit, or any persons whom they may appoint, to cause to be confined either in the county prison or other place of security all paupers *who are not of sound mind.*

The original Wayne County poorhouse was organized by a vote of the people of Detroit on March 8, 1832. It was removed to its present location in 1839.[1] The first reference to insane inmates of the poorhouse of Wayne County appears March 22, 1841, when one Bridget Hughes was admitted as crazy. Shortly after the year 1842 a "crazy house" was built at the Wayne County almshouse for the accommodation of the violent insane. For many years this building constituted the only provision for the insane in the state.

In 1840 the number of insane and idiots, as presented in the United States Census,[2] was but 65, only seven of whom were supported at public charge. In the next decennial census the number reported was 326; and from the census and statistical returns made to the Department of State in pursuance of an act of the Legislature the whole number of insane and idiots in May, 1854, was found to be 428. The following table shows the ratio of insane and idiotic to the existing population:

Year.	Number of insane.	Total population.	Proportion of insane and idiots to entire population.
1840	65	212,267	1 in 3,265
1850	326	398,654	1 in 1,190
1854	428	509,374	1 in 1,119

The subject of public provision for the insane of the State of Michigan was first introduced for legislative action in 1848. A joint resolution of the Senate and House of Representatives made it the duty of the assessors, in their annual assessment rolls, to report the number of the insane, deaf and dumb, and blind, in their respective townships. The laws of that session also established the asylums, and appropriated eight sections of "Salt-Spring Lands" (5120 acres) for the erection of buildings. The government of the proposed institutions was vested in a Board of

[1] See "History of Eloise Hospital" in this volume, page 824.

[2] The United States Census of 1840 is not reliable. See "The Census of the Insane," Vol. I.

Trustees, empowered to establish rules and regulations and appoint officers, and required to report to the Legislature annually.

In 1849 the amount of lands appropriated for asylum purposes was increased to 15 sections (9600 acres), and the immediate selection of the land required. The proceeds of the sale were to be placed to the credit of the "asylum fund," and it was made the duty of the Board of Trustees to select suitable locations on which to erect the proposed institutions. At the next session of the Legislature 10 additional sections of land were appropriated, making a total of 16,000 acres; also $5000 from the general fund, to be used by the trustees in the construction of the asylums and in defraying other expenses connected with them.

In 1851 the Board of Trustees reported to the Legislature that they had ascertained as nearly as possible the number and wants of the insane, deaf and dumb, and the blind, and recommended the erection of institutions for their care and treatment. They found in the state between 300 and 400 insane persons, some of whom were with their friends and relatives, but the greater number of whom were confined in county houses and jails. The wants of this class of persons being of pressing necessity, the Board of Trustees recommended the immediate erection of an institution capable of accommodating 200 patients; to have attached not less than 160 acres of land, located near some town or village, the institution to be built substantially and upon the general plan of the most perfected buildings in the country; to be warmed by steam or hot water, and ventilated upon the most approved modern plan.

The citizens of Kalamazoo had donated for the site of the asylum for the insane 10 acres of land in the central portion of the village and in addition the sum of $1380. The land donated being unsuitable for the location of an institution, it was disposed of and 160 acres about one mile from the village purchased. The Legislature of 1853 made another appropriation from the general fund of $20,000, and appointed a second Board of Trustees, whose duties were to adopt plans for the buildings and advertise for proposals for their erection.

The first Board of Trustees had presented to the Legislature the plans of two of the most approved institutions for the insane in the United States, but without making any specific recommendations. With the view of obtaining data which should govern their action the second Board of Trustees appointed one of their number to visit some of the Eastern asylums. In referring to this subject in their report for 1855, the board remarks:

> Of the existing institutions for the insane in the United States, that established at Trenton, N. J., a plan of which was submitted to the board, is probably best adapted in its general features to the wants of this state; but the present board came to the conclusion that none of the existing institutions combine all the improvements which are important to be adopted. It further seemed to them advisable to secure the early appointment of the medical superintendent in order that the building might be erected so far under his supervision as to secure his approbation when completed.

Acting upon these suggestions, the Board of Trustees in January, 1854, appointed Dr. John P. Gray, then acting superintendent of the New York State Lunatic Asylum, to the post of superintendent. As early as practicable in the following spring the erection of the center building was commenced. The asylum was finally opened for the reception of patients in August, 1859.

The Pontiac State Hospital was established under the title of the Eastern Michigan Asylum by Act 120, Laws of 1873. The building was begun in February, 1875, and the hospital was opened for the reception of patients in August, 1878.

During the period from 1870 to 1880 the State Care Act became effective in Michigan and, as a result, the care of insane persons in county houses, jails and other receptacles was prohibited. In consequence of this prohibition, further provision for the insane became necessary, which was met by the passage of an act in 1881 which provided for an additional asylum. The new asylum was located at Traverse City, under the name of the Northern Michigan Asylum, and was opened for the admission of patients on November 30, 1885. It is now known as Traverse City State Hospital.

The Ionia State Hospital was established in 1883 under the name of the Michigan Asylum for Insane Criminals, and was opened for the admission of patients in September, 1885.

A growing demand on the part of the people of the upper peninsula for an institution more accessible to them than one in the lower peninsula could be, finally induced the Legislature of 1893 to provide for an asylum in that territory. The new institution was located at Newberry under the name of the Upper Peninsula Hospital for the Insane, and was opened for patients in October, 1894. It is now known as the Newberry State Hospital.

The Legislature of 1901 passed an act[1] to provide for the construction and equipment of a psychopathic ward upon the hospital grounds of the University of Michigan at Ann Arbor, and appropriated the sum of $50,000 therefor. The State of Michigan thus became the first of the states to establish a university hospital for the care and treatment of mental diseases. The new hospital was opened on February 7, 1906, under the name of the State Psychopathic Hospital at the University of Michigan.

In addition to the various state hospitals there is, in connection with Wayne County, a county hospital for the care of the insane. This is the successor of the original Wayne County poorhouse already mentioned, which was organized in 1832. In 1839 it was moved to its present location at Nankin, 16 miles west of Detroit. In 1872 the name was changed to Wayne County Almshouse, which was again changed to Wayne County House in 1886. In 1911 the name Eloise Infirmary was adopted in place of Wayne County House, and Eloise Hospital for the group of buildings devoted to the treatment of mental diseases. This hospital cares for the insane of Wayne County only.

In 1895 the state established at Lapeer the Michigan Home and Training School, designed for the care and treatment of feeble-minded and epileptic. Its present capacity is 1200 beds.[2]

Previous to 1889 private patients had been allowed the benefit of the state asylums upon formal requests by friends and upon presentation of certificates of insanity from two physicians. Security for the cost of their maintenance was provided by bond. In 1889 a new law required that private patients should secure admission to the state institutions only by regular process of commitment.

No further changes in the law were made until 1897, when, by reason of the steady increase in the number of non-resident insane, the Legislature provided for the deportation from the state of all persons becoming insane who had not yet acquired a legal resi-

[1] Act 161, Public Acts of 1901.

[2] No history of the institution has been obtained.

dence in the state. This act subsequently received amendments whereby it was made more effective.

The Joint Board of Trustees of the Michigan institutions was created by an act of the Legislature of 1877. An act of the Legislature of 1885 amended, revised and consolidated the laws organizing the institutions for the insane, and repealed at the same time the laws of 1859, 1873 and 1877. Under this new organic act the principal function of the Joint Board of Trustees was to meet together for consultation twice each year and to fix annually the rate of support for the different institutions; also the board was invested with the power of transferring patients from one institution to another.

In 1903 a general revision and consolidation of the laws regulating asylums was effected. This revision was the work very largely of the Joint Board of Trustees.

The more important new features of this law were as follows: Monthly meetings were exacted from the various boards. Salaries of officers were fixed by the joint board and were made a charge upon the current expenses of the various institutions. The powers of the joint board were definitely prescribed with respect to the redistricting of the state from time to time and the transferring of patients from institution to institution; and the Governor was restricted in his appointments to each board to residents of the district. The establishment of training schools for attendants was made obligatory upon each board.

To the two classes of patients heretofore recognized by law—that is to say, public and private patients—there was added a third class, namely, voluntary patients. Voluntary patients were defined by the act as those who were not insane and were maintained without expense to the state. No commitment was required, merely a certificate from qualified examiners that the individual was affected mentally or had a serious nervous disability and needed asylum treatment, but was not insane.

Provision was made for the commitment upon temporary orders of urgent cases pending the determination of the question of support. Should the court decide to commit the alleged insane person as a private charge it was made incumbent upon the judge to see that the proper bond was provided. Until such bond was furnished the patient was to be regarded as a public charge. Thus security was given to the institution, and by the same section the superintendent of the institution was authorized at any time to call upon the judge of probate for the execution of a new bond when the sureties on the bond became uncertain. By this new law the old provision, whereby counties were liable for the maintenance of the patient for two years, was changed to make the period of residence at county expense one year, and at the same time the office of the Auditor General of the state was made the agency for the collection of all accounts against the counties.

No citation of court notice of any kind was permitted to be served upon an inmate of the institution except by the superintendent or by some one delegated by him for such duty. Inmates were forbidden to execute an instrument of any kind except by express orders from the probate court from which the patient was committed, and a copy of this order was to be sent to the superintendent.

All bills for the maintenance of public patients in each institution were rendered to the Auditor General, that officer collecting in turn from the county liable for the one year's support. Estates of patients committed were made liable to the state, and all prosecuting attornies of counties were made agents of the Attorney General in safeguarding the interests of the state in these commitments. Provision was made for reimbursing the state, particularly where the circumstances of the individual did not warrant commitment as a private patient.

Provision was made whereby an unrecovered patient might be removed under bond in any case in which the superintendent was unwilling to assume the responsibility of discharging the patient.

The cost of keeping patients and the amount which should be collected therefor from the state was, as heretofore, left to the joint board, the statute defining more specifically the items which should enter into the actual cost of maintenance of patients.

Subsequent to the passage of the Act of 1903, which is still the organic law of the state institutions, there have been certain amendments to the act, as well as new legislation, which may be summarized as follows:

In 1905 the psychopathic ward at the University Hospital was established by special act. In the same year the organic law was amended in such a manner that the Board of State Auditors was added to and became a part of the Joint Board of Trustees for the purpose of fixing annually the rate of maintenance to be charged by the various institutions for the support of patients. The action of this body was to be submitted to the Governor, who was given veto power over its decision; but by provision of the law it is required that his approval must be filed within 10 days of the date upon which the notice reaches him. In the event of his disapproval of the rate it becomes the Governor's duty to forthwith reconvene the joint board to readjust the rate.

In 1907 the act establishing the psychopathic ward at the University Hospital was repealed and a new act passed, organizing the State Psychopathic Hospital as an independent institution, with a governing board composed of a joint committee from the Board of Regents and from the various boards of trustees of the state hospitals. In the same year, by separate act, boards of trustees were required to submit any increase in salary of chief executive officers of institutions to the Governor for his approval before such increase could be audited. An amendment to the organic law of the state institutions provided for the admission of inebriates and drug habitues from Wayne County to the state institution of that district at public expense. This law was subsequently declared invalid by the Attorney General.

In 1909 a new enactment required the superintendent of institutions and the judges of probate to render to the Auditor General of the state full reports of all patients committed and received, with full information concerning the estate of the patient, date of admission and date of discharge. The object of such legislation was to secure for the Auditor General's department a complete check upon institutions, with full information concerning the estate of the committed person. In the same year an amendment to the organic law required the judges of probate to furnish to the Auditor General proof in writing of the financial circumstances of the alleged insane person.

In 1911 further effort was made to secure to the state institutions the admission of indigent alcoholics and drug habitues by the passage of an act which was again pronounced invalid by the Attorney General. In the same year the organic law was amended so as to change the title of all institutions for the insane from state asylums to state hospitals.

In Michigan the supervision of charitable, penal and reformatory institutions is in the hands of the Board of Corrections and Charities, consisting of five members, four appointed by the Governor for a term of eight years, the Governor being a member ex-officio. They serve without compensation.

Each general state hospital is under the control of a board of trustees, consisting of six members appointed by the Governor for a term of six years.

The Ionia State Hospital is under the control of a board of three trustees, appointed by the Governor for a term of six years.

The Board of Trustees for the State Psychopathic Hospital consists of eight members, four of whom are chosen from the trustees of the state hospitals, the remainder from among the regents of the State University.

The rate of maintenance in the several hospitals in the state as of March 30, 1912, was as follows: Newberry State Hospital, 50 cents per day; Kalamazoo State Hospital and Ionia State Hospital, 47 cents per day; Traverse City State Hospital and Pontiac State Hospital, 49 cents per day. In the State Psychopathic Hospital the state pays the rate which prevails in the asylum district from which the patient is committed. For the maintenance of patients in the Wayne County Asylum the state pays a rate not exceeding that which applies to the Pontiac State Hospital. The rate in the Home for the Feeble-minded and Epileptic is 46 cents per day. The rates in the several hospitals are fixed by the Board of State Auditors and the boards of trustees of the state hospitals subject to the approval of the Governor.

Classes Committed.—All insane persons residents of the state not feeble-minded or epileptics are committed.

Insane patients are of three classes: public patients, maintained at the expense of the state; private patients, maintained without expense to the state, and voluntary patients, who are not insane and are maintained without expense to the state. A non-resident of the state may be admitted for temporary care pending return to his home.

Procedure in Commitment.—The father, mother, husband, wife, brother, sister or child of a person alleged to be insane or the sheriff or superintendent of the poor or supervisor of any township or peace officer of the township in which the person is found may petition the probate court for his admission to an asylum. The petition must contain a statement of the facts. The court must fix a day for a hearing and appoint two reputable physicians to make examinations of the person, whose certificate must be filed with the court on or before hearing, and served personally on the person at least 24 hours before the hearing, if made by a sheriff or peace officer; also upon the father, mother, husband, wife or some one next of kin of the alleged insane person, residing within the county, and upon such of the relatives outside of the county and within this state as may be ordered by the court, and also upon the person with whom the alleged insane person may reside. The court may dispense with personal service or may direct substitute service. In such cases the court must appoint a guardian *ad litem* to represent the insane person. The court must institute an inquest and take proofs in writing of the financial circumstances of the relatives legally liable for his support. If no jury is demanded the probate court determines the question of insanity. If the court deems it necessary or if the alleged person or any relative or other person concerned demands it a jury must be summoned to determine the question. If it appears upon the certificate of two legally qualified physicians to be necessary, the court may order the alleged person to be placed in the custody of some suitable person or to be removed to the asylum of the district in which he resides, or to any hospital, home or retreat, pending the proceedings for commitment, but not for more than 30 days except by special order of the court. The alleged insane person has the right to be present at the hearing.

No resident may be held as a public or private patient in any asylum, public or private, or in any institution for the care or treatment of the insane, except upon certificates of insanity and an order for admission.

Certificates of insanity must be made by two reputable physicians under oath, appointed by the probate court. The physicians must be permanent residents of the state, duly registered, have the qualifications prescribed by the laws of the state for the practice of medicine and surgery and not related by blood or marriage to the insane person nor to the person applying for the certificate. Their qualifications must be certified to by the clerk of the county. Neither of the physicians may have any interest, directly or indirectly, in the institution to which it is proposed to commit the person. The physicians must make a personal examination of the alleged insane person to form an opinion as to his sanity or insanity, and no certificate of insanity may be made except after personal examination. A copy of the physician's certificate, together with a copy of the application for commitment of the patient, must accompany the order of commitment.

Voluntary Patients.—All residents of the state who are afflicted mentally or with serious nervous disability, but who are not insane, may be admitted to the hospitals connected with the asylums as voluntary patients under special agreement when there is room. No order of probate court is necessary. In the case of a voluntary patient a certificate signed by two reputable physicians having the qualifications prescribed by law, stating that the person needs asylum treatment, but is not insane, must be presented. The certificate must be accompanied by a certificate from the county clerk. Voluntary patients may be discharged at any time. Indigent patients may, by action of the Board of Trustees, be admitted as voluntary patients.

Appeal from Commitment.—Anyone in custody as an insane person is entitled to a writ of habeas corpus upon a proper petition to the circuit court of the county made by him or some friend in his behalf.

Cost of Commitment.—The expenses of committing a person are paid by the county.

KALAMAZOO STATE HOSPITAL.[1]

KALAMAZOO, MICH.

Previous to the year 1848 Michigan, then with a population of nearly 400,000, had made no provision for the special care and treatment of the insane, although the needs in this respect were general and urgent, if we may judge from the several petitions presented to the Legislature of that year asking for the adoption of some humane plan in behalf of this unfortunate class and also from the promptness with which Governor Ransom issued a special message, dated February 28, 1848, recommending that "provision should be made for the establishment of a hospital for the insane and an asylum for the deaf and dumb and blind at the earliest period consistent with the existing obligations of the state."

In response to this message the Legislature by Act No. 187 of the Public Acts of 1848 established such institutions, provided for the appointment of a Board of Trustees to select sites and erect buildings and appropriated eight sections of Salt Spring lands (5121 acres) for these purposes. But the reasons for associating under a single board three institutions so different in general object, construction, organization and management do not appear in any state paper or document.

Certain conditions influenced the Governor to delay the appointment of the Board of Trustees and to urge in the year 1849 that other provision in addition to that of the establishing act should be made. The Legislature increased the appropriation of land to 15 sections (9600 acres) and required the immediate selection of land, the proceeds of which were to be credited to the "asylum fund." It was further made the duty of the Board of Trustees to select suitable locations. The first Board of Trustees appointed by the Governor, consisting of Messrs. Elon Farnsworth, Charles C. Hascall, Charles E. Stuart, John P. Cook and Charles H. Taylor, held their first meeting at Detroit May 22, 1849. They presented their first report December 22, 1849, and made public their selection of a site for the asylum for the insane at Kalamazoo,

[1] By A. I. Noble, M. D., superintendent.

the citizens of that place donating as an inducement $1506 in conditional notes, payable in cash, work and material in 6, 12 and 18 months, and 10 acres of land for the buildings. The asylum for the education of the deaf, dumb and blind was located at Flint. The Legislature of that year appropriated 10 additional sections of land, making a total of 16,000 acres, and $5000 from the general fund, to be used by the trustees in the construction of the asylum and in defraying other expenses. Fortunately, however, sufficient money was not available and the erection of buildings was deferred, for the land given by the citizens was entirely inadequate in extent and was improperly located near the center of the village and in what is now a fashionable residential section of the city. The trustees by their investigations had ascertained that there were in the state in 1851 between 300 and 400 insane persons, "some of whom were with their friends and relatives, but the greater number confined in county houses and jails." Appreciating the pressing necessity, they recommended to the Legislature of that year "the immediate erection of an institution capable of accommodating 200 patients; to have attached not less than 160 acres of land, located near some town or village; built substantially, and upon the general plan of the most perfect building in the country; to be warmed by steam or hot water apparatus, and ventilated upon the most improved modern plan." They presented to the Legislature without specific recommendation, however, plans of two of the most recently constructed and approved institutions in the United States. They also urged upon that body a more liberal policy in the development of the asylum plan.

Acting under the authority granted them, the Board of Trustees purchased a tract of 160 acres of land about a mile from the village of Kalamazoo. The more liberal policy advocated by them was sanctioned in 1853 by Governor McClelland, who commended the asylums of the state to the favorable notice of the Legislature of that year. The result was an appropriation from the general fund of $20,000 to be used as a purchasing and construction fund in the years 1853 and 1854. There was also appointed a second Board of Trustees consisting of Sheldon McKnight, Bela Hubbard, Israel Kellogg, James B. Walker and John Barber. This board "fully concurred in the judicious course pursued by the first Board of Trustees in the purchase of 160 acres of land near

Kalamazoo, to be used as the site and for the purposes of the hospital for the insane, in lieu of the 10 acres originally donated, and in accordance with the provisions of the act the latter tract was offered for sale and a sale effected for $1280, being a full equivalent for the sum paid for the 160 acres, the title to which was secured and recorded."[1]

This original tract, subsequently increased by purchase to 240 acres, is conveniently located, and is by nature admirably adapted to institution purposes. The site of the main building is upon an irregular eminence about one mile from the business portion of the city and sufficiently elevated above the valley of the Kalamazoo River to afford an extensive prospect, yet well sheltered and easy of access from the plain below. On 50 acres of the land the original growth of oak, hickory and other trees was preserved, affording every facility that could be desired for beautifying the grounds. In the rear of the site the land falls by a series of ravines about 80 feet to the valley below, at the bottom of which flows a small but rapid stream of pure water. Along this valley extend the tracks of the Michigan Central Railroad.

Inasmuch as the public and the Legislature failed to fully appreciate the magnitude of the undertaking which the state had entered upon in establishing these institutions, considerable educational and missionary work had to be performed by those who were particularly interested in the beneficent enterprise; and even then the amount of money appropriated did not justify the inauguration of the building operations until April, 1854. In the meantime careful plans for the erection of the buildings had been prepared. The ground plan was drawn from suggestions made by Dr. John P. Gray and the work was begun under his direction. "The principles laid down in a series of propositions relative to the construction and arrangement of hospitals for the insane, unanimously adopted by the Association of Medical Superintendents of American Institutions for the Insane, were fully carried out in all of the details of its construction." In general the proposed structure followed what has come to be known as the Kirkbride plan. The main front of the building has an easterly outlook and consists of

[1] John Barber and Col. McKnight retired from the board and were succeeded by Luther H. Trask, of Kalamazoo, and Zina Pitcher, M. D., of Detroit.

a center building and six wings. Immediately behind the center or administration section were located the chapel, kitchen, laundry, fan-room, boiler and engine house and work shops. The style of architecture adopted was the Italian as "being the lightest, most cheerful and least expensive for the effect required in such an extensive range of building." The material used is brick, covered with Roman cement and sand and finished to represent freestone, and the window-caps, sills, brackets and belt courses are of Athens stone. The wards or halls are 16 in number, affording ample facilities for classification, and accommodating 300 patients, 150 of either sex. The single rooms for patients are 8 and 10 by 11 feet, so that the amount of cubic space allotted to each patient is one-third more than usual, and the number of patients accommodated in single rooms proportionately greater; there was provided for each sex a well-arranged infirmary, it being a detached building in the rear of the first transverse wings, but connected with the wards by a covered corridor. At the time, this addition was regarded as a very important feature and was an innovation in asylum construction in this country.

In order that the asylum might be erected under the supervision of some one having a practical and technical knowledge of the actual requirements of such a plant, the board in January, 1854, tendered the post of medical superintendent to Dr. John P. Gray, acting superintendent of the New York State Asylum at Utica. Dr. Gray accepted the position upon condition that a fixed and satisfactory salary should be given him from the time when he should assume full control, that is, after the completion of the necessary buildings for the reception of patients. In the meantime it was agreed that he should devote so much of his time and attention to the buildings and fixtures as should be important, at a compensation not exceeding $800 per annum for his services and expenses. All the plans were submitted to him, and by correspondence and visits to Michigan and elsewhere the interests of the institution were promoted. But at the end of two years he resigned to accept the superintendency at the Utica institution and his associate and acting first assistant there, Dr. Edwin H. Van Deusen, was appointed to fill the Michigan position, with the understanding that no salary should attach until his services were required as medical superintendent proper. Dr. Van Deusen nevertheless gave much attention to the completion and equipment of the asylum, although he did not assume his full duties until October, 1858, the year following the separation of the Asylum for the Deaf and Dumb and the Blind and the Asylum for the Insane at Kalamazoo by legislative enactment and the appointment of two distinct boards of trustees, Luther H. Trask, J. P. Woodbury and Henry Montague constituting the Kalamazoo board. The last named served two years and then was appointed steward, an office which he filled until 1884.

Previous to the year 1855 $17,487.48 had been expended in the work preliminary to the construction of buildings and in labor upon the center building, etc., and in 1855-6 the Legislature appropriated $67,000 as an asylum construction fund. The work, which had proceeded slowly because of these small and infrequent appropriations, sustained a serious set-back in the total destruction of the unfinished administration building by fire on the night of February 11, 1858, an estimated loss of nearly one-fifth of the portion erected. Nevertheless the trustees reported to the Legislature of 1859 that they were about ready to care for 90 men patients and asked for an appropriation of $90,500 to provide accommodations for 54 more of the opposite sex, to reconstruct the center building and to erect a chapel, general kitchen and other accessory buildings. More liberal appropriations were made, but unfortunately the money was not available. At this juncture the distressing lack of provision for the insane throughout the state impelled the management of the asylum to extend whatever relief was possible and to face the embarrassing situation of caring for both men and women patients in the south wing, the one completed portion of the building, where only living quarters for the officers could be provided. This part of the asylum was fully equipped for the reception of patients February 24, 1859, and the first patient was admitted April 23 following, although the formal opening of the asylum did not occur until August 29, 1859, that is, 11 years after the enactment of the law establishing the Michigan asylums.

Under the Organization Act passed by the Legislature in 1859 the entire management of the institution is committed to six trustees. Appointed by the Governor and confirmed by the Senate, they hold office for a term of six years. They choose as their executive officer a medical superintendent, and upon his recommendation the subordinate officers of the asylum. The first trustees to serve under this act were Luther Trask, William Brooks, J. P. Woodbury, Zina Pitcher, D. L. Pratt and Charles Coggeshall. The first meeting of the board was held on March 30, 1859, when David A. McNair was elected treasurer. At a subsequent meeting, April 28, the code of by-laws was adopted. The Civil War and the conditions leading up to it delayed the completion of the asylum buildings until 1869, when the work was consummated in accordance with the original plan and there were provided accommodations for 300 patients, 150 of either sex.

These provisions, however, were not sufficient to meet the demands of the rapidly increasing population of the state, and the institution had become so much crowded that Governor Baldwin recommended an appropriation for another building to be occupied exclusively by male patients. This was authorized and the sum of $220,000 appropriated for the purpose by the Legislature of 1871. Of this amount $80,000 was made available in 1871 and $140,000 in 1872. The building was completed in 1874.

This extension, really a complete hospital in itself, and called the male department, was located 40 rods south of and upon a line with the parent building, which was now designated the female department. The same general plan was observed in the second structure as obtained in the first, except that it had four wings instead of six. The center building, moreover, was cut down to less than half the size of that of the corresponding department, while the first wings from the center were made longer and three stories high. This building, substantial but much less ornate than the first, was constructed of brick with stone window seats and belt courses. The halls were ten in number, designed to accommodate 280 patients. The building was supplied with a separate heating and ventilating equipment, and had its own water supply and cooking apparatus.

The Michigan Asylum for the Insane was now considered complete. It had a capacity of 580 patients, possessed all the modern improvements, and took rank with the large and admirable institutions of the older states. The cost to the state for both buildings, with adjacent structures, all furnished and complete, together with 195 acres of land, was $727,173.90.

During the last four years of his connection with the Michigan Asylum Dr. Van Deusen was occupied in adjusting and perfecting the internal arrangements of the plant and in thoroughly reorganizing the institution. His administration had been an exceedingly arduous one and the tremendous activities and responsibilities of 20 years had so affected his general health that he, much to the regret of his Board of Trustees, felt obliged to retire from the service. What he had accomplished cannot be easily estimated. Counseled and sustained by his Boards of Trustees, made up of able and influential citizens, he practically completed and organized two hospitals for the insane and was a prominent factor in establishing and locating two others—the Pontiac and the Traverse City state hospitals. In a masterful way he had overcome the embarrassments and difficulties of the pioneer days of the institution, and long before his retirement in March, 1878, there had been created an enlightened public sentiment which resulted in the present comprehensive system of provision for the insane of the state.

Dr. George C. Palmer succeeded Dr. Van Deusen March 1, 1878, and Dr. Henry M. Hurd, assistant physician for eight years, was promoted to the position of assistant medical superintendent, resigning the same year, however, to accept the post of medical superintendent at the Eastern Michigan Asylum at Pontiac. Notwithstanding the relief Michigan Asylum experienced in the transfer of patients to the recently opened Pontiac institution, the problem of still further provision for the insane became a pressing one early in Dr. Palmer's administration, and it was not solved by the opening of the Northern Michigan Asylum at Traverse City and the Asylum for the Criminal Insane at Ionia in 1885, although some of the discomforts and dangers of overcrowding were for a time alleviated in this way.

In 1885 the trustees purchased for $16,000 a tract of 250 acres of land, now known as "Brook Farm" and located three miles north of the asylum. This farm is well adapted to grazing purposes and the object of the trustees was to produce the milk required at the institution and to increase the facilities for occupation of patients. The next year upon this land there were erected a two-story frame house with room for 40 men patients and a barn for 60 cows.

This was the first experiment in distant segregation of patients, and it proved so satisfactory that the Board of Trustees was prompted to adopt a similar but more ambitious plan to relieve the wards, more particularly those of the department for women. The excess of patients to accommodations was due to the accumulation of chronic cases, and the trustees in their report of 1886 presented to the Legislature the "colony plan" of caring for this class of patients and asked for an appropriation of $23,000 with which to build four "colony houses" and a cottage for a resident physician. The Legislature of 1887 authorized the purchase of 320 acres of land three miles southwest of the asylum for colony purposes and the erection thereon of two cottages to accommodate 50 patients each. Building operations were begun without loss of time, and upon the completion of two colony cottages the accommodations afforded for patients in the Michigan Asylum district were, for the first time in the history of the institution, equal to the demands.

The Legislature of 1889 granted an appropriation of $12,500 for a new chapel, since the old one was outgrown and the room was needed for other purposes. This building, comprising a chapel on the first floor and an amusement hall below and located between the two departments, is a plain brick one story and high basement structure, 73 x 44 feet in dimension, which was opened for use in May, 1891. An important feature in connection with the auditorium was the small room on either side of the chancel, designed for epileptic patients.

Dr. Palmer resigned June 1, 1891, to take charge of Oak Grove Hospital at Flint, Mich. As assistant physician and medical superintendent, he had been connected with the institution 27 years, and his associate and successor, Dr. William M. Edwards, in his first report paid a high tribute to Dr. Palmer's character and work and said: "His prudent administration of its affairs, his zealous and faithful devotion to every interest had placed the asylum on a high plane."

Dr. Edwards took up the work laid down by Dr. Palmer, and Dr. William A. Stone, promoted from the Northern Michigan Asylum, received the appointment of assistant medical superintendent. The asylum in the following 15 years maintained a steady growth, its population increasing during the time from

1000 to nearly 1700 patients. The immediate plans for the colony at the beginning of the period, namely, two additional cottages for patients and one for a resident physician, were faithfully carried out as fast as means were provided by the Legislature. It may be justly said, however, that the Board of Trustees as then constituted and the medical superintendent did not enthusiastically favor the plan conceived in the previous administration "to lay the foundation of a large colony for both sexes." The real purpose of these men was rather the development of the home plant and the firm establishment of the institution upon a hospital basis. What they actually accomplished cannot be recounted in detail; it can best be indicated by citing building operations and large improvements, among the more important of which are five detached brick cottages for the accommodation of patients. One of these, Fletcher Hospital, located south of the male department and opened in November, 1897, affords sufficient room for the treatment of 190 men of the infirmary class. The second of these buildings, opened in August, 1898, and located near the female department, with a capacity of 45 beds, was a well-equipped hospital for the reception and treatment of the recent and hopeful cases admitted to this department. The counterpart of this building at the male department, called Edwards Hospital, with a capacity of 76 beds, was practically completed under the direction of Dr. Edwards, but was not opened for patients until November, 1905. The third of the group of buildings erected in point of time is Burns cottage, located west of the male department and opened in August, 1900. It accommodates 125 working men patients. A building corresponding to this in size and purpose, Monroe cottage, was opened at the female department in May, 1902.

In the early part of this period there was also installed a central heating, power and electric lighting plant with all the accessory buildings, thus greatly enhancing the economy, efficiency and safety of operating the institution. A water tower erected at about the same time gave the first adequate supply of water for fire purposes and rendered possible water mains with hydrants about the buildings and standpipes within. Wooden stairways were replaced by others of fireproof construction. Important changes were made in the water supply and sewerage systems. A congregate dining room was provided for each department. A training school for nurses was established and vigorously maintained. Mechanical restraints, much restricted by Dr. Palmer, were still further reduced; and clinical work, therapeutic measures and laboratory methods were greatly stimulated by a scientific spirit carefully fostered by Dr. Edwards. "He was a close student of the methods employed in other institutions in this country and in Europe, and made use of any that he thought would be of advantage to him in his own field of work. He not only adopted the best methods of others, but he was the originator of many new ideas and methods in his specialty."[1] But for years he was handicapped by a serious heart affection and he succumbed to the disease April 26, 1905.

Following Dr. Edwards' death, Dr. William A. Stone acted as medical superintendent until January 1, 1906, when Dr. Alfred I. Noble, of Worcester, Mass., was appointed to that position. A Board of Trustees, made up of devoted and energetic men, experienced through long tenure of office and a thoroughly competent and loyal medical staff made it possible to continue the same wise and progressive policies in this administration as obtained in the previous one.

Edwards Hospital had not been occupied a great while when plans were drawn for a new building for women patients. This structure, called Van Deusen Hospital in recognition of the long and distinguished service of the asylum's first medical superintendent, was opened for use in June, 1908. It has a capacity of 104 beds. It was designed for a receiving hospital and is well equipped with modern appliances.

Among the extraordinary improvements of this period may be mentioned the transposition and enlargement of the general kitchen and the general dining room at the male department, completed in November, 1908, and the enlargement and re-equipment of the bakery in the latter part of the year 1911.

A modest wooden shack, with accommodations for 200 tubercular men, was completed and occupied February 3, 1910, thus securing the desired segregation and open-air treatment for this infected class of patients. A corresponding structure for 25 women patients, similarly afflicted, was first occupied October 13, 1911.

[1] Dr. Herman Ostrander Memorial Notice, Transactions Am. Medico-Psychological Assn., 1906.

At the colony "Rich Building," so designated in honor of ex-Governor Rich, was completed and opened for use September 21, 1910. This is a three-story brick structure, centrally located with reference to the cottages. It accommodates in its basement a general heating plant, a laundry, work room and bath room; upon the first floor a commodious general kitchen and congregate dining room, while upon the second and third floors are the nurses' sleeping rooms. It facilitates and economizes service, makes it possible to employ a much larger number of patients and indirectly increases the capacity of the cottages by 50 beds.

The old greenhouse, designed for conservatory purposes and located conspicuously in the foreground of the female department, fell into a state of decay and was replaced in November, 1910, by a new sectional house in a more favorable part of the grounds.

A pathological building of stucco construction, one story, with high basement, was completed in the spring of 1912. This comprises three laboratory rooms, a library, class room and lavatory on the ground floor, and mortuary rooms, with cooling facilities and autopsy rooms, in the basement.

The opening of Van Deusen Hospital made it possible to convert Potter cottage, previously used for hospital purposes, into an excellent and highly prized home for the nursing force at the female department. The retirement and comforts here afforded are the more appreciated because the eight-hour system for nurses is in successful operation and has been for several years. The building is in charge of the superintendent of nurses, who lives with her pupils and devotes her energies to maintaining an efficient and progressive training school.

Two new wards have been added at the male department by raising the roofs over the extreme wings. The classification of patients has been improved, apparatus for hydriatic treatment has been installed at both departments and mechanical restraints were abolished at the beginning of the period.

The institution, with name changed to Kalamazoo State Hospital by the Legislature of 1911, has now been established nearly 66 years. During all this time it has carefully followed the course marked out by its founders, and it has attained a measure of success worthy of its high mission. We may obtain some idea of its growth and of what it has accomplished if we note that its property value (1914), comprising 73 buildings and a tract of 1053 acres of land, is $1,585,189.15; that in its first biennial period there were 141 patients treated and in the last (ending June 30, 1914), 3036; that in all (July 1, 1914), 14,125 patients have been cared for since the first admission, and that of this number 2714 were discharged as recovered, 3086 as improved, 2027 as unimproved, 94 as not insane, while 4093 died and 2111 remained in the hospital June 30, 1914. Directly connected with the institution there is a staff of nine physicians, including a pathologist.

TRUSTEES.

Name	Years
Elon Farnsworth	1849-1853
Charles C. Hascall	1849-1853
John P. Cook	1849-1852
Charles E. Stuart	1849-1852
Charles H. Taylor	1849-1852
Sheldon McKnight	1853-1857
Bela Hubbard	1853-1857
Perly J. Spaulding (declined)	1853-
Israel Kellogg	1853-1857
James B. Walker	1853-1857
John Barber	1853-1855
Luther H. Trask	1855-1857 1858-1879
Zina Pitcher, M. D.	1856-1857 1859-1872
Charles T. Gorham	1857-1858
Jeremiah P. Woodbury	1857-1863
Henry Montague	1857-1859
Charles Coggeshall	1859-1860
William Brooks	1859-1865
Daniel L. Pratt	1859-1873
Erastus Hussey	1861-1863
Charles W. Penney	1863-1873
Wilson C. Edsell	1863-1865
Joseph Gilman	1865-1877
William A. Tomlinson	1865-1880
James E. Pittman	1872-1873
Charles T. Mitchell	1873-1891
Edward S. Lacey	1873-1880
James A. Brown	1873-1879
William H. Withington	1877-1879
E. O. Humphrey	1879-1885
Fitch R. Williams	1879-1885
George Hannahs	1879-1887
Robert Burns	1880-1881
Edwin C. Nicolls	1880-1881
Ira Grosvenor	1881-1893
Thomas R. Sherwood	1883-1883
Alva W. Nichols	1883-1889
Foster Pratt, M. D.	1883-1889
Charles J. Monroe	1887-1891
Erastus N. Bates	1889-1907
Niram A. Fletcher	1891-1896
Chauncey F. Cook	1891-
Nathaniel H. Stewart	1892-1893
William M. Robinson	1893-1896
Alfred J. Mills	1893-1899 1900-1911
Harris B. Osborne, M. D.	1895-1913
Henry Spring	1896-1899
William J. Stuart	1896-1897
Samuel Post	1897-1903
Henry S. Hadsall	1899-1903
Samuel N. Bickerstaff	1899-1899
C. S. Palmerton	1903-1909
Charles E. Belknap	1903-1905 1907-1913
Charles L. Edwards	1905-1911
Jason E. Hammond	1909-1915
Charles Clarage	1911-
Charles K. Warren	1911-
Thomas J. Cavanaugh	1913-
Ralph E. Balch, M. D.	1913-
Frank E. Pulte	1915-

MEDICAL SUPERINTENDENTS.

John P. Gray, M. D..... 1854-1856
Edwin H. Van Deusen, M. D. 1856-1878
George C. Palmer, M. D. 1878-1891
William M. Edwards, M. D. 1891-1905
Alfred I. Noble, M. D... 1906-

ASSISTANT MEDICAL SUPERINTENDENTS.

George C. Palmer, M. D. 1873-1878
Henry M. Hurd, M. D... 1878-1878
Edwin A. Adams, M. D.. 1879-1882
Halsey L. Wood, M. D... 1882-1885
Thomas R. Savage, M. D. 1885-1891
William A. Stone, M. D.. 1891-1910
Herman Ostrander, M. D. 1910-

ASSISTANT PHYSICIANS.

Park Loring, M. D...... 1859-1860
Dean M. Tyler, M. D.... 1860-1867
George C. Palmer, M. D. 1864-1873
Edward G. Marshall, M. D. .... {1865-1866, 1867-1870}
Justin E. Emerson, M. D. 1870-1878
Henry M. Hurd, M. D... 1870-1878
John H. Twombly, M. D. 1874-1878
Edward A. Adams, M. D. 1876-1879
William L. Worcester, M. D. 1878-1888
Halsey L. Wood, M. D... 1878-1882
Thomas R. Savage, M. D. 1878-1885
Helen W. Bissell, M. D.. 1879-1886
Henry S. Noble, M. D... 1882-1884
Wm. M. Edwards, M. D.. 1884-1891
Frederick H. Welles, M. D. 1885-1889
Mary S. McCarty, M. D.. 1886-1887
E. W. Fleming, M. D..... 1885-1886
Miles H. Clark, M. D.... 1887-1889
Herman Ostrander, M. D. 1888-1910
Charles Dunning, M. D.. 1888-1888
Mary H. Cullings, M. D. 1888-1888
Wadsworth Warren, M. D. 1889-1891
Bertha Van Hoosen, M. D. 1889-1890
George B. Tullidge, M. D. 1889-1890
Albert M. Haskins, M. D. 1890-1898
Irwin H. Neff, M. D..... 1891-1895
Herbert O. Statler, M. D. 1892-1896
H. J. Kennedy, M. D..... 1895-1895
Arthur MacGugan, M. D. 1895-1901
George F. Inch, M. D... 1895-
Eugene H. Robertson, M. D. 1895-1897
Emma W. Mooers, M. D. 1896-1896
Harriette O. McCalmont, M. D. 1897-1899
George M. Livingston, M. D. 1898-1901
A. D. Pollock, M. D..... 1898-1898
Florence E. Allen, M. D. 1899-1902
Frances E. Barrett, M. D. 1900-1908
Earl H. Campbell, M. D. 1901-1903
Charles W. Thompson, M. D. 1902-1905
William A. Evans, M. D. 1902-1903
Frank A. Shaver, M. D.. 1903-1904
Emory J. Brady, M. D.. 1904-1912
Geo. G. Richards, M. D.. 1904-1905
S. Rudolph Light, M. D.. 1904-1907
Albert E. Stripp, M. D... 1905-1906
Henry B. Carey, M. D... 1905-1906
H. R. Pitz, M. D......... 1906-1908
P. D. McCarty, M. D.... 1906-1908
A. Christine Iverson, M. D. 1907-1909
William Meyer, M. D.... 1908-1909
J. D. Heitger, M. D...... 1908-1909
Carl E. Holmberg...... 1908-1909
Melvin J. Rowe, M. D... 1909-1912

Maud M. Rees, M. D....	1909-1912	Edward M. Auer, M. D..	1912-1914
George C. Hardy, M. D..	1909-1911	Eva Rawlings, M. D.....	1912-
U. Sherman Gregg, M. D.	1909-1910 1914-	Gordon F. Willey, M. D..	1912-
Vincent A. McDonough, M. D.	1911-1913	Edmund M. Pease, M. D.	1912-1914
Margery J. Gilfillan.....	1912-	Edward M. Steger, M. D.	1913-1914
James A. Neville, M. D..	1912-1912	Roy A. Morter, M. D....	1914-
		Jerome F. Berry, M. D..	1914-

STEWARDS.

Henry Montague	1859-1884	Charles C. Cutting......	1892-1900
Stephen G. Earl........	1884-1889	John A. Hoffman.......	1900-1914
Willis W. Hodge.......	1889-1890	Howard H. Buckhout...	1914-

CHAPLAINS.

Daniel Putnam	1859-1884	R R. Claiborne.........	1898-1901
George F. Hunting.....	1884-1887	Robert W. McLaughlin.	1901-1902
F. Z. Rossiter..........	1887-1890	E. J. Blekkink..........	1902-1905
J. A. Johnston..........	1890-1898	Henry W. Gelston......	1905-

TREASURERS.

John P. Cook...........	1849-1852	Allen Potter	1880-1885
James B. Walker.......	1853-1857	S. S. Cobb..............	1885-1891
Henry Montague	1857-1859	Edward Woodbury	1892-1893
D. A. McNair..........	1859-1862	Melville J. Bigelow.....	1893-1895
F. W. Curtenius........	1862-1879	Edwin J. Phelps........	1895-
William A. Wood......	1879-1880		

PONTIAC STATE HOSPITAL.

PONTIAC, MICH.

The Pontiac State Hospital was established under the title of the Eastern Michigan Asylum by Act 120, Laws of 1873, Statutes of Michigan. The sum of $400,000 was appropriated for the purchase of a site and the erection of buildings.

This act required that the institution should be located in the eastern part of the State of Michigan, and that the site should be healthy and supplied with an inexhaustible supply of pure living water; that the farm should be ample and well suited to cultivation, and that the institution when built should be conveniently located to a railway line and be provided with a side-track for the reception of coal and other heavy freight. It was also provided that the institution should not be less than one mile from a city or village easily accessible in any season of the year. In view of the fact that fully one-third of the patients to be admitted to the institution would come from the City of Detroit, it was the desire of the commissioners to locate the proposed asylum at Detroit. But it was later found impossible to do so because of local opposition to the most available site.

The commissioners appointed to locate the hospital were Amos Rathbone, E. H. Van Deusen and George Hannahs, to whom were added W. M. McConnell, Samuel G. Ives and Michael Crofoot, to serve with them as building commissioners.

After a careful survey of many sites in the eastern part of the state, the commissioners decided to locate the new asylum upon the Woodward farm, about three-quarters of a mile from the City of Pontiac, 26 miles northwest of Detroit. The farm contained 307 acres and was obtained at an expense of $30,000. It consisted of excellent farming land, and provided a fine building site about 50 feet above the railroad line, which skirted the property on the north and east.

The citizens of Pontiac donated 200 acres of the farm which was purchased, and the state provided the remainder. The citizens of Pontiac also guaranteed an adequate supply of pure spring water and provision for ample sewerage and drainage. The

Detroit & Milwaukee Railroad also guaranteed the extension of a side-track from the railroad line to the institution.

As usually happens under similar circumstances, these guarantees were imperfectly executed. It was found impossible to utilize the water derived from an adjoining lake because of the expense; nor was the water of sufficient purity for the use of the institution.

There were also serious difficulties in the way of disposing of the sewage of the hospital, and it finally became necessary for the hospital to complete a system of sewage disposal at considerable cost.

The railroad line which had guaranteed the side-track went into bankruptcy, and the hospital was compelled to supply money to build the siding and to receive repayment in driblets by a rebate upon the freight delivered over it.

The ground plan of the hospital was furnished by Dr. E. H. Van Deusen, for many years superintendent of the Kalamazoo State Hospital, and a member of the Board of Commissioners.

The elevations and architectural features were furnished by E. E. Myers, an architect of Detroit. The building was erected on what is known as the Kirkbride plan. The building, which fronted east, was located on an elevation about 60 feet above Pontiac Creek, which flowed through the southern portion of the estate. It consisted of a central or administration building with wings for patients extending right and left *en echelon,* and the necessary buildings for cooking, heating, power, work shops and laundry were grouped in the rear of the administration building. The administration building served to divide the sexes. The longitudinal division consisted of a corridor with rooms on each side, each room designed for a single patient. The rooms were from 9 to 12 feet and 11 by 12 feet in size, and the clear space between the floor and ceiling was in each case 13 feet. The corridors were intended for day rooms and a large bay window in the center of each corridor afforded an abundance of sunshine and a pleasant view to the inmates. The large rooms in front of the transverse division were day rooms or parlors or associate dormitories. In the four main transverse divisions were baths, clothes rooms, water closets and clothes shafts, so that each ward had a group of these rooms readily accessible.

A four-inch brick arch formed the ceiling of each patient's room and of the corridor. This arched ceiling was plastered and served as a deafening of sound and provided great security in case of fire. The floor joists above were not in contact with the arches.

Iron sashes were used throughout the wards, but were of the same size as the window sashes and painted white to resemble them. The roofs were of slate. The construction was of brick with stone ornamentation, and the great variety of stone work formed a pleasing feature of the architecture. The administration building was surmounted by a tower and the wards had towers at each end; also peaks upon the bay projections and ornamental ventilators upon the roof; all of which increased the architectural effect of the building.

The heating was by low steam, mainly through indirect radiation. Ventilation was effected by a Sturtevant fan.

The capacity of the building as designed was 330 patients.

The building was begun in February, 1875, and was completed and opened for the admission of patients in August, 1878.

Meantime a Board of Trustees had been appointed, consisting of Henry P. Baldwin, Michael Crofoot, Willard M. McConnell, Warren G. Vinton and Samuel G. Ives. Henry M. Hurd was appointed medical superintendent and James D. Munson assistant physician.

The building was opened upon the 1st of August, 1878, with 222 patients—121 males and 101 females.

The cost of the hospital at the time the building was opened had been about $467,000. About 20 counties of the state had been assigned to the district of the hospital.

In view of the fact that the appropriation made by the Legislature for furnishing the hospital had been cut down fully $15,000 below the lowest estimate made by the commissioners, it was necessary to use the strictest economy in providing for the patients and many temporary fixtures were used. The furniture for the wards, the administration building and the chapel was much reduced in quality and quantity. The grounds were not graded or ornamented with trees or shrubbery. No outbuildings had been erected; no vehicle had been purchased for the use of the hospital, nor had any money been appropriated for a working capital. Under the circumstances great difficulties were experienced during the first year of the operation of the hospital.

In 1882 two new wings were added to the original hospital building; they were designed for the care of the excited patients, and each wing accommodated 75 inmates. Each wing was three stories in height and connected directly with the north and south wings of the hospital by means of an ornamental tower.

In 1882 special efforts were made to give employment to patients and with that end in view a committee of the Board of Trustees visited England to inspect institutions and to see what could be done to increase industrial pursuits in the hospital. As a result of the experience there obtained a provision of law was secured whereby authority was given to employ patients. It was considered that if labor was beneficial medical officers should have authority to prescribe it in any manner calculated to benefit the patient.

In the year 1885 two infirmary wards were built, each accommodating about 30 patients. These were two stories in height and were designed to care for recent cases on the first two floors and for infectious and contagious cases upon the third floor. They were connected with the other wards by a long corridor and were convenient to the laundry and power house.

An addition to the laundry was also erected and a new green house was built. A large brick stable and carriage house and a new brick settling basin for the sewage were also erected during the same biennial period.

In 1889 Dr. H. M. Hurd resigned as superintendent and was succeeded by Dr. C. B. Burr, who had been an assistant physician since 1879.

In 1890 the Legislature was memorialized by the Joint Board of Trustees to provide for the increase in the number of the insane by constructing accommodations for 100 patients at Kalamazoo, for 200 at Pontiac, and for 150 at Traverse City. In this same year the training school for attendants was established at Pontiac, the first of its kind in the state, and the eighth in order of priority in the country. An ice famine during the previous winter led to the construction of the first of two large ice houses for the storage of ice.

In 1891 the interior of the administration building was destroyed by fire. In addition three halls were burned out and a number of others were rendered uninhabitable. By the autumn of

1892 the damage had been repaired at a total cost approximately of $75,000.

In 1891 the Legislature authorized the erection of a building for 50 patients, to be paid for from surplus funds in the institution's treasury. This building was never constructed. The same Legislature authorized the purchase of 50 acres to be added to the farm, as a result of which two additions known as the "Hickey" and the "Mawwhinney" parcels were annexed. This same year saw the construction of a large store house. The construction of a slaughter house at the same time initiated a plan, followed for many years after, of slaughtering on the premises all the beef used by the asylum.

In 1893 the Legislature provided for two additional buildings for 50 patients each, at a total cost of $30,000. These buildings, the Baldwin and the Vinton, were occupied in 1894.

In the fall of 1894 Dr. C. B. Burr relinquished his position as medical superintendent to accept the medical directorship of the Oak Grove Hospital at Flint, Mich. He was succeeded by the present incumbent, Dr. E. A. Christian.

In 1895 there were added a granary with bins and elevators, and two surgical operating rooms. The farm was increased by the addition of 80 acres (west half of the Seeley farm).

In 1896 fire again visited the asylum, resulting in a partial destruction of a brick carriage barn.

In 1897 the Legislature authorized the installation of an electric lighting and power plant and the construction of a new laundry building. These improvements were completed in 1898. The electric light and power plant then installed is still in successful operation. In this same year the major portion of the asylum sewer in its course through the City of Pontiac was abandoned, in consequence of the construction of a city sewerage system.

In 1898 an isolation hospital for contagious diseases was improvised from the upper portion of the former laundry.

In 1899 the Legislature provided for two additional buildings for 100 of each sex, at a cost of $78,000. These buildings, the Stevens and the Kinney, were occupied in 1899. In the same year (1899) the bake shop was moved to the lower portion of the building formerly occupied by the laundry, whereby its quarters were greatly enlarged.

From 1891 on special attention had been given to the improvement of the herd of cattle. Thoroughbreds and registered stock had replaced grade animals. The attention given by the steward, Mr. C. E. Smith, to this subject resulted in a rapidly increased supply of milk, and in the creation of a herd that in time became famous among cattle breeders the country over.

In 1901 small hospital wards were set apart for the isolation of cases of tuberculosis, and a start was made upon the erection from year to year of verandas upon which disturbed and feeble patients could spend the greater part of their time in the open air. In the same year an autopsy room was added to the hospital, and the former silos of wood construction were replaced by substantial brick silos, the feeding of ensilage having become an established procedure.

In 1903 the former water supply was abandoned as inadequate, and new wells equipped with new pumping apparatus were sunk; the coal shed was greatly enlarged and two new water-tube boilers, the beginning of an entirely new installation, were erected. A central hot water plant for all buildings was also installed. Seventy acres (the Abbott farm) were added to the state property.

In 1905 the Legislature made provision for a complete fire-fighting equipment. This was secured by a pump connected with an independent high-pressure system of mains devoted entirely to fire-fighting purposes. This installation was such that the entire equipment could be used independently of or in conjunction with the city mains. The equipment was placed in commission in 1906. The same Legislature made provision for additional accommodations for the insane, as the result of which an infirmary building to care for 100 women patients and costing $40,000 was occupied in 1907.

In 1907 the remaining portion of the old asylum sewer lying within the city limits was abandoned, connection being made at the asylum boundaries.

The Legislature in 1907 made further provision for the insane in the erection of a new chapel and assembly hall. The former chapel was converted into a dining room and the ward dining rooms into dormitories. In March, 1909, the central dining room was opened with provision for 600 patients, both sexes eating within the same room. At the same time the new chapel and assembly hall were placed in commission. These changes cost in the neighborhood of $60,000. In the same year and by provision of the same Legislature (1907) the former water tanks in the attics were abandoned and an outside water tower erected, one more vertical water-tube boiler was installed, and a central heating plant connected with all of the detached buildings by tunnel was erected—all this at an expense of $40,000.

In the year 1908 the laundry building was partially destroyed by fire, with a loss of machinery and equipment of about $10,000.

The Legislature in 1909 made provision, at a cost of $8000, for a modern dairy barn, constructed on sanitary lines, for the now valuable herd of Holstein cattle. This new barn was placed in commission in 1910.

In 1911 money was appropriated by the Legislature to complete the rehabilitation of the boiler room. Two more vertical water-tube boilers were erected, replacing the last ones of the old horizontal type, and supplying the institution for the first time in many years with a reserve horse power.

In 1913 work was started on a building for 100 men, to be completed and occupied in 1915. This building is intended for the old and infirm. It is semi-detached from the main building, and consists of two floors, duplicates of each other. The building is divided into large dormitories and day rooms, and has its own culinary appointments.

In this same year building operations were started on a home for women night nurses.

The Pontiac State Hospital, like all other Michigan state institutions, has been put under a provision of the statute, passed by the Legislature of 1913, providing for employees' compensation in the event of accident. The hospital contributes, through its current expense account, a stated amount each year, which goes with the casualty liability fund administered by the State Treasurer.

In the same manner the hospital buildings and furnishings have been insured against loss by fire and tornado.

There has been established in Michigan, under the auspices of the Joint Board, a method of purchasing for the various state hospitals, through a stewards' association, which association performs the offices of a purchasing board.

COMMISSIONERS TO SELECT A SITE AND TO ERECT THE EASTERN MICHIGAN ASYLUM.

Edwin H. Van Deusen, M. D., Kalamazoo 1873-1875
Amos Rathbone, Grand Rapids 1873-1874
George Hannahs, South Haven 1873-1879
Michael E. Crofoot, Pontiac 1874-1879
Willard M. McConnell, Pontiac 1874-1879
Samuel G. Ives, Chelsea 1874-1879
Warren G. Vinton, Detroit 1876-1879

The work of the commission was closed in December, 1879.

TRUSTEES.

Samuel G. Ives, Chelsea 1878-1879
Warren G. Vinton, Detroit 1878-1897
Willard M. McConnell, Pontiac 1878-1885
Michael E. Crofoot, Pontiac 1878-1881
Henry P. Baldwin, Detroit 1878-1879
George Hannahs, South Haven 1878-1879
John P. Wilson, M. D., Pontiac 1879-1879
James A. Brown, M. D., Detroit 1879-1882
Jacob S. Farrand, Detroit 1879-1891
Norman Geddes, Adrian 1879-1891
Augustus C. Baldwin, Pontiac 1881-1899
Thomas Pitts, Detroit 1882-1883
Moses W. Field, Detroit 1883-1889
Joseph E. Sawyer, Pontiac 1885-1899
James A. Remick, Detroit 1889-1895
William W. Stickney, Lapeer 1891-1897
Frederick Schmid, Ann Arbor 1891-1895
J. J. Goodyear, Ann Arbor 1895-1896
Walter S. Eddy, Saginaw 1895-1901
William C. Stevens, Ann Arbor 1896-1901
Joseph Armstrong, Lapeer 1897-1903
Jane M. Kinney, Port Huron 1897-1903
Harvey S. Chapman, M. D., Pontiac 1899-1905
Harry Coleman, Pontiac 1899-1905
George Jay Vinton, Detroit (died in office) 1901-1910
Delbers E. Prall, Saginaw 1901-1907
George Clapperton, Grand Rapids 1903-1906
Fred E. Thompson, Columbiaville 1903-1907
Peter Voorheis, Pontiac 1905-1911
Edward M. Murphy, Pontiac (died in office) 1905-1909
I. Roy Waterbury, Highland 1906-1907
William C. Cornwell, Saginaw 1907-1913
Joseph F. Cartwright, Mayville 1907-1909

William J. Kay, M. D., Lapeer 1907-
John G. Clark, Bad Axe 1909-
Edward L. Keyser, Pontiac 1909-
Clement C. Yerkes, Northville 1913-
William G. Malcomson, Detroit 1910-1911
Stuart E. Galbraith, M. D., Pontiac 1911-
Charles W. Hitchcock, M. D., Detroit.......... 1911-1913
Horatio J. Abbott, Ann Arbor................ 1913-

MEDICAL SUPERINTENDENTS.

Henry M. Hurd, M. D... 1878-1889
C. B. Burr, M. D........ 1889-1894
Edmund A. Christian, M. D. 1894-

ASSISTANT MEDICAL SUPERINTENDENTS.

James D. Munson, M. D. 1878-1885
C. B. Burr, M. D........ 1885-1889
Edmund A. Christian, M. D. 1889-1894
Jason Morse, M. D....... 1894-1912
Frank S. Bachelder, M. D. 1894-

ASSISTANT PHYSICIANS.

C. B. Burr, M. D........ 1878-1885
Emma L. Randall, M. D. 1880-1885
Edmund A. Christian, M. D. 1882-1889
Charles W. Hitchcock, M. D. 1885-1886
Jason Morse, M. D...... 1885-1894
J. B. W. Lansing, M. D.. 1886-1889
W. Clark Pepper, M. D.. 1889-1891
Dwight B. Taylor, M. D. 1889-1894
Harry C. Guillot, M. D.. 1891-1895
Calvin R. Elwood, M. D. 1894-1896
James F. Breakey, M. D. 1894-1896
Louis J. Goux, M. D..... 1894-1898
Irwin H. Neff, M. D..... 1895-1908
Eugene H. Goodfellow, M. D. 1896-1897
Carlton D. Morris, M. D. 1896-1902
Claudius B. Chapin, M. D. 1897-1900
William G. Hutchinson, M. D. 1898-1899
Will Mac Lake, M. D.... 1899-1903
Anna Joy Clapperton, M. D. 1899-1904
Samuel C. Gurney, M. D. 1900-1901
Guy C. Conkle, M. D.... 1901-1904
Homer Clarke, M. D..... 1902-1907
Edward C. Greene, M. D. 1904-1911
Clarence E. Simpson, M. D. 1904-1906
Mary Elizabeth Morse, M. D. 1905-1906
Frank S. Bachelder, M. D. 1906-1912
Bertha M. L. Lyps, M. D. 1906-1908
Howard O. Osborn, M. D. 1906-1908
Clifford W. Mack, M. D. 1908-1913
Samuel A. Butler, M. D.. 1908-
Geneva Tryon, M. D..... 1909-1913
Margaret Hughes Bynon, M. D. 1913-1914
Henry L. Trenkle, M. D.. 1913-
Heinrich Reye, M. D..... 1914-
Alice Baxter, M. D. 1914-

TRAVERSE CITY STATE HOSPITAL.[1]

TRAVERSE CITY, MICH.

The decade from 1870 to 1880 marked a revolution in the methods of the care of the insane in Michigan. During this period the State Care Act became effective; the care of insane people in county houses, jails and other receptacles was prohibited, with the result that a very great increase in the accommodations of the state institutions was demanded. In 1879, at a meeting of the trustees of the two asylums of the State of Michigan, in joint session at Kalamazoo, resolutions were adopted to the effect that, owing to the overcrowded condition of the state asylums, several hundred insane persons were at that time still outside and denied admission, and that, as the insane population of the state was growing at the rate of about 170 per annum, they recommended to the Legislature the erection of an additional asylum, similar to the asylums already built.[2] They also called attention to the injustice done to many of the counties of the state by obliging them to support their insane by county tax, while paying their portion of the state tax for the maintenance of state patients.

The resolutions of the Joint Board of Trustees resulted in the passing by the Legislature of 1881 of Act No. 225, which provided for locating an additional asylum for the insane and selecting a site therefor. Under this Act Governor Jerome appointed Perry Hannah, of Traverse City, E. H. Van Deusen, M. D., of Kalamazoo, and M. H. Butler, of Detroit, as a Board of Commissioners to select a location for the proposed institution. The law from which this board derived its authority made no limits as to the

[1] By James D. Munson, M. D.

[2] Dr. Henry M. Hurd, superintendent of the Eastern Michigan Asylum, in his report to the Legislature for the biennial period ending September 30, 1880, commenting on these resolutions, says: "In this connection it is proper to refer to the cause of the crowded state of the asylums, and the necessity of increased provision for the insane. This necessity is not due, as many suppose, to the marked increase of insanity, or to the inefficiency of the present methods of treating it, but to the fact that sufficient provision has never existed to meet the requirements of the state or to keep pace with its remarkable growth in population."

portion of the state in which the additional asylum should be located. The Michigan Asylum at Kalamazoo was located in the extreme southwestern corner of the state, and the Eastern Michigan Asylum at Pontiac was located in the southeastern portion of the state. The center of the Upper Peninsula was about 300 miles from either of these hospitals, and the northern part of the Southern Peninsula of the state was almost as remote. The prevailing public sentiment seemed to indicate a general expectation that the new asylum would be located somewhere in the northern part of the state. Finally, by unanimous decision of the locating board, the asylum was located at Traverse City. In determining its location the board was largely influenced by the favorable climatic characteristics of the Grand Traverse region. These have made Northern Michigan a popular and delightful summer resort, and no better evidence of the attractiveness and healthfulness of this region can be adduced than the fact that thousands resort there annually in search of health and recreation. The extreme heat of summer and the severe cold of winter are each in turn modified by the large and deep bodies of water which nearly surround the Grand Traverse region and over which prevailing winds must pass. After the lapse of a quarter of a century the wisdom of the board in selecting Traverse City as the site of the new institution has been amply justified. For beauty and healthfulness it is doubtful whether a more desirable location could have been found anywhere within the borders of the state.

The site of the Northern Michigan Asylum, now the Traverse City State Hospital, is almost ideal. The buildings are at a distance of one and one-half miles southwest from the city. The hospital is located partly within the corporate limits of the city, but the nature of the grounds immediately in front is of such a character that it will remain permanently isolated.

The building plateau is 61 feet above the level of Grand Traverse Bay and three-fourths of a mile from it, with an extended view of the bay, the city and its surroundings. The grounds in the rear ascend in a series of heavily wooded hills, separated by ravines, and have complete protection from all westerly winds. These timbered ridges, overlooking the bay and the city, have proved an attractive feature in the outdoor exercise of patients, and are so secluded as to be adaptable to all classes of inmates.

The site has an abundant supply of pure water and easy communication by rail and water for both passengers and freight.

The hospital tract originally comprised 339.9 acres of land, little of which was cleared at the time the site was selected. It is well watered, susceptible to drainage throughout and of excellent soil. The lumber secured from some portions has more than paid the purchase price. The following additions have been made to the asylum domain by the Legislature, at a total cost of $30,077.83:

In 1887	56½	acres	$ 3,806.17
In 1892	2¼	"	225.00
In 1893	120	"	10,280.00
In 1896	29	"	2,900.00
In 1896	40	"	1,600.00
In 1900	40	"	2,000.00
In 1900	1⅓	"	66.66
In 1901	40	"	3,200.00
In 1907	60	"	6,000.00
			$30,077.83

The farm now consists of 729 acres, of which about 400 are under cultivation. Much attention has been paid to the development of orchards, gardens and grounds, and the dairy. The grounds fronting the institution are attractive, and have been carefully planted with trees and shrubs. Much attention was primarily given to the selection of trees, and an effort was made to plant all trees that would grow in this latitude. These trees have attained considerable size and lend beauty and interest to the grounds. A lake has been constructed in the grounds in front of the hospital and is a favorite spot with women patients.

The growth in size of the farm and increased value of its products have been marked. In the early planning of the farm, orchards and gardens received large consideration. During the past 25 years orchards containing over 5000 fruit trees have been planted, which furnish an unlimited supply of fruits for the hospital population. In addition to orchards, there are vineyards and large settings of currants, raspberries and strawberries. The gardens also yield abundant supplies of choice vegetables. Green houses were established soon after the institution was opened and are of economic value, as many flowers and vegetables are grown throughout the year, and stock is made ready for outside culture as early as the season will allow. Under about 10,000 square feet of glass, tomatoes, radishes, lettuce and many other vegetables are grown the year round.

The dairy herd of Holstein-Friesian cattle has been a source of pride and profit to the hospital, the breed being introduced 25 years ago. Much attention has been paid to the breeding and the herd has attained a reputation for purity, general good qualities and excellence throughout the country. Altogether $6035 has been spent for foundation stock. The sales in the meantime have amounted to nearly $7000 in a single year. Tuberculin tests of all the cattle have been made at least once each year; recently it has been decided to make tests twice a year; to receive no animal into the herd without a test within 30 days to be certified to by the State Veterinary Surgeon, and to sell no animal without furnishing with it a non-tuberculous certificate from the same state officer. Recently, also, the institution has been requested by the Live Stock Commission to sterilize all milk fed to young animals, with the hope that infection of the young stock from milk may be prevented.

After the selection of the site a building commission was constituted by adding to the locating board Alex Chapaton, Sr., of Detroit, and Henry H. Riley, of Constantine, making a board of five members. To this board was entrusted the responsibility of procuring and adopting plans for asylum buildings and for constructing, furnishing and equipping the same. At the first meeting of the building board C. M. Wells was appointed to fill the position of superintendent and secretary provided by law, and in January, 1882, Gordon W. Lloyd, of Detroit, was selected as architect.

The original hospital was built to accommodate 500 patients, and is substantial and durable in character, without extravagance, and of pleasing appearance. The original buildings were built upon the linear or Kirkbride plan. Four hundred thousand dollars were appropriated for site and buildings. Subsequently $125,000 were appropriated for furnishing the hospital. Additions have been made to the asylum by succeeding Legislatures as follows:

In 1887 completion of attics for 50 patients	$ 5,550
In 1887 Cottage 28 for 50 patients	13,000
In 1889 Cottage 32 for 30 patients	15,000
In 1889 north and south infirmaries for 60 patients..	30,000
In 1891 Cottage 25 for 50 patients	15,000
In 1893 Cottages 24 and 26 for 100 patients	25,000
In 1893 Cottage 29 for 75 patients	18,750
In 1899 Cottage 34 for 50 patients	20,000
In 1899 Cottage 21 for 50 patients	20,000
In 1899 Cottage 31 for 30 patients	7,300
In 1901 Cottage 30 for 50 patients	21,367
In 1901 Cottage 23 for 50 patients	21,367
In 1903 Cottage 36 for 60 patients	24,000
In 1903 Cottage 27 for 60 patients	24,000
In 1907 extension to north and south wings	90,000
Total	$350,284

In 1912 the institution had accommodations for 1500 patients. The experience gained from planning, building and using these cottages and extensions has demonstrated that separate heating plants and separate dining rooms and kitchens are expensive, and that the storage of coal for each isolated heating plant is not only unsanitary, but increases the danger of fire and costs more than in a congregate building. Experience has also demonstrated that the preparation of food is better in isolated kitchens, but much more expensive than in a central kitchen.

The original building contained 18 wards, nine for each sex, each ward distinct, complete in itself, possessing a dining room, clothes room, lavatory, bath room, water closet and exit at each end. Segregation is attained through the division of each ward into individual rooms from 8 feet 6 inches by 11 feet, to 9 feet 6 inches by 11 feet 8 inches, or larger rooms, each for two or three persons. Each ward, except those for disturbed patients, has one or two associated dormitories with floor space for five or six beds. The center building is devoted to administrative purposes, the second, third and fourth stories being occupied as living apartments by the officers, their families and employees.

The original system of heating and ventilating consisted of indirect radiators located in the basement and connected by flues with the various halls. The system was provided with two long tunnels connecting the basement with power house, where a large steam-driven fan was provided to deliver fresh air into the basement. This fan proved impracticable and its use was abandoned shortly after the plant was installed. The system was faulty. Ventilation was not constant nor was fresh air provided irrespective of the degree of heating required.

The Legislatures of 1909 and 1911 respectively made appropriations for installing a new system of heating and ventilating in the main building. The principle of this system is that the heating and ventilating are entirely separate, and consequently the best results can be secured with the greatest possible economy. The present heating system consists of radiators located so as to maintain proper temperatures in all of the various rooms, and these radiators are equipped with the vacuum system and automatic regulation. The new ventilating system is operated by motor-driven fans, which are capable of giving the guaranteed air supply to each and every room under all conditions of weather. This air supply is at the same temperature as the rooms. High pressure steam is supplied to direct radiators and tempering coils. The condensed water is returned to a surge tank, from which it is pumped back to the boilers. There are five boilers of 1350 horse-power capacity, all of the water-tube type and provided with automatic stokers. With one exception these stokers are of the chain variety, the exception being a Detroit stoker. These stokers are only adapted for non-coking coals and of a size not larger than nut or egg. The coal is supplied to and the ashes are removed from these boilers in part mechanically. The boilers are connected to the tempering coils in the basement and each of the tempering coils has a supply air fan, capable of handling 10,000 cubic feet of air per minute.

There are seven banks of tempering coils, with seven supply fans, located in the basement. Exhaust fans are located in the attic, which are capable of handling the same number of cubic feet of exhaust air as is furnished by the supply fans. For each of the supply and exhaust fans a 120 volt direct-current variable speed motor is furnished, of from 2½ to 5 horse-power. The tempering coils are controlled by thermostats, located at some neutral point in the wards above, which are usually maintained at from 68° to 70°. The apparatus is simple and works well with comparatively little attention. The heating system is known as the "Paul System," and has been in operation in the north wing of the main building for two years; occasionally the thermostats have to be cleaned.

concrete, covered with planking where the animals stand. There is stable room for 25 horses. The ice houses store about 1000 tons of ice and the cellars 30,000 bushels of roots. The refrigerator building was completed in 1911. It is furnished with up-to-date ice-making machinery and is arranged for the care of meats, butter, fresh and dried fruits, canned goods, cheese, eggs, etc. This is the most important improvement in recent years.

There have been 12 cottages for patients built and furnished since the opening of the institution. The struggle against tuberculosis at this institution commenced in 1890. The first effort was to isolate these patients on one ward. While this plan was better than having the cases scattered, yet it was impossible to maintain perfect isolation. Later separate cottages for men and women were converted into tuberculous hospitals, and have since supplied means of complete isolation and treatment for this class. The number of developing cases in the hospital has been lessened. New cases of tuberculosis are admitted from time to time, and new cases also develop in the institution. The number of deaths from tuberculosis during the last period was 16 per cent of the deaths from all causes, a decrease of 5 per cent over the former period. The greatest spread of the disease has occurred among male patients, as isolation could not be thoroughly carried out before the cottage for their care was constructed.

Of the cottages, one for men and one for women were designed for convalescent patients. For a number of years all convalescent cases were sent to cottages, but experience has demonstrated that this is no special advantage to the patient. In fact, many patients recover and are discharged from the hospital wards where they have resided during their entire period of treatment.

In 1906 a training school for nurses was established. Last year the training school had 62 pupil nurses, with 21 graduates. The experiment of employing women nurses for the care of men patients was tried, and, after two or three years' experience, was discontinued. The advantage of women nurses over well-trained men nurses was never very clearly demonstrated, and there were some objectionable features.

The employment of patients has been very carefully fostered and supervised. As the asylum property was originally largely a wilderness, its clearing and development have been a constant source of employment to a large number of male patients.

In 1898 the asylums of Michigan, in conjunction with the University at Ann Arbor, established a pathological department, out of which the present psychopathic ward and pathological laboratory, under the directorship of Dr. A. M. Barrett, were developed. Research work under Dr. Barrett's direction is carried on by all the institutions conjointly. A uniform classification of mental diseases has been adopted. A pathological museum has been established at the psychopathic ward, and already a valuable collection has been made of diseased brain conditions. The old cumbrous way of recording admissions, discharges, etc., of patients has been substituted by the card-index system wherever possible, and vertical filing of clinical notes, correspondence and everything relating to the patient has been adopted.

For several years a dietitian has had general oversight of the foods and their preparation. She teaches dietetics to the pupil nurses and especially directs the preparation of food for the sick. There are no fixed menus. Each day's food distribution is arranged. Foods are prescribed for the feeble and the sick and are specially prepared for their needs. Great attention is given to food requisitions in order to maintain a fairly well-balanced ration. The food nutrient principles of all foodstuffs supplied during one month of each year are accurately determined, and the results thus obtained are of economic as well as scientific value. It is hoped to make these analyses much oftener than once a year.

A domestic art department has been established, which up to the present time has been under the direction of the dietitian. A competent person will be put in charge of this department. All the needle work of the institution will be directed by this officer. In the recent extension to the north wing a sewing room with necessary conveniences was built, and it is hoped that practically all of the sewing of the institution may be done in this room, all the patients competent to assist with the work being brought to it. Passenger elevators have been built in connection with the building, so that patients can be transported without undue effort to themselves and without confusion on the wards.

Staff meetings are held sufficiently often to examine every new case, and also to determine the diagnosis of recovery or the mental status of patients at the time of discharge. Records are made of all examinations. The Wassermann test, both of the spinal fluid and of the blood, is made of all suspects. Lumbar punctures become part of the routine method of examination. The Nonne-Apelt test is made in all these cases. The technical part of the Wassermann test is made at the laboratory of the psychopathic ward at Ann Arbor.

Instead of the old plan of employing painters and helpers to clean and wax the floors, this work is now done under the direction of the chief attendant of each ward and mostly by the men patients. The head painter of the hospital prepares the materials. In this way the floors are kept in better condition than ever before and at a saving to the hospital. Wherever possible, wood floors are being replaced by tile, and doubtless within a comparatively few years all the main corridors of the asylum proper will be laid in tile.

In regard to general medical supervision, it will be only a short time before the old plan of congregating the medical officers in the administration building will be abandoned. Each and every medical officer will be assigned to the charge of a certain number of wards and patients, and will be required to spend as many hours per day as may be deemed necessary for the best interests of the patients and of the hospital. In this way it is believed much better insight will be obtained of the cases, much better treatment afforded them and better results obtained in every way. At the present time there are 1395 patients under treatment—779 men and 616 women. There has been a gradual decrease in the hospital population during the last three or four years. The hospital is now caring for overflow cases from the Eastern Michigan and Upper Peninsula districts. The general population of the hospital district has increased 5000 during the last ten years.

COMMISSIONERS.

Perry Hannah	1881-1885	H. H. Riley............	1881-1885
E. H. Van Deusen......	1881-1885	Thomas T. Bates.......	1885-1885
M. H. Butler...........	1881-1885		

TRUSTEES.

C. M. Wells (president 1885-1886)	1885-1887	H. H. Noble (president 1892-1897)	1885-1897
Alex. Chapaton, Sr.	1885-	Geo. A. Farr...........	1885-1891
J. W. French............	1885-1889	Varnum B. Cochran....	1887-1893
Thos. T. Bates (president 1886-1892; 1907-1910).	1885-	Lorin Roberts (president 1897-1899)	1887-1899

H. D. Campbell........ 1889-1901
G. A. Hart (president 1902-1907) 1889-1907
John Benjamin 1889-1891
C. L. Whitney.......... 1891-1895
W. W. Cummer........ 1895-1901
H. C. Davis (president 1899-1902) 1897-
John Maywood 1897-1901
C. F. Backus........... 1897-1905
W. W. Mitchell........ 1901-
H. D. Brigham.......... 1901-1901
D. B. Butler............ 1902-1903
A. F. Temple........... 1903-1908
M. F. Quaintance....... 1905-
William Lloyd 1907-
E. S. Wager............ 1909-

MEDICAL SUPERINTENDENT.

James D. Munson, M. D........................ 1885-

ASSISTANT MEDICAL SUPERINTENDENTS.

J. H. Dawson, M. D..... 1885-1890
C. G. Chaddock, M. D... 1890-1892
A. S. Rowley, M. D..... 1895-

ASSISTANT PHYSICIANS.

C. G. Chaddock, M. D... 1885-1890
W. A. Stone, M. D...... 1886-1891
Henry Hulst, M. D...... 1888-1889
J. F. Canavan, M. D. (died) 1889-1907
D. L. Harris, M. D....... 1899-1899
I. L. Harlow, M. D..... 1889-1891
G C. Crandall, M. D.... 1890-1894
A. S. Rowley, M. D..... 1891-1895
M. Rockwell, M. D....... 1891-1892
C. G. Speer, M. D....... 1892-1896
Robert Howell, M. D.... 1893-1898
H. J. Kennedy, M. D..... 1894-1895
L. C. Stillings, M. D..... 1894-1895
E. L. Niskern, M. D..... 1895-1898
G. L. Noyes, M. D....... 1895-1900
G B. Furness, M. D..... 1896-1897
F. P. Lawton, M. D..... 1898-1901
C. A. Good, M. D....... 1898-1900
Fonda Nadeau, M. D..... 1898-1899
W. D. Mueller, M. D..... 1900-
Minta P. Kemp, M. D... 1900-1903
W. J. Kirkbride, M. D... 1901-1902
F. H. Newberry, M. D... 1902-1904
Beatrice A. Stevenson, M. D. 1903-1909
B. F. Sargeant, M. D..... 1904-1905
H. D. Purdum, M. D.... 1906-1910
R. E. Wells, M. D....... 1907-
Guy M. Johnson, M. D... 1908-1910
Adah Epperson, M. D... 1910-
James A. J. Hall, M. D.. 1910-
E. G. C. Williams, M. D. 1910-1911
S. C. Niles, M. D........ 1911-
R. F. Wafer, M. D....... 1913-

STEWARDS.

J. D. Billings........... 1885-1886
John Goode 1886-1887
J. P. C. Church......... 1887-1894
C. L. Whitney.......... 1894-1911
G. B. Pike.............. 1912-

CHAPLAINS.

Rev. W. G. Puddefoot.. 1886-1888
Rev. D. VanAlstin...... 1888-1890
Rev. D. Cochlin........ 1890-

IONIA STATE HOSPITAL.[1]

IONIA, MICH.

The Ionia State Hospital was established in 1883 under the name of the Michigan Asylum for Insane Criminals by the Act of Legislature No. 190, Public Acts of 1883, which provided that the State Board of Corrections and Charities should locate an asylum for insane criminals in connection with or adjacent to the State House of Correction at Ionia, purchase the necessary land, and procure the desired plans and specifications, and that the Board of Managers of the State House of Correction should then proceed with the construction of the asylum at a total cost not to exceed $60,000. This act further provided for the internal organization of the institution and specified the different types of patients to be admitted and the legal formalities incident thereto.

The preliminary arrangements were speedily made and on June 24, 1885, the first buildings of the institution were formally accepted by the Board of Managers of the State House of Correction, which was to continue in charge of this new institution, although it was to maintain its integrity entirely separate from the prison. The first patients were admitted in September, 1885.

These first buildings were erected just outside the wall of the State House of Correction and connected with it by walls at both ends forming an airing court for the patients between the high prison wall and the asylum buildings. The unfortunate choice of the location immediately became apparent to all concerned and in the first biennial report, dated September 30, 1886, we note that the State Board of Corrections and Charities refused to recommend certain requests for appropriations to enlarge the capacity of these buildings because of its location adjoining the prison. As early as that time the institution was caring for 81 male patients in accommodations intended for only 76, and had only two vacancies in the female department, which provided for 16 patients.

In 1890, when the population had increased to 124 patients, with no relief beyond what increase could be had by making temporary sleeping quarters in what was intended as an attic, there were purchased 98 acres of land beautifully situated on a high bluff

[1] Sketch furnished by Dr. Robert H. Haskell, superintendent.

overlooking the original institution from the opposite side of the Grand River, and on this property was speedily built a cottage for male patients, the present Building No. 1. There were transferred here about 50 patients, care being taken so far as possible to choose such patients as would be suitable to work the farm which the institution had now come to have. Two years later another building to accommodate 75 male patients was built on the new location, with a service building containing kitchens and store rooms in the half basement, congregate dining room for the total 125 patients on the first floor and an amusement room, 32 feet by 42 feet, on the second floor. It is interesting for us to-day to note that this cottage plan building was at that time considered as a temporary expedient. In 1896, however, another cottage, now Building No. 3, was erected to accommodate 70 male patients, planned and still used to care for the more dangerous and scheming of the population. At this time also a central boiler and engine house and a special bakery building, with large brick oven, were built, and numerous other improvements in the buildings, grounds and farm were made. In 1903 another building was finished, the largest up to that time, of pleasing exterior and of airy and light internal arrangement and accommodating easily 100 patients. In 1909 a building for women patients was erected on the south side site with accommodations for 60 women patients and nurses, which was enlarged in 1913 by the addition of a wing, until now it can care comfortably for 94 patients. There is now (1915) approaching completion a new building for male patients, which was originally planned to accommodate 80 patients, but lack of funds made it possible to erect only the front of a U-shaped building with accommodations for only 36 patients. An attempt was made to obtain from the Legislature of 1915 a sufficient appropriation to allow the addition of the two wings in the original plans, but without success. The wisdom displayed by the Board of Corrections and Charities in 1886, only about a year after the original buildings had been put next door to and connected with the prison, which led them to refuse to recommend further appropriations for the north side group and to recommend the regrouping of these buildings in some other location, although not lying dormant wholly, has thus far failed to bring about the greatly desired concentration of all the forces in one spot and this notwithstanding that the present condition of affairs costs the state approximately $10,000 a year in unnecessary duplication of expenses.

At various times there have also been built the usual accessories of such an institution as a laundry building with modern appliances, a cold storage plant with its own refrigerating machinery, a milk house, carpenter shop, various barns and other out buildings, oil house, transformer building, etc. A separate administration building, with the offices and living quarters of the superintendent, was built in 1903. In 1915 an employees' building was finished, which provides living accommodations for 16 outside employees. On the ground floor is a large, well-furnished reading room and a billiard room. The basement, which has not been finished yet, will provide a small gymnasium. These quarters, the first attempt to furnish anything in the line of comfort for the employees, have become popular with all classes of workers, and should prove a potent agency in making them more contented. One side of the first floor of this building is devoted to the assistant physicians' offices and to the business offices. In the basement under this half are located the pharmacy, the clinical laboratory, photographic quarters and the X-ray room.

During the first years no provision was made for any farming activities, but with the purchase of the south side site land for such purposes became available. At the present time there are 135 acres under intensive cultivation. This furnishes the tables with green vegetables in the summer, nearly enough potatoes, onions and other vegetables for the year and sufficient ensilage to feed a large herd of Holsteins during the winter. The character of the patients is such that working parties cannot be given the freedom usually accorded them in civil institutions, but the farmer has constantly with him 15 patients, the number being augmented in busy times with special squads of 5 to 14 men under an outside attendant, and in the picking season with more, including groups of women patients.

The carpenter shop was sufficiently well equipped with modern machinery to undertake the complete installation of the interior finish in the new Building 6 and the present plan is to continue such work in any future building. The engineer's department has large, well-arranged and well-equipped work rooms for all usual repairs and changes in this department, such as installing a hot-water storage tank of 365 gallons capacity for laundry service, a Marsh automatic boiler feed pump and receiver to return the condensed water to the boilers at an average temperature of 180°, and a Marsh air compressor and storage tank with power to compress 50 cubic feet of free air per minute at 60 pounds pressure for use in the water system. All the buildings are heated with the exhaust steam. The same department has also done all the electrical work for the building now approaching completion and likewise all the heating, plumbing and sewage installations. As early as 1897 two Ideal engines connected direct to two Westinghouse generators of 40 kw. capacity were installed for lighting purposes, but they proved too small for the rapidly growing institution and were never used. The institution still buys its light and power from the local power company because it has never been possible to obtain an appropriation to enlarge and modernize the first plant. The mason, assisted by patients, recently made 130,000 concrete brick for the employees' building and all the artificial stone in the foundation and trimmings.

The problem of obtaining a sufficient water supply at all times in this institution, as in many others occupying an isolated position, has been a serious matter. Until the winter of 1914-15 the institution depended upon numerous springs situated on the property, but mainly upon two wells situated on the flats, 180 feet below the level of the institution and 1000 feet from the buildings. An electric pump of 30 horse power at this well forced the water to two reservoirs, one of 132,000 gallons capacity 70 feet above the level of the institution and the other of 366,000 gallons capacity at a slightly lower level. During the winter months of 1914-15 a three-inch well, 380 feet deep, which had been sunk in 1902 and immediately abandoned because it did not furnish sufficient flow by suction, was rediscovered within 65 feet of the boiler house.

The idea of a deep-well engine being discarded because of its inability to deliver the volume of water desired, a forced delivery of air under pressure was decided upon. The Marsh air compressor previously referred to was accordingly installed and a three-quarter inch air line carried from it 162 feet down the well inside the original three-inch casing.

This arrangement was a complete success from the first, when it delivered about 60 gallons per minute. Experimentation quickly showed the optimum pressure and side-hole relations and it now delivers without difficulty 75 gallons a minute. An underground reservoir, capable of holding 20,000 gallons, is now being built around the top of this well. There are now three satisfactory sources of water supply: three springs draining into one reservoir of 1000 gallons capacity to supply drinking water, the rediscovered "Eureka" well of sufficient flow to supply fairly soft water for all needs, including small fires, and the old reservoirs of 584,000 gallons capacity, filled by the electric pumps at the wells on the flats, which form a reserve fire supply. Through a well-arranged system of pipes and by-pass valves in the engineer's department, the two pumps, one of which is constantly in reserve, can switch instantly from one source of water supply to the other with no inconvenience.

As an integral part of the water supply should perhaps be mentioned the fire system. The ward buildings are well provided with stand pipes, hose and chemicals on each floor, which are frequently inspected. Numerous ordinary fire hydrants are located throughout the grounds. The two pumps in the engine rooms are capable of pumping 300 gallons a minute, sufficient to meet any ordinary requirements, but to meet extraordinary demands there are in Fire House No. 1 two Rumsey heavy-duty electric fire pumps which can deliver 500 gallons per minute at 100 pounds gauge pressure at the pumps. In this same fire house there are two man-hauled hose reels with 900 feet of two-inch Underwriters' rubber-lined hose. In Fire House No. 2, located in the neighborhood of the barns and work shops, where most of our fires occur, is a third hose reel with 500 feet of two-inch hose and a Champion chemical engine, furnishing 60 gallons of fire-fighting compound to the charge. A carefully worked out fire drill is held at frequent intervals.

The character of the patients makes it impossible to utilize the usual open-air walking party for recreation. In all but the stormiest weather they are given exercise daily in airing corridors connecting the different buildings. In the summer months they have the freedom of the airing court, which at the time of its establishment in 1900 was unique in its arrangement. From the outside it appears like any ordinary brick wall, 46 inches in height, surrounding a level plat of land 297 feet long by 198 feet wide. On the inside, however, this is seen to be a non-climbable stone and brick wall 13 feet 10 inches high, from the bottom of which on all sides runs a quick slope of land to a point 12 feet back from the wall. This furnishes a pleasant court where the patients can enjoy the fresh air and see at close hand the activities of the hospital grounds without the unpleasant features of a high prison wall and without danger of escape. This court is entered through a tunnel intersecting the main tunnel system.

For the use of such classes of patients as can be given greater freedom there is a beautiful grove of ten acres, well provided with rustic seats, benches, tables and swings and also a partially enclosed summer house with fireplace, where they can warm coffee and tea for their lunches.

At the present time there are 76 patients at work besides those who help on the wards. This number is distributed among the different departments as follows:

Engineer's department, 4; farm department, 15; carpenter shop, 7; garden and lawn department, 6; laundry department, 7; store room department, 1; kitchen department, 14; dining room department, 13; with teamster, 2; with attendant outside, 7.

During the winter of 1914-15 all working patients were brought together under one roof of Building No. 1 and there given additional privileges, such as staying up one hour later than the others, special tables in the congregate dining room with certain changes in their dietary and other slight table distinctions. The formation of this Working Men's Club, with its little privileges, appears to have had its stimulating effect throughout the entire institution. A sewing room with motor-driven machines is maintained in the women's building, where the women patients make all their own clothes and practically all the sheets, curtains and other household articles required in the institution, and do as well the general mending. Rug making and knitting machines keep a small number of patients occupied. It is the present intention to further extend such occupational activities until it will become possible as well as profitable to employ a skilled person to devote his entire energies to this line of treatment.

The medical staff is composed of the medical superintendent, the assistant physician and a junior assistant physician. Upon admission the patient is given a careful physical and neurological examination, a formal mental status is carefully drawn up and running ward notes are started. These notes are written at frequent intervals during the early part of a patient's residence, and at stated intervals throughout his stay in chronic cases. The recent introduction of semi-weekly clinical conferences, in which two or three cases are considered intensively along lines of modern psychiatrical and socio-criminological interest, together with a weekly ward walk throughout the entire group on each Sunday morning, has already resulted in a considerable development of interest in the work from an individualistic psychiatrical point of view and the consequent improvement in the character and volume of the clinical notes. This institution has the benefits of association with the State Psychopathic Hospital at Ann Arbor and its laboratories. A routine Wassermann examination is made upon the blood serum of each admission and in positive reactors and suspicious or organic cases lumbar puncture is done with the usual tests on the cerebro-spinal fluid.

The clinical laboratory is fairly well equipped, being provided with the apparatus and reagents necessary for the routine examinations of the urine, blood, cerebro-spinal fluid, milk, stomach contents, fæces, etc. An incubator allows of carrying cultures for Widal tests, etc. No histopathological work has ever been attempted, and, in view of the small number of deaths and the association with the laboratories at Ann Arbor, it hardly seems necessary to attempt such innovations at present. The X-ray laboratory is well equipped for making plates, fluoroscopic examination and also use of electricity in diagnosis and treatment. A modern operating room was built in a small separate unit back of Building 4 and connected with a quiet ward, where post-operative cases have satisfactory attention and care.

There has never been any attempt to establish a training school for attendants. A few of them stay long enough to become really valuable and fairly expert in their work, but for the most part the roving element is still uppermost here. With, however, additional attention to their interests, the recreation rooms, proper relief periods, more comfortable living quarters and the instruction planned to be given them, it is hoped that the history of other institutions will repeat itself here.

The institution has undergone frequent change of name. Because it was felt that the original name of the Michigan Asylum for the Insane Criminals worked some injustice upon those who were transferred here from civil institutions, this name was in 1891 changed by the Legislature to the Michigan Asylum for the

Dangerous and Criminal Insane. In 1899 it was again changed to the State Asylum. In 1911 the present name of the Ionia State Hospital was chosen.

In the original act the management of the institution was placed in the hands of the Board of Managers of the State House of Correction (now the Ionia Reformatory), although in all respects it was to be an entirely separate and distinct institution. On October 1, 1891, along with the penal and corrective institutions of the state, it passed into the control of what might be considered a central board, the State Board of Inspectors. This condition of centralized control was short-lived, and in June, 1893, it came under the control of its own Board of Trustees and was divorced from its original close connection with the penal institutions so thoroughly that in March, 1913, Hon. Grant Fellows, Attorney General of the state, ruled definitely that it was not a penal institution.

The Board of Trustees consists of three members, one member being appointed by the Governor each two years to serve a term of six years. The trustees receive only their actual travelling expenses. They hold regular meetings at the institution on the second Tuesday of each month, at which time they receive the report of the medical superintendent, the report of their own visiting committee of one member, discuss plans and other matters of importance, approve all bills before payment, and visit and inspect the buildings and grounds. The following persons have acted in the capacity of managers, inspectors or trustees of the institution:

MANAGERS.

A. H. Piper	Detroit	Dec. 5, 1883	Dec. 12, 1888
John Heffron	Detroit	Dec. 5, 1883	Feb. 7, 1889
Geo. W. Stevenson	St. Johns	Dec. 5, 1883	Feb. 4, 1885
Hampton Rich	Ionia	Feb. 6, 1885	Oct. 7, 1891
Moreau S. Crosby	Grand Rapids	Dec. 12, 1888	Feb. 5, 1891
Jerome Croul	Detroit	Feb. 7, 1889	Oct. 7, 1891
D. O. Watson	Coopersville	Feb. 5, 1891	Oct. 7, 1891

STATE BOARD OF INSPECTORS.

Milo D. Campbell	Coldwater	Oct. 7, 1891	June 5, 1893
Orlando M. Barnes	Lansing	Oct. 7, 1891	June 5, 1893
Francis F. Palms	Detroit	Oct. 7, 1891	June 5, 1893
Edward Duffy	Ann Arbor	Oct. 7, 1891	June 5, 1893

TRUSTEES.

C. C. Vaughan	St. Johns	June 5, 1893	Feb. 7, 1898
Edward C. Reid	Allegan	June 5, 1893	Feb. 1, 1901
A. B. Darragh	St. Louis	Feb. 1, 1898	Sept. 28, 1901
W. H. Mattison	Ionia	June 5, 1893	Feb. 1, 1905
J. W. Belknap	Greenville	Feb. 1, 1901	Oct. 31, 1911
J. H. Lancashire	Alma	Sept. 28, 1901	Dec. 1903
E. M. Hopkins	Detroit	Dec. 1903	Jan. 31, 1909
F. A. Washburn	Belding	Feb. 1, 1905	Jan. 31, 1911
J. K. Flood	Hart	Feb. 1, 1909	Jan. 31, 1915
C. F. Backus	Detroit	Feb. 1, 1911	
C. H. Gibson	Greenville	Dec. 5, 1911	Jan. 31, 1913
S. F. Kennedy	Lakeview	Feb. 1, 1913	
T. B. Preston	Ionia	Feb. 1, 1915	

As medical superintendent of the institution at its foundation, the Board of Managers chose Dr. Oscar R. Long, who had been for several years physician to the State House of Correction. Dr. Long continued in charge without change until his sudden death from heart failure on the night of September 9, 1914. He literally died in harness, for death came after an evening's business consultation with the president of the Board of Trustees over matters of considerable importance to be acted upon in the monthly meeting on the following day. In view of extensive building operations and matters of business reorganization which were being carried on at this time, it was deemed advisable that the president of the board, Hon. Charles F. Backus, who, from a previous experience of six years as trustee of the Traverse City State Hospital and four years of most active service on the board of this institution, was well acquainted with the intricacies of the general problem and particularly those features affecting this institution at that time, should be appointed acting superintendent. Mr. Backus continued in charge for seven months, during which period much progress was made in modernizing the institution along many lines, not omitting the care of the patients. In March, 1915, the Board of Trustees elected as medical superintendent Dr. Robert H. Haskell, who had been for the three years preceding first assistant physician at the State Psychopathic Hospital at Ann Arbor and instructor in psychiatry at the University of Michigan. He accepted and assumed the duties of the position April 15, 1915.

Patients under treatment here present many difficulties not met with to any large extent in civil insane practice. It is the constitutionally paranoid individual, the psychopathic personality, who cannot stand the burden of discipline under any circumstance and least of all in prison, and the schemer with a bad prison record, a long sentence, perhaps life, ahead of him with little prospect of pardon relief, who has feigned insanity in hopes of being able to escape from what he supposes is a less firmly built and less carefully watched institution than the prison. It is the presence of these classes that makes it necessary to enforce discipline of a somewhat different nature from most institutions. Yet seclusion and mechanical restraint are at a minimum. The dormitory system can be used here to only a very limited extent. Most patients sleep in single rooms.

The patients for whom this institution is provided may be roughly grouped into three classes: those from the penal institutions, from the courts, and from the civil insane hospitals. The first group does not require much discussion. The warden or other executive officer of a prison must, when the prison physician certifies to him that a prisoner is insane, transfer that inmate to this hospital. No other formalities are necessary. When this patient has recovered he may be transferred back to the prison from which he came. The time he may have passed in this hospital counts toward the expiration of his sentence as if he had continued in prison. No person can be paroled by the Pardon Board while he is a patient in this hospital. If the patient is still insane at the expiration of his sentence, two courses are open: If not dangerous to the community, in the opinion of the medical superintendent, he may, upon some responsible person providing a bond satisfactory to the superintendent that he will not become a public charge, be discharged to his family or other interested party. If still insane and not discharged according to the foregoing provisions, the medical superintendent shall, within five days following the expiration of his term of sentence, certify to the judge of the probate court of Ionia County (in which the institution is located) that this person, whose prison term has expired, is still insane, and pray for his commitment. The patient's family and the clerk of the county where he formerly resided are notified, and after notification papers have been served on the patient, he is examined by two outside physicians and the matter of hearing and commitment proceeds exactly as it would were the patient an ordinary member of the community gone insane. Where his maintenance as a transferred patient from the prison had continued as a state charge, it becomes under the new commitment a county charge for one year. In the original act there was no provision for the recommitment of a patient whose sentence had expired. This legal technicality was early seized upon and a patient under *habeas corpus* proceedings, though manifestly insane, was ordered by the Supreme Court discharged, not because he had not been or did not continue insane, but because at the end of his sentence there had been no judicial commitment.

To illustrate the group of cases which may be admitted directly from the courts, it is best to quote briefly from the statutes governing these cases:

> When a person accused of any crime shall have escaped indictment, or shall have been acquitted upon trial, upon the grounds of insanity, the court being certified by the jury, or otherwise, of the fact, shall carefully inquire and ascertain whether his or her insanity in any degree continues, and if it does, shall order such person into safe custody, and to be sent to the Michigan Asylum for Dangerous and Criminal Insane, or to any one of the state asylums for the insane. If any person in confinement under indictment for crime shall appear to be insane, the judge of the circuit court of the county where he or she is confined shall institute a careful investigation. He shall call two or more respectable physicians and other credible witnesses, and the prosecuting attorney, to aid in the examination; and if it be deemed necessary to call a jury for that purpose, is fully empowered to compel the attendance of witnesses and jurors. If it is satisfactorily proved that such person is insane, said judge may discharge such person from imprisonment, and order his or her safe custody and removal to the Michigan Asylum for Dangerous and Criminal Insane, or to any one of the state asylums, at the discretion of such judge, where such person shall be retained until restored to his or her right mind, and then, if the said judge shall have so directed, the superintendent of said asylum shall inform the said judge and prosecuting attorney, so that the person so confined may within 60 days thereafter be remanded to prison, and criminal proceedings be resumed, or otherwise be discharged.

Those patients admitted under the first part of this section may be discharged when recovered. Those to whom the second portion applies ordinarily must be returned to the court for its further action.

In the original act the provisions were not quite so general, but applied only to persons accused or under indictment for "the crime of murder, rape, attempt at rape, highway robbery or arson."

Patients may be transferred from the civil insane hospitals in various ways.

First. Any patient admitted to a civil institution that has previously been treated in the Ionia State Hospital shall be transferred to that institution.

Second. Whenever a patient is admitted to a civil insane hospital that has previously served one term in prison, he may, at the discretion of the superintendent and Board of Trustees of that hospital, be transferred, provided there is room to receive him.

Third. Whenever a patient is received in any of the asylums of the state who has served two or more terms in prison or but one term for murder, attempted murder, manslaughter, rape, or attempt at rape, or assault with intent to do great bodily harm, arson, or burglary, it shall be the duty of the medical superintendent of such asylum to transfer such patient to the Michigan Asylum for Dangerous and Criminal Insane.

Fourth. Apart from this ex-convict class, provision is further made that "the medical superintendent of any of the asylums for the insane in Michigan may, with the consent of their respective boards of trustees or governing boards, make application to the Board of Corrections and Charities for recommendation for the transfer of any or all criminal insane persons under treatment in any of the said asylums who have been guilty of an act of homicide previous to admission to the asylum, and whose presence is dangerous to others; likewise all insane persons who have committed any act of homicide while under treatment in any of the asylums. And the Board of Corrections and Charities shall investigate all of the facts and report to the Governor, who may in his discretion order the transfer of such person or persons to the Michigan Asylum for Dangerous and Criminal Insane.

Fifth. In case any patient under treatment in any of the asylums in the state shall commit any act of homicide or develop unmistakably dangerous or homicidal tendencies rendering his presence a source of danger to others, proceedings may be instituted as above.

The logical development in the law whereby persons under arrest or trial for crime, in whose case the question of insanity has been raised, could be sent here for a period of observation with report to the court, has not yet been reached.

The following table shows the number of admissions in the various classes above described up to June 1, 1915:

From prisons	911
From hospitals	291
From courts	146
Total	1348

NEWBERRY STATE HOSPITAL.[1]

NEWBERRY, MICH.

The Newberry State Hospital was authorized by an act of the Legislature of Michigan in the year 1893, under the name of the Upper Peninsula Hospital for the Insane. It was opened for the occupation of patients on November 4, 1895. It contemplates in the plan, when completed, 20 cottages, arranged in the form of a quadrangle and connected by covered porches or cloisters. These cloisters are continuous around the inside of the quadrangle, and in the winter time are enclosed in glass. The capacity of the 20 cottages is 1000 patients. The general kitchen and dining rooms are also included in this quadrangle. The heating plant, laundry, storerooms and other industrial buildings are situated in the rear. The institution is governed by a Board of Trustees, composed of six members, appointed by the Governor, by and with the consent of the State Senate, each for a term of six years. The first medical superintendent of the institution was Dr. Samuel Bell, who served from the opening of the institution until April 1, 1899. He was succeeded by Dr. George L. Chamberlain, assistant medical superintendent, who served from April, 1899, until April 1, 1905. He was succeeded by Dr. Earl H. Campbell, assistant medical superintendent. The hospital is now fairly well equipped. It has a receiving ward for each sex, also hydrotherapeutic and electrical apparatus, laboratory and operating rooms. All male bed cases and infirm patients are cared for by women nurses. All patients, excepting the bed patients and recent cases, are fed in a congregate dining room. Training schools for nurses and attendants are maintained, with a superintendent of nurses in charge of the training schools. The present population of the hospital is 880 patients. There are four physicians and 143 employees.

Occupation work is carried on among the women patients, there being a room fitted up for this purpose, under the charge of a special teacher. Patients are taught raffia and basket work, embroidery and plain sewing. On one afternoon of each week they are given calisthenic exercises and instruction in various folk dances.

[1] By E. H. Campbell, M. D., superintendent.

BOARD OF TRUSTEES, 1914.

STEWARD.

R. C. Bradley.

MEDICAL SUPERINTENDENTS.

Name	Years
Samuel Bell, M. D.	1895-1899
George L. Chamberlain, M. D.	1899-1905
Earl H. Campbell, M. D.	1905-

ASSISTANT MEDICAL SUPERINTENDENTS.

Name	Years
George L. Chamberlain, M. D.	1895-1899
Henry E. Perry, M. D.	1899-1903
Earl H. Campbell, M. D.	1903-1905
Charles W. Thompson, M. D.	1905-1913
Emory J. Brady, M. D.	1913-

ASSISTANT PHYSICIANS.

Name	Years
T. M. Cunningham, M. D.	1899-
Maud B. Martin, M. D.	1899-1903
Flavius J. Downer, M. D.[1]	1902-1905
Frances E. Rutledge, M. D.	1903-1909
Eugene W. Mullen, M. D.	1905-1911
Minta P. Kemp, M. D.	1909-
William R. Tutt, M. D.	1911-1912
George G. Smith, M. D.	1912-1913
Festus C. Bandy, M. D.	1913-

[1] Deceased.

STATE PSYCHOPATHIC HOSPITAL.[1]

ANN ARBOR, MICH.

The State of Michigan has the creditable position in the history of psychiatry in America of being the first to establish a university hospital for the care and treatment of mental diseases and of providing adequate facilities for the instruction of medical students of the university regarding insanity. The achievement of this hospital is almost entirely due to the late Dr. Wm. J. Herdman, for many years at the head of the department of nervous and mental diseases in the State University. Influenced by the general awakening throughout this country to the needs of such institutions, Dr. Herdman took a warm interest in the establishment of a psychopathic hospital in connection with the general hospitals of the State University. As a result of his interest and initiative there was passed by the Michigan State Legislature in 1901[2] an act to provide for the construction and equipment of a psychopathic ward upon the hospital grounds of the University of Michigan and to appropriate the sum of $50,000 therefor.

It must be borne in mind that there were no precedents to follow in drafting a comprehensive set of provisions for the organization and administration of the new hospital. The problem was to establish an institution of the type desired in the usual state organization for the care of the insane. It was essential that there should be harmonious cooperation with the asylums of the state, and at the same time the new hospital should be an integral part of the University Medical School. The state had been divided into districts, each sending its insane to an asylum. The best method would be for the Psychopathic Hospital to draw its patients from a district of its own, but this was not possible. Accordingly it was provided that the institution should be of such a special type of organization that its patients could come from any part of the state. It should also be in such relation with the asylums of the state that patients could be sent from the asylums to the psychopathic ward, and be transferred from this hospital to the asylums.

[1] By Dr. A. M. Barrett.

[2] Act 161, Public Acts of 1901.

As stated in the act, patients could be admitted to the psychopathic ward under any of the following provisions:

I. In cases where application is made to send persons claimed to be insane to any of the insane asylums in the State of Michigan, "the judge of probate before whom said application is pending may require the assistance of three competent and skilled physicians, who shall investigate the condition of the patient and report the same to the judge of probate in writing; and if said judge of probate shall, upon such investigation, ascertain that there are present in the condition of the patient such features as render detention in a suitable psychopathic hospital advisable as a precautionary or curative measure, or if, from such investigation, said judge of probate shall be of the opinion that the case requires the services of trained and well-recognized specialists in the treatment of disorders other than those of the nervous system, he shall pass a decree or decretal order, directing such afflicted person to be transported for treatment to said Psychopathic Ward or Hospital of the University of Michigan, and shall further order that in case the said patient, while in said psychopathic ward, shall recover, said patient shall be forthwith discharged, but in case said patient shall not recover, then, upon certificate of the head of the department of nervous diseases of the Hospital of the University of Michigan, that said person is insane and should be confined in one of the asylums of the State of Michigan, the said afflicted person shall be transported to and confined in such insane asylum as said judge of probate shall designate in his said decree or decretal order.

II. In case the superintendent of either of the asylums for the insane shall be of the opinion that the condition of mind of any person who shall have been, or who shall hereafter be, confined in such asylum, is caused by some malady or disease that, under treatment of a specialist, might be cured, and the patient restored to sanity, he shall cause such person to be conveyed to said psychopathic ward, and in case such patient shall, while confined in said ward, be restored to sanity, such patient shall be discharged, but in case such patient shall be found incurable, the superintendent of the University Hospital, of which said psychopathic ward is a part, shall cause said insane person to be returned to the asylum from which such patient was received, the charges for the care, maintenance and transportation to be paid by the respective counties or by the state as the patient may be a county or a state charge.

Private patients could be admitted to the ward in the same manner as public. The charge for their maintenance was to be fixed by the regents of the State University.

The psychopathic ward was to be an additional ward of the General Hospital of the University and under its management, control and regulation. The superintendent of the University Hospital was to be the administrative officer of the psychopathic ward.

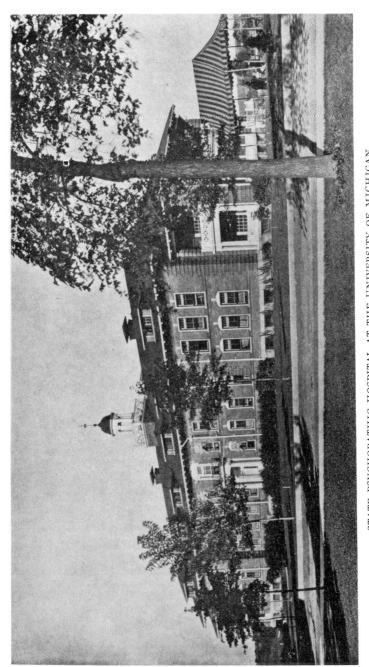

STATE PSYCHOPATHIC HOSPITAL AT THE UNIVERSITY OF MICHIGAN.

The bills for the per capita cost of maintenance of public patients were to be rendered monthly by the treasurer of the university to the county of which the patient was a resident.

By the above provisions the psychopathic ward was entirely under the control of the university. No provision was made for its medical control, apart from the department of nervous and mental diseases of the university, except that the superintendents of the several asylums of the state were to be members of the clinical staff of the psychopathic ward.

The erection of the building was placed in charge of a committee of the Board of Regents, and in 1902 work was begun. The plans for the building were prepared by architects Mason & Kahn, of Detroit. It is a brick building, two stories and a half high, with a high basement. It is 188 feet long, 47 feet wide, and is of fireproof construction. The internal arrangement of the building consists of a central division, with wards on either side. The center of the building on the first floor contains the medical offices, reception rooms, general office and a room now used as a psychological laboratory. On the second floor are the living rooms of the resident physician and the head nurse. The wards on the north side of the center are for men, and those on the south for women. Each ward on the first floor has 7 beds and on the second 13 beds. The only division it has been possible to make, with such limited facilities for classification, is to reserve the lower floor wards for the more disturbed patients, while all others are cared for on the second floor. Each ward has its dining and serving rooms, closets, toilet and bathrooms. The wards for the more disturbed patients have two tubs arranged for giving prolonged warm baths. One end of each ward has a large sun room, which serves as a general sitting room. The third floor contains living rooms for the male attendants and for the domestics of the hospital.

The basement has in its south half the kitchens, store rooms and dining rooms for employees. The north end is occupied by the hydrotherapeutic room and laboratories. The hydrotherapeutic room is very completely equipped with a Baruch apparatus, and is extensively used in the treatment of the patients. Several rooms are devoted to laboratory purposes. The equipment consists of the necessary apparatus for conducting research into the problems connected with the study of insanity and diseases of the nervous system. A psychological laboratory has been arranged and equipped for clinical and experimental investigations in the problems of abnormal psychology.

The progress of the building was delayed by many complications resulting from the failure of the original act to provide for a medical director and to appropriate money for the payment of his salary and for the research work which would naturally be a function of such an institution.

It had become evident that some closer affiliation with the asylums of the state would be necessary, in view of the intimate relations which must necessarily exist in the interchange of patients. The plan, which was developed during the years before the legislative session of 1905, was to make the psychopathic ward an institution where a laboratory for the investigation of problems in relation to insanity could be maintained in which all of the state asylums for the insane could cooperate, but still keep the entire organization in as close relation with the university as possible. These difficulties were remedied by the passage of an act by the Legislature of 1905.[1] This act provided that the joint boards of trustees of the asylums for the insane of this state, in conjuction with the Board of Regents of the State University, should select and employ " an experienced investigator in clinical psychiatry who should be placed in charge of the psychopathic ward," " and whose duty it shall be to conduct the clinical and pathological investigations therein, to direct the treatment of such patients as are inmates of the psychopathic ward, to guide and direct the work of clinical and pathological research in the several asylums of the state, and to instruct the students of the medical department of the university in diseases of the mind." The title chosen was to be " Pathologist of the State Asylums for the Insane and Associate Professor of Neural-Pathology." There was to be established and maintained in the psychopathic ward a clinical laboratory of research, " in which investigations shall be continuously carried on with a view of determining the nature and causes of insanity and of perfecting the means of prevention and cure of diseases of this nature."

To meet the expenses for salaries and the maintenance of the laboratory there was to be annually appropriated $5000. The act

[1] Act 140, Public Acts of 1905.

further provided for an appropriation of $14,000 for the equipment of the ward and laboratory.

By the provisions of this act of 1905 the asylums shared with the Board of Regents of the State University in the control of the new ward. From the beginning Dr. Herdman had taken personal direction of the carrying out of the plans for the arrangement of the building, and these were adopted with but slight changes by the committee in control.

In accordance with the act of 1905 a committee from the joint asylum boards of trustees was appointed to act with a similar committee from the Board of Regents. This joint committee met on August 9, 1905, in the regents' room of the university. There were present from the boards of trustees of the state asylums, Trustees Chauncey F. Cook, of the Michigan Asylum; F. S. Case, of the Upper Peninsula Asylum, and G. Jay Vinton, of the Eastern Michigan Asylum. From the Board of Regents there were present Regents C. D. Lawton, L. E. Knappen and H. W. Carey. The committee took charge of the building, which had been practically completed under the direction of the Board of Regents, and entered upon its equipment and the organization of its medical work.

At a second meeting on September 13, 1905, a formal organization of the committee was made with Chauncey F. Cook as chairman and E. S. Gilmore, superintendent of the University Hospital, as secretary. At this meeting the committee appointed as pathologist of the state asylums for the insane and associate professor of neural-pathology in the psychopathic ward, Dr. Albert M. Barrett, who was then pathologist of the Danvers (Mass.) Hospital for the Insane and assistant in neural-pathology in the Harvard University Medical School. Dr. Barrett began his work on January 1, 1906.

On agreement with the superintendents of the state asylums and on the authority of the provisions allowing patients to be transferred from the asylums to the psychopathic ward, there were sent to the ward on February 7, 1906, 37 patients from the asylums at Kalamazoo and Pontiac, and on the above date the work of the hospital was formally begun.

In the administrative work new problems were continually presenting themselves, and it soon became evident to those in control that the difficulties could be remedied only by new provisions authorized by the Legislature. These difficulties came about through the failure of the acts relating to the ward to provide for certain contingencies which arose, especially in matters pertaining to the admission and discharge of patients. It also seemed advisable that the controlling organization should be a board of trustees rather than a committee. It seemed that these and other administrative difficulties could be solved in a satisfactory manner only by making the psychopathic ward an institution organized as an independent hospital, but yet in such close relations to the university that they should be mutually helpful. The most important difficulty related to the provisions for the support of patients at the psychopathic ward. It was evident that an institution carrying on the specialized work for which the psychopathic ward was organized could not care for the patients at as low a cost as could the asylums. With careful administration the daily per capita cost for maintenance was more than one dollar. The rate of maintenance in the asylums of the lower peninsula was 49 cents per diem. The effect of this soon showed itself in a progressive decrease in the number of public patients sent to the psychopathic ward. It was very evident that some change in the method of supporting patients would be necessary. The county authorities could not be expected to send patients to the ward when they could be sent elsewhere for at least half the cost. As it was essential to have these provisions at least, changed by legislative action, it was thought best by the committee in control of the psychopathic ward to embody them in an act which should also provide for other matters, and establish the psychopathic ward in as ideal a way as seemed possible under the conditions which existed in this state. A bill with this end in view was prepared by the pathologist and approved by the committee in control of the psychopathic ward. This was introduced in the Legislature of 1907 by Senator Bates, and after its passage was approved by Governor Warner on June 27, 1907.

By this act the former act was repealed and the psychopathic ward became the State Psychopathic Hospital at the University of Michigan. It was to be a "state hospital especially designed, equipped and administered for the care, observation and treatment of insanity and for those persons who are afflicted with abnormal mental states, but are not insane." Its control was placed in a board of trustees composed of four members chosen from the boards of trustees of the Michigan asylums for the insane, and four members chosen from the Board of Regents of the State University. This provision gives in one governing board a most satisfactory union of university and asylum interest. This board has all the powers which legislative action has assigned to boards of trustees of the state asylums.

The administrative head of the Psychopathic Hospital is the medical director, who is, by virtue of his position, the pathologist of the state asylums for the insane, and, with the approval of the Board of Regents of the State University, shall hold the position of professor of psychiatry in the department of medicine and surgery of the State University. The medical director of the Psychopathic Hospital is the pathologist of the state asylums for the insane, and it is his duty to advise regarding the clinical and pathological research in the several asylums of the state and to maintain a systematic cooperation between the several asylums and the Psychopathic Hospital. He shall from time to time visit the asylums of the state and may advise and instruct the medical officers of such asylums in subjects relating to the phenomena of insanity. The expenses incurred in these visits shall be charged to the account of the asylum visited.

The provisions for the admission of patients are enlarged over those in the former act. Patients may be admitted to the Psychopathic Hospital by any of the following procedures:

I. Any judge of probate may commit any insane person to the Psychopathic Hospital whom the director regards as a suitable patient for the hospital.

II. A person may be sent to the Psychopathic Hospital as an observation patient for a period not longer than 35 days for any of the following reasons:

1. When the judge of probate may have doubt as to whether the person is insane and desires such data as could be furnished by an observation under such conditions as the Psychopathic Hospital can furnish.

2. When the mental condition of the person is associated with complicating physical disease, which may be benefited by treatment by the physicians and surgeons of the General Hospital of the university.

3. When the judge of probate regards a decree of insanity as inadvisable, as when the disease will be of such short duration as to recover within the period of 35 days.

In the order sending a person for observation to the Psychopathic Hospital, the patient is described as a person afflicted with some nervous or mental disease and is not declared to be insane. It further states that the person shall be confined and treated in the Psychopathic Hospital for a period not to exceed 35 days. Before this time expires the director of the hospital shall return to the judge of probate the results of the observation and treatment and an opinion stating whether the patient is insane or sane. If the observation shall show that the patient is insane, then the judge may commit the person as insane to the Psychopathic Hospital, or to any of the state asylums, or any other institution in the state for the care of the insane, or he may take any other action which is provided for by the general insanity laws of the state. If the observation shows that the patient is sane or if the patient becomes sane before the expiration of the period of observation, the patient must be discharged from the Psychopathic Hospital.

III. The superintendent of any one of the asylums for the insane in the State of Michigan may transfer any patient in his institution to the Psychopathic Hospital whenever it is his opinion that the patient may be benefited by the special facilities which the Psychopathic Hospital offers.

IV. Any person who is afflicted mentally or with serious nervous disorder, but who is not insane, may be admitted to the Psychopathic Hospital as a voluntary private patient at the discretion of the director of that hospital. In all orders committing patients to the Psychopathic Hospital the judge of probate specifies that in case such a patient shall not recover after a satisfactory period of observation and treatment, or whenever, in the opinion of the director of the Psychopathic Hospital, further residence in this hospital is inadvisable, such a patient shall be transferred to the state asylum for the insane designated in the order of committal.

Provision is made that patients may be transferred from the Psychopathic Hospital to the wards of the General Hospital, for special medical or surgical treatment, such treatment to be furnished by the staff of the hospital without charge, except for maintenance. The expenses for the maintenance of public patients at the Psychopathic Hospital are paid by the state, and during the first year of the patient's confinement as a public patient the state collects from the county in which the patient resides the daily rate which has been fixed for the maintenance of public patients in the asylum located in the district of which the patient was a legal resident. Private patients must pay for their maintenance whatever rate the Board of Trustees may fix. The rate has been $15 per week since the hospital was opened. In addition, those responsible for the support of a private patient must make an advance payment of $50 at the time the patient is admitted, and file an approved bond to the treasurer of the Psychopathic Hospital in the sum of $1000 as a guarantee of payments for the maintenance of the patient.

The superintendent of the General Hospital of the university is the business officer of the Psychopathic Hospital, and the treasurer is the treasurer of the University of Michigan.

The laboratory work at the Psychopathic Hospital and the relation of the hospital to the scientific work in the asylums are provided for as follows:

> There shall be maintained as a part of the Psychopathic Hospital a clinical pathological laboratory, which shall be a central laboratory for the Michigan state asylums for the insane, and a laboratory in which research into the phenomena and pathology of mental diseases shall be carried on.
>
> It shall be provided by rules of the trustees and the joint asylum boards that the medical officers of the several asylums shall from time to time receive instruction at the Psychopathic Hospital at the expense of the asylums respectively.

The support of the laboratory work and the payment of the salaries of the physicians are provided for by an annual appropriation of $10,000.

The medical and administrative work is in charge of the director and two assistant physicians, one of whom resides in the hospital.

The nursing of the patients is under the supervision of a trained nurse of much experience in caring for the insane. Graduate nurses are in immediate charge of the wards, and on the women's wards are assisted by pupil nurses of the General Hospital Training School, who spend three months of their course at the Psychopathic Hospital. The men are cared for by experienced male attendants.

Since its opening the hospital has at all times been well filled and the demand for admission far exceeds the ability of the hospital to satisfy. At the present time the monthly admissions to the hospital average about 20 new cases.

Since the opening of the hospital students of the medical department have enjoyed unusual opportunities in the study of mental diseases. Clinical lectures have been given each week to the senior class and groups of students have been given bedside work in the wards of the hospital. In the laboratories, courses have been given in the pathological anatomy of mental diseases, and systematic research has been carried on into the pathology of insanity, some of which has already appeared in publication.

The maintenance of a helpful relation of the hospital and its laboratories to the larger state hospitals for the insane has been an important part of the work. From the first the medical officers of the several institutions have shown a warm interest in the hospital, and there has been a systematic cooperation established between it and the various institutions caring for the insane. The hospitals for the insane send a considerable amount of anatomical material to the laboratories of the Psychopathic Hospital, accompanied by full clinical records. The results of the study of this material have been communicated to the institutions on routine visits of the director of the Psychopathic Hospital.

The hospital has passed out of the period of experiment and has become firmly established as an intimate part of Michigan's system for the care of the insane.

ELOISE HOSPITAL.

NANKIN, MICH.

"Eloise" is the name used to designate the various Wayne County buildings, located on Michigan Avenue, Nankin, 16 miles west of Detroit. There are three distinct groups of buildings, known as Eloise Infirmary, Eloise Sanitarium, and Eloise Hospital.

The original Wayne County Poorhouse was organized by a vote of the people of Detroit on March 8, 1832. It was moved to its present location in 1839.

In 1872 its name was changed to Wayne County Almshouse, and continued as such until 1886, when it was changed to Wayne County House. On June 2, 1911, the name "Eloise Infirmary" was officially adopted in place of "Wayne County House" and "Eloise Hospital" for the group of buildings devoted to the treatment of mental diseases, then known by the name of "Wayne County Asylum."

The first reference to insane inmates of the poorhouse of Wayne County appears March 22, 1841. At this time Bridget Hughes was admitted and the entry "crazy" was placed beside her name in the register. She remained only 13 days and disappeared, to be readmitted January 5, 1842, with five other persons and to remain until her death March 8, 1895, after a residence of 53 years. She is spoken of as a "harmless old soul," who was never sent to the "crazy house," but remained an inmate of the poorhouse building all her days.

The books of the county almshouse, especially the entry in the repair account, indicate that the so-called "crazy house" was built for the violent insane soon after 1842. Some years later a frame building two stories high was built for "colored paupers" on the first floor and "other persons," undoubtedly insane, on the second floor. The upper floor was constructed with strong cells, in which were chains fastened to the walls for securing the insane.

An order is recorded that the judge of the circuit court had directed that two insane criminals, then in the house of correction, should be accommodated in the Wayne County Almshouse. For several years this building was the only provision for the insane in the state.

In 1858 the statement is made by the superintendents of the poor that 29 cases of insanity had been treated during the year, and that 17 still remained under treatment, of which number 12 required to be confined continuously in cells.

The first institution for the insane, that at Kalamazoo, known as the Michigan Asylum, was not opened until August, 1859, and when opened the amount of accommodation was so small it was not possible to receive any great number of the insane who required treatment.

In 1867 the superintendent of the poor of Wayne County sent a letter to several eminent physicians residing in Detroit, informing them that there were in the almshouse 48 incurable cases of insanity, who required care and treatment, and asked that a committee of physicians be appointed to visit the almshouse at an early day to suggest the best course to pursue in regard to cases of incurable insanity. The physicians complied with the request and within a few days a committee visited the institution and made a thorough examination. They recommended that a separate asylum be built to provide for these patients, which was accordingly done, and $10,000 was appropriated, after a great deal of discussion, for the purpose. A building for them was finally constructed in connection with the county house, which cost with furnishings about $25,000. It was opened for patients in August, 1869.

For a few years everything went smoothly. In October, 1872, however, when the superintendents of the poor presented their estimates for the coming year, they requested the purchase of an adjoining farm of 157 acres for the use of the so-called asylum. The matter was referred to a committee, which made an unfavorable report and asked for the appointment of a committee to visit the institution to look into its general management. The report complained of the lack of ventilation, the absence of bathing facilities, the untidy habits of the patients, the need of better clothing and food, and concluded with the recommendation that all the insane be sent to the State Asylum. No action was taken, however, and in 1875 an appropriation of $7000 was asked for from the supervisors for the erection of an extension to the asylum. The addition when completed cost rather more than $15,000. In 1879, however, it became necessary to ask for an appropriation for another building. The sum of $41,000 was asked for.

In 1881 the crowded condition at the Wayne County institution was met by the transfer of patients to state hospitals. During this year an important change took place in the management of the asylum. Previous to this time the institution had been under the care of a keeper, but by a resolution of the board of superintendents in 1881 he was requested to resign, and a resolution was adopted that in the future the keeper of the asylum should be a physician in good standing, who should also be physician to both the almshouse and asylum. At the same time Dr. E. O. Bennett and wife were appointed as medical superintendent and matron and during the next 19 years they filled their positions in a creditable manner.

as made for an extension
...mpleted at a cost of $4000 and
... female patients. A laundry was
...000. The remainder of the appropria-
... in providing for an extension of the male
...struction enabled them to do away with all the
ce... basements and increased the capacity of the establish-
me... y 58 patients.

In 1890, by act of the Legislature, the Wayne County Asylum was legalized and it was provided that patients might be committed to the Wayne County Asylum instead of the State Asylum, and if they were supported in this institution at the expense of the county for two years, the expense for their support should be transferred to the State of Michigan. This action placed the institution on the same footing as other state hospitals and gave a broader field for its activities.

In the early winter of 1892, owing to the destruction by fire of one wing of the Eastern Michigan Asylum, 75 patients from Wayne County were transferred from that institution. It accordingly became necessary to erect a building for 70 patients and to buy an additional 200 acres of ground for use in connection with the Wayne County Asylum. During the year a new building, called the women's building, was erected at a cost of $35,000. In 1899 the old asylum was remodeled at a cost of $33,000.

In 1900 Dr. E. O. Bennett, who had been connected with the hospital for 19 years, resigned and was succeeded by Dr. John J. Marker, who had been a house physician of the County House, and assistant medical superintendent of the asylum.

In 1903 a new building was erected at a cost of $68,000. The number of patients in the institution June 25, 1913, was 576—287 were men and 289 were women.

The institution is housed in a substantial building, provided with all essentials of good heating, adequate ventilation, a good water supply and pumping plant, and a power and electric light plant.

ST. JOSEPH'S RETREAT.

Dearborn, Mich.

In the early history of Michigan prior to the construction of a single state institution the Sisters of Charity, who were then connected with St. Mary's Hospital, Detroit, began to receive acute cases of insanity at that hospital. The location of St. Mary's being not well adapted to the care of the insane, the Sisters of Charity established themselves in a farm house on a tract of 20 acres, on what is now West Boulevard and Michigan Avenue, and began to take care of their insane patients at their new location.

At first the work was conducted in a small way, but during the Civil War the government paid liberal sums of money to St. Mary's Hospital for the care of soldiers who were sent to Detroit. These funds were used to construct on the above-mentioned site a brick building for 80 insane persons, which was opened in 1870, and from this time forward all connection with St. Mary's Hospital was terminated.

In 1874 a part of the original tract of 20 acres was changed for 100 acres in the vicinity of Dearborn, about ten miles from the City of Detroit, and ten years later 40 additional acres were purchased.

Here, within easy reach of Detroit, could be had freedom from noise and dust, pure country air, spacious grounds for the patients, and, not least, direct supervision of the fields, gardens and animals depended upon to yield necessaries not easily procurable in a fresh state in urban markets. Steps to effect the change were taken speedily, and the corner-stone of the great structure in which the work is being carried on to-day was laid November 1, 1885.

At first what might be called the main building—now known as the "center"—and the first east wing, with detached steam power and electric plant, were erected. The house was blessed October 28, 1886, and the Sisters and 99 patients were installed in it a few days later.

The following year the property at Michigan Avenue and Twenty-fourth Street was sold, the proceeds being added to the resources of the Retreat.

So rapidly did the number of patients increase that in 1887 the construction of the first west wing was begun; this was completed in February, 1888. In the same year was built a commodious and thoroughly equipped laundry. A model brick barn and stable, a large kitchen addition and pavilions in the recreation grounds were erected in 1894.

By 1896 the women's quarters were filled, so the second east wing was added. The same congested condition on the men's side in 1905 made a second west wing necessary, and the chapel was built in the same year.

A cold storage plant, with ice machine, was put in operation in 1909, and the ice house which had done service from the beginning was demolished. In the following winter a greenhouse was built.

There are no wards. Every room is separated from those adjoining it and from the corridors upon which it opens by a solid brick wall two feet thick, which has its foundation below the basement and extends to the attic, so that each tier of rooms is practically a separate building. Metal lath is used in the ceilings; the floors are of hardwood; in every attendant's apartment and in the wardrobe of every hall is a fire hose attached to pipes which run from huge tanks of water in the attic; there are seven of these tanks, and they contain at all times 44,000 gallons of water supplied by pumps that never stop; steam is kept up in the boiler house day and night, summer and winter; scores of chemical fire extinguishers are distributed about the house.

The arrangement of the building, with long wings extending from the imposing center, is such that every room is flooded with sunshine during a part of the day. Every room has its own ventilating shafts, and a copious supply of fresh air comes through flues equipped with steam coils.

The patients are classified according to the nature or extent of their affliction, and provision is made for keeping each class by itself. To this end 15 halls, with broad corridors, spacious apartments and high ceilings, are arranged on each side of the building.

The halls occupied by men have smoking rooms and sunny alcoves, while for those who can enjoy them there are billiards, cards and other games. In the women's halls are large sitting rooms and alcoves, with pianos, house plants and the knick-knacks dear to the feminine heart. Here the patients beguile the time with music, reading or sewing.

Every hall is in charge of a Sister, who aims at making it a home and under whose direction the paid attendants must strive for the same end.

Even the mildest form of restraint is regarded as undesirable, and is resorted to only when absolutely unavoidable.

No patient, whatever his status or condition, may be treated otherwise than with respect, and even a slighting word from an attendant is held to justify summary discharge.

A source of great pleasure for the patients is the entertainment hall, which has a seating capacity of 300, with stage, scenery and all other necessary appurtenances. Concerts, dramas, moving pictures, etc., are presented at frequent intervals.

The present premises consist of 140 acres, 22 of which are natural woods. They are situated on the River Rouge, from which the water supply is conducted and purified by filtration. The present value of the plant is $1,225,000.

There are no work-shops or special methods of employment, but many facilities for outdoor life.

From 1855 to 1873 the medical department was under the charge of Dr. Hugo Gilmartin, with Drs. Zina Pitcher and David Farrand as consultants. From 1873 to 1908 the medical work was under the direction of Dr. J. G. Johnson, associated with whom, from 1890 until 1908, was Dr. J. E. Emerson; from 1908 until 1914, Dr. David R. Clark. Dr. Johnson died in 1908 and Dr. Emerson became chief of the staff, with Dr. Clark as physician-in-charge, assisted by a house staff.

The Retreat has a well-equipped laboratory for all clinical examinations, and facilities are also furnished to outside investigators for research work.

The nursing of the Retreat is under the executive care of 31 Sisters of Charity, assisted by trained nurses and orderlies.

The food is prepared in a central kitchen and transferred to 15 ward dining rooms by steam-jacketed electric elevators. There are six special diet kitchens in connection with the wards.

There is no training school, but lectures are given by the members of the executive staff to graduate nurses on special topics.

The large cold storage plant renders it possible to purchase perishable supplies in large quantities. Beef is purchased by the car-load and butter is the whole product of a creamery in a neighboring county.

As a reform in the management of the insane, it must be added that hydrotherapy has been substituted for mechanical restraint. It is also an assistance in the abrupt withdrawal of drugs and liquors and the treatment of toxæmias of this character.

The present name, St. Joseph's Retreat, was adopted November 1, 1883, when the Sisters filed new articles of incorporation. In July, 1885, Sister Mary De Sales resigned, and she was succeeded by the present superior, Sister Mary Borgia.

OAK GROVE HOSPITAL.[1]

Flint, Mich.

Oak Grove,[2] a hospital for the treatment of nervous and mental diseases, located in Flint, Mich., incorporated under " An Act to Authorize the Formation of Health Institutions, Approved March 16, 1867; Chapter 185 of Howell's Statutes," was organized " for the purpose of establishing an institution for the treatment of insanity and imparting instruction in the principles of hygiene."

The articles of association, dated April 28, 1890, were recorded in the office of the Secretary of State May 5 of the same year. Under the original articles, the capital stock was placed at $100,000. On August 9, 1905, in order that additions to the then existing hospital group might be built, it was increased to $125,000.

Among the signers of the original articles and those to whom the first certificates of stock were issued are comprised the names of a justice of the United States Supreme Court, who was the first president of the association, two former Governors of Michigan, four superintendents, a treasurer and five trustees of state institutions for the insane, a member of the State Board of Corrections and Charities, a physician in active practice in Detroit, and the principal owner of a general sanitarium then in operation in

[1] By C. B. Burr, M. D.

[2] Originally Oak Grove Sanitarium, name changed by vote of the stockholders, June 18, 1891.

Michigan. Seven of the foregoing were closely related to mental invalids for whom treatment at home was impossible or inexpedient, and several others of the stockholders bore near or remote relation to patients for whom public hospitals were not available or who, excluded therefrom when room was deficient, were compelled to seek shelter in some institution in a remote part of the country.

It will be observed how compelling were the sentiments which dominated these men in the new undertaking, and the enthusiasm with which the enterprise was begun and carried on may be inferred from the urgent need which its founders believed it would supply. At the time of its inception there was no hospital, so far as the writer is aware, in the United States which was planned, built and equipped to care for a few patients on a liberal scale of expenditure. Private establishments for a limited number there were elsewhere, to be sure, but these had been country places transformed, and were not purposefully built for the end to which they were eventually placed.

The locating committee carefully inspected several proposed sites. Almost by chance the one selected came to its attention, and it is perhaps not too much to claim that the location of the buildings has preserved to Flint and to Michigan a natural oak park of more than 60 acres which, in the rapid development of a progressive and commercial city, would surely have been annihilated. As it is, this beautiful grove, containing in the neighborhood of 1000 native forest trees, many of which are of immense size, has been conserved for the public benefit. There has been up to this time practically no restriction laid upon its use within the bounds of reason and expediency by the people of Flint and the nearby country.

Happily little has been done in the way of "ornamental" landscape work. Vines and flowering shrubs of luxuriant growth are in close proximity to buildings; but in its depth the grove remains in natural loveliness.

Through the wise vision of the late James A. Remick, of Detroit, an ideal location of the buildings was affected. These were fronted southeast as to the administration building, nearly east as to the department for women and almost south as to the department for men. The buildings form an artistic group, are practically free from dark corners, and although located in the

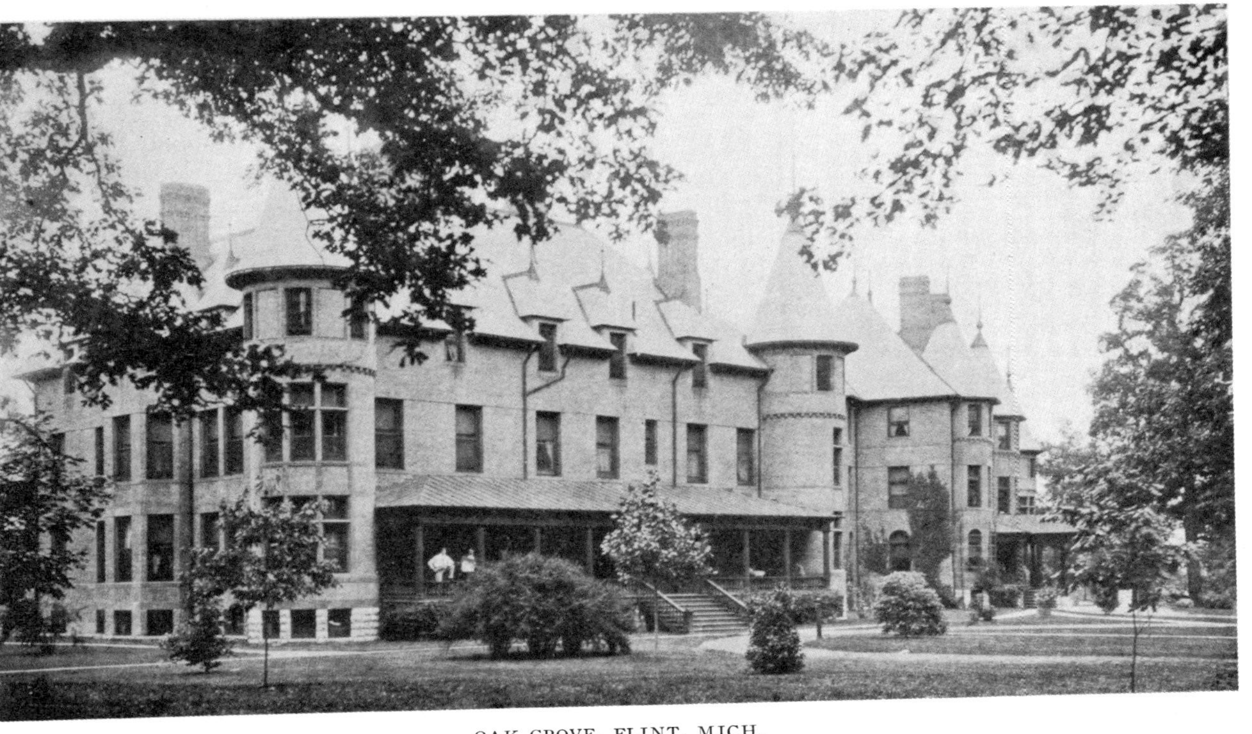

OAK GROVE, FLINT, MICH.

midst of a grove, have the benefit of direct sunlight in practically every room at some time during the day.

There were associated in the incipiency of the movement to establish Oak Grove James A. Remick and W. G. Vinton, of Detroit; Charles T. Mitchell, of Hillsdale, and Dr. George C. Palmer, then superintendent of the Michigan Asylum for the Insane, at Kalamazoo. Of these the moving spirit and the practical founder of the hospital was James A. Remick. He was a practical lumberman, but an idealist and philanthropist. He had served as a member of the Board of Trustees of the Eastern Michigan Asylum, at Pontiac, and was looked upon by its officers as one of the most liberal and dependable in the board's membership. He lived to enjoy the knowledge of Oak Grove's prosperity, its management determined by the broad policies which he furthered.

The original buildings were erected by the Vinton Company, of Detroit, whose president, W. G. Vinton, was also president of the Board of Trustees of the Eastern Michigan Asylum. He had been for three years a member of the building commission of that institution, and served as trustee from the organization in 1878 until 1897.

Mr. Vinton succeeded Justice H. B. Brown as president of Oak Grove Corporation and was himself succeeded by George B. Remick, of Detroit. Mr. Remick was a cultured and scholarly man, of cordial manners and gentle disposition. He died in 1913 and was succeeded as president by Dr. W. H. Sawyer, of Hillsdale, a regent of the University of Michigan.

Of the original stockholders of Oak Grove but six are living at the present writing (January, 1914), and of this number none are of the early boards of directors, which latter have included James A. Remick, W. G. Vinton, G. J. Vinton, George B. Remick and Thomas Pitts, of Detroit; C. T. Mitchell, of Hillsdale; Wm. L. Smith and Wm. Hamilton, of Flint. The composition of the present board is as follows: Dr. W. H. Sawyer, Hillsdale, president; Jerome H. Remick, Detroit, vice-president; Dr. C. B. Burr, Flint, secretary; Walter O. Smith, Flint, treasurer; C. M. Begole, Flint; Dr. H. R. Niles, Flint; Wm. A. Butler, Jr., Detroit; Dr. E. A. Christian, Pontiac, and S. T. Crapo, Detroit.

Dr. Geo. C. Palmer, who had been medical superintendent of the Michigan Asylum for the Insane, at Kalamazoo, was upon its organization unanimously elected medical director of Oak Grove. He died on the 8th of August, 1894, much lamented by patients, by the directors and employees of Oak Grove and by the medical profession in Michigan.

During Dr. Palmer's illness Dr. W. L. Worcester was elected acting medical director. He was succeeded in November, 1894, by Dr. C. B. Burr, who had spent 11 years as assistant physician and assistant superintendent, and five years as medical superintendent of the Eastern Michigan Asylum, at Pontiac. He organized the training school of the Eastern Michigan Asylum in 1890 and wrote for convenience in teaching "A Primer of Psychology and Mental Disease."

The staff of the hospital is composed of two besides the medical director. There have served Oak Grove in the capacity of assistant physician or assistant medical director with conspicuous efficiency and fidelity, Dr. Wadsworth Warren, of Detroit; Dr. H. R. Niles, of the Michigan School for the Deaf, in Flint; Dr. C. B. Macartney, of Thorold, Ontario; Drs. F. B. Miner and C. P. Clarke, Flint; Dr. J. A. Elliott, of Battle Creek; Dr. E. R. Johnstone, of Bancroft; Drs. H. L. Trenkle and Samuel Butler, of the Pontiac State Hospital; Dr. H. E. Clarke, formerly of the Pontiac State Hospital, and Dr. P. M. Crawford, formerly of Chicago. The two latter are still members of the staff. The medical work is supervised by the medical director, the detail being in charge of the assistant.

The site, original buildings and equipment cost in the neighborhood of $135,000, $35,000 of which was met by the issue of bonds. In 1895 Noyes Hall, containing billiard rooms, assembly hall, gymnasium, bowling alley, electrical room and hydrotherapeutic rooms, was completed from funds in part provided by the bequest of Dr. James F. Noyes, of Detroit, and in part from the revenues of the hospital.

The Parterre Building was built in 1900 to accommodate patients of the restless class. The arrangement of this building and that of the Ormeau, built in 1906, providing accommodation for acute cases among men, has been most satisfactory. An important feature of these buildings is the opening of the rooms for patients who are noisy upon an enclosed vestibule. Free circulation of outside air as necessary is provided through tilting windows located at the ceiling. The Ormeau is provided with a tub for continuous baths and both buildings have shower baths.

The dietary is liberal and varied. The dining rooms communicate with the kitchen, which is equipped with a modern cold storage system provided by brine circulation. Ice in sufficient quantities for the use of the hospital is made daily.

The nursing is directed by head nurses, a man for the men's, a woman for the women's departments respectively. No training school has been organized, it being thought undesirable in view of the small clinic.

There is a detached boiler house and electric light plant (built in 1906) and a 1200-ton brick coal shed (built in 1907). There is a large and well-equipped basement laundry.

It has been the aim of the medical staff to introduce as much of the home spirit as possible into the lives of patients. To this end friends living in Flint are invited to the hospital's house parties and patients are interested in society and church matters in the city. The "apart" feeling which in the early days of the hospital was noticeable is no longer in existence, and in theatrical, church and social activities patients have a large place. The nursing force is large, special nurses are in frequent requisition, and vigilance must make up for the noticeable lack of window guards and other "safety first" appliances.

The daily average of patients is in the neighborhood of 50.

APPENDIX A.

Report of Commission.

In connection with the history of the insane in Michigan, it is interesting to note that in the year 1913 a commission was appointed, consisting of the medical director of the State Psychopathic Hospital, the Superintendent of Public Instruction, the secretary of the State Board of Health, and the secretary of the State Board of Corrections and Charities, to investigate the extent of insanity, feeble-mindedness and epilepsy in the State of Michigan, and the causes productive of it.

The commission made a careful study of conditions in the state and published in 1915 the following general conclusions as to insanity:

> In Michigan the ratio of insane in institutional care is 27 per 10,000 of the general population. This ratio is about the same as that of states having the same general geographic position and less than in certain older states, with larger facilities for the care of the insane.

60

There has been an increase of 145.2 per cent of the insane in institutional care in the past 24 years. In large part this increase is due to an increase of institutional capacity.

There has been an increase of 43.7 per cent in the total admissions to the Michigan state hospitals for the insane in the past 14 years.

The annual admission of new cases of insanity has increased 62.7 per cent between 1901 and 1914.

The fact that the ratio of admissions estimated to 10,000 of the population has increased from 4.5 in 1901 to 5.9 in 1910 indicates that the character of the population has changed.

Between 1901 and 1910 the population has increased 16.1 per cent and the annual admission of new patients has increased 51.3 per cent.

The foreign-born population furnishes a much larger proportion of the annual admissions to the state hospitals for the insane than does the native born, the ratio for 10,000 foreign-born being 8.9 and for native born, 5.4.

Native born of foreign parents have a rate of admission 166 per cent greater than a native born of native parents.

Of the foreign population, Russia (including Poland), Finland, Scotland and Ireland have a higher rate in relation to their numbers in the state than other foreign nationalities.

The highest rates of admission are in districts having a population of 2000 to 5000.

All counties having large state hospitals for the insane have the highest ratio of admissions, in proportion to their population. It is supposed that fewer insane individuals in these counties escape commitment to institutions, owing to their proximity and greater familiarity with institutional administration.

There is reason to believe that the rate in these counties approaches the truer number of insane needing commitment than in counties having lower rates.

The counties of the upper peninsula have relatively higher rates in proportion to the population than those of the lower peninsula. Insanity is most liable to occur between the ages of 30 and 39. The age of greatest frequency in Michigan has changed in the past 20 years from the ages between 25 and 30 to the ages between 35 and 40. Within recent years there has been a great increase in the proportion of admissions of individuals above the age of 50.

In general, males contribute a relatively larger proportion of insane individuals than do females. There has been in recent years a relatively larger increase in the proportion of male admissions than females.

Alcohol is the direct cause of insanity in 8.4 per cent of all admissions to Michigan state hospitals for the insane. Alcoholic insanity is 6.5 per cent as frequent in males as females. This form of insanity is, however, relatively frequent among females, this sex contributing 13.2 per cent of all cases of this disease. Of the insane, 31.2 per cent are more than moderate in their use of alcoholic drinks.

Drug habits are productive of only a small proportion of the cases of insanity admitted to the state hospitals.

Syphilis is the cause of 12.9 per cent of the cases of insanity annually admitted to the Michigan state hospitals. It was the direct cause of insanity in 17.5 per cent of all males and 6.65 per cent of all females admitted. As shown by the Wassermann test, 21.6 per cent of all insane have syphilis.

The conjugal mates of 38.18 per cent of all individuals having paresis have syphilis.

In 44.8 per cent the marriages of paretics are childless and their number of living children is abnormally low.

Heredity is the most important and far-reaching influence in the production of insanity.

Of the insane, 65.4 per cent have insanity or nervous abnormalities present in their ancestors or families. In 58.3 per cent the transmission was from parent to child. The most frequent hereditary influence is insanity, this being present in 58.7 per cent of those who had any hereditary influence.

The total number of abnormal individuals is strikingly high in families of the insane.

A study of epilepsy and defective mentality showed that out of 1141 individuals under treatment in the Home and Training School at Lapeer 324 were epileptic. Out of 165 persons on the waiting list of the insane institutions, 34 were epileptic. At the Michigan Farm Colony 24 were epileptic; in the state hospitals for the insane, including the Wayne County Asylum, 268 men and 148 women were epileptic. There were also at St. Joseph's Retreat 8 men and 14 women epileptic; in the county infirmary 114 were epileptic. Although these figures of epilepsy and feeble-mindedness are given, the list is incomplete and it is impossible to present the percentage.

As a result of this study the following recommendations are made:

1. That a more effective control and supervision be made by the state and federal authorities over foreign immigration.

2. That the state, rather than the individual counties, should exercise a more centralized control and supervision of all institutions having the care of the insane or mentally defective or epileptic.

3. To look after discharged patients from hospitals for the insane who live at home and continue in an unrecovered state, there should be a field-worker appointed in connection with each institution to give them systematic supervision.

The other recommendations made related to the better care of those suffering from venereal diseases and alcoholic excesses, and the laws relating to the prevention of marriage of the insane be enforced.

THE CARE OF THE INSANE IN MINNESOTA.

Prior to the establishment of the St. Peter State Hospital in 1866 the insane of the State of Minnesota were cared for in insane hospitals in Iowa and St. Louis. On the opening of the temporary hospital at St. Peter on December 6, 1866, the patients from Minnesota remaining in the hospitals of Iowa and St. Louis were removed thereto, and shortly afterwards the hospital buildings were made permanent.

Rochester State Hospital, designed originally as an inebriate asylum in 1874, but later changed to the Second Minnesota Hospital for Insane, was opened for the reception of patients on January 1, 1879.

Fergus Falls State Hospital was established by an act of the Legislature of 1885 and opened on July 29, 1890. The Legislature of 1887 designated this hospital to be of the school of homeopathy, and directed that all medical appointments be made in accordance therewith.

The Legislature of 1899 established two state asylums, and located them at Anoka and Hastings, respectively. They were opened in 1900, and are designed for the care of chronic and incurable cases or such cases as are deemed unfit for hospital treatment.

The Hospital Farm for Inebriates, opened at Willmar in 1912, was established at the request of the State Board of Control in 1910.

In 1879 the State of Minnesota established and opened at Faribault the Minnesota School for Feeble-minded and Colony for Epileptics.

These institutions, which constitute the equipment of the State of Minnesota for the care of its mentally diseased, were from their establishment up to the year 1901 managed by individual boards of trustees.

In 1901 Minnesota made radical changes in its methods of managing the public institutions of the state by establishing a State Board of Control.

This board was to manage and control the charitable reformatories and penal institutions of the state and also, by an unfortunate combination of duties, to assist in the management of the State University and the State Normal School.

The act of organization of the board abolished the Board of Corrections and Charities, which previously had done an important work in connection with the institutions of Minnesota.

The Board of Control was appointed by the Governor by and with the advice of the Senate and consisted of three members, with a term of service of six years. The salary of each member was to be $3500 a year. The members of the board were required to give bond individually in the sum of $25,000. They were required to meet the superintendents, wardens and executive officers of the institutions under their care in conference at regular intervals. The officers, in fact, were to be appointed by them and might be removed by them for cause.

Fortunately the board very wisely decided to leave the appointment of subordinate officers to the heads of the different institutions and not to meddle in the details of institutional management.

The Board of Control was required to take charge of all building operations, the purchase of supplies and the payment of bills. It was required to make monthly visits to the institutions under its charge and also to investigate any complaints which might be presented with power to send for books and papers.

Authority was given to pay bills directly from the State Treasury. All standing appropriations for institutions were abolished and all funds on hand belonging to the different institutions were conveyed back to the State Treasury. The board purchased all supplies, made estimates for special appropriations and suggested to the Legislature such changes or improvements as were needed in the different institutions. It had power to transfer inmates of hospitals for the insane from one institution to another—in fact, their powers were more ample than has usually been given to a similar Board of Control.

Under ordinary circumstances such legislation would have been followed by serious misunderstandings on the part of the officers of institutions, but, fortunately, the Board of Control wisely notified every superintendent that he was retained in office and that his powers to appoint his assistant medical officers would in no manner be abridged.

The organization of this board was due to the work of a commission which had visited the States of Iowa, Wisconsin, Michigan and Illinois and formally reported its conclusions and recommendations. The commission found that in Iowa and Wisconsin the organization of such a board had decreased the cost of maintenance and had eliminated politics from the state institutions; also that officers of state institutions had been given a wider latitude to display their personality and increase their efficiency by being relieved from routine duties in the financial management of their institutions; that local controversy as to appropriations from the Legislature had been eliminated, and, finally, that the humane objects of the institutions had been much extended by the action of a wise, intelligent and far-seeing board which could act for the whole state as well as any district of the state.

The act establishing the Board of Control provided that all money should be paid directly from the state treasury and that no institution should have a local treasurer charged with the custody and payment of money. It was also provided that there should be no political interference with the management of state institutions and no contributions for political purposes.

The Board of Control could appoint the superintendents, wardens and matrons only of state institutions and these officers, once appointed, were free to make their own appointments and discharge for cause all persons neglecting any duty.

At the close of the first biennial period the Board of Control announced that the cost of maintenance of the institutions under its control had been decreased; that the superintendents had been given power to manage their own institutions without dictation and control; that all state institutions had been treated as the property of the state; that the local interests did not possess any proprietary rights in their management or the control of the revenue; and, finally, that the resident officers had been required to bear constantly in mind the duty of preserving and extending the humane purposes for which their institutions had been founded. It had adopted a uniform system of records and accounts to be kept in the state institutions. It had provided for the care and custody of the state property and supplies and had established methods of receiving, inspecting and paying for them.

It had also established a system of accountability for the property and supplies of the institutions so that it was possible for every institution to know what had been purchased, what articles were on hand and to what uses the goods purchased had been appropriated. A settled policy was established that no relation of any member of the board, either by blood or marriage, should be appointed to any position in any state institution, and that no superintendent or warden should employ or retain in his employ any relation, either by blood or marriage. It was further provided that political control should have no voice in the appointment of officers.

The board did not escape criticisms on the part of persons residing in the vicinity of the different state institutions. Many complaints were made that money was being expended outside of the state in the large markets and that supplies were purchased away from home. The board pursued an extremely wise course in relation to these complaints; it painstakingly showed that supplies were only purchased elsewhere when it was for the interest of the institution to do so, and that, all things being equal, 90 per cent of the supplies for the state institutions came from Minnesota.

It was also possible for the Board of Control to show that the foodstuffs purchased for the different institutions were better and cheaper than they had been under any system of local control; that the dietary was fresher and more varied, and that the flour, butter and meats were all of a higher grade than had formerly been purchased for the use of the state institutions.

Farming industries and industries requiring increased labor for female patients had also been fostered to the great advantage of institutions.

Quarterly conferences had been held between the members of the board and superintendents of the state institutions; carefully prepared papers had been read and discussed at these conferences, to promote the education of both board and superintendents, and other officers in charitable methods. The topics discussed were practical in character and related to the routine work, to merit systems for employees, to the treatment of inmates, to what industries should be established and the like.

In the purchase of supplies estimates were required by the superintendent one month in advance of the beginning of each quarter. These were sent to the office of the board and there reviewed, revised and classified, after which schedules were sent out to the different bidders. At the next quarterly conference meeting the superintendents met to examine the samples, to study the proposals and to make the awards. This course, it is claimed, saved the state thousands of dollars, besides providing a higher standard of supplies, provisions and foodstuffs for institutions.

In a succeeding report the statement was made that during the previous biennial period 141 non-resident insane patients and feeble-minded people had been deported from the state, and that out of 144 jails, lockups, etc., inspected, 42 had been condemned; that the cost of maintenance of the institutions for food, clothing, etc., had been materially decreased and the character of the supplies had invariably been improved; that the salary list of employees had been increased from an average salary of $407 per year to one of $486 per employee.

In the same report the erection of dormitories for nurses and attendants was urged upon the ground that the duties of the nurse in institutions for the insane are so arduous and exacting that there is an obligation on the part of the institution to furnish her, when off duty, a complete rest and change from the proximity of patients.

The succeeding report announced that 153 non-resident and feeble-minded dependents had been deported at a saving of about $150,000 to the state.

In the report for the period ending 1908 it was stated that an effort had been made to develop a system of after-care of the insane and two agents had been appointed to visit the insane patients who had been able to leave the hospital and to acquaint themselves with their condition. It was hoped in this manner to extend and develop a system of parole and cottage-care for the insane in the various communities.

The institution at Anoka was changed in the character of the patients admitted, so that in future it was to be used exclusively for women and the asylum at Hastings was to be used exclusively for men—the latter institution being extremely well adapted for agricultural operations and the former being so situated as to not permit of much work for men. There are no commitments direct to these institutions. All inmates are transferred from the state hospitals by authority of the State Board of Control.

A law passed in 1901 provided for the commitment of doubtful cases of insanity to certain wards in county or city hospitals for the sick, to be designated by the State Board of Control as places of detention for the insane until the State Board of Examiners shall determine that "he is cured or a fit subject for a state insane hospital." In 1907 the law was amended so as to provide for the establishment of detention hospitals at the three state hospitals. The first detention hospital was opened at Fergus Falls on August 1, 1910. The second detention hospital was opened at St. Peter on August 1, 1911. The detention hospital at Rochester was opened in 1912.

The most noteworthy use of detention hospitals, as an essential part of the machinery of the state care of the insane, seems to be found in Minnesota.

In the report of the Board of Control for 1910 it is stated to be a matter of congratulation that the establishment of a detention hospital in connection with each state hospital places it on the same footing as the general hospital in a city, so that admission to the detention hospital may not occasion any more remark than the admission of patients suffering from any acute disease to a general hospital.

The new law of 1909 covering the admission of patients to the detention hospital provided for the admission of the patient without any forms resembling the trial of a prisoner and permits a voluntary entrance on the part of any person who feels himself in need of treatment.

It was also enacted that the judges of the district courts at each location of a detention hospital should appoint a State Hospital Commission of three persons, one of whom shall be a physician to examine all unrecovered voluntary cases recommended for transfer from the detention hospital to the state hospital. All cases, however, regularly committed to the detention hospital by a judge of probate are transferred by a written order from the Board of Control without the formality of a new examination. The opinion is expressed by one who is familiar with the conditions in Minnesota that a state psychopathic hospital should be established closer to the larger cities of the state for voluntary and uncommitted patients, to save the expense of commitment and to relieve the patient from a fatiguing journey. Prior to the establishment of the state detention hospitals the state paid a weekly rate for the care of patients who were detained in the wards of general hospitals.

At the present time every acute case of insanity is first admitted to a state detention hospital. The State Board of Control in one of its reports speaks of the purpose which the detention hospital was designed to serve in the care of the insane as follows:

We believe it is a matter for congratulation that the detention hospital has been made a feature in the care of the insane in this state. It marks a step toward the time when hospitals for the insane will be on the same plane in the minds of the public as the general hospitals—simply a place where persons who have a certain malady are to be cared for and cured if possible; not a place where admission involves in the minds of many the idea of disgrace. This feeling that there is something of disgrace in mental affliction is one of the heritages of many years in many lands, when the insane were thought to be accursed and were treated and cared for as criminals. In the arrest, the placing of insane in jail for safekeeping and their transportation to the hospital by the chief peace officer of the county (the sheriff) is still to be seen a relic of former customs. Those features of the new law covering the detention hospital which provide for the admission to the hospital without the forms resembling the trial of the prisoner and the voluntary entrance on the part of anyone who feels himself in need of treatment are great steps in advance. When all the detention hospitals are established and sufficient time has elapsed to give the general public acquaintance with the results accomplished it will be found that a wider knowledge of the splendid work that has been and is being done by state hospitals for the insane will help to eradicate the inherited prejudices. Much has been done in this direction through the system of looking after the paroled insane by reliable and experienced agents, and the work of the detention hospitals will aid materially.

Previous to 1893 the commitment laws in Minnesota were comparatively simple. The constitution of the state provided that the probate court only could commit a person to an institution for the insane. On complaint to the probate court the sheriff apprehended a person believed to be insane on a warrant issued by the probate court. The probate court had a hearing, and the law provided that there should be called in one layman and one physician to examine the alleged insane person and report their findings to the court, when the court might, in its discretion, commit the person to a hospital.

At the session of the Legislature in 1893 the laws governing the public institutions and the patients in the hospitals were codified, and the provisions for commitment were altered with the object of removing the apparent stigma connected with the commitment. The probate court was authorized to appoint a commission, consisting of two physicians, to examine an alleged insane person and, in the discretion of the court, the patient might be committed without legal formality or without his appearing in court.

In 1894 a paranoiac, through his attorney, questioned the legality of his commitment, and the Supreme Court, ignoring the statute of 1893, released the patient. The existence of the statute was then recognized by the Supreme Court and the law was declared to be unconstitutional because it conflicted with that section of the Constitution of the United States that provided for a jury trial.

In 1895 the law was amended by calling the "commission" a jury, and patients were committed under the statute thus amended until the statute now in force was enacted in 1909.

Classes Committed.—All insane persons who have a settlement in a county, town, city or village must be admitted to an institution for the insane.

Legal Procedure.—Whenever the probate judge or, in his absence, the court commissioner of any county receives information that an insane person in the county needs care and treatment, he must order the person to be brought for examination and appoint two examiners in lunacy, who, with a judge or court commissioner, constitute a jury to examine him. The county attorney must be notified of the examination and appear on his behalf. Upon the request of the county attorney the judge or court commissioner must issue subpœnas for the attendance of witnesses. If the examiners find the person to be insane and a fit subject for hospital treatment they must certify to the fact within 24 hours after the examination, whereupon the judge or court commissioners must issue a duplicate warrant committing the person to the superintendent of the proper state hospital or to the superintendent of any private licensed institution for the care of the insane. If the jury finds the person sane or disagrees it must certify to the fact, and the person must thereupon be discharged. In any county having a population of 150,000 inhabitants the judge of probate may refer the examinations of alleged insane persons to the court commissioner of the county for action with the examiners in lunacy appointed by the judge of probate. When the alleged insane person is found to have a legal residence in some other county he may, nevertheless, be examined and committed to a state hospital if found insane.

The board of examiners may, when the question of insanity is doubtful, commit an alleged insane person to a place of detention, but not for more than six weeks. If then they determine that he is cured he must be discharged, but if he has not improved and they deem him a fit subject, he must be conveyed to a state hospital.

The above provisions, while still in force, are practically superseded by the laws in regard to commitment to detention hospitals.

Each person found to be insane, except the criminal insane, must be committed to the proper detention hospital, to be kept and treated until the superintendent determines and certifies either that he is not insane or that he is a fit subject for a state hospital for the insane. If he is found to be sane he must be discharged. If the superintendent deems him a fit subject for a state hospital and so certifies to the State Board of Control, it must transfer him to a hospital or asylum.

Any husband, wife, parent, son, daughter or guardian, believing a wife, husband, father, son, daughter, mother, brother, sister or ward to be afflicted with mental disease for which such person should be treated at a detention hospital, may apply to the judge of probate of the county of his residence for the appointment of a board of three physicians, one of whom must be a female physician if there be such. The judge of probate must appoint such board to determine whether the patient is in need of treatment at a detention hospital, and if a majority of the board so determine the patient may be placed in a detention hospital by the relative, who must sign the necessary application therefor, in the same manner and under the same restrictions and provisions as for detention in a hospital for the insane. When information is filed with any judge of probate that a resident of his county is in need of treatment at a detention hospital he must make investigation and appoint a board to determine whether he is in need of treatment and, if he so determines, the patient must be placed in a detention hospital under the same restrictions that govern voluntary commitment.

Voluntary Patients.—Any person believing himself to be afflicted with mental disease and desiring to receive treatment at a detention hospital may voluntarily place himself therein. He must make and sign a written application as provided by the Board of Control. Should the patient demand release from the detention hospital and it is deemed unsafe, the superintendent must, within three days, call in the State Hospital Commission to take charge of the case and determine whether the patient is insane. If adjudged insane he must be committed to the hospital. If found to be sane, he must be required to leave the hospital.

Where a state hospital for the insane is located, a state hospital commission composed of three reputable persons, at least one of whom is a duly qualified physician, must be appointed by the judge or judges of the district court of the county to hold office for two years. The commission has power to examine alleged insane persons to determine whether they are insane. The State Hospital Commission must meet at the detention hospital as often as may be requested by the superintendent, but not oftener than twice each month, except in cases requiring immediate action.

Appeal from Commitment.—Every person restrained of his liberty may prosecute a writ of *habeas corpus.*

Cost of Commitment.—The expenses of the examination and commitment of an insane person are chargeable to the county.

MEMBERS OF STATE BOARD OF CONTROL SINCE 1901.

Name	Term	Name	Term
Silas W. Leavett	1901-1903 1903-1909	Peter M. Ringdal	1907-1913
		Charles Halvorson	1909-1911
William E. Lee	1901-1902	Charles E. Vasaly (in office)	1909-
Charles A. Morcey	1901-1901	Carl J. Wendson (in office)	1911-
Ozro B. Gould	1901-1907	Ralph W. Wheelock (in office)	1913-
James A. Martin	1902-1904		
Jacob F. Jacobson	1904-1905		
Leonard A. Rosing	1905-1909		

ST. PETER STATE HOSPITAL.

St. Peter, Minn.

The St. Peter State Hospital was organized and begun by the state as a hospital for the care of the insane. The first insane patient recognized by the state commitment, according to the records, was adjudged insane on April 28, 1862, and from that time until the fall of 1866, 62 patients were sent away and cared for outside of the state, 55 being sent to the insane hospital in Iowa and seven to St. Vincent's Institution in St. Louis. In 1866 urgent requests for a state hospital became prevalent, and on March 2, 1866, an act of the Legislature established an institution for the insane in Minnesota. On the 1st of July, 1866, a building in the town of St. Peter was selected and arranged for temporary use. On October 2, 1866, Dr. Samuel E. Schantz, of Utica, N. Y., was elected medical superintendent, and he arrived at the hospital November 1, 1866. As an institution it was opened December 6, 1866, and the patients who had been boarded in Iowa were sent for and placed in this temporary building.

In 1867 the board, under authority given by the act of the Legislature, decided to provide further temporary accommodation by erecting a building in St. Peter, and $40,000 was provided for that purpose. This building was occupied October 23, 1867, and furnished accommodations for 100 patients; during that year 97 patients were admitted.

The site selected was on sloping ground overlooking the Minnesota River in the outskirts of the City of St. Peter. The location is quite scenic in natural beauty, probably equalling that of any similar institution in this or adjoining states. During the year, Dr. Schantz, the superintendent, died, his death occurring August 20, 1868. Dr. Jacob E. Bowers, who in the early part of the year had been appointed assistant physician, became acting superintendent until the arrival of Dr. C. K. Bartlett, who came to the hospital as superintendent from Northampton, Mass., December 20, 1868. Forty-seven more patients were admitted during the year.

The plan selected for the buildings was that of the so-called Kirkbride type; indeed, Dr. Kirkbride was consulted as to the form of the building and its plan. A central administration por-

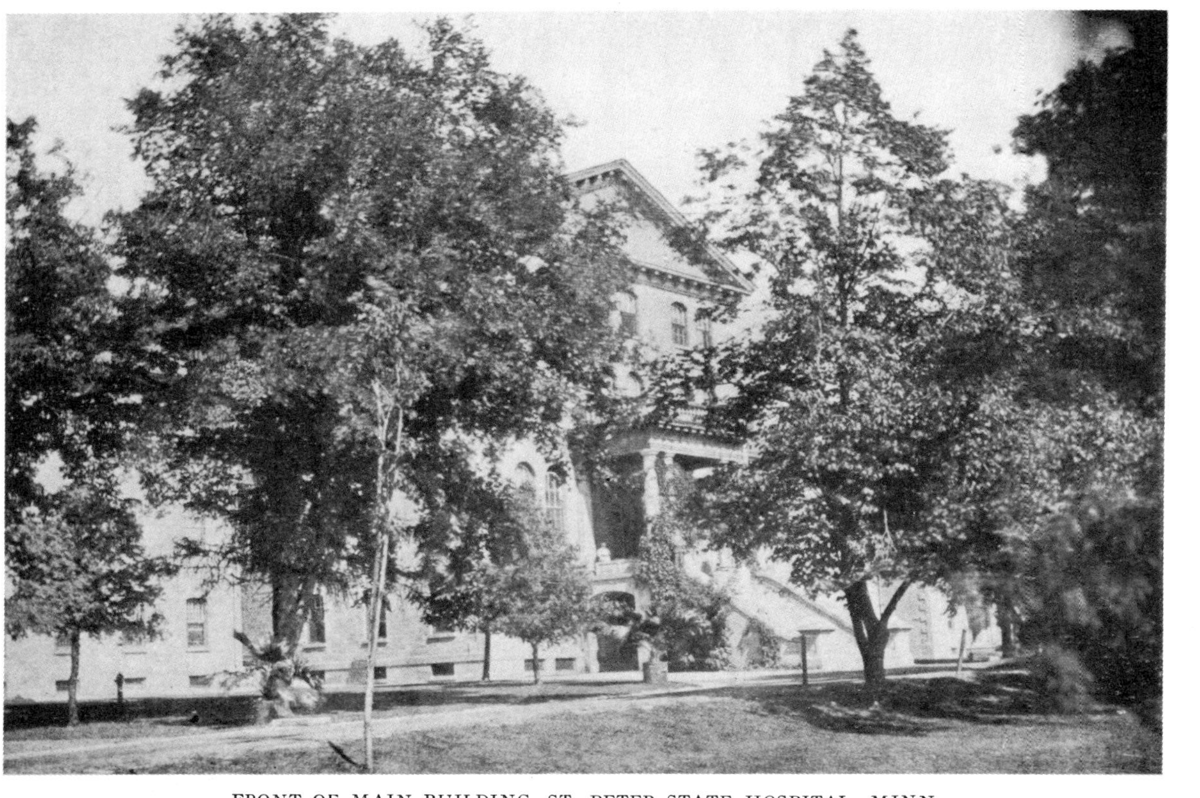

FRONT OF MAIN BUILDING, ST. PETER STATE HOSPITAL, MINN.

tion, with diverging wings upon either side, each broken by one or two cross halls, was designed; behind the central building the service buildings, including kitchen, heating plant and laundry, were to be placed. This original plan was substantially carried out during the next six or eight years. About 12 or 15 years later two annex buildings, one for men and the other for women, entirely separated from the main building, were built, designed at that time as a more economical way of grouping working patients and those mostly needing custodial care. The idea seems to have been fairly well justified, and these buildings are still in use in practically this way. In the early nineties additions were made to the rear of each wing, which served to form congregate dining rooms. This gave six congregate dining rooms, one for each flat of the two sides of the three-story building. This may be said to be a compromise upon, or a modified form of, the idea of one large congregate dining room.

The buildings so constructed still constitute the main buildings. These were not originally of distinctly fireproof design in any portion. A disastrous fire occurred in the men's wing of the building on the night of November 15, 1880—disastrous not only on account of the financial loss, but in that 18 people were known to have been burned and that six more were unaccounted for. The night was severely cold, and the disaster was very distressing to everyone. This marked the beginning of attempts to secure fireproof buildings in future hospital construction in the state. It is, however, the only large and disastrous fire which the State of Minnesota has had in its state hospitals.

Dr. C. K. Bartlett continued as superintendent of the hospital up to the year 1894. He was always considered a very capable man and was universally liked by patients and employees. He might be characterized as genial, courteous and respected, and as especially fitted to carry out the relation of superintendent to the patients and to the hospital in a way which was satisfactory to the board, to his associates and to the patients.

Dr. Bartlett was succeeded by Dr. H. A. Tomlinson in 1894, who for a couple of years had been acting as assistant physician in the hospital. Dr. Tomlinson entered upon his duties with the enthusiasm of a younger man and with the distinct endeavor to introduce and carry out "medical" aims and purposes. That which most characterized his superintendency was this endeavor to make the institution a hospital as much like other hospitals as could be done. He insisted upon advanced medical ideas and methods, and he introduced, as soon as was possible, the practice of laboratory work, even though he was not allowed a nominal pathologist. After a while, however, he secured the services of Dr. H. D. Valin, who for many years supervised the work of the laboratory and did a large share of it himself. Dr. Tomlinson's pursuance of medical aims led him continually to insist, in writing and in speech, upon the disregarding of the custodial portion of hospital work and in the bringing into prominence of the medical study of the patients. Dr. Tomlinson was a member of the American Neurological Association, and as far as possible brought to the aid of insane patients the neurological studies more or less peculiar to that Association. He also made prominent the training school for nurses and insisted upon the employment of the graduates as trained nurses in outside and private work. A very large number of these nurses are still doing the work of trained nurses in this and other states.

Dr. Tomlinson continued in the service as superintendent until October 1, 1912, at which time he resigned to accept the superintendency of the Hospital for Inebriates at Willmar, Minn. A few months after making this change his death occurred, following a cerebral hemorrhage. He left upon record quite a number of articles, in which he maintained strongly the value of a biological study of insane patients. He insisted upon the prominence of kidney disease as an element in the degeneration and death of the insane. His reports show that he declined to accept and make use of any one of the classifications offered by the different authors—seeming to insist upon the idea of grouping the insane with very little of formal separating lines of division.

On October 1, 1912, upon the resignation and departure of Dr. Tomlinson, Dr. R. M. Phelps received the superintendency of this institution and holds the same at the present time (1914).

There has never been very great variation in the per capita cost of keeping insane patients in Minnesota. This has been largely because they were under common management, first by the Board of Trustees, and later, during the last 14 years, under a Board of Control; also because full and detailed accounts of every movement were reported, and because sufficient allowances of money were not made that would enable one institution to become more expensive than another. The per capita cost has usually been from $160 to $200 per year.

Patients are received at the present time in a special hospital located on the same grounds as the state hospital, and under the same management. This is called a Detention Hospital, and is somewhat peculiar to this state. There may be a special warrant of ordinary form committing the patient to the hospital, or, if it be so desired, the patient can commit himself "voluntarily" without warrant, or can be "placed" by relatives. Those who are "placed" by relatives, and those who are "voluntary" can be discharged by the superintendent without ever coming to the State Hospital if they are judged to be recovered. If, however, it is judged desirable that they should go to the State Hospital, the voluntary and placed patients must necessarily be re-examined and a special commitment made to place them in the State Hospital. The patients under ordinary warrant can be transferred to the State Hospital by the approval of the Board of Control.

It is the plan of this detention hospital to pay particular attention to hospital methods in caring for patients; to care for them in a rather more thorough and better way than could be done in the main hospital, and to make them feel as much as possible that they are in a hospital, and are not as yet fully committed as insane. It is thus quite different from what is usually termed a "recovering ward."

This detention hospital is one of the notable features of the later years of this hospital. Another element is that of the nurses' home, which is a fine building and probably as good as any erected of late years. It is for the women nurses. Another prominent feature of later years is the asylum for dangerous insane (usually going by the name of the "Criminal Building") to which are sent not only patients who have come from the state prison, but other patients who have been under indictment and have been acquitted on the ground of insanity; also an occasional insane patient who has dangerous or criminal tendencies. This institution at present accommodates men only and has a capacity for 60. Whether this plan and method are to be continued in the future is at present considered doubtful; it being judged in this state that it would be more useful and more appropriate as an adjunct to the state prison than as an adjunct to one of the state hospitals.

During later years the institution has been made almost completely fireproof. In the years 1906 to 1908 the central portion was rebuilt, an excellent laboratory established in three large rooms, and a large and fine operating room constructed; several special diet kitchens were established along the idea of more complete hospital methods.

A special building out of the ordinary, besides the detention hospital, the asylum for dangerous insane and the nurses' home, which have been mentioned, is a hospital building for the tubercular insane. This is of rather peculiar design and method, incorporating ideas advocated by Dr. Tomlinson.

The present medical work includes full records, arranged by means of Tengvall files so as to form a removable leaf system. It includes a full and complete examination of all the bodily organs on the admission of every patient, together with the examination of blood and urine. The post-mortem work has always received considerable prominence, and a room for the purpose is quite fully fitted out.

BOARD OF TRUSTEES.

Name	Term	Name	Term
C. T. Brown	1867-1879	A. Barto	1883-1893
Rev. A. H. Kerr	1867-1878	M. R. Tyler	1887-1893
Solomon Blood	1867-1871	C D. Wright	1887-1893
Ruben Butters	1867-1874	A. T. Stebbins	1889-1893
H. B. Strait	1867-1889	J. F. Fulton	1889-1893
Wm. Schimmell	1867-1891	John Peterson	1891-1893
Luke Miller	1867-1872	J. W. Mason	1891-1899
L. Fletcher	1870-1880	T. H. Titus	1893-1899
Wm. L. Lincoln	1872-1874	W. A. Jones	1893-1895
James E. Child	1874-1875	Robt. A. Smith	1893-1895
Nathaniel Stefft	1874-1875	J. H. Block	1895-1899
Freeman Talbott	1875-1880	C. L. Wells	1895-1897
Burr Deuel	1878-1889	John A. Coleman	1897-1899
Thomas Brooks	1879-1883	D. N. Jones	1897-1901
Rev. K. O. Cavallin	1880-1883	A. W. Daniels	1900-1901
A. L. Sackett	1880-1891	John Heinen	1900-1901
M. J. Daniels	1881-1889	Joseph H. Wagoner	1900-1901
John F. Meagher	1881-1893		

SUPERINTENDENTS.

Samuel E. Shantz ....Nov. 1, 1866, to Aug. 20, 1868 (died).
Cyrus K. Bartlett ....Nov. 1, 1868, to Jan. 1, 1893 (resigned).
Harry A. Tomlinson ....Jan. 1, 1893, to Oct. 1, 1912 (resigned).
Robert M. Phelps ....Oct. 1, 1912-in office.

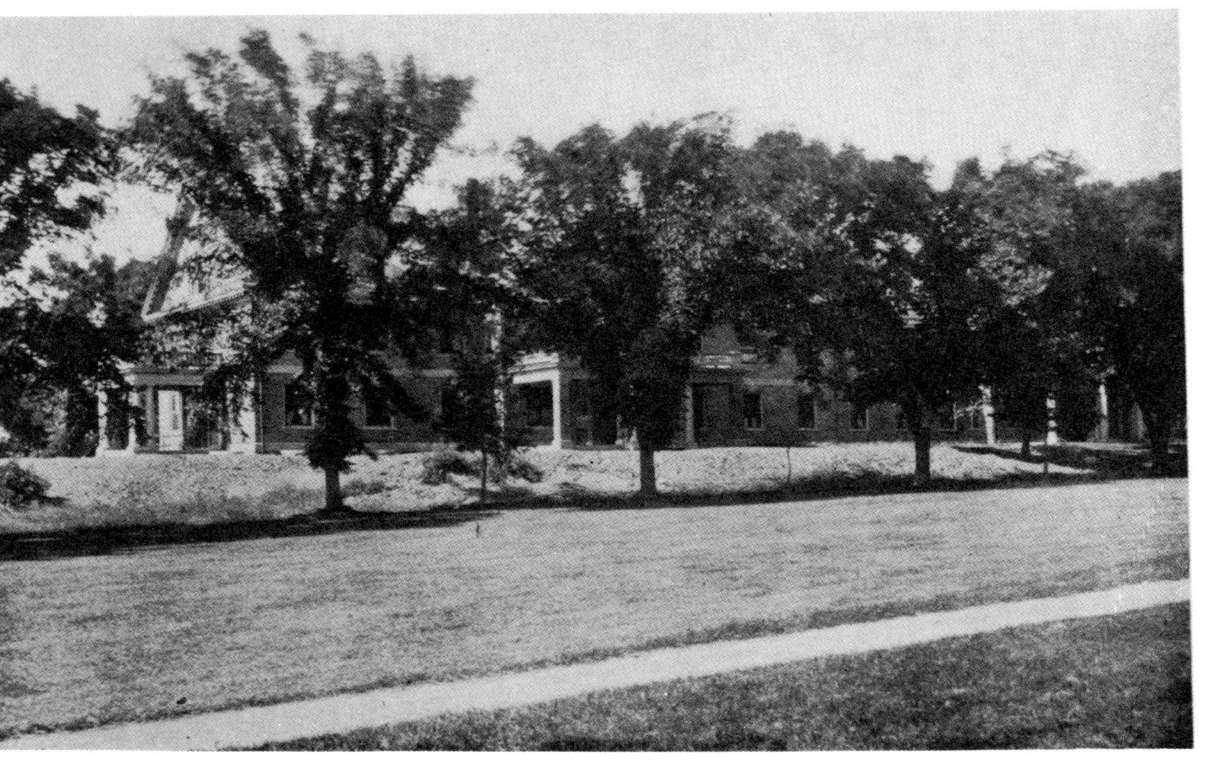

NURSES' HOME, ST. PETER STATE HOSPITAL, MINN.

91

1881

t., 1883

y, 1884, to July, 1889-May, 1893

, to June, 1889

90, to May, 1893

, 1890, to May, 1893

Ha .... ec., 1891, to Jan., 1893

Nath .... May, 1893, to Aug., 1895

C. A. E .... May, 1893, to June, 1893

Gustav A. .... June, 1893 to Aug., 1898

Ella B. Eve .... Sept., 1893, to Sept., 1896

Thomas K. Fo .... Oct., 1893, to May, 1905

W. H. Darling .... July, 1895, to Jan., 1908

Mary E. Bassett .... Sept., 1896, to July, 1898

O. M. Justice .... May, 1897, to May, 1898

Abraham A. Strickler .... June, 1898, to May, 1899

Clark Tuomy .... Sept., 1898, to Sept., 1906

M. E. Ransome .... July, 1898, to June, 1900

Donald A. Nicholson .... May, 1899, to Dec., 1904

Rose Marie Merrill .... July, 1900, to June, 1901

Mary F. Hopkins .... Oct., 1901, to May, 1907

Charles F. Burleson .... Dec., 1904, to Oct., 1905

John Hoyt .... Oct., 1905, to Oct., 1906

George H. Freeman .... Nov., 1906, to Nov., 1912

Frank Winter .... Apr., 1907, to May, 1907

Mary McMillen .... July, 1907, to Aug., 1907

Mary Blakeledge .... Aug., 1907, to Feb., 1908

W. A. Dorsey .... Nov., 1907, to Mar., 1908

B. C. Dorsett .... Mar., 1908, to Oct., 1908

Arthur Huzzar .... June, 1908, to Aug., 1908

George T. Baskett .... July, 1908, to July, 1910

Holland T. Ground .... Oct., 1908, to Aug., 1909

Olive Thorne .... Feb., 1908, to Aug., 1910

A. S. Sanderson .... Oct., 1909, to Nov., 1909

B. L. Wickware .... Dec., 1909, to Apr., 1910

Lindsey W. Baskett .... May, 1910, to Oct., 1913

Clara Hayden .... Aug., 1910, to Oct., 1911

Herman Covey .... Nov., 1910, to-

Audry Goss .... Oct., 1911, to Mar., 1912

Clement C. Blakely .... Jan., 1911, to-

Margaret Fleming .... Apr., 1912, to Dec., 1913

George T. Baskett .... Nov., 1912, to-

Holland T. Ground .... Nov., 1913, to-

Clara Eirley .... Feb., 1914, to-

ROCHESTER STATE HOSPITAL.

ROCHESTER, MINN.

This institution is located at Rochester, Olmsted County, and the history of its organization is as follows:

By a special law passed by the Legislature of 1873 and amended in 1874 a tax of $10 on all liquor dealers was assessed to raise a fund for the establishment of a state inebriate asylum which, when completed, was to be maintained by a continuation of the same tax. As soon as a sufficient fund was accumulated the Inebriate Asylum Board purchased a farm of 160 acres, within a mile and a half of the City of Rochester, for $9000, secured plans and began building in 1877. Strong opposition was raised by liquor dealers against this tax as discriminating and unjust. Test cases were tried in the courts and the constitutionality of the law was sustained. At the same time it became apparent and was admitted generally that additional room was much more urgently needed for the care of the rapidly increasing insane of the state than for the care of inebriates. The Legislature of 1878, in view of this and of the determined opposition to an inebriate asylum to be built and maintained on such a plan, repealed the act levying the tax and changed the inebriate asylum to the Second Minnesota Hospital for Insane, which title was later changed to the Rochester State Hospital, with the proviso, however, that inebriates should be admitted and cared for and treated at the expense of the state on the same basis as the insane. Accordingly a separate ward was maintained for inebriates until the department was abolished by the Legislature in 1897.

The building was in an unfinished condition, and consisted of a center and small east wing, then only under roof, without inside finish, and without outbuildings, such as laundry and engine house.

When the trustees examined the property they recognized its unfitness for the purposes of an insane hospital and the fact that it would necessarily require many changes to adapt it to this new use. Owing to these objections they hesitated to accept the transfer; but the urgency for room was so great they reluctantly concluded to do the best they could with it. An appropriation of $15,000 accompanied the transfer as a fund to be used to prepare the building for the accommodation of patients. This was in the summer of 1878.

Dr. J. E. Bowers, with over 10 years' experience as first assistant physician at St. Peter, was elected superintendent, and the Rev. A. H. Kerr, who had been a trustee from the beginning of the St. Peter Hospital, was chosen steward. On January 1, 1879, the institution was opened for the reception of patients. Transfers were made from St. Peter and new cases were admitted, and accommodations for 100 men were soon filled.

The Legislature of 1880 granted $20,000 for the erection of a wing on the west side for women. This was erected in the summer of 1880, and was ready for the furniture and heating apparatus when a disastrous fire occurred at St. Peter. Money for furnishing and heating was immediately provided. The building was hastily completed, and furnished room for over 100 women, who were transferred to relieve the crowded condition of the first hospital. In 1882 a large extension was built on the men's side, accommodating 200 patients, and costing when furnished $76,000. In 1883 and 1884 a similar wing was built on the west side for women, costing when furnished $83,000, thus completing the original design of the main structure, with a capacity for 600 patients. The building of a detached ward for women, authorized by the Legislature of 1887, was completed and accepted for occupancy on the 12th of February, 1890.

A modern and complete power plant is under process of construction at the present writing. Within the past few years a home for women nurses has been built and a club house for the men nurses is planned. The Legislature of 1909 appropriated $55,000 for the detention hospital and at the same time passed a voluntary commitment act. Into this building all the new patients are received.

The hospital estate contains 1720 acres. The total number of inmates remaining in the hospital January, 1914, was 602 men and 519 women. Owing to the transfer of patients to the Hastings State Asylum and Anoka State Asylum, the population of the Rochester State Hospital has reached the lowest point it has attained during the past 12 years.

SUPERINTENDENTS.

Dr. Jacob E. Bowers....	1879-1889	Dr. Arthur F. Kilbourne (in office)	1889-

ASSISTANT PHYSICIANS.

Dr. W. A. Vincent......	1881-1883	Dr. Oscar C. Heyerdale (in office)	1899-
Dr. A. Brodie Cochrane	1883-1884	Dr. Chas. L. Chapple....	1899-1911
Dr. Homer Collins......	1884-1889	Dr. Ernest Z. Wanows..	1899-1902
Dr. Robert M. Phelps...	1885-1912	Dr. Laura Linton (in office)	1900-
Dr. Harry Randall......	1889-1889	Dr. W. P. Broderick....	1899-1899
Dr. N. M. Baker........	1890-1893	Dr. A. F. Strickler......	1899-1899
Dr. Sarah V. Linton....	1890-1890	Dr. Graham M. Lisor....	1911-1912
Dr. E. Franchere......	1890-1892	Dr. Ethel R. Beede (in office)	1912-
Dr. Erick O. Giere.....	1892-1892	Dr. Wm. B. Linton (in office)	1912-
Dr. G. W. Moore.......	1892-1893		
Dr. Cyrus B. Eby.......	1893-1899		
Dr. Rose A. Bebb.......	1893-1900		
Dr. H. H. Herzog......	1893-1899		
Dr. Mary E. Bassett....	1894-1896		

STEWARD.

John Miner

FERGUS FALLS STATE HOSPITAL.[1]

FERGUS FALLS, MINN.

In 1885, the two existing state hospitals for the insane of Minnesota being overcrowded with patients, it became necessary to take steps for the erection of a third institution. Consequently the Legislature of 1885 passed an act to establish a commission to locate a third hospital for the insane and prepare plans for its construction. This act authorized and required the Governor to appoint a commission to consist of five persons, who should locate a site for said hospital at some point in the northern part of the state, cause plans to be made, and present an estimate of the cost under said plans. The act was approved by the Governor, Lucius F. Hubbard, on March 2, and shortly afterwards he appointed R. B. Langdon, of Minneapolis; C. K. Bartlett, superintendent of the St. Peter Hospital; H. H. Hart, of St. Paul, secretary of the Board

[1] By G. O. Welch, M. D., superintendent.

of Corrections and Charities; H. G. Stordeck, of Breckenridge, and F. S. Christensen, of Rush City, as members of the commission. The commission looked over the various sites suggested and finally selected one in the northern part of the City of Fergus Falls. An estimate was prepared covering the cost of land and the erection of ward buildings for 300 patients, with boiler house, laundry, etc. The report and recommendations of the commission were laid before the Legislature of 1887 and that body passed an act locating and establishing a third hospital for the insane at the City of Fergus Falls and placing the institution under the charge and control of the Board of Trustees for the insane of Minnesota. Later in the session an appropriation of $24,280 was made for the purchase of 596 acres of land, and $70,000 for the buildings recommended by the commission.

As soon as it was known that a new institution for the insane was contemplated the homeopathic physicians of the state, believing that their school deserved some recognition, took active steps to secure the proposed hospital. As a result of their efforts the Legislature of 1887 passed the following act:

> That the superintendent and corps of physicians appointed for the third hospital for the insane, located at Fergus Falls, shall be of the school of homoeopathy, and the Board of Trustees of the hospitals for the insane of Minnesota are hereby directed to make appointments in accordance herewith as soon as the hospital is ready for patients.

Shortly after the Board of Trustees took control of the affairs of the new hospital Warren B. Dunnell, of Minneapolis, was appointed architect. During the fall of 1887 he visited many of the Eastern hospitals and on his return plans were prepared for the new institution, upon which work was begun in 1888. The ward buildings are of the congregate plan, with a main wing 430 feet long, and a detached wing 200 feet long for each sex. The buildings are three stories high, with a finished attic; they are built of cream brick with sandstone trimmings and a slate roof; are of fireproof construction, and are of pleasing and artistic appearance.

There was considerable delay in completing the first buildings contracted for, as the money appropriated was not sufficient for the purpose. The Legislature of 1889 made an additional appropriation of $65,000 and the first ward building was at length ready for occupancy. On July 29, 1890, the hospital was declared open and on the 30th 90 men were transferred thereto from the St. Peter State Hospital.

Since the opening of the hospital each succeeding Legislature, realizing the necessity of relieving the overcrowded condition of the other institutions for the insane, has been very generous in its appropriations. The ward buildings proper and all the outside buildings as contemplated in the original plans were completed in 1899. Since then the farm acreage has been largely increased, several new buildings have been erected, some of the older ones have been enlarged in order that they may be better adapted to the purposes for which they were intended, and many improvements have been made in various parts of the plant in order to bring it up to the highest state of efficiency.

The total cost of the plant up to the present time has been approximately $1,252,000, divided as follows: Land (1075.61 acres), $51,365; ward buildings, $750,000; administration building, $57,000; kitchen and storeroom buildings, $91,000; heating and lighting plant, $90,000; barns and live stock, $30,500; laundry, $32,000; water supply, $12,000; nurses' home, $80,000; amusement hall and congregate dining room, $32,000; shops, $8500; library, $1000; subways, $5000; improvement of grounds, $4500; electric and surgical apparatus, $5000; fire alarm system, $2000.

In September, 1887, the Board of Trustees appointed Captain O. C. Chase, of Fergus Falls, as general overseer of the work. In February, 1890, Captain Chase was appointed to the position of steward, which office he has held since that time, having proved himself a faithful and efficient officer.

During the spring of 1890 the Board of Trustees selected Dr. Alonza P. Williamson as superintendent, and he took charge of the institution on the 4th of May. Dr. Williamson was a graduate of the Hahnemann Medical College of Philadelphia. After graduation he served for a time at Ward's Island, New York, and afterwards accepted a position at the Middletown State Hospital, New York, where he served for a number of years as assistant superintendent. Coming to the new hospital in Minnesota in its infancy, he was instrumental in establishing the work upon a solid foundation, to which much of its future success was due. Dr. Williamson resigned his position on November 9, 1892, and opened an office in Minneapolis, devoting himself to special work in mental and nervous diseases. On the day of his resignation Dr. George O. Welch was appointed superintendent. Dr. Welch was a native of Massachusetts and a graduate of the Boston University. In June, 1887, he was appointed to a position on the staff of the Westborough State Hospital of Massachusetts and resigned that position in February, 1892, to take a post-graduate course in mental and nervous diseases in Europe. While abroad he was appointed to the position of superintendent at the Fergus Falls State Hospital, which position he has held since that time.

As soon as the institution was ready for patients the Board of Trustees divided the state into three hospital districts. The Fergus Falls district includes practically all of the state north of the City of Minneapolis, a much larger area than the other two districts combined, but not nearly so thickly populated. As the state is growing fast, the hospital is beginning to suffer from the usual overcrowded condition, having now (1912) a population of 1650 patients, with a normal capacity of 1500. Since the opening of the hospital over 8000 patients have been admitted. The results of treatment have been very satisfactory, a large proportion of the recently admitted cases being sent out each year in a normal mental condition.

A training school for nurses was organized in 1894. The two years' course at first required by the school was later changed to three. The school has always been open to both sexes, but entrance therein has never been obligatory. Since the opening of the school 103 men and 114 women have been graduated. The school has helped materially to raise the standard of efficiency among the nursing force, and many of the graduates now hold responsible hospital positions elsewhere.

The following named gentlemen served upon the Board of Trustees from the opening of the hospital until 1901, when all institutions were placed under the Board of Control: A. L. Sackett, J. F. Meagher, A. Barto, M. R. Tyler, C. D. Wright, A. T. Stebbins, Dr. J. F. Fulton,. John Peterson, J. W. Mason, T. H. Titus, Dr. W. A. Jones, R. A. Smith, J. H. Block, Dr. C. L. Wells, T. D. O'Brien, Dr. D. N. Jones, Dr. A. W. Daniels, J. H. Wagoner, J. A. Coleman, John Heinen, C. J. Hanson.

SUPERINTENDENTS.

Dr. Alonzo P. Williamson 1890-1892
Dr. George O. Welch (in office)..............................1892-

ASSISTANT SUPERINTENDENTS.

Dr. A. S. Dolan.........	1890-1893	Dr. Franklin S. Wilcox..	1904-1912
Dr. G. R. Ball..........	1893-1895	Dr. Clarence C. Burlington (in office)........	1912-
Dr. Wm. O. Mann......	1895-1899		
Dr. Henry M. Pollock...	1899-1904		

ASSISTANT PHYSICIANS.

Dr. E. P. Taft..........	1891-1893	Dr. Ralph Deming......	1914-
Dr. Hamilton Meade....	1893-1895	Dr. W. L. Patterson....	
Dr. W. D. Kirkpatrick..	1895-1897	Dr. Emile Young........	1893-1895
Dr. H. H. Bingham.....	1895-1899	Dr. Addie F. Fitzpatrick	
Dr. Addie F. Gilman....		Dr. Bertha A. Hughes...	
Dr. G. H. Cobb..........		Dr. Oskar L. Bertelson..	
Dr. Bertha A. Frost....	1895-	Dr. Jennie G. Erdman...	
Dr. L. A. Williams......	1897-	Dr. DeEtte Brownell...	
Dr. Edwin Waite.......	1900-	Dr. Bertha G. Dressner..	
Dr. J. B. Brown........	1900-	Dr. Cora M. Johnson....	
Dr. N. F. Doleman......		Dr. Olive E. Smith......	
Dr. T. M. Thayer.......		Dr. A. W. Ogden (in office)	1912-
Dr. F. R. Sedgley.......		Dr. C. M. Jared (in office)	1914-
Dr. I. H. Kiesling.......			
Dr. L. R. Clapp..........			
Dr. J. F. Lovell.........			

STEWARD.

O. C. Chase (in office) 1889-

ANOKA STATE ASYLUM.

Anoka, Minn.

The Anoka State Asylum was established in 1899, with the purpose of accommodating the overflow consequent upon the overcrowding of the various state hospitals. It is designed for the care of chronic or incurable cases, or such cases as are deemed unfit for hospital treatment. No other classes of patients are received.

The institution was opened March 10, 1900, with 100 patients in residence. This number has been gradually increased as additional buildings have been erected, until in 1915 the capacity of the hospital is 900 patients.

The asylum is built on the cottage plan and consists of an administration or main building, which accommodates 300 male patients, and nine cottages, which accommodate between 60 and 75 women patients each. A central heating, lighting and pumping plant furnishes power and heat for all the buildings by means of underground tunnels.

A farm of 680 acres is maintained in connection with the institution, the work being done by patients, directed by competent overseers.

The officers of the institution are (1915):

John Coleman ....Superintendent.
Lloyd Boxwell ....Steward.
Dr. J. H. Frank ....Physician.

HASTINGS STATE ASYLUM.

Hastings, Minn.

Under an act of the Minnesota Legislature the second state asylum at Hastings for the care of the chronic insane was established in 1899. The main building was first occupied in April, 1900. Since that date seven additional cottages, all of them fireproof, have been erected and occupied, while two more are now in course of construction, making a total of nine cottages. The main building, consisting of four wards, is at present housing about 300 patients; the number of inmates of each cottage varies between 65 and 70. On May 1, 1915, the total population of the asylum was 750, and the full capacity of the institution, including the two new cottages, will be about 900.

Patients at the Hastings asylum are not received by direct court commitments, but by transfer from larger hospitals.

The reservation connected with the Hastings asylum comprises an area of 683 acres, 450 of which are under cultivation. Besides its main building and nine cottages, the institution has a complete farming and dairy department, power house, general laundry and several repair shops. After the completion of the two new cottages, at an expense of about $115,000, the total value of land and buildings will be about $634,538.

The management of the Hastings Asylum is headed by W. J. Yanz, superintendent; W. F. Hicks, assistant superintendent; Dr. A. M. Adsit, resident physician.

HOSPITAL FARM FOR INEBRIATES.

WILLMAR, MINN.

The Hospital Farm for Inebriates, located at Willmar, Minn., was opened for the reception of patients December 26, 1912.

The State Board of Control had requested, in its report for the period ending July 31, 1910, legislation giving authority to issue certificates in anticipation of special tax collections for the Inebriate Hospital Farm fund. This authority having been granted, contracts aggregating a total of $211,230 were awarded in June, 1911. These included the main administration building with two wings for male and female patients and hospital, superintendent's cottage, power plant, laundry and equipment, complete electrical system, heating, ventilating, plumbing and water supply, and septic tank and sewerage system. The time of completion was fixed as of August 1, 1912.

The institution is situated on a farm of 500 acres, of which 477 consist of tillable land. There are 23 acres of meadow, and 10 in use for a pasture. The buildings and grounds cover approximately 33 acres, which include a grove of cottonwoods of about six acres.

Since the opening of the hospital in 1912 various improvements and additions have been completed. These include the Tomlinson cottage for women patients, an ice house, blacksmith shop, farmer's cottage and engineer's cottage at a cost of $12,600, the installation of full-sized electrical and plumbing equipment in the new tunnel for $9986, a cow barn for $4891, a silo and houses for hogs for $662, a water softener for $3290, an addition to power plant costing $3223, and various minor improvements costing $2031. In addition considerable grading and laying out of roads has been done, various shrubs and trees planted and an apple and plum orchard laid out.

The institution has been planned comprehensively, so that its growth in the future will be simply the adding of units to a main system already complete. The cost of the buildings originally constructed was met by the 2 per cent tax on liquor licenses. This tax, however, amounting to about $50,000 per annum, is insufficient to cover future development and current expenses, and, therefore, appropriations will be necessary from time to time to cover deficiencies.

The law creating the Inebriate Hospital provides for voluntary commitments and that persons so received shall pay such sum for maintenance as shall be fixed by the board. The percentage of these patients is, however, very small. In the superintendent's report for the biennial period ending July 31, 1914, there appear a total of 241 committed and 21 voluntary patients during a period of 18 months. This makes the percentage of voluntary patients but 8. A little over 13 per cent of those admitted were women.

As yet the hospital is prepared to care for only the presumably hopeful cases. As a rule the treatment consists of a fairly rapid reduction in the amount of alcohol or drug used, depending entirely upon the patient's condition. Hydrotherapy is employed and every possible endeavor is made to improve the patient's physical and mental health. In this upbuilding of body and character the following are essential: time, regularity of habit, discipline, work, food and recreation, together with the personal influence of the physician.

On July 31, 1914, there were under care at the hospital 279 males and 35 females, a total of 314.

The first superintendent was Dr. H. A. Tomlinson, for many years in charge of St. Peter Hospital for the Insane. He died May 31, 1913, and was succeeded by Dr. George H. Freeman.

RESIDENT OFFICERS (1914).

George H. Freeman, M. D. ....Superintendent.
J. R. Ward ....Steward.
Lulu Healey ....Matron.

MINNESOTA SCHOOL FOR FEEBLE-MINDED AND COLONY FOR EPILEPTICS.

Faribault, Minn.

Under date of November 30, 1868, Dr. J. L. Noyes, a superintendent of the Minnesota Institution for the Education of the Deaf, Dumb and Blind, reported that two weak-minded children had been dismissed from that institution, there being no facilities for their training and the law limiting the privileges of the institution to those of a "capacity to incur instruction." The act of

1879 established a commission to visit the hospitals for insane and among other duties they were required to select idiotic and feeble-minded persons found there and turn them over to the trustees of the deaf, dumb and blind institution. The latter were authorized to establish a school for their training. Five thousand dollars was appropriated for this purpose for 1879 and $6000 for the year 1880. This school was spoken of as the "experimental school" and the work was begun in a frame building belonging to George M. Gilmore, situated on the east side bluff between Second and Third streets, formerly used as a private school for young ladies and known as the "Fairview House." The school was organized by Dr. Henry M. Knight, from Lakeville, Conn., a veteran in the care and training of the feeble-minded. His son, Dr. George H. Knight, was elected superintendent on June 1, 1879, under the general superintendence, however, of Dr. Noyes, at the head of the school for deaf. On July 18, 1879, Dr. George Knight arrived to take charge of the work and on July 28 of the same year 14 children (nine boys and five girls) selected by the commission (consisting of Dr. George W. Wood, of Faribault; Dr. W. H. Leonard, of Minneapolis, and Dr. C. H. Boardman, of St. Paul) from the St. Peter Hospital for Insane, were received at the institution at Faribault.

On March 7, 1881, the Legislature passed a bill introduced by R. A. Mott, from Faribault, establishing a permanent school at the latter place, termed a "Department for the Training of Imbeciles and the Custody of Idiots," in connection nominally with the institution for the deaf, dumb and blind, although to be located in new buildings, for the construction of which the Legislature provided $25,000. The contract for the new permanent quarters was let on May 2, 1881. On May 19, 1881, Dr. George Knight was made superintendent of this department, the administration being entirely separate from that of the school for the deaf. On February, 1882, the inmates were moved into their new quarters, which are now the north section of the north wing of the present administration building. On April 20, 1884, the Legislature having provided for the same, contract was let for an additional building attached to the one mentioned above and of equal capacity. These two sections provided, when completed, for about 100 children.

April 20, 1885, Dr. Knight resigned as superintendent and on July 6 following Dr. A. C. Rogers, at the same time physician to the government training school for Indians near Salem, Ore., was elected to the position and took charge September 1 of the same year. Dr. Rogers' previous experience in this work had been at the School for Feeble-minded at Glenwood, Iowa, for five years.

Until 1901, when the Legislature adopted a central board of control for state institutions, this institution was under the general management of a board of directors, consisting of five members appointed by the Governor, the latter and the Superintendent of Public Instruction being ex-officio members thereof. Politics have never affected the organization of the institution itself, and the governing board changed but little in personnel, except during a short time just before the board of control organization. The members who were in control of this institution at its beginning had already served long periods in charge of the schools for the deaf and blind. Rodney A. Mott, appointed in 1863, served till 1903; Hudson Wilson, appointed in 1866, served till 1899 (when he was succeeded by Edgar H. Loyhed). Thomas B. Clement served from 1875 till 1900 (B. B. Sheffield succeeding him). George E. Skinner, of St. Paul, appointed in 1876, served until his death in September, 1895. Rev. George B. Whipple, who was appointed in 1882, served until his death, in 1888, created a vacancy, filled by Anthony Kelly, of Minneapolis.

In April, 1901, the Board of Control of State Institutions took charge of the school.

In 1894 "Sunnyside" was first occupied as a distinct custodial or asylum building for those children unable to profit by school room training. The corresponding building, known as "Skinner Hall," was constructed in 1896 and named in honor of George E. Skinner, of St. Paul, a former trustee of the institution and whose influence had been exerted strongly in support of a better classification of the inmates, realized by the construction of these buildings.

In 1900 the first building distinctively for epileptics was erected as the beginning of the epileptic colony, which now has five cottages devoted to the care of this class of patients, in one of which a modern hydrotherapeutic equipment is installed and is in regular use in their treatment.

The original administration building, with the various additions made thereto since 1881, has been devoted to the work of school training.

A corps of 20 teachers conduct a well-organized school, in which manual and industrial training are predominant features. For the girls there is training in netting, basketry, plain and fancy sewing, as well as mending and darning, lace making, ironing, domestic work and gardening. And to the trained girls comes the opportunity to do work for which each has an aptitude. Such helpers, often quite independent, are found in the dressmaking and tailor shops, in mending room, kitchen and dining room, in the laundry and at the chicken ranch.

Boys are schooled in netting, basketry, sloyd work, mat braiding and sewing, and brush making, and become valuable helpers in the care of their own departments about the institution, mattress and cabinet shops, the barn, laundry, green-house, garden, farm and dairy.

In 1909 the board purchased for the school a colony farm in the town of Walcott, its nearest point being one and one-half miles south of the administration building. Here is established a colony home for boys, who are helpers in the cultivation of 507 acres of land and assist in the care of stock.

In 1915 an additional colony building for 50 boys was opened on this tract of land.

In 1909 the Legislature created a department for incurables, certain cases of those who are not mentally affected but are physically permanently helpless as a result of disease, such as rheumatoid arthritis, etc.

At the present time there are about 74 buildings of all kinds pertaining to the institution; about 1058½ acres of land, all of which, with the furnishings and equipment, have cost about $1,440,000.

The population of the entire institution the first week in June, 1915, was as follows: First, feeble-minded department school: male, 240; female, 260; total, 500; farm colony: male, 95; custodial: male, 368; female, 370; total, 738. Second, epileptic colony: male, 98; female, 126; total, 224. Third, incurables: male 2; female, 3; total, 5. Total, 1562.

The last four buildings at the center plant are of fireproof construction and each is planned for the particular type of "children" to be housed in it, viz., one for adult males, one for adult females—both representing working groups—one for custodial women and one for custodial men. These last two are planned with open center courts, where the children have the freedom of the air with sunshine and shade, screened from the gaze of the curious outsider.

The institution is a village community for the classes indicated, with the same activities as pertain to a community of normal people, with its regular duties, recreation and pleasures, where they can be protected from the results of their own mistakes and the slights and rebuffs of a cold world too busy to be patient with their peculiarities, and yet where their efforts, be they much or little, contribute towards their maintenance.

OFFICERS AND LENGTH OF SERVICE FROM 1885 TO 1915.

Dr. A. C. Rogers, superintendent (in office)	1885-
Dr. W. F. Wilson	1891-1894
Dr. C. F. Groff	1894-1894
Dr. John W. Bailey	1894-1894 1895-1897
Dr. Lucy A. Wheeler	1894-1895 1896-1900
Dr. F. S. Warren (non-resident)	1897-1902
Dr. A. R. T. Wylie (dispensary clerk)	1898-1903 1904-1904 1905-1905
Dr. Fred Huxley	1900-1902 1903-1904
Dr. W. P. Baldwin	1902-1903
Dr. D. B. Kriedt	1902-1903
Dr. H. A. Lamoure	1903-1907
Dr. F. C. Sheeran (pharmacist)	1904-1907
Dr. E. P. Campbell	
Dr. A. R. T. Wylie, first asst.	1906-1910
Dr. J. Walter Warren	1906-1909
D. E. McBroom	1907-1911
Dr. Oscar F. Lang	1909-1912
Dr. A. C. Tanner	1910-1911
Dr. Fred Kuhlman (in office)	1910-
Dr. A. B. Moulton	1911-1911
Dr. Alice M. Patterson	1911-1914
Dr. W. G. Stroebl	1912-1913
Dr. E. H. Trowbridge (in office)	1913-
Dr. B. A. Finkle (in office)	1913-
Dr. L. A. Lane	1914-
Dr. Elizabeth Barnard (in office)	1914-

THE CARE OF THE INSANE IN MISSISSIPPI.

In a memorial presented to the Legislature of Mississippi in 1850 by Miss Dorothea L. Dix the following statement occurs:

> It will be seen that Mississippi is one of the few states in which no provision has yet been supplied for the recovery of the demented and the maniac. Such as have received the advantages of hospital treatment have under very difficult and painful circumstances of fatigue and expense been conveyed to institutions in other states, more or less remote; but there are many who languish in inappropriate habitations, in wretched poverty-stricken dwellings, in ill-directed poorhouses, in exposed pens, or dreary, unlighted and unventilated cells; and in those most unfit departments, the solitary strong rooms or the dungeons of your county jails; guiltless of crime, chargeable only with incapacity for self-care, and irresponsible by reason of sickness, physical infirmity and the breaking down of the fortress of reason.

Miss Dix stated further that, according to the census of 1840, there were in the State of Mississippi 198 cases of insanity. These did not include the wealthier patients who had been placed in hospitals in other states, such as Tennessee, Kentucky, Ohio and Pennsylvania. She estimated that, according to the most reliable data, the lowest possible number of insane in the state was 400, and that there was substantial reason for believing that this estimate was below the standard, and that the census of 1850, if correctly made, would show from 450 to 500.[1]

The question of an asylum for the insane had previously been agitated in the Legislature of 1846, but without result. In 1848 an act was passed appropriating $10,000 to arrange and locate an institution on a tract of five acres of land at Jackson. This was manifestly insufficient, and the appeal of Miss Dix was successful in securing an additional appropriation of $50,000, with which the building of an institution on a larger tract of land was begun.

The asylum was opened for the reception of patients in 1856, and is now known as the State Insane Hospital, Asylum, Miss. Its capacity in 1914 was 1450 beds.

[1] The census of 1850 gives the number of insane in Mississippi as 129.

In 1882 the crowded condition of the State Insane Hospital at Asylum necessitated the building of a second institution. The Legislature accordingly made an appropriation for the erection of a hospital on land donated by citizens of Meridian. This institution is now known as the East Mississippi Insane Asylum, Meridian, Miss. Its capacity in 1914 was 650 beds.

The State Insane Hospital at Asylum is governed by a board of five trustees, of whom three must be physicians; they are appointed by the Governor for a term of two years, and he is ex-officio president of the board. The superintendent must be a skilled physician, and is appointed by the Governor for a term of four years.

The East Mississippi Insane Hospital is governed by a board of five trustees, appointed by the Governor for a term of two years. The superintendent must have the same qualifications and is appointed in the same manner as the superintendent of the State Insane Hospital at Asylum.

Classes Committed.—All insane persons who are *bona fide* residents of the state and have not been brought into the state as insane within five years and non-residents in special cases by the consent of the Governor are admitted.

Legal Procedure in Commitment.—The chancery courts have jurisdiction of writs of lunacy, to be exercised by the clerks at any time, subject to the approval of the court. Any relative of an insane person may have him so adjudged, but if relations and friends neglect or refuse to place him in an insane hospital and permit him to go at large the clerk of the chancery court must, on application in writing and under oath of any citizen, direct the sheriff by a writ of lunacy to summon the person to contest the application and six free holders to sit at the hearing. The result of the inquisition must be returned to the clerk. If he is adjudged insane by the jury or a majority of its members, and the jury finds that he should be confined, the clerk must direct the sheriff to arrest him and place him in one of the insane hospitals if there is a vacancy, and if not, to confine him in a county jail pending such vacancy. A person may be admitted who has never been adjudged insane; if he is in fact insane he may be detained; but the superintendent and trustees of the asylum do this at their peril.

There is also a provision in the law that the chancery judge may issue an order to confine an habitual user of morphine or whiskey, and on such an order the hospitals are authorized to receive patients for the drug or whiskey habit.

If a person has been declared insane by a jury he loses his right in regard to transfer of property, and if he has no property a guardian must be appointed.

If the superintendent discharges a patient as having been fully restored, and gives a certificate to that effect, any business transaction made by this party will be legal. But in some cases, to avoid any controversy, juries are sometimes called to pass on the question so as to have records in the courts, and if a jury declares a person to be sane, then he is restored to all his rights and privileges.

Appeal from Commitment.—The writ of *habeas corpus* extends to all cases of illegal confinement or detention by which any person is deprived of his liberty.

Cost of Commitment.—The cost of an inquest is to be paid by the estate of the insane person; if he have none, by the persons required by the pauper laws to support him.

STATE INSANE HOSPITAL.

ASYLUM, MISS.

It was not until 1846 that Mississippi proposed to do anything for her insane people, and then the ideas of the Legislature were exceedingly contracted. The bill for the establishment of a hospital consequently failed, but two years afterwards it was passed. The Governor suggested an appropriation of $3000, thinking that would be sufficient, and the people of Jackson offered a lot of five acres. The Legislature, however, had more liberal views and appropriated $10,000 and arranged to locate the new institution on this tract of five acres. The Board of Commissioners, however, who had been appointed to consider and prepare plans and erect the institution decided that it would not be possible for them to overlook the true interests of the state by attempting to build on such a site, and accordingly secured 140 acres of land about two miles from Jackson for the sum of $1750, and wisely concluded to wait for another appropriation.

In 1850 Miss Dix appeared before the Legislature and presented a memorial in which she urged the needs of the insane in her usual forceful and convincing fashion.[1]

Her appeal resulted in securing an appropriation of $50,000, with which the building of an institution on the larger tract of land was begun. As this was not sufficient the Legislature in 1852 gave the commission $75,000 additional. Then $30,000 more was found to be needed and finally the $10,000 intended for the running expenses of the asylum was expended on these buildings. The buildings were at last ready, but there was no money for the maintenance of the patients. The trustees, however, came to the rescue, and giving the Governor sufficient bond to indemnify him in case the Legislature refused to reimburse the treasurer, he consented to make the needful advance, and the asylum was opened for the reception of patients in 1856.

The first superintendent was Dr. W. S. Langley, who resigned after three years of service and was succeeded by Dr. W. B. Williamson, who served only one year. Dr. Robert Kells succeeded

[1] See "The Care of the Insane in Mississippi."

him and served for a period of six years and during the Civil War. During his service the City of Jackson was besieged by Federal soldiers, while the Confederates, under the impression that the Federals had removed the patients and had entrenched themselves in the institution, began to fire upon the building, thus placing the unfortunate patients between two fires. Fortunately the mistake was found out in time to prevent any personal damage being done to the patients or the institution.

Dr. Kells was succeeded by Dr. H. B. Cabaniss, who served for three years, but was compelled to resign because he could not take the oath required for the office of superintendent during the Reconstruction period. He was followed by Dr. W. B. Deason, who was affiliated with the dominating party in the state at that time, and after a service of one year was succeeded by Dr. W. M. Compton, a competent and faithful officer, who, during his term of eight years, greatly enlarged the institution and placed it in a proper position to do the work for which it was founded.

In 1876, following a general political upheaval throughout the South, he was removed and Dr. T. J. Mitchell appointed in his place. Dr. Mitchell's term of service was for 34 years, and during his administration many improvements were made. The institution was enlarged in capacity and the name was changed from asylum to hospital.

Colored patients are received in this hospital and are cared for in separate buildings on the same grounds as the white patients. An effort has been made to induce the Legislature to establish a separate hospital for the negro patients, but so far without success. The present arrangement is considered by all not to be free from objections.

Dr. Mitchell resigned on account of age in 1910 and was succeeded by Dr. Roland Stewart, who served for a period of three years and was succeeded by Dr. W. W. Smithson in 1913, who continues in office.

The capacity of the institution is 830 patients, of whom nearly 400 are colored people. During the year 1892 the administration building was burned, but was afterwards rebuilt.

EAST MISSISSIPPI INSANE HOSPITAL.[1]

MERIDIAN, MISS.

This institution was established in 1882 on account of the necessity of larger accommodations for the insane. The appropriation for the erection of the building was made by the Legislature of the state, but the grounds and land, consisting of 500 acres, were donated by citizens of Meridian.

The original structure was a three-story building on the Kirkbride plan, with an administration building in the center, and two wings, of three wards each, which furnished an accommodation of 250 patients.

Since that time the development of the institution has been on the cottage plan, and there are now six cottages, one tuberculosis building and one hospital for the treatment of the acute sick, making nine buildings in all for the accommodation of the insane.

In addition to these buildings, there is one three-story building, containing the kitchen and bakery on the first floor; a congregate dining room on the second, and an assembly hall on the third floor. There is a power plant, including rooms for the boiler, engine and laundry combined. In addition there is a building for manufacturing purposes, known as the industrial building. These buildings have been erected from year to year, as the necessity for more room demanded them, and the hospital now has an accommodation for 650 patients, with a total population on June 30, 1913, of 640 patients.

The institution is supported entirely from appropriations made by the Legislature, which are now on a basis of $150 per capita for each patient.

The hospital is fast being filled with a helpless and incurable class. Applications for the reception of dotards and senile dements are constantly being received, and unless these old people are admitted they are confined in jails, as the counties will make no provision for their keep in county almshouses. This same condition applies to idiots and imbeciles. The hospital also cares for the criminal insane.

[1] By J. M. Buchanan, M. D., superintendent.

A hydrotherapy department was installed in September, 1911, and has been of much benefit in the treatment of patients. In addition there is a chemical and microscopic laboratory.

Amusement and recreation have been provided for as far as practicable. Dances and concerts are given during the winter and the usual Christmas and Fourth of July entertainments are provided. Many patients are taken to the circus, and baseball, volleyball and croquet afford recreation during the spring and summer months.

While the farm is not a paying proposition the garden furnishes the institution with fresh vegetables in season.

On July 1, 1913, the hospital represented the following values:

649 acres of land	$58,410.00
Administration building	100,000.00
Kitchen, dining room and amusement hall	12,000.00
Cottages A, B, C, D, E	68,000.00
Annex building	20,000.00
Hospital building and tubercular pavilion	27,000.00
Ice plant	12,000.00
Laundry	6,000.00
Various out-buildings	14,385.00
Cottages, etc., for employees	12,500.00
Furnishings, supplies, etc.	48,545.78
Total	$378,840.78

TRUSTEES.

M. H. Whitaker	1884-1886
W. W. George	1884-1888
W. S. Harris	1884-1886 1892-1896
G. W. Myer	1884-1886
A. H. Smith, M. D.	1884-1886
M. J. Lowery, M. D.	1886-1888 1900-1902
W. G. Stevenson	1886-1888
B. F. Quarles	1886-1888
S. B. Watts	1886-1906
W. F. Brown	1889-1906
G. S. Covert	1888-1890
John Stinson	1888-1902
H. M. Threefoot	1890-1906
C. M. Rubush	1894-1908
C. C. Miller	1896-1904
K. Threefoot	1896-1898
J. F. Parker	1896-1904
E. B. McRaven	1896-1904
W. E. Jones	1898-1904
H. M. Street	1888-1890 1904-1908
B. F. Cameron	1904-1908
E. C. Cunningham	1904-1908
W. N. Ray	1904-1906
N. M. Collins	1906-1908
F. L. Walton, M. D.	1908-1910
J. M. Harwell	1908-1912
G. C. Kendall	1908-1912
W. A. Nall	1908-1912
W. D. Cameron	1908-1910
J. W. Waldrop	1910-1912
W. F. Wilcox	1910-1912

SUPERINTENDENTS.

C. A. Rice, M. D.	1884-1890	J. M. Buchanan, M. D.	1890-

ASSISTANT PHYSICIANS.

J. M. Buchanan, M. D.	1884-1886	T. B. Bordeaux, M. D.	1901-1902
G. S. Johnson, M. D.	1886-1888	W. R. Card, M. D.	1902-1907
H. S. Gully, M. D.	1888-1890	W. G. Stephens, M. D.	1908-1911
W. O. Porter, M. D.	1890-1892	J. H. Dameron, M. D.	1909-1913
J. R. Tackett, M. D.	1892-1895	G. F. Douglas, M. D.	1911-
T. L. Dobson, M. D.	1895-1899	T. G. Cleveland, M. D.	1913-
E. G. Denson, M. D.	1899-1901		

STEWARDS.

H. D. Cameron	1884-1886	J. F. McBeath	1904-1910
Lily Smith	1886-1901	A. G. Lyle	1910-
R. E. Moody	1901-1904		

GULF COAST SANATORIUM.

LONG BEACH, MISS.

Gulf Coast Sanatorium was opened by Dr. Rives A. Manker as a private sanatorium for the treatment of neurological and narcotic cases on October 1, 1913. It is located at Long Beach, Miss., three miles from Gulfport.

The sanatorium faces the Gulf, and consists of a ten-room colonial mansion, with a ten-room cottage annex; its capacity is 13 patients. It is equipped with approved electrical and hydrotherapeutic appliances, has all modern conveniences, a private bathing pier, and is supplied with artesian water.

Patients are under the care of trained nurses and there is a separate cottage for convalescents.

OFFICERS.

Dr. Rives A. Manker	Superintendent and resident physician.
Dr. W. A. Dearman	Bacteriologist.
Mrs. Nellie Cummings	Matron and head nurse.

THE CARE OF THE INSANE IN MISSOURI.

There are four state hospitals for the care of the insane in Missouri. State Hospital No. 1, located at Fulton, was established in 1848, and opened for the reception of patients in August, 1851. State Hospital No. 2, located at St. Joseph, was established in 1872, and opened in 1874. State Hospital No. 3, located at Nevada, was erected in 1885-1887. State Hospital No. 4, located at Farmington, was established in 1899, and opened for patients in January, 1903.

The same Legislature that established State Hospital No. 4, at Farmington, created the Missouri Colony for the Feeble-minded and Epileptics, which was established at Marshall, and opened for the reception of patients in 1901.

The City of St. Louis maintains its own asylum for the care of its insane. This institution was established in 1864, and was known as the St. Louis County Insane Asylum until the separation of city and county in 1877. Since that year it has been the property of the City of St. Louis and is under the jurisdiction of the Hospital Commissioner, who reports to the Director of Public Welfare of St. Louis. The institution is now known as City Sanitarium, St. Louis.

The investigation of the system of public charities and corrections and the inspection of all charitable and correctional institutions and insane asylums receiving state, county or municipal aid are duties of the State Board of Charities and Corrections. This is an unpaid board of seven members; six appointed by the Governor for a term of six years, the Governor a member ex-officio.

In addition there are individual boards of managers for each of the four state hospitals. These boards consist of five members appointed by the Governor for a term of four years; they receive a salary for their services.

The cost of maintenance of indigent patients at the state hospitals is paid by the county from whence they have been committed. The counties pay $3 per week for each patient.

There are no voluntary patients. A patient committed to a hospital for the insane in Missouri has no legal rights except through a guardian. After the patient has been discharged " restored " his legal rights and citizenship are restored to him by court proceedings.

Classes Committed.—Persons afflicted with any form of insanity may be admitted to the state hospitals. A pay patient or one not sent to a hospital by order of the court may be admitted on request to the superintendent. Accompanying the request must be a sworn certificate of insanity, dated within two months, by two physicians.

Legal Procedure.—When a citizen files with the clerk of the court a statement that a person is insane and in need of hospital treatment the clerk must issue subpoenas for the witnesses and such other persons to appear at a specified time, which must be the first day of the first session of the court thereafter. The county clerk must convene the county court forthwith for the purpose of passing upon the sanity or insanity of the person The court must have witnesses examined before the court or a jury if one be ordered. One of the witnesses must be a respectable physician. If the court or the jury is satisfied of the truth of the statement it must enter an order that the person is a fit subject to be sent to the state hospital, and require the medical witness to make out a detailed history. The clerk of the court must send a certified copy of the order to the superintendent of the hospital, accompanied by a request for the admission of the person. Indigent patients must be given preference over pay patients.

Appeal from Commitment.—Any person restrained of his liberty may prosecute a writ of *habeas corpus.*

Cost of Commitment.—The cost of examining patients is a charge upon the county of their residence.

STATE HOSPITAL NO. 1.[1]

FULTON, MO.

On December 9, 1847, Carty Wells introduced a resolution in the Senate of the Fourteenth Assembly of Missouri which provided for the appointment of a committee to take into consideration the necessity of the erection of a lunatic asylum. The resolution was adopted and a committee of seven, with Carty Wells as chairman, was appointed. As a result of the investigation of this committee a bill was passed on January 15, 1848, which provided for the election by the Legislature of three commissioners to select a site by purchase or donation for the erection of an asylum for the insane. It was required that the site should consist of from 100 to 500 acres, and the location was confined to one of eight counties named in the act.

On February 13, 1848, Robert E. Acock, James M. Hughes and Charles F. Woodson were selected as commissioners.

The commissioners reported to the Legislature January 3, 1849, that they had selected for a site a tract of 500 acres of land near the town of Fulton, at a cost of $11,500, and that they had adopted plans for buildings modelled after those of Indiana. The commission at that time was composed of James M. Hughes, W. J. McElheney and M. Horner.

On April 16, 1849, the contract for the erection of the buildings was awarded to Solon Jenkins, of St. Charles, at a cost of $44,950. Several changes were made, bringing the total cost up to $47,450. The commissioners then asked a further appropriation of $50,000 for fittings, furnishings, additions and support for two years, and a joint committee of the Legislature which visited Fulton reported in favor of such an appropriation. The commissioners made a report on the construction of the buildings to the Sixteenth General Assembly, January 4, 1851, James Baskett then being one of the commissioners in place of James M. Hughes.

The Board of Managers was organized in March, 1851, but during the summer two of its number, George C. Sibley and James L. Minor, resigned, and George K. Budd failed to qualify. David

[1] By F. A. Sampson, secretary of the State Historical Society of Missouri.

McKee and E. B. Cordell were appointed in their stead, the other members being J. B. Leiper, Thos. B. Harris and Charles H. Hardin, the latter afterwards Governor of Missouri. The building was delivered as finished in August, 1851, but it was not in condition to receive patients until the spring of 1852, though a few were admitted during the winter.

In the *American Journal of Insanity* for July, 1852, the statement is made that the Missouri State Hospital, as it was then called, located at Fulton, was opened in May, 1852, under the superintendency of Dr. T. R. H. Smith.

The building consisted of a four-story brick structure, 80 by 42 feet, with porticos in front, supported by massive columns. The front portion was used by the officers of the institution, the rear of the administration building being used as dining rooms for men and women, whose sleeping rooms were provided for in two wings on either side.

The center building was heated by stoves and grates, but the wings for the accommodation of patients were heated by steam, generated from boilers in a special building erected for them.

The water supply came from a creek three-fourths of a mile distant, and the water was pumped into a reservoir holding 200,000 gallons.

The institution was said to accommodate 100 patients. The first report of the superintendent was made November 29, 1852, at which time there had been 70 admissions.

In the second biennial report, November 27, 1854, the board asked for $146,000 for further improvements and additions, and the superintendent's report showed 193 patients under care.

Dr. T. R. H. Smith, for many years superintendent of the asylum, died at the institution December 21, 1885.

Dr. Smith seems to have been deprived of the superintendency of the institution during the Civil War, when Dr. C. H. Hughes was placed in charge of it. When Dr. Hughes was displaced Dr. Smith was re-instated. The change seems to have been made in consequence of political changes in the state.

It has not been possible to obtain further details of the history of State Hospital No. 1, nor the names of the medical officers prior to the years 1911-1912.

The daily average population of the hospital for the year ending December 31, 1912, was 1027. The daily average cost per capita for two years was 50 cents.

A training school for nurses was established in 1912, and a building for tubercular patients completed and occupied.

Moving picture shows are given weekly and such patients as are able are given employment on the farm and about the grounds and in industrial work.

BOARD OF MANAGERS, DECEMBER 31, 1912.

R. M. White, President.
John H. McDonald, Secretary.
Fred. D. Williams, Treasurer.
R. R. Buckner. J. B. Hereford.
Samuel Sharp. E. B. Clements, M. D.

RESIDENT OFFICERS, DECEMBER 31, 1912.

George Williams, M. D. .... Superintendent.
Frederick Walter, M. D. .... Assistant physician.
H. G. Dallas, M. D. .... Assistant physician.
D. E. Singleton, M. D. .... Assistant physician.
L. S. Smith .... Steward.
Mrs. M. R. Brown .... Matron.
Mrs. Elsie Binder .... Supt. training school.
C. J. Smith .... Farm superintendent.

STATE HOSPITAL NO. 2.

St. Joseph, Mo.

State Hospital No. 2 was brought into existence in response to the urgent need of the state for more extended facilities for the care of its insane, and was made possible by a legislative act approved March 28, 1872. This statute carried with it an appropriation of Missouri state bonds to the value of $200,000, which were to be sold and the proceeds applied to cover the expense of construction.

Prior to the opening of the institution the following officers were selected for medical service: Dr. George C. Catlett, superintendent, and Dr. A. P. Busey, assistant physician.

The hospital was opened for the reception of patients on the 9th day of November, 1874. It contained 76 small rooms, 9 by 12 feet, and 32 dormitories, 12 by 18 feet, which were constructed to accommodate 275 patients, but which, under a proper classification of patients, housed comfortably but 250 persons. On account of the increase in population the institution was soon filled to its utmost capacity.

On the night of January 25, 1879, the entire plant was destroyed by fire. Two hundred and seventeen patients were under treatment in the hospital at the time, and, as the calamity came in midwinter, but for the kindness and generosity of the citizens of St. Joseph the emergency could not have been met without serious consequences. The helpless wards of the state were housed in temporary quarters until the 5th of May following, when a temporary building was provided for their reception on the asylum grounds, east of the ruins of the destroyed building, where they were made reasonably comfortable.

Since that time the institution has made steady growth, keeping pace with scientific advancement.

Under the administration of Dr. C. R. Woodson the open-door system and the open-toilet room, to which patients might have access day and night, were put into use.

Many men who are eminent in the field of psychiatry have had service in this institution, and have had part in the good name that it has achieved.

There are at present 47 wards in the institution, with a capacity of 1525 patients, and with the average increase in growth the vacancies will all be filled by the end of the biennial term ending January, 1915. Through the concerted action of its boards of managers and medical officers the hospital is well equipped for service to the insane. Its sanitary arrangements are as nearly perfect as money and intelligent effort can make them. The installation of apparatus for hydrotherapeutic treatment of patients has proven eminently satisfactory. The abolition of all forms of mechanical restraint within the past few years has given excellent results and has proven that it is possible to control the most maniacal patients, except in rare instances, without the use of the straight jacket, the locked chair or any other form of mechanical restraint.

One of the crying needs of this institution is more land. It has been the plea of superintendents of this hospital for the past 20 years to the General Assembly to make an appropriation to buy land for the institution, but, through lack of funds and lack of appreciation of the importance of the matter, these pleas were not affirmatively answered, so that instead of owning 1000 acres of land, as all such institutions should do, State Hospital No. 2 has a little more than 200 acres and finds it necessary to rent 800 acres in addition in order to find employment and to raise food stuff for its population of nearly 1700 people.

The Forty-sixth General Assembly appropriated $84,200 for repairs and improvements during 1911-1912.

On February 1, 1913, all the officers, with the exception of Mary E. Miller, the matron, were removed from office. Dr. A. C. Pettijohn was succeeded as superintendent by Dr. George R. Thompson, of St. Joseph.

The total appropriation for salaries, repairs and improvements for 1913 and 1914 was $110,540. This included, besides general repairs, painting, etc., a new heating plant at a cost of $21,660, an ice plant for $12,000, and twin reservoirs for fire protection at $15,000. The hospital has a pathological laboratory, and special wards for tubercular cases.

The number of patients enrolled December 31, 1914, was 1629.

MANAGERS.

Allen H. Vories	1874-1883	G. W. Davis	1887-1889
R. L. McDonald	1874-1883	J. P. Kirschner, M. D.	1889-1895
John C. Evans	1874-1877	John H. Carey	1889-1893 1901-1909
Silas Woodson	1874-1882		
Joseph Malin, M. D.	1874-1885	Wm. C. Wells	1889-1893
E. A. Donelan, M. D.	1874-1879 1883-1885	Edward P. Gates	1889-1893
		J. W. Alexander	1893-1897
James C. Roberts	1874-1877 1881-1885	Richard L. Waller	1893-1897
		H. Clay Arnold	1893-1895
John Doniphan	1877-1885	J. S. Rust	1895-1897
Arthur Kirkpatrick	1877-1883	W. C. Ellison	1895-1901
Waller Young	1883-1889	L. C. Christian	1897-1901
W. W. Ramsay	1885-1889	David R. Atchison	1897-1899
W. K. Debord	1887-1889	W. P. Stapleton	1897-1901
A. V. Banes, M. D.	1887-1889	C. N. Solman	1899-1901
J. W. Heddens	1887-1899	E. M. Harber	1901-1905
T. R. Valiant	1887-1889	C. C. Biggs	1901-1907

John C. Dawson........	1901-1905
L. E. Miller, M.D.......	1903-1905
P. E. Field.............	1905-1909
E. M. Miller, M.D.......	1907-1909
Richard L. Spencer.....	1907-1911
Jacob Geiger, M.D......	1909-1913
W. C. Pierce............	1909-1913
H. D. Faxon...........	1909-1913
W. K. Amick...........	1909-1911
John E. Frost..........	1911-
E. M. Lindsay..........	1911-
Dr. J. A. Postlewait (in office)	1913-
Smith A. Penney (in office)	1913-
George B. Baker (in office)	1913-

SECRETARY, 1914.

Fred. Hornkohl.

TREASURER, 1914.

Beverly R. D. Lacy.

SUPERINTENDENTS.

Dr. George C. Catlett...	1874-1886
Dr. Robert E. Smith....	1886-1890
Dr. C. R. Woodson.....	1890-1907
Dr. Wm. F. Kuhn......	1907-1909
Dr. F. A. Patterson (acting) (died)	1909-1910
Dr. A. H. Vandivert (acting)	1910-1910
Dr. Abram C. Pettijohn	1910-1913
Dr. George R. Thompson (in office)	1913-

ASSISTANT PHYSICIANS.

A. P. Busey, M.D......	1874-1884 1895-1899
C. H. Wallace, M.D.....	1884-1894
C. F. Knight, M.D......	1885-1891
F. C. Hoyt, M.D........	1887-1891
J. C. Smith, M.D.......	1891-1893 1899-1909
C. O'Ferrell, M.D.......	1893-1901
J. J. Field, M.D.........	1895-1897 1899-1901
C. B. Simcoe, M.D.....	1897-1899
E. B. Bagby, M.D......	1899-1901
B. H. Smith, M.D......	1901-1907
G. R. Thompson, M.D...	1901-1909
W. L. Whittington, M.D.	1901-1903
T. E. Graham, M.D.....	1903-1909
W. E. McKinley, M.D...	1907-1909
A. H. Vandivert, M.D...	1909-1913
H. P. Miles, M.D.......	1909-1913
W. E. Carey, M.D......	1909-1911
F. A. Lindsay, M.D.....	1909-1911
V. R. Hamble, M.D.....	1909-1911
W. H. Heuschele, M.D...	1909-1911
E. H. Trowbridge, M.D.	1911-1913
Henry Snure, M.D......	1911-1912
A. C. Cravens, M.D.....	1911-1912
H. W. Davis, M.D.......	1912-1913
W. J. Hunt, M.D.......	1912-1913
B. A. Finkle, M.D.......	1912-1913
Wm. L. Whittington, M.D. (in office)......	1913-
C. L. Woolsey, M.D. (in office)	1913-
R. O. Lienallen, M.D. (in office)	1913-
Amos T. Fisher (in office)	1913-

STATE HOSPITAL NO. 3.

NEVADA, MO.

State Hospital No. 3 was erected in 1885-1887. The crowded conditions of State Hospitals 1 and 2 made another hospital necessary.

Chapter 72, Art. I, Sec. 4898, provided that—There shall be established as soon as practicable after the passage of this act an insane asylum for the treatment of lunatic and insane persons in this state, to be located south of township line 44, and west of range 15, in Southwest Missouri, and to be known as State Lunatic Asylum No. 3.

The General Assembly of 1887 appropriated $200,000 therefor, the succeeding Legislature $149,000, and a subsequent Legislature $215,375; a total of $564,375, which has been used in completing the institution. In addition to the original main buildings there have been erected two new wings, chapel, electric light plant, carpenter shop, machine shop, cold storage, ice plant, butcher shop, water system, tool house, three barns, vegetable and ice house, dairy and store rooms, cow sheds, two tubercular buildings, industrial building, boiler room, engine house, new laundry and garage.

The institution has an industrial department, an occupation department and a training school for nurses and attendants. The industrial department manufactures many articles, such as mattresses, brooms, brushes, etc. The occupation department is conducted by an occupation teacher, and many valuable and useful articles are made in this department. The training school for nurses and attendants is under the supervision of a superintendent of nurses and is affiliated with the General Hospital of Kansas City. The length of training in this training school is one year for attendants; two and a half years for nurses. By the aid of this training course a much better class of attendants and nurses can be secured and retained.

During the years 1911-1912 the total number of patients under treatment was 1791. Of this number 216 died and 333 were discharged as restored, improved or stationary. There were remaining January 1, 1913, 1234 patients in the hospital and on parole. Since the establishment of the institution to January 1,

1913, the admissions aggregated 6651. Of that number 2578 have been discharged as recovered, 621 as improved, 573 as unimproved, 8 as not insane, and 1605 have died. One thousand two hundred and forty-nine patients were under care on June 1, 1913. The annual per capita cost per patient, including clothing, is $173.34.

BOARD OF MANAGERS.

H. C. Moore	1886-1892, 1897-1904
J. F. Robinson, M. D.	1886-1892
Daniel C. Kennedy	1886-1892
J. K. Cole	1886-1890
Wm. M. Bunce	1886-1890
W. H. Jopes, M. D.	1891-1904
J. B. Latimer	1891-1892
George Carstarpher (secretary)	1891-1896
J. S. Grosshart	1893-1894
J. L. George	1893-1896
D. F. Brown, M. D.	1893-1900
C. R. Creasey	1895-1896
J. D. Ingram	1897-1900
J. B. Jewell	1897-1902
James R. Allen (secretary)	1897-1900
C. R. Walters	1901-1906
R. E. Ball	1901-1904
A. E. Rogers (secretary)	1901-1904
E. F. Mann	1903-1904
John Montgomery, Jr.	1905-1906
T. F. McDearmon	1905-1910
L. F. Murray	1905-1906
J. A. Daugherty	1905-1908
E. W. Mitchell (secretary)	1905-1908
S. A. Wight	1907-1908
John M. Hale	1907-1908
R. M. Kemp	1907-1908
W. E. Clark	1909-1912
G. M. Smith	1909-1912
F. A. Howard, M. D.	1909-1910
Fred. George (secretary)	1909-1910
W. J. Sewell	1910-1912
C. P. Bouden, M. D.	1910-1912
J. J. Alford (secretary)	1910-1912

SUPERINTENDENTS.

R. E. Young, M. D.	1886-1892
J. F. Robinson, M. D.	1893-1904
L. H. Callaway, M. D.	1905-1906
G. Wilse Robinson, M. D.	1907-1908
J. W. Lampson, M. D.	1909-1910
M. P. Overholser, M. D.	1910-1912
Will P. Bradley, M. D. (in office)	1912-

ASSISTANT PHYSICIANS.

James Gordon, M. D.	1886-1892
G. P. True, M. D.	1886-1896
J. L. Warden, M. D.	1893-1894
S. A. Johnson, M. D.	1895-1900
R. Gillaspy, M. D.	1897-1900
L. M. Thompson, M. D.	1901-1902
J. W. Angle, M. D.	1901-1906
C. B. Simcoe, M. D.	1903-1904
H. Unterberg, M. D.	1905-1906
V. O. Williams, M. D.	1905-1906
J. G. Love, M. D.	1907-1912
S. T. Mead, M. D.	1907-1908
E. F. DeVilbliss, M. D.	1907-1908
R. P. Price, M. D.	1909-1910
O. R. Rooks, M. D.	1909-1912
C. L. Sellers, M. D.	1910-1912
C. B. Simcoe, M. D. (in office)	1912-
J. W. Dawson, M. D. (in office)	1912-
W. R. Summers, M. D. (in office)	1912-

STATE HOSPITAL NO. 4.

FARMINGTON, MO.

This hospital was established because of the necessity for another state hospital in Southeast Missouri, and a commission was appointed for its location at the session of the General Assembly of 1899. Three hundred and twenty-six acres of land were purchased near Farmington, the state paying $13,889.90, and the citizens paying $6110.10. The original appropriation was $150,000. At first there were constructed five cottages, a kitchen, dining room, power house and superintendent's residence, and since that time the following have been constructed: Administration building, infirmary, Cayce cottage, cottage for disturbed patients, and an auditorium and employees' quarters. There are four deep wells and a steel water tank of 50,000 gallons capacity. A great deal of work and money have been expended on the roads and granitoid walks, which are in good condition.

Hospital No. 4 was opened for patients in January, 1903. Since opening the hospital there have been admitted 1749 patients. At the close of the biennial period, December 31, 1910, there were enrolled in this institution 308 men and 270 women, making a total of 578.

The hospital is located in the foothills in the Ozarks, in the southeastern part of Missouri, and has many advantages in climatic, water and hygienic surroundings. Its capacity is 600 patients. It is built on the cottage plan. There are eight cottages, an infirmary, a tuberculosis ward, one general dining room and two special kitchens.

The administration building was erected at a cost of $50,000. There is also an entertainment hall and a home for nurses. The institution is equipped with a hydrotherapeutic outfit, pathological laboratory and the modern domestic equipments of a good hospital.

The institution has a special district allotted to it for the reception of patients. It receives both acute and chronic patients from 31 counties of Southeast Missouri.

Insane poor, under sentence as criminals, may be also sent to this hospital by the Governor at any time.

Private patients are sometimes committed here by probate courts, but if the institution at any time becomes crowded preference must be given to county patients.

A discharge of a patient as recovered, by the proper officer of this institution, viz., the superintendent, is *prima facie* evidence of his recovery and restores said patient to the control of his property and his rights as a citizen. A commitment to this hospital for the insane suspends for the time committed all legal rights of the patient so committed.

This institution is governed by a Board of Managers, composed of five men appointed by the Governor of the state for a term of four years. The following gentlemen have held such office since the institution was established:

Theodore Frazier.	Paul B. Moore.
C. M. Whitmer.	B. B. Cahoon, Sr.
R. A. Anthony.	Green B. Greer.
M. P. Cayce.	W. R. Lang.
Hina Schultz.	Byrd Duncan.
R. C. Jones.	Samuel Ulen.
John A. Hope.	H. D. Evans.
Paul B. Hinchey.	Charles R. Pratt.
Thomas Higginbotham.	F. F. Frazier.
Merrell Pipkin.	Samuel McMinn.
J. P. Clarke.	Byrd Ulen.
T. P. Russell.	G. C. Vandover.

The superintendent is in charge of this hospital and is appointed by the Board of Managers for a term of four years. The following list of gentlemen have held such office since the beginning of the institution:

Dr. L. T. Hall.	Dr. J. F. Harrison.
Dr. F. L. Kieth.	Dr. R. E. Kenney.
Dr. W. F. Kuhn.	Dr. J. A. Waterman.

Dr. G. E. Scrutchfield, in office.

The assistant physicians of this hospital are elected for a term of two years by the Board of Managers. The gentlemen whose names are given below have held such office since the beginning of the institution:

Dr. Charles A. Wells.	Dr Henry Lloyd.
Dr. F. S. Vernon.	Dr. W. S. Hutton.
Dr. Frank Long.	Dr. J. A. Tiller.
Dr. F. S. Weber.	Dr. W. G. Patton.

Dr. Frank L. Long.

MISSOURI COLONY FOR THE FEEBLE-MINDED AND EPILEPTIC.

Marshall, Mo.

The material furnished for the history of this institution is meager. It was created by an act of the Legislature of Missouri in 1899, for the purpose of receiving feeble-minded and epileptic persons between the ages of 6 and 45 years. Patients are received at the expense of the state or as private patients. There are also patients whose expense is divided between the state and individuals.

All patients are received by an order of court, even when they are private patients, and once received they presumably make their home in the institution during the remainder of their lives. It consequently seems to be more for custodial care than for educational or curative work.

As might be anticipated in a state where there are fully 20,000 feeble-minded and epileptic persons, the institution is constantly overcrowded. It has a capacity of 470 patients, and in May, 1913, more than 400 applications were on file in behalf of urgent cases waiting admission.

The institution was opened in 1901. No account is given of the character of the buildings, the size of the estate in which it is located, nor of the arrangements which exist for care, education or occupation.

The superintendent is Dr. H. D. Quigg. The assistant officer is Dr. James R. Davis; E. E. Barnum, steward; J. P. Huston, treasurer; Mrs. Julia A. Gleason, matron.

The Board of Managers are S. P. Houston, president; John R. Hall, M. D., vice-president; Miss Alice Welborn, secretary; Miss Kathryn Gordon and L. D. Murrell.

CITY SANITARIUM.[1]

ST. LOUIS, MO.

The City Sanitarium, formerly the St. Louis Insane Asylum, was originally called the St. Louis County Insane Asylum, and was, until the separation of the county and city in 1877, a county institution.

The first suggestion as to the erection of an asylum for the insane by the County of St. Louis occurs in a resolution submitted to the St. Louis County Court by Judge John H. Fisse in 1863. At that time the county sent such of its insane charges as were deemed fit subjects for asylum treatment to the State Lunatic Asylum at Fulton, Mo., then the only institution of its kind in the state. The resolution called for the erection of a county asylum, on the poorhouse grounds, with ample provision for the accommodation of 150 patients; the cost of the building not to exceed $50,000.

On April 20, 1864, this resolution was adopted by the County Court, but with an amendment changing the capacity of the proposed asylum to 100 patients. On August 23, 1864, plans having been drawn by the County Architect, William Rumbold, and approved by the court, work on the buildings was begun. On December 1, 1864, the cornerstone was laid with appropriate ceremonies.

Twenty-three acres of the County Poorhouse tract had been set aside for the asylum site, and on June 20, 1864, the county purchased eight and three-tenths acres additional on the south line of the tract for $7012.

Early in 1865 the court established a brick yard on the grounds, where all the bricks used in the construction of the buildings were made. During this same year Edward Mortimer was appointed as architect and superintendent of construction at a salary of $2500 per annum. In 1867 the court appointed a new building committee, consisting of Judge Cronenbold and Messrs. Farrar and Brannon. At this time the architect was instructed to finish the east wing as soon as possible. The iron work of the asylum was finished during this year, and some iron beds were purchased and

[1] Extracts from The Annals of the City Sanitarium, compiled under the direction of the superintendent, St. Louis, March, 1915.

installed, but a fund of $60,000 which had been appropriated for furnishing the institution was diverted by an order of the court to the purpose of completing the east wing. Contracts were made this same year for the construction of a rear building of brick, to be used for employees' quarters, engine room, kitchen and laundry. In February, 1868, the asylum grounds were laid out and roads and walks constructed. This work was not completed for more than a year. In December, 1868, the work on the building was so nearly completed that the court appointed an engineer, William H. Lamoureau, who appears to have been the first person to be given a position at the asylum. Dr. Turner R. Smith was shortly afterward appointed physician and superintendent, but seems not to have served, his appointment having been revoked for reasons not stated. Early in 1869 David Henderson was appointed steward, and the first patients were admitted by transfer from the poorhouse. In March, 1869, the furnishing of the asylum was completed.

During the same month Dr. Charles W. Stevens was appointed superintendent and physician and came with his family to reside at the asylum.

A week or so after the appointment of Dr. Stevens 127 St. Louis County patients were brought from the Fulton asylum and lodged in the new institution. From the county farm, city hospital, county jail, city workhouse and St. Vincent's Asylum 80 cases were admitted and the new institution was formally opened.

The institution when completed represented an outlay for buildings alone of $750,000; its capacity was then 300 patients. It is situated on a hill commanding an extensive view of the surrounding country and on the east the City of St. Louis.

The main building consists of a center building, with east and west wings. The center building is five stories high and provides living quarters for the superintendent and a number of officers and employees. On the fourth floor is located the sewing room; on the fifth, the ball room, chapel and quarters for the night watch. The second and third floors are occupied by the assistant physicians and the superintendent and his family. On the first floor are the general office, the superintendent's private office, the reception room and the drug store. In the basement, which extends under the center building, are store rooms. In the east and west wings are the quarters for the patients; in the east the males, in the west the females. These wings are each four stories high, except for an angle at each end, which affords an additional story. Each floor constitutes a hall or ward, with its own bed rooms, dining rooms, closets, etc. The bed rooms are on either side of the hall, north and south, and the hall extends the whole length of the wings. There were in all 10 such halls, each with a capacity of about 30 patients and two attendants.

The middle of the center building is surmounted by a large dome. The main entrance originally consisted of a stone porch, with large stone steps and heavy marble supporting columns. This porch alone cost $21,000. In the rear of the main building was a building constructed of brick and given over to the outside employees as their living quarters, dining room, etc.; on the first floor were located the general store room and laundry; in the basement were the engine room and kitchen, and these departments were connected with the center building and wings by means of a tunnel, which is still in use. This rear building was torn down to make room for a new and larger engine room and kitchen.

From the date of its inception until 1877 the County Court exercised supervisory authority over the asylum. When the institution was turned over to the City of St. Louis in 1877 this authority was vested in the Health Commissioner and Board of Health. In 1910 the office of Hospital Commissioner was created and that official, with a Hospital Board, supervised the asylum management. On the adoption of the new city charter in 1914 the Hospital Board ceased to exist, and the institution has since been under the jurisdiction of the Hospital Commissioner, who reports to the Director of Public Welfare.

The superintendents from 1877 to the present time have been appointees of the Mayor. The term of office is for four years. Prior to 1877 the salary was $2500 per annum; from 1877 to 1910, $2000 per annum. At present it is $3000 per annum, and the superintendent once more holds the additional title of resident physician.

Early in the life of the asylum an artesian well was bored on ground now occupied by the kitchen. It was sunk at great expense, but was a failure, as no water was found. It was at that time deeper than any other boring of its kind in the world, with the exception of one in Belgium, being 3850 feet in depth.

On March 16, 1873, Dr. J. K. Bauduy assumed medical control of the asylum. In 1875 Dr. N. deV. Howard became superintendent and resident physician.

In January, 1877, the asylum was transferred to the City of St. Louis, and it was provided that St. Louis County patients should be maintained at the asylum and poorhouse, the county to pay the city for their support the amount of the actual cost of keeping them.

From January, 1877, to June, 1877, the city and county authorities wrangled over the terms of transfer of the asylum.

In July, 1877, Charles W. Francis received the appointment of Health Commissioner, and entered into his duties of exercising supervisory authority over the asylum, poorhouse and sanitary department generally.

During this year the name of the asylum was changed from the St. Louis County Insane Asylum to the St. Louis Insane Asylum.

In 1879 a residence for the carpenter was erected, as well as one for the engineer. Other improvements included a porter's lodge at the front entrance to the asylum grounds; a store house; hot beds and green houses, and the installation of gas for lighting. Frequent complaints are made in the annual reports as to the overcrowding due to the greatly increased population of St. Louis.

On June 4, 1880, a large part of the roof of the east wing was torn off by a tornado and much other damage done to the buildings and grounds, necessitating an expenditure of $4000 for repairs.

Dr. G. W. Hoover, assistant physician, died at the asylum during 1881.

During this same year the center building was converted into an infirmary and a boiler house was installed near the eastern gate.

In 1884 Dr. Howard retired as superintendent and was succeeded by Dr. Charles W. Stevens, who was reappointed after an absence of 11 years.

On December 8, 1885, a cottage, located just west of the asylum, was completed and opened by the transfer of 70 patients from the halls of the asylum. The cost of this cottage was $7529. The number of patients in the asylum April 1, 1884, was 428—150 men and 278 women. The expenditures for the year were $74,583.02.

In the superintendent's report for 1886 is found a complete list of the names of the patients remaining at the asylum at the close of the year, with their former street addresses, their ages, duration of residence in the city prior to admission to the asylum, and also the length of time they had been confined in the asylum. This is the only instance of the publication of information of this character.

Dr. Charles W. Stevens, in consequence of his advanced age, retired from the superintendency at the close of the year 1886. He was succeeded by Dr. LeGrand Atwood.

On May 30, 1889, a reporter of the St. Louis *Republic* was admitted to the asylum by feigning insanity, and after remaining eight days published an account of his experience. He reported that the institution was frightfully overcrowded, and that the patients lacked ordinary accommodations.

The report for 1890 records the death of Dr. Charles W. Stevens, who had served two terms as superintendent, being the first to hold that position.

At the expiration of his term of office Dr. Atwood retired, in order to accept the position of superintendent of the State Lunatic Asylum at Fulton. Dr. Gustav A. Herrmann, under the title of "First Assistant Physician-in-Charge," conducted the asylum for 10 months after Dr. Atwood's resignation, or until the appointment of Dr. Ernest Mueller as superintendent.

In 1892 electric lights were substituted for gas at the asylum.

In 1894 a large number of patients were transferred to the insane department of the poorhouse, reducing the population of the asylum from 553 to 360.

Dr. Mueller during his term of office had charge of the insane department of the poorhouse; he was the only asylum superintendent to have such authority.

In 1895 Dr. Mueller was succeeded as superintendent by Dr. Edward C. Runge.

On the afternoon of May 27, 1896, a tornado, which caused great damage to St. Louis, injured the asylum slightly.

On January 31, 1904, Dr. Runge tendered his resignation, with the expectation of resuming private practice. A few weeks after his retirement from the superintendency of the asylum he took pneumonia and died, being but 46 years old.

He was succeeded as superintendent by Dr. Henry S. Atkins

On March 23, 1905, the chief engineer, John McGovern, was killed by accidental contact with a live wire.

In 1910 additional buildings authorized in 1907 were completed and occupied. These buildings consisted of additional east and west wings, and a separate building for acute cases. The buildings, when completed, afforded room for 2000 patients and 300 employees; their cost was $962,000.

The new wings are three in number, similar in design to the old wings, and are four stories high. The maniacal or observation building is three stories high and stands a short distance southeast of the main building. All told the institution has 54 wards or halls, with a capacity for 2100 patients and 250 employees and officers. The grounds embrace an area of 50 acres.

On April 31, 1911, Dr. Atkins was succeeded as superintendent by Dr. G. A. Johns.

Among the improvements for the year 1913 the superintendent mentions the completion of a well-equipped laboratory; new store room completed; chapel enlarged and improved; new morgue completed; park improved, etc. The amusements consist of moving pictures, bowling, billiards, music and dancing, etc., as in former years.

The number of patients on March 31, 1914, was 2006—947 men and 1059 women. The expenditures for the year were $229,161.35. The per capita cost for one year, $140.13.

PHYSICIANS AND SUPERINTENDENTS.

Dr. Turner R. Smith[1]..	1868-
Dr. Charles W. Stevens.	1869-1873
Dr. J. K. Bauduy[2]......	1873-1875
Dr. N. deV. Howard....	1875-1884
Dr. Charles W. Stevens (reappointed)	1884-1886
Dr. LeGrand Atwood....	1886-1892
Dr. Gustav A. Herrmann (pro tem)	1892-1892
Dr. Ernest Mueller.....	1892-1896
Dr. Edward C. Runge...	1896-1904
Dr. Henry S. Atkins....	1904-1911
Dr. George A. Johns (in office)	1911-

[1] Did not serve as the appointment was revoked a few weeks after being made, for reasons not given.

[2] Non-resident.

ASSISTANT SUPERINTENDENTS.

Dr. Charles W. Thiery.	1901-1902	Dr. F. L. Whelpley.....	1904-1908
Dr. Theodore Greiner...	1902-1903	Dr. G. A. Johns.........	1908-1911
Dr. Garrett Hogg.......	1903-1904	Dr. O. J. Raeder (in office)	1912-
Dr. H. Unterberg......	1904-1904		

VISITING PHYSICIANS.

Dr. E. S. Frazier.......	1875-	Dr. S. H. Frazier........	1875-

ASSISTANT PHYSICIANS.

Dr. H. S. Leffingwell[4]..	1868-	Dr. Harry H. Meyer....	1898-1899
Dr. Hazzard[4]	1868-	Dr. Eugene Scharff......	1898-1898
Dr. Harry L. Fitchekam.	1872-	Dr. C. M. Gilbert.......	1898-1899
Dr. C. D. Kemble.......	1875-	Dr. C. W. Molz.........	1898-1898
Dr. Henry S. Geresch...	1878-	Dr. Charles W. Thiery..	1899-1901
Dr. Gib. W. Carson....	1878-	Dr. Theodore Greiner...	1899-1901
Dr. G. W. Hoover......	1878-1881	Dr. F. A. Lane.........	1900-1901
Dr. F. D. Mooney......	1881-	Dr. A. S. Bleyer........	1901-1901
Dr. H. L. Wolfner......	1881-	Dr. C. E. Gimbel.......	1901-1902
Dr. M. E. Haase........	1884-	Dr. M. O. Steinmler....	1902-1902
Dr. Frank Heitzig......	1884-	Dr. Garrett Hogg......	1902-1903
Dr. E. A. Junkin.......	1885-	Dr. H. B. Miller........	1902-1904
Dr. F. W. Lowry.......	1886-	Dr. H. Unterberg......	1903-1904
Dr. Ernest Mueller......	1886-1892	Dr. F. L. Whelpley.....	1904-1904
Dr. Gustav A. Herrman.	1888-1892	Dr. W. J. Loler.........	1904-1905
Dr. Hugh A. Jones......	1888-1891	Dr. W. J. Johnson......	1905-1905
Dr. Given Campbell....	1891-1892	Dr. A. M. Painter......	1905-1905
Dr. George L. Kearney..	1892-1894	Dr. K. K. McAlpine....	1905-1905
Dr. Wm. M. Banks.....	1892-1893	Dr. W. Richardson.....	1905-1906
Dr. Charles L. Gorton..	1893-1894	Dr. G. A. Johns........	1905-1908
Dr. Joseph J. Meredith..	1894-1895	Dr. P. Newman........	1908-1909
Dr. Jacob Jacobson.....	1894-1895	Dr. C. C. Nash..........	1908-1908
Dr. Louis J. Oatman....	1895-1897	Dr. G. W. Flinn........	1908-1909
Dr. J. M. Epstein......	1895-1895	Dr. Collins	1908-1908
Dr. C. A. Newcomb....	1895-1895	Dr. G. A. Schmid........	1909-1909
Dr. F. W. Jelks.........	1895-1896	Dr. C. R. Castien........	1909-1910
Dr. A. E. Horwitz......	1895-1895	Dr. D. L. Fish.........	1909-1911
Dr. J. G. Parrish.......	1896-1897	Dr. O. J. Raeder........	1910-1912
Dr. Henry W. Curtin...	1896-1898	Dr. B. Lemchen........	1910-1911
Dr. Conrad Baumgartner	1896-1898	Dr. A. Garlitz (in office)	1911-
Dr. J. H. Farrar........	1897-1898	Dr. C. L. Sellers........	1911-1911
Dr. Nelson J. Hawley...	1897-1898	Dr. H. W. Fay..........	1911-1912
Dr. L. H. Hempelman..	1898-1898	Dr. J. P. Kissel........	1911-1912
Dr. W. E. Sauer........	1898-1898	Dr. J. P. Kein..........	1911-1912

[4] Date of service uncertain.

Dr. C. H. Wachenfield..	1912-1912	Dr. C. H. Hecker.......	1912-1914
Dr. T. C. Lorton.......	1912-1912	Dr. J. Lewald (in office)	1912-
Dr. A. H. Deppe........	1912-1913	Dr. C. H. Shumaker (in office)	1913-
Dr. A. C. Vickery.......	1912-1913	Dr. F. J. Riordan.......	1913-1913
Dr. D. L. Penny........	1912-1912	Dr. C. H. Burdick (in office)	1913-
Dr. A. S. Heitkaus......	1912-1912		
Dr. T. B. Butler........	1912-1912		

STEWARDS.

David Henderson	1868-1873	A. S. Tayon............	1879-
B. P. Taaffe............	1873-1879	Henry Stevens (in office)	1911-

ST. VINCENT'S INSTITUTION.

St. Louis, Mo.

St. Vincent's Institution is a private institution for mental and nervous diseases, and is conducted by the Sisters of Charity of St. Vincent de Paul.

Some 56 years ago the Sisters in charge of the St. Louis Mullanphy Hospital had among their patients some who were mentally afflicted. Their condition was detrimental to the other patients and it became necessary to provide other quarters for them. A home was secured for this purpose at Ninth and Marion Streets, St. Louis, and in August, 1858, was occupied by four Sisters and 15 patients.

After some years the growing patronage of St. Vincent's necessitated increased accommodations, and, in 1891, 97 acres of land were purchased on the St. Charles Rock Road, St. Louis County, about a mile and a half beyond the city limits. Here under the supervision of Sister M. Magdalene, Superior, plans for a massive structure were soon in readiness, and in the fall of 1895 the Sisters with their patients moved to the new home. This was indeed providential, for, a few months later, in May, 1896, the great cyclone that swept over the City of St. Louis occurred, and the house so recently vacated was entirely destroyed.

The institution is beautifully located on an eminence sufficiently far removed from the city's noise and foul air, and with ample grounds. The building is of modern construction, well heated and ventilated, and possesses accommodations for 500 patients under the sole charge of the Sisters of Charity in each department.

The institution is provided with conveniences calculated to afford patients all the comforts of home with medical attendance and careful guarding and nursing.

Since its erection, among other improvements, a spacious and well-equipped entertainment hall and gymnasium have been added. All cases of mental and nervous diseases are received. During the year from 500 to 600 are treated, the usual number under treatment being upwards of 300. Where the mental breakdown is due to lack of proper mental hygiene the fault is corrected, as far as possible, by instruction and proper changes in the mode of living. The sympathy and co-operation of the patient are sought in every case. The percentage of cures has averaged about 20 to 25 per cent, while the percentage of improvements has reached as high as 60 per cent.

MEDICAL OFFICERS, 1914.

H. W. Herman, M. D. .... Attending neurologist.
J. J. Kehoe, M. D. .... Assisting physician.

MENTAL ILLNESS AND SOCIAL POLICY

THE AMERICAN EXPERIENCE

AN ARNO PRESS COLLECTION

Barr, Martin W. Mental Defectives: Their History, Treatment and Training. 1904.

The Beginnings of American Psychiatric Thought and Practice: Five Accounts, 1811-1830. 1973

The Beginnings of Mental Hygiene in America: Three Selected Essays, 1833-1850. 1973

Briggs, L. Vernon, et al. History of the Psychopathic Hospital, Boston, Massachusetts. 1922

Briggs, L. Vernon. Occupation as a Substitute for Restraint in the Treatment of the Mentally Ill. 1923

Brigham, Amariah. An Inquiry Concerning the Diseases and Functions of the Brain, the Spinal Cord, and the Nerves. 1840

Brigham, Amariah. Observations on the Influence of Religion upon the Health and Physical Welfare of Mankind. 1835

Brill, A. A. Fundamental Conceptions of Psychoanalysis. 1921

Bucknill, John Charles. Notes on Asylums for the Insane in America. 1876

Conolly, John. The Treatment of the Insane Without Mechanical Restraints. 1856

Coriat, Isador H. What is Psychoanalysis? 1917

Deutsch, Albert. The Shame of the States. 1948

Dewey, Richard. Recollections of Richard Dewey: Pioneer in American Psychiatry. 1936

Earle, Pliny. Memoirs of Pliny Earle, M. D. with Extracts from his Diary and Letters (1830-1892) and Selections from his Professional Writings (1839-1891). 1898

Galt, John M. The Treatment of Insanity. 1846

Goddard, Henry Herbert. Feeble-mindedness: Its Causes and Consequences. 1926

Hammond, William A. A Treatise on Insanity in Its Medical Relations. 1883

Hazard, Thomas R. Report on the Poor and Insane in Rhode-Island. 1851

Hurd, Henry M., editor. The Institutional Care of the Insane in the United States and Canada. 1916/1917. Four volumes.

Kirkbride, Thomas S. On the Construction, Organization, and General Arrangements of Hospitals for the Insane. 1880

Meyer, Adolf. The Commonsense Psychiatry of Dr. Adolf Meyer: Fifty-two Selected Papers. 1948

Mitchell, S. Weir. Wear and Tear, or Hints for the Overworked. 1887

Morton, Thomas G. The History of the Pennsylvania Hospital, 1751-1895. 1895

Ordronaux, John. Jurisprudence in Medicine in Relation to the Law. 1869

The Origins of the State Mental Hospital in America: Six Documentary Studies, 1837-1856. 1973

Packard, Mrs. E. P. W. Modern Persecution, or Insane Asylums Unveiled, As Demonstrated by the Report of the Investigating Committee of the Legislature of Illinois. 1875. Two volumes in one

Prichard, James C. A Treatise on Insanity and Other Disorders Affecting the Mind. 1837

Prince, Morton. The Unconscious: The Fundamentals of Human Personality Normal and Abnormal. 1921

Putnam, James Jackson. Human Motives. 1915

Russell, William Logie. The New York Hospital: A History of the Psychiatric Service, 1771-1936. 1945

Sidis, Boris. The Psychology of Suggestion: A Research into the Subconscious Nature of Man and Society. 1899

Southard, Elmer E. Shell-Shock and Other Neuropsychiatric Problems Presented in Five Hundred and Eighty-Nine Case Histories from the War Literature, 1914-1918. 1919

Southard, E[lmer] E. and Mary C. Jarrett. The Kingdom of Evils. 1922

Southard, E[lmer] E. and H[arry] C. Solomon. Neurosyphilis: Modern Systematic Diagnosis and Treatment Presented in One Hundred and Thirty-seven Case Histories. 1917

Spitzka, E[dward] C. Insanity: Its Classification, Diagnosis and Treatment. 1887

Supreme Court Holding a Criminal Term, No. 14056. The United States vs. Charles J. Guiteau. 1881/1882. Two volumes

Trezevant, Daniel H. Letters to his Excellency Governor Manning on the Lunatic Asylum. 1854

Tuke, D[aniel] Hack. The Insane in the United States and Canada. 1885

Upham, Thomas C. Outlines of Imperfect and Disordered Mental Action. 1868

White, William A[lanson]. Twentieth Century Psychiatry: Its Contribution to Man's Knowledge of Himself. 1936

Willard, Sylvester D. Report on the Condition of the Insane Poor in the County Poor Houses of New York. 1865